HEALTH AND HUMAN DEVELOPMENT

PUBLIC HEALTH YEARBOOK 2009

HEALTH AND HUMAN DEVELOPMENT

JOAV MERRICK - SERIES EDITOR –

NATIONAL INSTITUTE OF CHILD HEALTH
AND HUMAN DEVELOPMENT,
MINISTRY OF SOCIAL AFFAIRS, JERUSALEM

Adolescent Behavior Research: International Perspectives
Joav Merrick and Hatim A. Omar (Editors)
2007. ISBN: 1-60021-649-8

Complementary Medicine Systems: Comparison and Integration
Karl W. Kratky and Joav Merrick (Editors)
2008. ISBN: 978-1-60456-475-4 (Hardcover)
2008. ISBN: 978-1-61122-433-7 (E-book)

Pain in Children and Youth
Patricia Schofield and Joav Merrick (Editors)
2008. ISBN: 978-1-60456-951-3

Challenges in Adolescent Health: An Australian Perspective
David Bennett, Susan Towns, Elizabeth Elliott and Joav Merrick (Editors)
2009. ISBN: 978-1-60741-616-6 (Hardcover)
2009. ISBN: 978-1-61668-240-8 (E-book)

Behavioral Pediatrics, 3rd Edition
Donald E. Greydanus, Dilip R. Patel, Helen D. Pratt, Joseph L. Calles, Jr. and Joav Merrick (Editors)
2009. ISBN: 978-1-60692-702-1 (Hardcover)
2009. ISBN: 978-1-60876-630-7 (E-book)

Health and Happiness from Meaningful Work: Research in Quality of Working Life
Søren Ventegodt and Joav Merrick (Editors)
2009. ISBN: 978-1-60692-820-2

Obesity and Adolescence: A Public Health Concern
Hatim A. Omar, Donald E. Greydanus, Dilip R. Patel and Joav Merrick (Editors)
2009. ISBN: 978-1-60456-821-9

Poverty and Children: A Public Health Concern
Alexis Lieberman and Joav Merrick (Editors)
2009. ISBN: 978-1-60741-140-6

Living on the Edge: The Mythical, Spiritual, and Philosophical Roots of Social Marginality
Joseph Goodbread and Joav Merrick (Editors)
2009. ISBN: 978-1-60741-162-8

Alcohol-Related Cognitive Disorders: Research and Clinical Perspectives
Leo Sher, Isack Kandel and Joav Merrick (Editors)
2009. ISBN: 978-1-60741-730-9 (Hardcover)
2009. ISBN: 978-1-60876-623-9 (E-book)

Rural Child Health: International Aspects
Erica Bell and Joav Merrick (Editors)
2010. ISBN: 978-1-60876-357-3 (Hardcover)
2010. ISBN: 978-1-61324-005-2 (E-book)

Children and Pain
Patricia Schofield and Joav Merrick (Editors)
2009. ISBN: 978-1-60876-020-6 (Hardcover)
2009. ISBN: 978-1-61728-183-9 (E-book)

Conceptualizing Behavior in Health and Social Research: A Practical Guide to Data Analysis
Said Shahtahmasebi, Damon Berridge and Joav Merrick (Editors)
2010. ISBN: 978-1-60876-383-2

Chance Action and Therapy: The Playful Way of Changing
Uri Wernik and Joav Merrick (Editors)
2010. ISBN: 978-1-60876-393-1 (Hardcover)
2011. ISBN: 978-1-61122-987-5 (Softcover)
2011. ISBN: 978-1-61209-874-6 (E-book)

Adolescence and Chronic Illness. A Public Health Concern
Hatim Omar, Donald E. Greydanus, Dilip R. Patel and Joav Merrick (Editors)
2010. ISBN: 978-1-60876-628-4 (Hardcover)
2010. ISBN: 978-1-61761-482-8 (E-book)

Adolescence and Sports
Dilip R. Patel, Donald E. Greydanus, Hatim Omar and Joav Merrick (Editors)
2010. ISBN: 978-1-60876-702-1 (Hardcover)
2010. ISBN: 978-1-61761-483-5 (E-book)

International Aspects of Child Abuse and Neglect
Howard Dubowitz and Joav Merrick (Editors)
2010. ISBN: 978-1-60876-703-8 (Hardcover)
2010. ISBN: 978-1-61122-049-0 (Softcover)
2010. ISBN: 978-1-61122-403-0 (E-book)

Positive Youth Development: Evaluation and Future Directions in a Chinese Context
Daniel T.L. Shek, Hing Keung Ma and Joav Merrick (Editors)
2010. ISBN: 978-1-60876-830-1 (Hardcover)
2010. ISBN: 978-1-61668-376-4 (E-book)
2011. ISBN: 978-1-62100-175-1 (Softcover)

Positive Youth Development: Implementation of a Youth Program in a Chinese Context
Daniel T.L Shek, Hing Keung Ma and Joav Merrick (Editors)
2010. ISBN: 978-1-61668-230-9 (Hardcover)
2010. ISBN: 978-1-61209-091-7 (E-book)

Pediatric and Adolescent Sexuality and Gynecology: Principles for the Primary Care Clinician
Hatim A. Omar, Donald E. Greydanus, Artemis K. Tsitsika, Dilip R. Patel and Joav Merrick (Editors)
2010. ISBN: 978-1-60876-735-9

Understanding Eating Disorders: Integrating Culture, Psychology and Biology
Yael Latzer, Joav Merrick and Daniel Stein (Editors)
2010. ISBN: 978-1-61728-298-0 (Hardcover)
2011. ISBN: 978-1-61470-976-3 (Softcover)

Advanced Cancer Pain and Quality of Life
Edward Chow and Joav Merrick (Editors)
2010. ISBN: 978-1-61668-207-1 (Hardcover)
2010. ISBN: 978-1-61668-400-6 (E-book)

Bone and Brain Metastases: Advances in Research and Treatment
Arjun Sahgal, Edward Chow and Joav Merrick (Editors)
2010. ISBN: 978-1-61668-365-8 (Hardcover)
2010. ISBN: 978-1-61728-085-6 (E-book)

Environment, Mood Disorders and Suicide
Teodor T. Postolache and Joav Merrick (Editors)
2010. ISBN: 978-1-61668-505-8

Social and Cultural Psychiatry Experience from the Caribbean Region
Hari D. Maharajh and Joav Merrick (Editors)
2010. ISBN: 978-1-61668-506-5 (Hardcover)
2010. ISBN: 978-1-61728-088-7 (E-book)

Narratives and Meanings of Migration
Julia Mirsky and Joav Merrick (Editors)
2010. ISBN: 978-1-61761-103-2 (Hardcover)
2010. ISBN: 978-1-61761-519-1 (E-book)

Self-Management and the Health Care Consumer
Peter William Harvey
2011. ISBN: 978-1-61761-796-6 (Hardcover)
2011. ISBN: 978-1-61122-214-2 (E-book)

Sexology from a Holistic Point of View
Soren Ventegodt and Joav Merrick
2011. ISBN: 978-1-61761-859-8 (Hardcover)
2011. ISBN: 978-1-61122-262-3 (E-book)

Principles of Holistic Psychiatry: A Textbook on Holistic Medicine for Mental Disorders
Soren Ventegodt and Joav Merrick
2011. ISBN: 978-1-61761-940-3 (Hardcover)
2011. ISBN: 978-1-61122-263-0 (E-book)

Clinical Aspects of Psychopharmacology in Childhood and Adolescence
Donald E. Greydanus, Joseph L. Calles, Jr., Dilip P. Patel, Ahsan Nazeer and Joav Merrick (Editors)
2011. ISBN: 978-1-61122-135-0 (Hardcover)
2011. ISBN: 978-1-61122-715-4 (E-book)

Climate Change and Rural Child Health
Erica Bell, Bastian M. Seidel and Joav Merrick (Editors)
2011. ISBN: 978-1-61122-640-9 (Hardcover)
2011. ISBN: 978-1-61209-014-6 (E-book)

Rural Medical Education: Practical Strategies
Erica Bell, Craig Zimitat and Joav Merrick (Editors)
2011. ISBN: 978-1-61122-649-2 (Hardcover)

Advances in Environmental Health Effects of Toxigenic Mold and Mycotoxins
Ebere Cyril Anyanwu and Joav Merrick (Editors)
2011. ISBN: 978-1-60741-953-2

Child and Adolescent Health Yearbook 2009
Joav Merrick
2011. ISBN: 978-1-61668-913-1 (Hardcover)

Public Health Yearbook 2009
Joav Merrick
2011. ISBN: 978-1-61668-911-7 (Hardcover)

Child Health and Human Development Yearbook 2009
Joav Merrick
2011. ISBN: 978-1-61668-912-4 (Hardcover)

Alternative Medicine Yearbook 2009
Joav Merrick (Editor)
2011. ISBN: 978-1-61668-910-0 (Hardcover)

The Dance of Sleeping and Eating among Adolescents: Normal and Pathological Perspectives
Yael Latzer, Joav Merrick and Orna Tzischinsky (Editors)
2011. ISBN: 978-1-61209-710-7 (Hardcover)

Child and Adolescent Health Yearbook 2010
Joav Merrick (Editor)
2011. ISBN: 978-1-61209-788-6 (Hardcover)

Child Health and Human Development Yearbook 2010
Joav Merrick (Editor)
2011. ISBN: 978-1-61209-789-3

Public Health Yearbook 2010
Joav Merrick (Editor)
2011. ISBN: 978-1-61209-971-2

Living on the Edge: The Mythical, Spiritual, and Philosophical Roots of Social Marginality
Joseph Goodbread (Editor)
2011. ISBN: 978-1-60741-162-8 (Hardcover)
2011. ISBN: 978-1-61122-986-8 (Softcover)

Alternative Medicine Yearbook 2010
Joav Merrick (Editor)
2011. ISBN: 978-1-62100-132-4 (Hardcover)
2011. ISBN: 978-1-62100-210-9 (E-book)

The Astonishing Brain and Holistic Conciousness: Neuroscience and Vedanta Perspectives
Vinod D. Deshmukh and Joav Merrick (Editors)
2011. ISBN: 978-1-61324-295-7 (Hardcover)

Translational Research for Primary Healthcare
Erica Bell and Joav Merrick (Editors)
2011. ISBN: 978-1-61324-647-4 (Hardcover)

Drug Abuse in Hong Kong: Development and Evaluation of a Prevention Program
Daniel T.L. Shek, Rachel C.F. Sun and Joav Merrick (Editors)
2011. ISBN: 978-1-61324-491-3 (Hardcover)

Human Development: Biology from a Holistic Point of View
Søren Ventegodt, Tyge Dahl Hermansen and Joav Merrick (Editors)
2011. ISBN: 978-1-61470-441-6 (Hardcover)
2011. ISBN: 978-1-61470-541-3 (E-book)

Our Search for Meaning in Life
Søren Ventegodt and Joav Merrick (Editors)
2011. ISBN: 978-1-61470-494-2 (Hardcover)
2011. ISBN: 978-1-61470-519-2 (E-book)

HEALTH AND HUMAN DEVELOPMENT

PUBLIC HEALTH YEARBOOK 2009

JOAV MERRICK
EDITOR

Nova Science Publishers, Inc.
New York

For permission to use material from this book please contact us:
Telephone 631-231-7269; Fax 631-231-8175
Web Site: http://www.novapublishers.com

Library of Congress Cataloging-in-Publication Data

ISSN: 2164-716X
ISBN 978-1-61668-911-7

Published by Nova Science Publishers, Inc. † New York

CONTENTS

PREFACE*

The 2009 Public Health Yearbook compiles articles published in the International Public Health Journal, a peer-reviewed journal which provides an international multidisciplinary forum with a holistic approach to public health issues, health and medicine, health and social policy, service aspects, developmental aspects, epidemiology, rehabilitation, family and social issues, quality of life and all other aspects of public health over the whole age spectrum.

Chapter 1 - Adolescence is a period of tremendous growth and represents a time of transition from childhood to adulthood. Youth who do not experience typical development as a result of chronic illness may experience psychological problems. Adolescents with chronic illness versus typically developing adolescents may need a greater degree of support, resources and guidance to ensure that they grow into psychologically healthy adults. Those youth who receive such help have a greater chance of developing the ability to live relatively healthy and productive lives. Youth who do not experience typical development as a result of chronic illness may experience psychological problems.

Chapter 2 - Context: Malaria is known as a disease of poverty, but there is a dearth of evidence to collectively summarize how social and demographic factors predict its incidence among pregnant women.

Objective: To summarize evidence on socio-demographic determinants of malaria in pregnancy.

Data sources: Electronic databases of OVID, MEDLINE, LILACS, EMBASE, PsycINFO, Science Citation Index and Social Science Citation Index, ERIC and reference lists of articles were searched for 1998-2008. Selection criteria: Two independent reviewers selected studies for inclusion if they expressly investigated or included investigation of social and/or demographic determinants of placental malaria or parasitemia in pregnancy. Data extraction: Data on study settings, designs, methods, population characteristics, relationship between socio-demographic variables and malaria were assessed. Data synthesis: Of the 98 studies found, 19 met the inclusion criteria. Overall, socio-demographic determinants of malaria in pregnancy were found to be age (less than 21 years), parity (more than 1 child), socioeconomic status (measured by absence of electricity in the house), trimester of pregnancy, seasonality (rainy season), geographic location (rural residence), HIV infection,

* Versions of these chapters were also published in the *International Public Health Journal,* Volume 1, Issues 1-4, edited by Joav Merrick, published by Nova Science Publishers, Inc. They were submitted for appropriate modifications in an effort to encourage wider dissemination of research.

and use of malaria prophylaxis. One study found an association with ethnicity. Conclusion: Given that age, parity, rural residence, low socioeconomic status, and HIV infection were found to be strong predictors of malaria in pregnancy, maternal and child health programs as well as malaria control programs must pay special attention to women with these characteristics if their interventions are to have optimum impact. Programs that target prevention of mother-to-child transmission of HIV should incorporate effective malaria prophylaxis and treatment to counter the effects of HIV on pregnant women with malaria.

Chapter 3 - The aim of this study was to investigate the effect of developing problem-solving abilities on depressive symptoms of women in primary care settings. Study subjects consisted of women with complaints of physical health problems not caused by a well-defined medical disease. The study was performed on 76 women randomized into the study group ($n = 38$) and controls ($n = 38$). The data of the research were obtained by using the interview form, Beck Depression Inventory and Problem-Solving Inventory at baseline and three and six months later. The study group and controls were comparable with regard to demographic data ($p > 0.05$). Depression and problem-solving scores of the study group and controls were comparable at baseline ($p > 0.05$). Overall, depression and problem-solving scores of the study group were significantly lower than those of the controls ($p < 0.05$). In the study group, depression and problem-solving scores at month 6 were significantly lower than those at baseline and month 3 ($p < 0.05$) and depression and problem-solving scores at month three were significantly lower than those at baseline ($p < 0.05$). In the control group, there were no significantly differences in depression and problem-solving scores measured at baseline and three and six months later ($p > 0.05$). The findings of our study demonstrated that with increase in problem-solving abilities of women, the depressive symptoms decreased. In primary care settings, there is need to implement programs to increase problem-solving skills of women, who have physical symptoms such as gastrointestinal, reproductive and neurologic symptoms in order to decrease depressive symptoms.

Chapter 4 - Parent-reported values for children's heights and weights are routinely collected in national, state, and school surveys in the United States. Our purpose was to examine the accuracy of those values for children 2–11 years old. Z scores, means and standard errors, paired t-tests and Spearman rank order correlations were calculated for three age and three ethnic groups to estimate reliability and validity of values. Few parents accurately reported their child's height, weight, and calculated BMI (15.0%, 13.7%, and 5.6%, respectively). Many parents responded 'Don't know' to questions about their children's weight (25%) and height (53%). The typical parent of 2-5 years olds under-reported height by about 4.6 cm. The magnitude and direction of the BMI bias or error for 2-5 years olds was +2.3 BMI units. The decreasing relative bias for height and BMI indicated increasing accuracy as children age. Height and BMI bias was greatest for children in the 2-5 year group; here, the sex-specific bias for non-Hispanic black and Mexican-American boys and girls exceeded the bias for non-Hispanic white preschoolers ($p = 0.05$). Regarding random error, the coefficients were smaller for height compared to weight indicating that height was a greater source of this error. For clinical and public health environments, use of parent reports introduced random and systematic errors to reported heights and weights particularly height and calculated BMI. The magnitude and direction of the errors varied by child's age and ethnicity.

Chapter 5 - Chronic fatigue syndrome (CFS) poses many socioeconomic, psychosocial, disability and quality of life difficulties for people with CFS in Canada. The self-reported prevalence of CFS was 0.78%, 1.22% and about 201,900, 331,500 Canadians have reported having CFS in 2000 and 2005 respectively. Canadians aged 40-64 years old (57.87% in 2000, and 58.59% in 2005) were the most frequently infected. More female Canadians (71.41% in 2000, and 68.44% in 2005) were affected than males (28.59% and 31.56%). Both physical and mental fatigue caused by CFS cost the Canadian economy an estimated $3.5 billion per year, and the annual lost productivity in Canada is estimated at $2.5 billion in 2003. However, the capacity in Canada for prevention and management of CFS is limited. Currently, there are only few medical doctors using the Clinical Working Case Definition, diagnostic and treatment protocols. Therefore, we need more research in the surveillance, diagnosis, treatment, and evaluation of CFS management in Canada.

Chapter 6 - To estimate the prevalence and associated factors of tobacco use among school-going adolescents in Himachal Pradesh, India. Data from the Global Youth Tobacco Survey (GYTS) 2004 was used to determine tobacco use prevalence, determinants, attitudes, and exposure to tobacco advertisements among adolescents. Frequencies and their 95% confidence intervals (CI) were calculated. Odds ratios (unadjusted (OR) and adjusted (AOR)) and their 95% CI were obtained using logistic regression analysis. Of the 1,976 respondents for whom gender was recorded, 6.4% males and 3.9% females reported current tobacco use ($p = 0.021$). After controlling for age, gender, parental tobacco use status, and perception of risks of tobacco use, 'having some friends who were tobacco users' was associated with tobacco use (AOR = 4.65; 95% CI [2.85, 7.58], the association being stronger if all their friends were tobacco users AOR=11.78; 95% CI [4.84, 28.63]. Participants reported high exposure to tobacco advertisements on billboards (71.0%), and television (53.3%). Nearly one in seven respondents (14.7%) reported possessing an item with a tobacco brand on it. The proportion of males who felt that tobacco use was harmful was higher than that for females ($p=0.002$). Findings from this study emphasize the critical role of friends, and the media in influencing adolescent tobacco use behaviours and the need for considering social and domestic environments in planning gender-specific interventions for this vulnerable population subgroup.

Chapter 7 - Child focused anti-smoking programs are almost non-existent in preschool education, despite the fact that a large number of young children are being brought up in environments, which are not tobacco free. The main purpose of the present study was first to record the perceptions, attitudes and familiarization of 4 to 6 year-olds about smoking and, second, to design, implement and assess the effectiveness of an innovative psycho-educational preventative program, focusing on smoking and its effects on health. Fifty-four preschool children attending state-run kindergarten schools in Central Greece participated in the study. Their perceptions, attitudes and familiarization with smoking were first assessed using an especially designed questionnaire. Approximately half of the children (experimental group) participated in a series of especially designed psycho-educational activities regarding smoking, immediately after the above assessment. All children were once again assessed with the same questionnaire after the psyco-educational activities were completed. The implementation and assessment of the program showed that it was suitably and effectively designed for preschoolers. Our results indicated that preventative programs could change young children's ideas regarding tobacco use and Environmental Tobacco Smoke and could, potentially, contribute to the formation of anti-smoking attitudes.

Chapter 8 - In Israel, the Office of the Medical Director of the Ministry of Social Affairs is responsible for the medical service in residential-care centers for persons with intellectual disability (ID). During 1997-1998 a standard annual questionnaire was developed and the first national survey study conducted in 1998. This present paper presents the findings of the fifth national survey in 2002, for which the following information was gathered via questionnaires: information on the age, gender, and level of intellectual disability of persons served at the residential care center in question, status of the population served, profile, nursing, medical, and allied professional staff, number of annual examinations, preventive medicine aspects, medications, number of annual cases of infectious disease, annual unintentional injury, number of deaths, number of hospitalizations, internal residential center hospitalization, ambulatory out-patient use, use of outside laboratory examinations and dental care. In 2002, 6,352 persons were served in nine government, 36 private and 12 public centers. The average number of persons per center was 111.44 (range 16 to 398). Of the patient population, 78.4% were between 20 and 60 years old, 50.4% had severe or profound intellectual disability, and 41.9% moderate disability. 25% were nursing patients, 18.7% were confined to a wheelchair, 28.9% suffered from epilepsy. Of the total population, 80.3% were receiving medication daily for chronic illness and 50.8% received psychotropic medication.

Chapter 9 - Black market medicine contradicts the ethical and moral codes obligating every physician to act ethically and not accept bribery for care provided or to accept compensation for a service that should be provided equally and without charge. The phenomenon is not new and has been described by various professionals working within the health and medical system in Israel. This paper is a short overview of black market medicine. We believe that if physicians are made aware of the issue of black market medicine and its immorality, emphasizing the harm that it causes them and the entire population due to its avaricious portrayal, perhaps in the future this practice will be reduced and more easily eliminated

Chapter 10 - Eosinophil granulocytes (eosinophils) are white blood cells that develop from bone marrow precursor cells. Their major morphological characteristic is eosinophilic granules within the cytoplasm, which are divided into specific and small granules. Four cationic proteins have been recognized within the eosinophil specific granules that include eosinophil cationic protein (ECP). It displays a variety of biological activities, most notably cytotoxicity that is due to its ability to make pores in cell membranes. ECP exerts this action on parasites, viruses, bacteria, tumor cells, and even respiratory epithelial cells. Other biological functions include stimulation of mucus production in the airway, interaction with the coagulation and complement systems, and immunomodulation. The role of ECP as a marker of eosinophil activity has been investigated in a variety of body fluids and diseases, particularly in wheezing children. The role of ECP has been investigated in acute viral bronchiolitis of infants and preschool wheezing in reference to both pathogenesis and prognosis of the disease. There is evidence that ECP can be used in asthma to evaluate severity, patient compliance to anti-asthma treatment, and to step-down inhaled corticosteroid dosage in stabilized patients. Further studies are required in order to elucidate its role as a diagnostic and prognostic tool in pediatric asthma.

Chapter 11 - In the World Health Report of 2000 a new concept was introduced, which gained acceptance among health policy scientists and the various World Health Organization agencies. This concept has been called the Four Health System Framework Functions: resource generation, financing, stewardship and service provision. These functions are interlinked and suppose to determine the way inputs are transformed to outcomes in health systems and have become the working language of policy makers and scholars, while they are not common for public health professionals. In this paper we deal with the applicability of the Four Health System Framework Functions for assessing and reforming Public Health Services (PHS). We suggest a model for this application in order to allow a discussion, which could provide a practical frame for systematic PHS assessment and planning of specific goals, objectives and interventions for efficient use of outputs and reform interventions at the public health level.

Chapter 12 - Tobacco use is a major public health concern among youth in developing countries, and it is a leading cause of behavior-related morbidity and mortality. Although youth tobacco use cessation efforts appear to almost double quit rates among youth, and have increased in the United States and some European countries, few cessation efforts have been initiated in developing countries. This paper provides general guidelines for initiating and advancing teen tobacco use cessation research and practice in developing countries. Initially, countries' larger social climate needs to be prepared for youth tobacco use cessation efforts, which requires recognition that tobacco use cessation programming is needed, and adequate resources such as funding and training. Subsequently, effective cessation programming targeting tobacco-using youth needs to be developed, implemented, evaluated, and institutionalized. Guidance and examples are provided for each step.

Chapter 13 - During the last two decades there has been an increase in research focusing on the effects of maternal depression on the developing child. Research in this field has apparently developed out of the recognition of a relatively higher prevalence of postpartum maternal depression than once believed and recurring observations of differences in mother/offspring relationships or child behavior associated with maternal postpartum depression. The offspring behaviors that have been implicated have included slight, transient effects to longer term deficits. Some researchers have argued that even in to young adulthood, individuals who experienced interactions with depressed mothers are at significantly greater risk of experiencing a variety of psychological symptoms, including depression, anxiety, and problems with addiction. Again, this view is controversial and others in the field link these increased risks to alternative factors such as low socioeconomic status or marital discord. While there appears to be consensus among most researchers in recognizing that there are likely effects of maternal postpartum depression on offspring, there is little consensus regarding the specific details of these effects. In our review, we will systematically analyze research focusing on the effects of postpartum depression on the offspring and those variables that are believed to be affected from potential difficulties in this bond.

Chapter 14 - Crying, which represents the very first communicative channel infants can use to communicate with their environment, plays an important role in child development. Crying is a biological signal that alerts those in the caregiving environment about the needs and wants of the infant and motivates them to respond. Cries act to release specific and appropriate patterns of caregiving actions, thereby ensuring the infant's survival. The aim of this study was to review research that has investigated expressions of distress, specifically crying, during early stages of development in infancy. We have emphasized on the importance of cry evaluation in specific psychopathology, particularly Autism Spectrum Disorders (ASD). First the neurobiological activation that takes place during an episode of crying, both in the caregiver and the infant brain, is described. A description of the function of crying episodes and their evolution, starting from the fetal stage through childhood, follows. Finally, how anomalies in the expression of cry can bias the caregiver's perception of them, and how parents' reactions to pathological crying can be qualitatively different from their reactions to typical crying of same-aged children, is described. Such differences can confound parental attempts to share feelings and develop inter-subjectivity with their children.

Chapter 15 - The study was inspired by general allegations against the preventive child health services of failing to take into account problems faced by modern families, e.g. attachment difficulties and stress. Objective: In order to improve the psychosocial effectiveness of the health services for preschool children, a comprehensive programme was tested. Study group and setting: Mothers of 1,963 children participated. 967 were recruited at 18 months (Cohort I, baseline, no intervention), 996 shortly after birth and followed until 18 months (Cohort II) in two arms: intervention – non-intervention. Thirty-six child health centres within primary care in Uppsala county (experiment) and 36 centres in five other Swedish counties (control) were enrolled. Methods: Quasi-experimental controlled trial under routine conditions. The intervention included screening for postpartum depression, a curriculum for attachment and interaction, book gifts, parent groups, encouragement to participate in network activities, and extended home visits if needed. Main outcome measures: management of postpartum depression, mother-child interaction, child vocabulary, group participation, stress in parents. Results: The programme was not implemented according to the plans. Apart from more invitations to parent groups and higher participation in parent groups, there were no effects attributable to the intervention. The experiences are discussed with a view to general recommendations for intervention research put forward in the literature. Conclusions: Intervention trials in primary care should not be launched without extra resources in terms of financial support, manpower, and monitoring. Recommendations of careful pre-planning and development of interventions in several stages should be followed.

Chapter 16 - The aim of this study was to examine the relationship between watching health content on television news programs and fear of health problems, risk perceptions and health behavior intentions. We explored the possibility that television exposure may not only be directly related to perceptions of risk, but also indirectly trough fear. 923 randomly selected adult respondents completed a Health and Media Interview Survey. Structural Equation Modeling confirmed that fear was an intervening variable between television news exposure and risk perception about health problems. There was a direct link between watching health content on television news and risk perception, but this was only true for rarely experienced health problems. While risk estimates were not related to intended health behavior, both fear of health problems and news exposure directly predicted respondents' intentions to engage in positive health actions.

Chapter 17 - Body esteem is an important variable that has been linked to a range of negative health outcomes including depression, negative affect, obesity and increased risk of suffering from eating disorders. However, little information is available regarding ethnic differences in body esteem in British children. Objective: To examine gender, ethnic and weight status differences in body esteem in a sample of British children. Methods: The study was cross sectional in design and assessed body esteem and weight status in 756 children (394 boys, 362 girls, mean age 11.4 ± 1.6 years). Body esteem was determined using the body esteem scale for children. Height and body mass were measured directly. Body mass index was determined as kg/m2. Overweight/obesity status was determined using child-specific, International Obesity task force cut-off points. Results: A 2 (gender) X 3 (ethnicity) X 2 (weight status) ways analysis of variance (ANCOVA) controlling for age indicated that body esteem was higher for normal weight boys compared to girls whereas body esteem scores were similar for boys and girls in the overweight/obese category (P = 0.044). Body esteem scores were higher in boys compared to girls from white and black ethnic groups but this pattern was reversed for Asian boys and girls (P = 0.039). Conclusions: Findings of this study indicate that body esteem interacts with weight status and ethnicity across gender groups in British children after controlling for age. In the context of the current study overweight children and Asian boys may be particular populations where future research needs to focus.

Chapter 18 - Childhood burn in Bangladesh is a significant public health problem. Uncovered kerosene-lamp ("Kupi") for lighting and traditional earthen oven for cooking is commonly used in rural areas. The study was conducted to reveal the epidemiology of childhood burn and thereby help in planning future strategies for prevention of child burns in Bangladesh. Methods: A prospective study was conducted on a total of 100 consecutively enrolled patients admitted in the burn unit of Dhaka Medical College Hospital between January and June 2005. Data extracted included demographics; burn related causes as well as treatment related variables. Results: The results revealed preponderance of older girls burnt by flame, mainly from uncovered, kerosene-oil lamp used for house hold lighting in rural areas. There were two deaths in the series, both were victims of massive flame burn. The mean duration of hospital stay was 34 +/- 15 days, with higher treatment cost than the monthly income of the families. Almost all the cases had some sort of permanent disfigurement as the treatment outcome. Conclusion: Kerosene lamp, cooking in open oven, loose attires and lack of parental supervision and awareness were the most important risk factors identified in childhood burn.

Chapter 19 - The objective was to explore the attitude of the secondary school children toward persons living with HIV/AIDS. Methods: This report is based on a cross section survey of the secondary school children in Barbados. Representative samples of these children were selected from the secondary schools across Barbados using a two stage randomization. The survey instrument consisted of a structured self administered questionnaire. Results: Respondents varied proportionately between 10 and 18 years coming from form (class) 1 to 5 of the secondary schools, 53% being males. Nearly a sixth of the respondents personally knew someone living with HIV/AIDS and nearly a third personally knew someone, who had died of AIDS. Around 50% of the respondents answered "ÿes", when asked whether HIV infected students and teachers should be allowed to attend school to learn and teach respectively. However, only a tenth were willing to buy food from a vendor who was HIV infected. Majority of the children were willing to take care of relatives or get close to a class mate infected with the HIV. However, over a half of the respondent would prefer to maintain secrecy about one of their family member being HIV infected. Conclusions: It is clear that the issues of stigma and discrimination remain important in Barbados. However, compared to our previous survey of the same population, attitudes toward persons with HIV/AIDS have softened.

Chapter 20 - To investigate a possible relationship between the way milk is consumed (defined as only bottle, only cup or combined both cup and bottle use) and obesity indexes among preschool children. Study Design: Cross-sectional. Methods: Body Mass Index (BMI), waist circumference (WC) and waist to length ratio (WtLR) where combined with parameters from a lifestyle questionnaire (n=1,755) and a 3-day dietary recall questionnaire (n=855) from preschool children (4-7 years old) in Crete, Greece. Results: Taking into account age, sex, nationality, mothers level of education, current energy intake and expenditure, children who consume milk only from a cup, were found to have lower mean BMI (16.44, 16.95 and 16.96 kg/m2, respectively, p=0.047), WC (55.5, 55.8 and 56.8 cm, respectively, p=0.024), and WtLR (0.480, 0.482 and 0.491, respectively, p=0.014) when compared to those who drank milk from either only a nursing bottle or from both a cup and nursing bottle. Prolonged bottle use was significantly related to obesity (OR of 2.14 [95%CI: 1.21 - 3.78]) and to having a waist circumference over the 90th percentile (OR of 1.88 [95%CI: 1.12 - 3.15]). Conclusions: Childhood obesity may be affected by prolonged bottle use during preschool years independently of current energy intake and expenditure. These current findings stress the imperative need for parental education on the effects of prolonged bottle use on child weight and health.

Chapter 21 - In a large scale European study of 1,250 adults, subjective reports of obsessive thinking was assessed using anonymous self-ratings. The incidence of frequent compulsive thinking was 3 percent, and a further 9.5% of the sample reported "often" experiencing compulsive thoughts. There were significant differences associated with age (obsessiveness decreased with age), gender (1:1.6 males to females) and educational status (obsessionals were likely to have higher educational status). There was no evidence that compulsivity rating was related to weekly hours worked nor with hours invested in physical exercise, or number of hours slept per night. An array of physical ailments emerged as major determinants of compulsivity including mental fatigue, sleeplessness, migraine and sickness or nausea. The mood predictors of compulsivity encompassed depression, apathy and fearfulness (as well as irritation, anger and anxiety). Persons rating themselves high on compulsive attitudes were more likely to display inferior mental well-being, dissatisfaction with physical health and with work relationships and job content. Despite inferior subjectively perceived physical health, persons displaying a high frequency of obsessive thoughts were not more likely to have been ill during the last year than those "free" of obsessive thinking. The implications of these findings for a better understanding of compulsive thinking/behaviour are discussed.

Chapter 22 - This study examines differences in knowledge of and the attitude toward anorexia nervosa among Israeli women. Methods: This study used data from a survey questionnaire answered by 360 Israeli women during the years 2007-2008. Data was split from two groups of 180 women, ages 45-65 and 15-25 years of age. Results: In contrast to the older age group the younger age group had a poorer understanding of the symptoms of AN; a more positive conception of being thin and a lower opinion of their body self-image. The younger women displayed higher percentages of socially beneficial elements considered outcomes of AN: finding jobs, having more friends, being popular and accepted and being the object of admiration. Discussion: Younger women viewed AN more positively than the older women. The distorted views of self and of the disease of AN among young Israeli women, warrants further investigation and implementation of intervention established.

Chapter 23 - In the normal newborn infants, human fetal hemoglobin (Hb F) is readily replaced by the adult hemoglobins A and A2, and at the age of about six months only a small percentage of fetal hemoglobin is detectable. The failure of normal process of switching off the production of γ-chains during neonatal period leads to a high level of fetal hemoglobin in adult life without causing any anemia. This is called as a hereditary persistence of fetal hemoglobin (HPFH). The Hb F in general delivers less oxygen to tissues, shortens the life span of red cells, and makes red cells unsuitable to cope with physiological stress of life. The HPFH is an autosomal co-dominantly inherited condition of rare occurrence. The present study reports for the first time a Paraja-Bhuyan (tribal) family having HPFH in four members, i.e. a mother with her three children from Sundargarh district of Orissa. These four cases showed no apparent clinical or hematological abnormality except mild pallor observed in two younger children. The acid elution test revealed pancellular distribution of fetal hemoglobin in all cases of HPFH in the erythrocytes. The findings of the present study have been discussed in the light of a few case reports available in the literature.

Chapter 24 - In the Tier 1 Program of the Project P.A.T.H.S., teaching units based on different positive youth development constructs are covered. A total of 24 experimental schools and 24 control schools were randomly selected to participate in a randomized group trial. Subjective outcome evaluation at posttest showed that the program participants generally had favorable perceptions of the program, workers and benefits of the program. Analyses of covariance and linear mixed models controlling for differences between the two groups in terms of pretest scores, personal variables and random effects of schools showed that participants in the experimental schools who perceived the program to be beneficial (N=1,888) had significantly higher positive youth development levels than did participants in the control schools (N=3,358) at posttest based on different indicators derived from the Chinese Positive Youth Development Scale. Both objective outcome and subjective outcome evaluation findings suggest that the Tier 1 Program of the Project P.A.T.H.S. was effective in promoting the holistic development of the program participants.

Chapter 25 - Nine focus groups involving 61 instructors recruited from nine schools were conducted to understand the perceptions of the program implementers of the Tier 1 Program of the Project P.A.T.H.S. via a qualitative approach. The informants generally described the program in a positive manner, although suggestions for improvement were proposed. When the informants were invited to name some metaphors that could stand for the program, the related metaphors and related explanation were generally positive in nature. Finally, the program implementers perceived many beneficial effects of the program in different domains. Intra-rater and inter-rater reliability analyses revealed that the coding of the positive or negative nature of the responses and the categorization was reliable. The present study provides qualitative support for the effectiveness of the Tier 1 Program of the Project P.A.T.H.S. in promoting holistic development among Chinese adolescents in Hong Kong.

Chapter 26 - Four schools participating in the Experimental Implementation Phase of the Project P.A.T.H.S. (Secondary 2 Level) were randomly selected to join this qualitative evaluation study. After completion of the Tier 1 Program, 260 secondary 2 (Grade 8) students in these four participating schools were invited to write a reflective journal in the form of weekly diary to reveal their perceptions and feelings regarding the Tier 1 Program and the related benefits. Results of the qualitative data analyses showed that most of the respondents (a) had positive views on the program, (b) had positive views on the instructors, and (c) stated that they had acquired competencies at societal, familial, interpersonal and personal levels after joining the program. The present qualitative findings based on students' weekly diaries are generally consistent with the previous evaluation findings using students' diaries and other evaluation strategies.

Chapter 27 - To evaluate the implementation quality of the Tier 1 Program (Secondary 2 Curriculum) of the Project P.A.T.H.S. in the Full Implementation Phase, 100 schools were randomly selected and participated in personal and/or telephone interviews regarding the implementation details of the Tier 1 Program. In the interviews, participants expressed their views on the students' responses and benefits of the program, appraisal of the positive and negative features of the program, and difficulties encountered during program implementation. Participants generally perceived that students had positive responses to the program and the program was perceived to be beneficial to the students, though negative comments and difficulties of program implementation were observed. They also perceived the Co-Walker Scheme to be beneficial. Consistent with previous findings, the present findings showed that the Tier 1 Program is generally perceived as helpful to the students and has positive global evaluation.

Chapter 28 - An interim evaluation was conducted to understand the implementation quality of the Tier 1 Program (Secondary 3 Curriculum) of the Project P.A.T.H.S. in the Experimental Implementation Phase. Twenty-five schools were randomly selected to provide information on the implementation details of the program via interviews and/or self-completed questionnaires. Results showed that a majority of the workers perceived that the students had positive responses to the program and the program was helpful to the students, although negative comments on the program design and difficulties in the implementation process were also recorded. In conjunction with previous findings, the present findings suggest that the three-year Tier 1 Program of the Project P.A.T.H.S. is well-received by different stakeholders and the program implementers perceive that the program can promote the holistic development of secondary school students in Hong Kong.

Chapter 29 - To understand the implementation quality of the Tier 1 Program (Secondary 2 Curriculum) of the Project P.A.T.H.S. in the Full Implementation Phase, observers carried out process evaluation in the form of systematic observations of 21 units in 14 randomly selected schools. Results showed that the overall level of program adherence was generally high, ranging from 70% to 100%, with an average of 89.3%. The implementation quality of the program regarding student interest, student participation and involvement, classroom control, use of interactive delivery method, instructors' familiarity with the students, degree of achievement of the objectives, time management, lesson preparation, overall implementation quality, and success of implementation was also found. The present findings are consistent with those based on the Experimental Implementation Phase, suggesting that the implementation quality of the Tier 1 Program (Secondary 2 Curriculum) was generally high.

Chapter 30 - This study examined the implementation quality of the Tier 1 Program (Secondary 3 Curriculum) delivered in the Experimental Implementation Phase of the Project P.A.T.H.S. (Positive Adolescent Training through Holistic Social Programmes). Process evaluation was conducted in the form of systematic observations of curriculum units in four randomly selected schools. Results indicated that the overall level of program adherence was high, ranging from 80% to 100%, with an average of 90%. The mean ratings of the program implementation quality were high, and the inter-rater reliability on these ratings across the observers was highly reliable. Despite limitations, the findings of this study suggest that the implementation of the Secondary 3 Program (Tier 1 Program) of the Experimental Implementation Phase was of very high quality. This provides strong evidence to account for the successful and encouraging outcomes of a major positive youth development program in Hong Kong.

Chapter 31 - This study examined the implementation quality of the Secondary 2 Program of the Project P.A.T.H.S. in the Experimental Implementation Phase. Classroom observations of 15 units implemented in ten schools were conducted under the Co-Walker Scheme, an initiative which attempts to provide support for the program implementers.

Results showed that the overall level of program adherence was generally high (mean = 81.9%) and implementation quality of the program in terms of students' interest and involvement, instructors' use of time, classroom management and interactive teaching strategies as well as their relationship with the students was good. Results also revealed that different aspects of program implementation were significantly correlated amongst themselves.

Chapter 32 - The Tier 2 Program of the Project P.A.T.H.S. is designed and implemented primarily by school social workers which attempts to help adolescents with greater psychosocial needs. After completion of the Tier 2 Program in the Experimental Implementation Phase (Secondary 2 level), 1,898 Secondary 2 students in 49 schools responded to the Subjective Outcome Evaluation Form (Form C) to assess their views on the program, instructors and perceived effectiveness of the program. Results showed that a large proportion of the respondents had positive perceptions of the program and the instructors and roughly four-fifths of the respondents regarded the program as helpful to them. Pearson correlation analyses showed that perceptions of the program and instructors were significantly correlated with perceived effectiveness of the program. Participants joining programs that adopted both adventure-based counseling approach and volunteer training activities generally perceived higher levels of program effectiveness and had better global views on the program than did participants attending programs adopted either approach only.

Chapter 33 - This article identifies various psychosocial factors influencing children and adolescents who are involved in sports. The emphasis is on lessons learned from being part of highly organized sports programs in the United States which have a primary emphasis on winning. We start with developmental issues and then proceed to the effects of (over) training, chronic illness or disability and intrinsic or extrinsic influences on sport participation experience by youth. This review also considers such concepts as psychological reactions to injury, stress and anxiety, depression and suicidal ideation, substance use and aggression. We conclude that sports participation by children and adolescents can have beneficial effects. However, these effects can be lifelong and potential adverse results of a highly competitive system must also be understood. This article reviews some of the psychosocial issues observed in American youth participation in highly organized sports programs. It is hoped that the lessons learned may be of help to others who develop and expand these programs for their children and adolescents.

Chapter 34 - Use of different drugs and supplements is a world-wide phenomenon in athletics. Drugs and nutritional supplements are used for many reasons, in hopes of feeling good, promoting good health, preventing illness, improving overt illness, reducing fatigue or enhancing muscle development, strength and appearance. Though unproven to be effective, various substances are popular with adolescent athletes of all types--cyclists, distance runners, soccer players, weight lifters, figure skaters, judo athletes, tennis players, football players and many others. A society which emphasizes winning over positive benefits of sports activity sets up its youth to try various chemicals to enhance sports performance as well as to relieve the stress that such pressure for winning inevitably brings. Much is not really known about how these substances affect the health of our youth, since research is often limited and typically only adult males in competitive sports are studied. Relating a known effect of drugs can also be difficult because there are multiple confounding variables found in the research studies and minimal information is available regarding long term effects of these drugs, especially in adolescents. This article reviews selected drugs and supplements used for doping by young athletes. It is important to note that the popularity and use of different substances change over time, sometimes rapidly, as new ones come to the market and old ones fade out of fashion. Also popular agents may vary in different countries and sports setting in which the athlete participates.

Chapter 35 - Doping in sports brings up not only ethical issues of fairness in competition, but also highlight the health hazards that the athletes may be at risk for. Many substances have been used for doping in sporting competitions since the ancient times. Growth hormone has been in use by elite athletes for the last several decades. Easy accessibility coupled with inadequate methods of detection available has made human growth hormone a logical option for doping in sports. Recent research work has established methodologies for detection of doping with growth hormone possible and ongoing work continues to refine these procedures.

Chapter 36 - Sudden death of a young athlete ($\leq$ 35 y of age) is always disconcerting. In the United States, the incidence of sudden cardiac death (SCD) is 2 in 100 000 among high school athletes and 1 in 65000 amongst collegiate athletes. The most common cause of SCD in a young athlete in the United States is hypertrophic cardiomyopathy (26%). Other main causes include commotio cordis (20%), anomalous origin of the coronary artery (14%), myocarditis, valvular heart disease, premature atherosclerotic heart disease, arrythmogenic right ventricular dysplasia, and aortic dilatation and rupture (5%-8% combined incidence). In athletes $\geq$ 35 years of age, coronary artery disease is the most common cause of sudden cardiac death. The pathophysiology of SCD is explained by and is a direct extension of the physiologic remodeling of the heart. Remodeling is characterized by chamber dilation and hypertrophy and precipitates fatal ventricular fibrillation. The main aim of pre-participation screening is to identify athletes at risk for SCD. In the United States, the screening is based on personal and family history and focused cardiovascular examination. In the United States, an electrocardiogram (ECG) is not recommended for mass screening of asymptomatic young athletes. Management of SCD includes prompt recognition and initiation of cardiopulmonary resuscitation (CPR), defibrillation, and early mobilization of emergency medical services (EMS). This article reviews screening and prevention of SCD in young athletes.

Chapter 37 - The incidence of systemic hypertension among adolescents and young adults has been on the rise. Several factors have contributed to this including, obesity, physical inactivity, unhealthy food habits, drug abuse, and familial tendencies. Early onset hypertension in children and adolescents has been associated with premature atherosclerosis and subsequent cardiovascular mortality and morbidity thus placing a huge economic burden on the individual family as well as the society in general. This article reviews the beneficial effects of exercise both aerobic and resistance training on blood pressure and the current recommendations for sports participation by adolescents who have hypertension.

Chapter 38 - Back pain in adolescent athletes is common. The most common cause of acute low back pain in adolescent athletes is musculotendinous injury. It is also the most common cause of back pain overall. The most common identified structural anomaly is in adolescents who present with chronic or recurrent activity related low back pain is spondylolysis. In all adolescents with back pain psychosomatic disorder must be considered in the differential diagnosis. Other significant causes of low back pain in adolescent athletes include scoliosis, kyphosis, diskitis, slipped disk, and inflammatory spondyloarthropathies. Evaluation is mostly based on history and physical examination. Imaging studies are indicated in some cases based on findings on history and examination. Management is non-operative in most cases and includes a short period of rest from sports, followed by physical therapy and conditioning. This articles reviews common causes of low back pain in adolescent athletes such as musculotendionus injuries, psychosomatic pain, spondylolysis, diskitis, scoliosis, kyphosis, and ankylosing spondylitis.

Chapter 39 - Ankle is a complex joint with many ligaments stabilizing the joint. Ankle sprains are commonly seen in sports in which jumping and landing, and sudden cutting are involved, as exemplified by American football, soccer, volleyball and gymnastics. The majority of ankle sprains are to the lateral ligaments resulting from an inversion type injury. Clinical assessment mainly depends up on history of the mechanism of injury and initial symptoms, and a careful physical exam of the ankle as well as for any associated injuries. Routine use of X-rays is not always useful. Treatment is generally conservative with early ice, rest, elevation, and protective weight bearing, followed by complete rehabilitation with physiotherapy. Delayed recovery and chronic pain should prompt further investigation and orthopedic consultation.

Chapter 40 - The knee is the most commonly injured joint from sport participation. Estimates of knee injuries range from 10-60% in various sports, and 50% of adolescent athletes present with sport-related knee pain. Most injuries in the adolescent athlete are due to overuse. Idiopathic anterior knee pain, Osgood-Schlatter disease, patellar tendinitis, osteochodritis dissecans, pathologic plicae, and bursitis are some of the many causes of chronic or recurrent symptoms. Referred pain from the hip, spine, abdomen, or pelvic pathology should always be considered in any athlete presenting with knee pain. Acute trauma is less common and can result in ligament injuries, meniscal tears, and fractures. In the adolescent athlete with acute trauma, injuries of the distal femoral and proximal tibial physes should also be considered in the differential diagnosis. This article reviews common overuse and acute injuries in young athletes.

Chapter 41 - Cricket is a popular sport worldwide. It is a non-contact sport, with moderate dynamic and low static demands on the energy systems. Many children and adolescents begin playing cricket at an early age and continue to participate for a number of years with increasing level of intensity. The incidence of injuries varies depending upon the age of the player and level of competition. Between 30% and 50% of the players report some injury during peak season. The most common significant injury in cricket is to the thoraco-lumbar spine in fast bowlers, because of repetitive, rotation, extension, and lateral flexion movements. Other acute injuries include soft tissue contusions, abrasions, and eye injuries from impact with the ball. Overuse injuries include shoulder impingement, elbow overuse injuries, patellar tendinitis, and stress fractures. This article reviews the epidemiology, mechanisms and prevention of cricket injuries in youth.

Chapter 42 - Martial arts are becoming increasingly popular among children and adolescents in many countries. Thousands of young children and adolescents are involved in taekwondo, karate, mixed martial arts, and other less well-known disciplines. Increasing media coverage has drawn attention to this growing trend and its potential benefits for youth. Proponents cite many benefits from participation, including self-defense, cardiovascular fitness, flexibility, improved self-esteem, and improved concentration. Some studies have reported on the role of martial arts in treating psychological and behavioral disorders. Injury rates have decreased with increasing awareness and preventive measures, such as padded floors and mandatory equipment. This article provides an overview of medical aspects of martial arts participation, injuries, and prevention strategies.

Chapter 43 - Musculoskeletal overuse injuries result from excessive stress to normal connective tissues and supporting structures. These injuries can affect bone, tendon, muscle, joint, bursa, and growth cartilage. Sport-related overuse injuries are the most common injuries seen in adolescents and account for half of all sport-related injuries in this age group. Rapid increase in the intensity and volume of physical activity is the most consistent risk factor for overuse injury. Data on other risk factors such as anatomical variations are equivocal. Most athletes present with pain localized to the affected area. Diagnosis is generally obvious based on clinical findings and routine laboratory or imaging studies are not indicated. Modification of the level of physical activity is the most important element of treatment. Other considerations in the treatment include use of anti-inflammatory and analgesic medications, therapeutic exercises, physical therapy modalities, and identification and modification of risk factors. This article reviews the general principles of diagnosis and management of overuse injuries in adolescents.

Chapter 44 - The objective was to investigate the differences between sexes in the two most common injuries in the young female athlete: anterior cruciate ligament injury and lower extremity stress fracture. Design: PubMed was searched for articles in the last fifteen years, from 1994-2009, with the terms “sport injuries in females,” “anterior cruciate ligament injury in females,” “lower extremity stress fracture,” and “stress fracture in female athletes.” Data: Young female athletes have a significantly increased risk of noncontact ACL injury and lower extremity stress fractures over male athletes. Studies over the last fifteen years have focused on identifying the differences between male and female athletes in mechanism of injury, biomechanics of injury, treatment and prevention strategies. Conclusion: As female participation in competitive sports increases, the physician needs to be aware of the underlying causes of increased ACL injury and lower extremity fractures and prevention strategies for these athletes.

Chapter 45 - Joav Merrick, MD, MMedSci, DMSc, is professor of pediatrics, child health and human development affiliated with Kentucky Children’s Hospital, University of Kentucky, Lexington, United States and the Zusman Child Development Center, Division of Pediatrics, Soroka University Medical Center, Ben Gurion University, Beer-Sheva, Israel, the medical director of the Division for Mental Retardation, Ministry of Social Affairs, Jerusalem, the founder and director of the National Institute of Child Health and Human Development. Numerous publications in the field of pediatrics, child health and human development, rehabilitation, intellectual disability, disability, health, welfare, abuse, advocacy, quality of life and prevention. Received the Peter Sabroe Child Award for outstanding work on behalf of Danish Children in 1985 and the International LEGO-Prize (“The Children’s Nobel Prize”) for an extraordinary contribution towards improvement in child welfare and well-being in 1987.

Chapter 46 - The National Institute of Child Health and Human Development (NICHD) in Israel was established in 1998 as a virtual institute under the auspicies of the Medical Director, Ministry of Social Affairs and Social Services in order to function as the research arm for the Office of the Medical Director. In 1998 the National Council for Child Health and Pediatrics, Ministry of Health and in 1999 the Director General and Deputy Director General of the Ministry of Health endorsed the establishment of the NICHD.

INTRODUCTION

Public Health Year Book 2009

Joav Merrick, MD, MMedSci, DMSc[1,2,3,4,5]

[1]National Institute of Child Health and Human Development, [2]Office of the Medical Director, Division for Mental Retardation, Ministry of Social Affairs and Social Services, Jerusalem, [3]Zusman Child Development Center, Soroka University Medical Center, Beer-Sheva, Israel, [4]Interuniversity College for Health and Development, Castle of Seggau, Graz, Austria, [5]Kentucky Children's Hospital, University of Kentucky, Lexington, United States

Correspondence: Professor Joav Merrick, MD, MMedSci, DMSc, Medical Director, Division for Mental Retardation, Ministry of Social Affairs, POBox 1260, IL-91012 Jerusalem, Israel. E-mail: jmerrick@zahav.net.il

Charles-Edward Amory Winslow (1877-1957), an American bacteriologist and public health professional, who in 1915 established the Yale Department of Public Health within the Yale Medical School defined public health as the science and art of preventing disease, prolonging life and promoting health through the organized efforts and informed choices of society, organizations, public and private, communities and individuals.

This department later became the Yale School of Public Health and most medical schools today also have schools of public health covering the areas of health epidemiology, biostatistics, health service issues, environmental, social, behavioral and occupational health.

The focus and goal of public health is to prevent rather than treat a disease, which can be done through surveillance and the promotion of healthy behaviors. and distribution of condoms are examples of public health measures. Many diseases can be prevented through simple, non-medical methods with hand washing to prevent disease as an easy example.

HISTORY

Public health aspects can be found from early sources (like the Bible) and for example man recognized early that water can be polluted and spread diseases. The Romans realized that proper diversion of human waste was a must in urban areas and the Chinese developed the practice of variolation following a smallpox epidemic. Vaccination was only much later introduced when Edward Jenner (1749-1823) in 1796 inoculated an eight year old boy with cowpow and this way paved the way for smallpox vaccination.

John Snow (1813-1858) was another pioneer, who became know for anaesthesia, medical hygiene and the father of epidemiology. He was one of the first to use ether and chloroform, which he administered to Queen Victoria at birth of two of her nine children. He identified the source of the 1854 cholera outbreak in London by talking to local residents and mapping out the spread of the disease. He found the source of the outbreak at the public water pump on Broad Street (now Broadwick Street) and even though his chemical and microscope examination of a sample of the Broad Street pump water was not able to conclusively prove its danger, his studies of the pattern of the disease were convincing enough to persuade the local council to disable the well pump by removing its handle and this way stop the further spreading of the disease. Afterwards Heinrich Hermann Robert Koch (1843-1910), Nobel Prize winner in medicine (1905) for his discovery of tuberculosis and Louis Pasteur (1822-1895) introduced the germ theory and the production of artificial vaccines. They are together with Ferdinand Julius Cohn (1828-1898) seens as the founders of modern microbiology and medical hygiene (1).

PUBLIC HEALTH IN OUR TIME

When infectious disease declined during the last century, public health became more focused on chronic illness, prevention and health promotion issues. Population health has broadened the focus of public health from individual behaviors and risk factors to population issues such as inequality, poverty, education and the social determinants of health.

The International Public Health Journal is a peer-reviewed journal published by Nova Science (New York) aimed at the scientific community interested in the broad area of public health. This journal provides an international multidisciplinary forum with a holistic approach to public health issues, health and medicine, health and social policy, service aspects, developmental aspects, epidemiology, rehabilitation, family and social issues, quality of life and all other aspects of public health over the whole age spectrum.

It is our hope that the 2009 Public Health Yearbook will provide interest for the reader and we hope it will induce directions and new research in the field of public health.

REFERENCES

[1] Detels R, McEwen J, Beaglehole R, Tanaka, eds. Oxford textbook of public health, 4th ed. Oxford: Oxford Univ Press, 2002.

Section one
Public health aspects

In: Public Health Yearbook 2009
Editor: Joav Merrick

ISBN: 978-1-61668-911-7

Chapter 1

Mental Health Aspects of Chronic Illness in Adolescence

Helen D Pratt, PhD*

Pediatrics and Human Development, Behavioral Developmental Pediatrics, College of Human Medicine, Michigan State University, East Lansing Michigan, Kalamazoo, Michigan, United States of America

Abstract

Adolescence is a period of tremendous growth and represents a time of transition from childhood to adulthood. Youth who do not experience typical development as a result of chronic illness may experience psychological problems. Adolescents with chronic illness versus typically developing adolescents may need a greater degree of support, resources and guidance to ensure that they grow into psychologically healthy adults. Those youth who receive such help have a greater chance of developing the ability to live relatively healthy and productive lives. Youth who do not experience typical development as a result of chronic illness may experience psychological problems.

Keywords: Adolescents, chronic illness, psychological issues.

Introduction

Adolescence is a period of tremendous growth and represents a time of transition from childhood to adulthood (1-8). Youth who do not experience typical development as a result of chronic illness (see table 1) may experience psychological problems (3,5,9-13). They may also need a greater degree of support, resources and guidance to ensure that they grow into

* Correspondence: Professor Helen D Pratt, PhD, Behavioral Developmental Pediatrics, Pediatrics Program, Michigan State University/Kalamazoo Center for Medical Studies, 1000 Oakland Dr, Kalamazoo, Michigan 49008 United States. Tel: (269) 337-6450; Fax: (269) 337-6474; E-mail: pratt@kcms.msu.edu (email)

psychologically healthy adults as compared to "typically" developing adolescents (10-15). Those youth who receive such help have a greater chance of developing the ability to live relatively healthy and productive lives.

Psychological development

Psychological development deals more specifically with the progressive organization of cognitive, emotional, and social aspects of function (see table 1). The synthesis of physical, biological, hormonal factors in the individual with the functional domains produces predictable types of behavioral and personality characteristics in each individual, the expression of which is unique (2-4,7,15-17). Research by noted personality theorist provides us with models of how these general expressions can be categorized (17-20).

Table 1. Sample Of Chronic Illnesses And Disorders That May Have A Psychological Impact On Adolescent Development [9-13]

Medical		Mental /Behavioral
AIDS	Muscular Dystrophies	Anxiety Disorders
Asthma	Neurological Disorders	Attention Deficit/Hyperactivity Disorder
Chronic pain	Non Migraine Headaches	Body Dysmorphic Disorder
Cancer	Neurocutaneious Syndromes	Chronic Depression
Crohn's Disease	Obesity	Disruptive Behavior Disorders
Congenital Heart Disease	Osteoid Osteoma	Eating Disorders
Cystic Fibrosis	Psoriasis	Elimination Disorders
Diabetes Mellitus	Scoliosis	Communication Disorders
Epilepsy	Seizures	Learning Disorders
Guillain-Barr'e Syndrome	Sickle Cell Disease	Mental Retardation
Hemophilia	Sleep Disorders	Motor Skills Disorders
Hepatitis	Spina bifida	Other Psychotic Disorders
Hypertension	Syncope	Personality Disorders
Juvenile Rheumatoid Arthritis	Thyroid Disorders	Pervasive Developmental Disorders
Leukemia		Reactive Attachment Disorders
Lupus		Schizophrenia
Migraine Headaches		Sexual and Gender Identity Disorders
Multiple Sclerosis		Tic Disorders

Individuals manifest emotional reactions and coping skills that are governed by their a) cognitive capacity, b) intelligence, c) mental flexibility, d) temperament, e) attachment to family, peers, community, f) sense of autonomy, g) social competence, h) problem solving skills, i) coping skills, and j) exposure to violence, substance, and poverty (see table 3) (8,15). Psychological development continues well into adulthood. During middle and late adolescence cognitive capacity expands to include abstract thinking and more complex thinking skills. Youth who had chronic illnesses during childhood, may not have mastered age appropriate psychological skills (cognitive, emotional, social, integrative adaptive) (see table 4) (13,19,22). This means that these youth must expend their energy in skill acquisition versus refinement of their psychological development. Cognitive and emotional responses to their environment may appear "childish" and parents may complain that they are not being responsible.

Table 2. Stages of Adolescent Development [1, 2,3 4, 5, 8, 13, 16]

Early Adolescence 10 – 14 year of Age Onset of puberty Neurobiological changes in the brain impact: speech, language Psychological Components Cognitive Growth results in major changes in mental abilities and thought processes: Preoccupation with rapidly changing events of puberty Increased abilities to perform more complex mental tasks (thinking skills and problem solving skills) Improved mental processing speed and alertness Longer attention span Better judgment Better ability to adopt another person's spatial perspective A clear sense of their own body image Clear sense of social standing with peer Comparison with peers and worry over perceived abnormalities Development of initial abstract thought The process of emancipation begins Establishment and maintenance of same-sex friendships Exposure to bullying and teasing (perpetrator, victim, or both)
Middle Adolescence 14 – 18 year of Age Somatic growth spurt. Females, and males who engage in body image activities may find it difficult to maintain a personally desired weight or body size; this may result in dieting, excessive exercise, purging or other pathogenic weight control measures or body image problems. Psychological Components" • Significant symbolic movement away from the home environment • Considerable need for independence • Strong reliance on peers setting personal rules • Heterosexual experimentation predominates • Altruistic nature emerges • Identification with non-parental adult role models • Experimentation with sex, substance use or abuse • Major changes in cognitive abilities and fantasy life • Can engage in fantasy • May become preoccupied with comparing their physical characteristics with peers • Is developing theories about life • Able to independently weigh consequences of decisions before taking action • Ability to engage in inductive and deductive reasoning is expanding • Can think about what they would like to do when they become adults • May know and understand the consequences of risk taking behaviors, but their caution may be overridden by their stronger need for popularity and peer recognition • May experience sexual fantasies • These fantasies may occupy much of their time • Some youth will fantasize about same sex peers and become very disturbed over these events • Beginning to development of a positive self-image and increased confidence occurs as he or she consistently experiences success • Is highly sensitive to negative comments from others and peer rejection, bullying, and traumatic personal experiences

Table 2. (Continued)

Late Adolescence 18 – 21 Final pubertal changes physiologic fine tuning) occur Psychological Components" • Issue of emancipation from parents are essentially resolved • Finalization of secure, acceptable body image and gender role • Establishment of adult versus narcissistic sexual relationships • Acquisition of adult lifestyle • Considerable energy spent in establishment of vocational skills for training • Cognitive abilities are more complex. ▫ Abstract thought has been established ▫ Empathy skills are well developed ▫ Personal values clearer and well defined. ▫ Is future oriented ▫ Perceives and reacts upon long range options. ▫ Beginning to resolve conflicts between themselves and their parents. ▫ Continuing to develop th ability to think and function independently ▫ Less influenced by peers ▫ Uses own judgment for setting personal rules. ▫ More actively participating is sexual experimentation ▫ Predominate altruistic nature emerges. ▫ Relationships with romantic partners are less narcissistic and more geared towards mutual respect and gratification. ▫ Prefers the association with groups and or couples and prefers intimacy versus isolation. ▫ Most adolescents at this stage of maturation have developed a strong sense of personal identity. ▫ Capable of establishing and maintaining stable, mutually caring and satisfying interpersonal (including sexual) relationships.

Impact of puberty/sexual maturation

All youth matriculate through three major stages (early, middle and late) of adolescence which occur in a dynamic, sequential, orderly and time-dependent manner (see table 2) (1-5,8,13,18). However, there is considerable individual variation in the onset, rate, and progression of an adolescents move through this process. That variation is significantly impacted by many factors: a) internal (including biological, neurological, physical growth, mental development) or external (changes in the adolescent's personal, family, peer, school, and neighborhood environment, exposure to violence, trauma, chemicals, etc.) (1,3-7,13,15). The effects can result in changes in any one of the essential components in the domains of function (see table 3) (8,15). The presence of a chronic illness can cause many of the factors mentioned above to impact psychological development of the adolescent.

The hallmark of adolescence is the onset of puberty, which can begin as early as age 8 or as late as age 15 years in females and as early as age 9.5 years and as late as age 15 years in males. Puberty ends when the adolescent reaches full physical and developmental maturity (which can be as late as age 21 years) (see table 2). Youth diagnosed with chronic illnesses such as intellectual disability, malnutrition, diabetes mellitus (when glycemic control is poor) cystic fibrosis, sickle cell disease, or anorexia nervosa may experience delayed sexual maturation (23).. This may mean that the adolescent becomes emotionally distressed over not experiencing physical changes in their bodies similar to those of their typically developing peers. Adolescents who do not experience the hormonal changes of puberty may not experience co-occurring changes in brain function (23).

Table 3. Domains of Function [8, 15]

Psychological Components	*Social/Emotional*
Cognitive Attention The ability to focus selectively and generally on events, actions and or information in the environment Mental Processing Speed (alertness) The ability to respond in an effective manner to physical, mental, emotional and physiological events in self to process information in a manner that allows for the appropriate adaptation of behavior to maximize positive outcomes and minimize negative outcomes Memory The ability to acquire, store, and recall recent, remote, and long term events, actions, information in an organized and useful manner. Thinking Knowledge of specifics, Comprehension, Application, Analysis, Synthesis, Evaluation, Decision Making, Problem Solving, Ability to monitor multiple events & people simultaneously	Ability to regulate, modulate and control emotions Ability to establish new friendships Ability to maintain peer relationships Ability to establish and maintain healthy family relationships Integration and coordination of all of these skills *Integrative/Adaptive* Ability to adapt skills and functions to meet demands of specific situations or conditions *Other Domains of Function* Auditory Language Motor Perceptual Motor Visual

Table 4. Psychosocial Issues that may be experienced by Chronically Ill Youth [13, 19, 28]

Personal	Parents	Siblings	Peers
Being disappointed in their bodies.	Feeling parents are angry at they because their chronic illness monopolizes parent's lives	Feeling stress of sibling because of their adjustment and stigmatizing guilt and fear of having a chronically ill sibling	Social Rejection
Dealing with complex medical procedures	Detecting parental stress because of adjustment to chronically ill teen and stigmatizing guilt and fear about having a chronically ill teen	Detecting their siblings' anger at them for monopolizing parental attention	Being made fun of because of their chronic illness

Table 4. (Continued)

Personal	Parents	Siblings	Peers
Feeling vulnerable	Realizing their parent's fatigue from having to deal with acute and chronic stressors of implementing daily medical regimes	Realizing their siblings are embarrassed about their condition	Acceptance
Feeling illness is unfair	Recognizing their parent's financial distress	Being rejected by healthy sibling	Collegial relationships
Having to continuously adapt	Knowing their parents are unhappy because of their inability to meet needs of spouse or their other children	Acceptance	
Lack of esteem	Rejecting their parent's over-protectiveness	Collegial relationships	
Lack of confidence	Feeling rejection from parents because they are not what their parents expected		
Loss of life freedoms that are associated with excellent health	Acceptance		
Periodic, and often unpredictable, crisis events.	Collegial relationships		
Permanent lifestyle changes	Loving parental relationship		
Problems with emancipation			
Slowed or altered physical development and appearance			
Social limitations			
Social stigma			
Unpredictable course of illness			
Self Acceptance			
Joy of living			
Self Confidence			
Success			

As adolescents work to adjust to physical and hormonal changes caused by puberty, the presence of a chronic illness may significantly alter their ability to master the tasks of adolescence: Individuation, emotional and behavioral regulation, ability to initiate and maintain reciprocal intimate relations, development of skills that support independence (4,9,21,24,25). Chronic illness may also result in over involvement of parents in to personal functioning (especially when bathing and toileting are involved) impeding the adolescent's ability to develop self confidence, feeling of independence, and opportunities for healthy sexuality development.

Impact on the adolescents relationships with family

The impact of chronic illness on family relationships is dependent the specific illness, its severity, how it affects the adolescent's body, how and if the functional limitations are perceived, what kinds of treatments are involved, and whether the symptoms of the illness or the results of treatment are manifested publically. For instance, spina bifida may impair an adolescent's ability to walk; siblings who see their "sick" sibling on crutches or in a wheel chair may be embarrassed by the visual images when they are around peers and the public. Those siblings may then treat the "sick" sibling differently; the adolescent with chronic illness may feel angry or saddened by this reaction. Youth who have loss their hair because of their chronic illness (alapegia) or chemotherapy also presents visuals for the individuals that can result in rejection, embarrassment and other emotions in sibling and thus cause reciprocal emotions in the chronically ill teen. Members of the family, especially parents may restrict/limit the ability of their teen to individuate and move towards emancipation. Parents may also become overprotective and limit their teen's access to activities that may give them opportunities to be with other youth of similar interests. The well intentioned family members may actually cause frustration for the teen and impede possibility of "typical" development.

Although the illnesses of asthma or diabetes may not be readily visible, if the teen has public displays of their illness in front of peers (i.e. a) an asthma attack, or b) the teen with diabetes begins to shake and get confused as the result of hypoglycemia) those illnesses also become visible or public. If the teen has to go to the office to take shots or use an inhaler before exercise or an outing, the illness becomes public. Other teens will "know." Most adolescents between ages 10 and 16 years will become very upset about these events because being different or a public spectacle is something to be avoided at all costs. Younger adolescents may be too embarrassed to return to the setting of a psychologically traumatic event (public display of their illness). However, if these same events occur when the teen is 17 years of age, he or she might be less psychologically traumatized and simply ask for help and explain to peers what just happened (see case example1).

Psychological development may also be impeded when there are visible signs of chronic illness - such as the loss of hair from chemotherapy, obesity due to medications (such as corticosteroids), or congenital conditions or injuries; these signs may result in the adolescent retreating from social situations. She may avoid contact even with former friends. Older adolescent may be helped to rationalize emotions about these visible signs of their illness and be prepared to address them with peers and others. Youth who appear younger than their chronological age may face various forms of discrimination or be treated like a younger child by adults who interact with them (case example 2).

Case story 1

For instance the youth who develops type I or insulin dependent diabetes at age 9 years usually adjusts well at this age and displays very responsible eating and exercise habits (with supportive parental help). Then at age 15 years, Mark begins to eat extra unhealthy foods, does not tell his parents; he also does not adjust his fast acting insulin to compensate for the extra foods. He said it he did not want to be different from his peers, he wanted to be like everyone else. He hated having diabetes. Mark is told he can adjust his insulin to allow some variation in his diet, yet he lies to his parents and physician about his diet and blood sugar levels. When his parents find out, they are livid, scared, and distressed. Many arguments result. Mark becomes very moody and resentful. Yet he repeatedly engages in this behavior and suffers the wrath of his parents and physician. When his parents present in the physician's office with Mark, they describe their son as a liar, a sneak, and an irresponsible teen who is killing himself.

The physician referred the family for counseling. A comprehensive psychological evaluation that includes developmental assessments. Results of testing and interviewing show that the Mark has above average intellectual function (verbal and non verbal), is mildly depressed but basically he is a very mentally healthy person who responds cognitively to emotional distress as a 9 or 10 year old. The psychologist tells Mark and his family that Mark's resistance to parental direction and non-compliance with his medical regime is the result of Mark's emotional development. Mark had not yet gotten past a concrete stage of intellectual development because when he was at that stage, he experienced the psychological trauma of being diagnosed with a chronic illness. When he acted out, Mark was not able to understand the long term consequences of not controlling his blood sugars. He could only focus on not wanting to be different from his peers.

Most of the literature on treatment responsibility (self efficacy) recommends that parents help their children be as independent with treatment regimes as possible. However, parents may need assistance in identifying when they have turned over too much care or have decreased their emotional involvement too much. Mark's parents were encouraged to make shot time and glucose testing times opportunities to spend "quality" time with their teen. They did not have to administer the procedures, but might sit with the teen and ask him about various events in his life or tell him about events in their lives. Mark was encouraged to help make these pleasant times also. Mark's parents were told to have the end goal of fading that level of involvement as their teen complied with treatment.

Psychoeducation was used as a major technique to help Mark. This included the teaching of coping skills, nurturing abstract thinking and helping him understand the relationship between his everyday behavior/actions and his long-term health. Mark was also helped to understand the motives of his parents and their fears about his long-term health. The clinician pointed out that his parents were reacting out of fear for their son's life, not because they hated him. With education, Mark's parents were able to view their son's emotional needs, and understand his behavior as a part of normal adolescence development; they were given strategies to intervene with Mark that respected their teen's chronological age and met his emotional need of more concrete instructions and more parental attention to the medication regime

Case story 2

Charles is a 15 year old male diagnosed with cystic fibrosis. Charles was short stature, had a high pitched voice, no facial hairs, and had not yet started to experience puberty. He was being seen by a clinician for help with anger management. Charles is short stature, has a slight frame and facial feature more like a nine or ten year old. At their first meeting the clinician greeted Charles as she does most "children" his perceived age. She bent down to shake his hand, leaned in and said "Hello, young man. How are you today?" When she escorted Charles and his mother to their respective seats, she told him he was welcome to sit any where he liked or could stay close to his mother if he felt safer. Charles began to get angry, he glared at the clinician. The clinician had not read his referral letter in a couple of weeks and went by her perceptions of his age and developmental stage. Next, she said: "Now, I am going to ask you some hard questions (she was joking) that most kids your age might struggle with, but I bet you know the answers."

Charles had enough! He said, "Look, stop being condescending to me! I am not a child, I am 15 years old and would appreciate you respecting me as a young man and not treating me like a child!" The clinician, realized the error of her ways, quickly apologized and told Charles she had read his referral letter a couple of weeks ago and was treating him inappropriately. She asked for his forgiveness and said, "Charles, would allow me to start over?" Charles agreed and the rest of the meeting went well. He completed evaluation and therapy and at follow-up, he said he was able to effectively employ the anger management techniques he learned. His mother supported the claim. Charles complete therapy with the clinician and both he and his mother gave her high satisfaction rating.

Developing psychologically healthy adolescents with chronic illness

Youth who are born with chronic illnesses can grow up to be psychological healthy if they have all of the characteristics and factors in their lives that researchers have found to be present in resilient youth. Those youth that develop a chronic illness a different stages in their lives may experience psychological problems because of the loss of function, However some researchers have found that those youth who do not perceive a loss of function and who have peer acceptance, will be able lead socially and emotionally healthy lives. Research on resilience in adolescents (with and without chronic illness) shows that resilient youth are better able to handle the complexities of growing up (see table 5) (26-29).

Table 5.Characteristics of Resilient Youth [25, 26, 29, 31]

Internal
Gender Being male
Psychological
Sense of Autonomy Positive sense of independence • Emerging feelings of efficacy • High self-esteem • Impulse Control • Planning and goal setting • Belief in future

Table 5. (Continued)

Social Competence • Responsiveness to others • Conceptual and intellectual flexibility • Caring for others • Good communication skills • Sense of humor
Problem-Solving Skills • Ability to apply abstract thinking • Ability to engage in reflective thought • Critical reasoning skills • Ability to develop alternative solutions in frustrating situations
External
A. Family • A healthy family environment • Parental acceptance of and ability to cope with their adolescents chronic illness • (es) both emotionally and financially. • Strong family connectedness and cohesion • Socio-economic class (access to and possession of resources to meet family an • chronically ill adolescent's needs)
B. Community/School • Acceptance by classmates and peers of the adolescents special needs. • Positive peer relationships • Lack of exposure to violence
• Lack of exposure to substance • Minimal exposure to trauma • Teachers who provide academic adaptations that meets adolescent's needs • A supportive social network • Peers who do not engage in maladaptive behavior

Youth with chronic illnesses who are also resilient show the same qualities. The ability to be resilient is a very important component of survival for all youth but especially those with chronic illness. Resilience is the capacity to successfully undertake the work of each successive developmental stage (see table 4) in the face of significant factors that predispose to vulnerability and adapt to those conditions in a manner that improves their trajectory (13,15,21,22,25-27).

Intimate relationships

Peer relationships provide the second most important influence on adolescent development (15). Peer interactions afford the opportunity to interact in an equal status relationship and reinforce cultural norms. The support network of chronically ill youth usually includes parents, siblings, peers, counselors, caring health care professionals; however, a survey of these youth supported that chronically ill youth said their pets also played an important role in providing a listening ear and emotional comfort (11). They further reported that they need direct communication from their doctors, teachers and other care givers; and benefited best from honesty, attention to their reports of physical and emotional pain. The researchers concluded that they teens understand both the value of the scientific and interpersonal aspect of care (12,28,31,32).

Impact on experimentation and risk behavior

Adolescence is a time where youth begin to experiment with making personal decisions, challenging the religious beliefs of their parents, making a variety of friends, defying parental rules and beliefs, trying different styles of dressing, hair, makeup, and talking. Some youth will want to get tattoos or body piercings, experiment with their sexuality, engage in sexual acts, use substances (smoke or chew tobacco, marijuana, heroin, cocaine, drink alcohol) , and or other drugs (10,32). Having a chronic illness does not prevent experimental behaviors during adolescence; these youth can be expected, as will their peers, to test their own limits. The opportunities to have access to peers, purchase items, go shopping without parental supervision, be alone with a sexual partners, or be alone with peers may be impeded by the severity of their illness and their physical limitations; however experimental behaviors are not rarer in adolescents with a chronic condition (31,32). It is important that these youth be afforded privacy to experiment so that they do not get involved in experimenting sexually with age inappropriate youth or public masturbation.

Conclusions

Youth who do not experience typical development as a result of chronic illness may experience psychological or psychosocial problems (see table 1) (3,5,9-13). As adolescents work to adjust to physical and hormonal changes caused by puberty the presence of a chronic illness may significantly alter their ability to master the tasks of adolescence: Individuation, emotional and behavioral regulation, ability to initiate and maintain reciprocal intimate relations, development of skills that support independence. External factors such as family support and resources, peer acceptance, and academic support and resources can have a major impact on the psychological development of these teens. When working with youth who have chronic illnesses, it is vital that clinicians remember that these youth are subject to the same statistical risk from experimentation with sex, drugs, and other risk taking behavior. They must also be aware of the impact of those chronic illnesses on the psychological development of each individual adolescent. Youth diagnosed with chronic illness can lead very psychologically healthy lives given a) individual strengths of cognitive flexibility, intelligence and hope (see table 5); b) a supportive family environment and resources; and c) peers who accept and value them; and d) teachers and classmates who provide a positive learning environment with resources to meet or adapt to the needs of these youth.

References

[1] Acosta M, Gallo V, Batshaw ML. Brain development and the ontogency of developmental disabilities. Adv Pediatr 2002;49:1-57.

[2] Erickson EH. Identity, youth and crisis, New York: WW Norton, 1968.

[3] Gemelli R. Normal child and adolescent development. Washington, DC: Am Psychiatr Press, 1996.

[4] King A. Adolescence. In: Lewis M, ed. Child and adolescent psychiatry. A comprehensive textbook, 3rd ed. Philadelphia, PA: Lippincott Williams Wilkins, 2002:332-42.

[5] Kreipe RE. Normal somatic adolescent growth and development. In: McAnarney ER, Kreipe RE, Orr DP, Comerci GD, eds. Textbook of adolescent medicine. Philadelphia, PA: WB Saunders, 1994:4-67.

[6] Sarnat HB. Normal development of the nervous system. In: Coffey CE, Brumback RA, eds. Textbook of pediatric neuropsychiatry. Washington DC: Am Psychiatr Press, 1998:26-36.

[7] Werry JS, Zametkin A, Ernst M. Brain and behavior. In: Lewis M, ed. Child and adolescent psychiatry. A comprehensive textbook, 3rd ed. Philadelphia, PA: Lippincott Williams Wilkins, 2002:120-5.

[8] Pratt HD, Patel DR, Greydanus DE. Sports and the neurodevelopment of the child and adolescent. In: Delee JC, Drez DD, Miller MD, eds. Orthopaedic sports medicine, 2nd ed. Philadelphia, PA: WB Saunders, 2002:624-43.

[9] LeBlanc LA, Goldsmith T, Patel DR. Behavioral aspects of chronic illness in children and adolescents Pediatr Clin North Am 2003;50(4):859-78.

[10] Brener ND, Kann L, Garcia D, MacDonald G, Ramsey F, Honeycutt S, Hawkins J, Kinchen S, Harris WA. Youth Risk Behavior Surveillance. Selected steps communities, 2005. Surveillance Summaries, 2005;56/SS-2.

[11] Kyngäs H. Support network of adolescents with chronic disease: Adolescents' perspective. Nurs Health Sci 2004;6:287-93.

[12] Britto MT, DeVellis RF, Hornung RW, DeFriese G, Atherton HD, Slap GB. Health care preferences and priorities of adolescents with chronic illnesses. Pediatrics 2004;114(5):1272-80.

[13] Dixon SD. Gender and sexuality: normal development to problems and concerns. In: Behrman RE, Kliegman RM, Jenson HB, eds. Nelson textbook of pediatrics, 17th ed. Philadelphia, PA: WB Saunders, 2004:470-6.

[14] Miauton L, Narring F, Michaud PA. Chronic illness, life style and emotional health in adolescence: results of a cross-sectional survey on the health of 15-20-year-olds in Switzerland. Eur J Pediatr 2003; 162(10):682-9.

[15] Pratt HD. Neurodevelopmental issues in the assessment and treatment of deficits in attention, cognition, and learning during adolescence. Adoles Med 2002;13(3):579-98.

[16] Piaget J. Intellectual evaluation from adolescence to adulthood. Hum Dev 1972;15:1-12.

[17] Greydanus DE, Pratt HD, Patel DR. The first three years of life and the early adolescent: Comparisons and differences. Lessons for child rearing. Int Pediatr 2004;19(2):68-80.

[18] Blos P. On adolescence. Glencoe, NY: Free Press, 1962.

[19] Boeree CG. Personality theories. 1997. Accessed on 2008 Jul 28. http://www.ship.edu/~cgboeree/perscont ents.html

[20] Millon T, Davis RD. Disorders of personality: DSM-IV and beyond, 2nd ed. New York : Wiley, 1996.

[21] Minuchin P. Families and individual development: provocations from the field of family therapy. Child Dev 1985;56:289-302.

[22] Kaplan MS, McFarland BH, Huguet N, Newsom JT. Physical illness, functional limitations, and suicide risk: A population-based study. Am J Orthopsychiatry 2007;77(1):56–60.

[23] Rosen DS. Pubertal growth and sexual maturation for adolescents with chronic illness or disability. Pediatrician 1991;18:105-20.

[24] Bandura A. Influence of model's reinforcement contingencies on the acquisition of imitative processes. J Pers Soc Psychol 1965;1:589-95.

[25] Resnick MD. Protective factors, resiliency, and healthy youth development. Adolesc Med 2000;11:157-64.

[26] Blum RW, McNeely C, Nonnemaker J. Vulnerbility, risk and protection. J Adolesc Health 2002;31S(1):28-39.
[27] Masten AS, Hubbard JJ, Gest SD, Tellegen A, Garmezy N, Ramirez M. Competence in the context of adversity: pathways to resilience and maladaptation from childhood to late adolescence. Dev Psychopathol 1999;11(1):143-69.
[28] Mandleco BL, Peery JC. An organizational framework for conceptualizing resilience in children. J Child Adolesc Psychiatr Nurs 2000;13(3):99-111.
[29] Masten AS. Ordinary magic. Resilience processes in development. Am Psychol 2001;56(3):227-38.
[30] Luthar SS, Cicchetti D. The construct of resilience: implications for interventions and social policies. Dev Psychopathol 2000;12(4):857-85.
[31] Wirrell E, Cheung C, Spier S. How do teens view the physical and social impact of asthma compared to other chronic diseases? J Asthma 2006;43:155-60.
[32] Wyman PA, Cowen EL, Work WC, Hoyt-Meyers L, Magnus KB, Fagen DB. Caregiving and developmental factors differentiating young at-risk urban children showing resilient versus stress-affected outcomes: a replication and extension. Child Dev 1999;70(3):645-59.

Submitted: November 03, 2008.
Revised: December 30, 2008.
Accepted: January 07, 2009.

In: Public Health Yearbook 2009
Editor: Joav Merrick
ISBN: 978-1-61668-911-7

Chapter 2

SOCIO-DEMOGRAPHIC DETERMINANTS OF MALARIA IN PREGNANCY

Faisal Shuaib, MD, MPH, Pauline Jolly, PhD, MPH and John Ehiri*, PhD, MPH

Department of Epidemiology and Department of Maternal and Child Health, University of Alabama at Birmingham, Ryals Public Health Building, Birmingham, Alabama, United States of America

Abstract

Context: Malaria is known as a disease of poverty, but there is a dearth of evidence to collectively summarize how social and demographic factors predict its incidence among pregnant women.
Objective: To summarize evidence on socio-demographic determinants of malaria in pregnancy.
Data sources: Electronic databases of OVID, MEDLINE, LILACS, EMBASE, PsycINFO, Science Citation Index and Social Science Citation Index, ERIC and reference lists of articles were searched for 1998-2008. Selection criteria: Two independent reviewers selected studies for inclusion if they expressly investigated or included investigation of social and/or demographic determinants of placental malaria or parasitemia in pregnancy. Data extraction: Data on study settings, designs, methods, population characteristics, relationship between socio-demographic variables and malaria were assessed. Data synthesis: Of the 98 studies found, 19 met the inclusion criteria. Overall, socio-demographic determinants of malaria in pregnancy were found to be age (less than 21 years), parity (more than 1 child), socioeconomic status (measured by absence of electricity in the house), trimester of pregnancy, seasonality (rainy season), geographic location (rural residence), HIV infection, and use of malaria prophylaxis. One study found an association with ethnicity. Conclusion: Given that age, parity, rural residence, low socioeconomic status, and HIV infection were found to be strong predictors of malaria in pregnancy, maternal and child health programs as well as malaria control programs must pay special attention to women with these characteristics if their interventions are to have optimum impact.

* Correspondence: Associate professor John Ehiri, PhD, MPH, Department of Maternal and Child Health, University of Alabama at Birmingham, 1665 University Boulevard, Ryals Public Health Building, Suite 320, Birmingham, Alabama, 35294-0022 United States. Tel: (205) 975-7641; Fax: (205) 934-8248; E-mail: jehiri@uab.edu

Programs that target prevention of mother-to-child transmission of HIV should incorporate effective malaria prophylaxis and treatment to counter the effects of HIV on pregnant women with malaria.

Keywords: Malaria, pregnancy, social determinants, maternal health, pregnancy outcomes, demographic factors.

Introduction

Malaria is responsible for disproportionately large morbidity and mortality worldwide. Every year, 300 million people suffer from the disease and its complications. Annually, an estimated 400,000 women suffer severe anemia as a result of malaria infection (1). Pregnant women, their unborn fetuses, and infants account for most of these preventable deaths from malaria (2). Ninety percent of the mortality from malaria occurs in sub-Saharan Africa. It has been estimated that 1.3% of the Gross Domestic Product (GDP) is lost to malaria annually by endemic countries in Africa. This is equivalent to $12 billion annually for the continent (3). Maternal anemia causes an estimated 10,000 maternal deaths per year, while malaria is responsible for 20% of infant deaths in Africa (3). The fact however, is that many of these children are either never born due to intra-uterine growth retardation and death or are born prematurely with low gestational weights (4).

The underpinning factor for the high incidence of malaria is the predominance of a very effective vector, the Anopheles mosquito in sub-tropical and tropical parts of the world. The efficiency of Plasmodium falciparum and its particular placental pathology makes it a viable vehicle of devastating consequences for mothers and their children. While the literature is replete with evidence on the accentuating relationship between pregnancy and malaria, the evidence has not been fully reviewed to elucidate the socio-demographic determinants of malaria in pregnancy. This review attempts to summarize studies on predictors of malaria in pregnancy in order to contribute to advocacy and priority setting for programs that seek to prevent malaria in pregnancy.

Methods

We searched online databases, scanned reference lists and hand-searched journals for potentially eligible studies. Specifically, we searched PubMed, OVID, MEDLINE, LILACS, EMBASE, Combined Health Information Database (CHID), National Research Register, PsychINFO, ERIC, Science and Social Science Citation Index, Dissertation Abstracts, Online Computer Library Centre (OCLC) and other bibliographic databases. The search covered articles published in English between January 1998 and September 2008. Among the terms and concepts searched were: determinants of malaria in pregnancy, predictors of malaria in pregnancy, economic status and malaria in pregnancy, education and malaria in pregnancy, social status and malaria in pregnancy, urban-rural differentials in malaria in pregnancy, ethnicity and malaria in pregnancy, parity and maternal malaria, gestational age, malaria and pregnancy, HIV and malaria in pregnancy, bednets and malaria in pregnancy, malaria prophylaxis and malaria in pregnancy, and seasonality and malaria in pregnancy. To identify studies published in the "gray" literature, we systematically reviewed the bibliographies of all relevant publications, searched the System for Information on Gray Literature in Europe database (SIGLE), the Grey Literature Database of the New York Academy of Medicine, and Grey Literature Network Service (GreyNet) which covers information produced on all levels of government, academia, business and industry in electronic and print formats not controlled by commercial publishing. We also explored online resources (Google and Google Scholar) extensively.

Two reviewers (Shuaib and Ehiri) screened titles and abstracts to assess their eligibility for inclusion in the review. Hard copies of studies that were potentially relevant were retrieved for further assessment. In assessing the quality of studies, we used the Cochrane Collaboration's standard method for study quality assessment (5). The search yielded 98 potential studies. Of these, 19 studies involving 25,647 participants qualified for inclusion and were retained for the review. The excluded studies were unclear regarding how the authors controlled for blinding of assessors (6) and for cohort and case-control studies, baseline comparability between study and control groups with respect to the socio-demographic variables of interest was unclear. They were also unclear with respect to contemporaneous data collection (data collected at similar time periods) for both control and study sites.

Results

Outcome measures for malaria in pregnancy included thick or thin film microscopy showing asexual forms of the parasite, peripheral malaria, placental malaria, parasitemia or Polymerase Chain Reaction (PCR). Of the 19 studies, thirteen (7-19) assessed malaria based on thick or thin film microscopy showing asexual forms of the parasite; two examined placental malaria alone (19,20), while one used a combination of peripheral and placental malaria (21); two used peripheral parasitemia and Polymerase Chain Reaction (PCR) (22,23). Only one study used submicroscopic malaria diagnosis using RCR. The following section summarizes findings of the review. Key results are highlighted in table 1.

Age

Nine studies (7-10,18-20,24,25), which were all conducted in sub-Saharan Africa examined the influence of age on malaria prevalence/incidence among 958 women under 21 years of age and 845 women above the 30 years of age. Of these, seven demonstrated an inverse relationship between maternal age and maternal placental or peripheral malarial parasitemia. One study (25) found no significant relationship between maternal age and malaria while the other (7) found increasing maternal parasitemia with increasing maternal age. Among the afore-mentioned seven studies, the measures of effect ranged from an odds ratio of 1.98 (CI =1.70-2.31) in the case of Van Eijk et al (9) in Kisumu, Western Kenya to 2.48 (CI=1.19-5.16) in Bandiagara, Mali (10).

Parity

Fifteen studies (7-10,12-14,16,18-20, 22, 24-26) investigated the relationship between parity and malaria in pregnancy. Of these, two (12,13) were in the Indian subcontinent and their findings were similar to studies conducted in Africa. Higher parity was found to protect against malaria infection in eleven of the fifteen studies. The strength of this association ranged from an adjusted odds ration of 1.66 (CI= 1.27-2.17)21 to 2.29 (CI=1.60-3.26) (18). From Southern Mozambique, Saute et al (24) showed that age and not parity was significantly associated with increased risk of parasitemia. Further corroborative evidence was provided by three other studies Adam et al (25,26) and Elghazali et al (22), which showed that malaria was not associated with parity in Eastern Sudan, an area of unstable malaria transmission. In one study done in the Jayapura provincial Hospital of Indonesian Papua New Guinea (16), pregnant women showed no higher risk of severe malaria (P=0.643) or death (P=0.771) compared to non-pregnant women.

Gestational age of pregnancy

Six studies investigated gestational age and the role of malaria, with conflicting results. While two studies (22,25) in North Africa and one in India (12) found the 3rd trimester to be more hazardous, two others in West Africa (7,10) (found the 1st trimester to have a higher incidence of maternal malaria. Interestingly, one study conducted in Southern Mozambique (24) found the 2nd trimester to be the riskiest.

HIV status

Five studies, all in East Africa (9,15,21,23,27) investigated the relationship between maternal malaria and HIV status. They all showed that the relative risk (RR) for parasitemia in HIV+ positive pregnant women was higher than in HIV- pregnant women (RR range: 1.54 (95% CI=1.05-2.26) to 2.40 (1.64-3.53). Van Eijk et al (21) stratified parasite density by gravidity, and demonstrated a loss of protection with increasing parity when pregnant women were HIV+. Their comparison of malaria parasitemia in 1st pregnancy among HIV+ women with malaria parasitemia in HIV- women demonstrated a relative risk of 2.40 (CI=1.64-3.53). For the 2nd pregnancy, the relative risk was 2.54 (CI=1.32-4.86), and RR=2.66 (1.10-6.43) for 3rd pregnancy,

Use of malaria prophylaxis and bednets

Three studies investigated the effect of malaria prophylaxis on peripheral parasitemia. Brentlinger et al (18) and Van Eijk et al (21) assessed the use of Sulfadoxine-pyrimethamine (SP).

Table 1. Summary of findings

Study ID	Objective	Design	Population	Outcomes	Results		Remarks
					<20 year	*30-39 years*	
Age					*Adj. OR (95% CI)*	*Adj. OR (95% CI)*	
Saute et al. 2002 (Southern Mozambique) (8)	To assess the prevalence of Malaria parasitemia and anemia in relation to age and parity in pregnant women	Cross-sectional	686 pregnant women	Malaria peripheral parasitemia and anemia	Ref	0.3 (0.1-0.8)	P<0.05
Tako et al. 2005 (Yaoundé, Cameroon) (9)	To evaluate the prevalence of placental malaria with respect to gravidity and maternal age	Cross sectional	1,944 pregnant women	Placental parasitemia and anemia	2.0 (1.3-3.0)	1.0 (0.7-1.4)	Prophylactic antimalarials used by 76.3% of participants
van Eijk et al. 2002a (Kisumu, Western Kenya) (14)	To assess risk factors for malaria in pregnancy	Cross-sectional	2,502 women who delivered in hospital and included in analysis	Peripheral malaria parasitemia	1.69 (1.43-2.00)	Ref.	Age group <20 includes <21 years P<0.05
Dicko et al. 2003 (Bandiagara, Mali) (12)	To identify risk factors for malaria infection in pregnant women	Cross-sectional	235 pregnant women	Malaria parasitemia in thick blood film	2.5 (1.19-5.16)	Ref.	Age comparing ≤27 years to ≥27 years
Brentlinger et al. 2007 (Central Mozambique) (13)	To find out factors associated with maternal peripheral parasitemia	Cross-sectional	5,528 pregnant women	Maternal peripheral parasitemia	0.96 (0.94-0.99)	Ref.	
Adam et al. 2005a (Eastern Sudan) (15)	To demonstrate the prevalence and risk factors for malaria	Cross-sectional	744 pregnant women	Malaria parasitemia in thick and thin blood film	0.90 (0.52-1.6)	Ref.	Age comparing ≤25 years to ≥25 years
Adam et al. 2005a (Eastern Sudan) (15)	To demonstrate the prevalence and risk factors for malaria	Cross-sectional	744 pregnant women	Malaria parasitemia in thick and thin blood film	1.1 (0.7-1.7)	0.96 (0.62-1.4)	Multi-gravidae =3 to 5 pregnancies

Table 1. (Continued)

Study ID	Objective	Design	Population	Outcomes	Results	Remarks	Study ID
Saute et al. 2002 (Southern Mozambique) (8)	To describe the prevalence of Malaria parasitemia and anemia in relation to age and parity in pregnant women	Cross-sectional	686 pregnant women	Malaria peripheral parasitemia	Ref.	0.7 (0.3-2.0)	Multi-gravidae≥5 pregnancies
van Eijk et al. 2002a (Kisumu, Western Kenya) (14)	To assess risk factors for malaria in pregnancy	Cross-sectional	2,502 women who delivered in hospital and included in analysis	Peripheral malaria parasitemia	1.23 (0.91-1.67)	Ref.	P<005
Tako et al. 2005 (Yaounde, Cameroon) (9)	To evaluate the prevalence of placental malaria with respect to gravidity and maternal age	Cross-sectional	1,944 pregnant women	Placental parasitemia and anemia	1.5(1.0-2.2)	Ref.	Among 1,016 women ≥25 years, prevalence of placental malaria is not significantly different

Keys: Ref.= Reference Group.

Both studies demonstrated a reduction in parasitemia associated with use of malaria prophylaxis OR=0.49 (95% CI=0.48-0.50) for Brentlinger et al (18), and OR=0.32 (95% CI=0.14-0.67) for Van Eijk et al (9). One study (10) found that Chloroquine was protective (OR=0.66 (CI=0.21-2.03). It should be noted that only Brentlinger et al (18) objectively assessed the number of doses and frequency of anti-malarials use.

While the frequency of bednets use was not clearly defined by the two studies that assessed them (14,18), they both showed protective effect for bednet use among study participants. Brentlinger et al (18) found an OR=0.49 (CI=0.48-0.50), while Marchant et al (14) found that parasitemia among bednet users and non-bednet users was 25% and 33% respectively (P=0.006).

Rural/urban residence

Two studies examined the relationship between living in a rural or urban area and malaria infection among a total of 2,737 pregnant women. Dicko et al (10) found that living in a rural area is associated with a two-and-half fold increase in malaria infection: OR=2.49 (CI=0.99-6.27). Van Eijk et al (9) found a risk ratio of 1.27 (CI 0.99-1.63) for pregnant women living in peri-urban areas of Kisumu, Kenya.

Seasonality

Four studies (10,24,9,26) investigated the relation between seasonality and malaria in pregnancy. Dicko et al (10) found a significant association between rainy season and the rate of malaria infection among pregnant women, OR=4.85 (95% CI= 2.42-9.75). Saute et al (24) showed that the end of the rainy season was a risk factor, OR=2.2 (CI 1.4-3.0, P<0.05) for parasitemia in pregnancy in a cross sectional study of 686 pregnant women in Southern Mozambique. Van Eijk et al (9) did not demonstrate any difference in the level of peripheral parasitemia based on seasonality RR=0.97 (95% CI =0.84-1.13). Adam et al (26) using PCR to detect submicroscopic parasitemia also found no statistically significant difference between the rainy and dry seasons.

Ethnicity

Only Dicko et al (10) and Van Eijk et al (9) assessed the relationship between ethnicity and maternal malaria. Among 2,502 pregnant residents of Kisumu in Western Kenya, Luo ethnicity was found by Van Eijk et al (9) to be associated with an 80% odds of malaria parasitemia compared to the other ethnicities, Luhya, Kissii, Kikuyu, Kalenjin and Nandi, (RR=1.81 (CI= 1.38-2.39)). The Luo people live within an area that stretches from Southern Sudan, through northern Uganda and Eastern Congo (DRC), into Western Kenya, and ending in the upper tip of Tanzania. Dicko et al (10) in the semi arid areas of Bandiagara, Mali found no statistically significant association between Dogon ethnicity and non-Dogon ethnicity in univariate or multivariate analysis.

Socioeconomic status and education

One study in central Mozambique (18) investigated the role of socioeconomic status and education. They demonstrated that among 4,157 pregnant women in a syphilis study site, socioeconomic status (as measured by absence of electricity at home) was associated with maternal peripheral malaria parasitemia (OR=1.71 (CI=1.19-2.47). The same study showed that not having school education was associated with increased risk of malaria among pregnant women, OR=1.38 (95%; CI=1.15-1.66).

Discussion

The position of randomized controlled trials (RCTs) as the gold standard with regard to study design quality is widely acknowledged. It is also known that there are many challenges in conducting such studies in less developed countries, including resource, logistical and ethical constraints. It is therefore, not surprising that none of the included studies was an RCT. Most were cross-sectional studies, and a few were cohort and case-control studies. In interpreting the results therefore, readers should take adequate cognizance of the limitation of these studies. For example, questions about use of bednets, malaria prophylaxis and treatment relied on self-reports (28), that are known to be subject to recall bias (29) and social desirability (30). Nevertheless, the consistency of the associations across studies in different settings points to the validity of the results.

Age

An overwhelming majority of studies found that age was a strong determinant of the prevalence and severity of maternal malaria (7,8,10,18-20,24). These studies show that in areas of stable, high malarial transmission, maternal age is an independent predictor of malaria in pregnancy. Young primigravidae and multigravidae, especially those under 20 years of age are at greater risk of malaria and its adverse effects than older primigravidae and multigravidae (18). Tako et al (20) demonstrated this relationship in a study in Yaoundé, Cameroon. After adjusting for confounding variables, they found that age and not gravidity was a major risk factor for placental malaria (P=0.008). Corroborative evidence was provided by a similar study in Mali where the over-riding risk factors for malaria were not gravidity but age, rural residence and season (10). Likewise, Okwa et al (7) found that women aged 30-39 years had a higher rate of parasitemia compared to those aged less than 20 years. The study however had a disproportionately larger number of participants in the 30-39 years age bracket (n=559; 70%) than those in the under 20 years age group (n=15; 1.8%).

In interpreting results of this study, it is important to note that participants were all on various types of malarial prophylaxis. Participants were likely to have had variable adherence to their prophylactic regimens. The anti-malarials also have different efficacies, thus making it inaccurate to conclude based on the data that the older women have a higher prevalence. It is important to note that while evidence abounds on the inverse relationship between age and malaria in pregnancy, there are studies that have failed to demonstrate this association. For example, Nnaji et al (8) working in Nnewi, Eastern Nigeria, found that though there was a higher prevalence of malaria parasitemia in pregnant women under 20 years of age compared to those aged between 30 and 39 years, the difference was not statistically significant. Similarly, in their study in Eastern Sudan, an area characterized by unstable malaria transmission, Adam et al (25) found no significant association between malaria and age.

In interpreting the effects of age on malaria in pregnancy, it is important to consider the role of socioeconomic factors (18). Compared to teenage and young adult mothers, older women are more likely to be of higher socioeconomic status (as measured by education and income) and may have more experience of managing health issues during pregnancy, including nutrition and malaria prophylaxis (31). Thus, malaria control program planners and implementers should consider pregnant teenagers and young adults as at-risk populations with special need for protection against malaria. Oftentimes, these groups of mothers may be unmarried and either in school or out of school. Typical clinic based reproductive health services for older, married women will not work for them (32). Where pregnancies are out of wedlock, very few of the young women are likely to present for prenatal care (33). Insecticide treated bednets which by priority are distributed through prenatal clinics will therefore not reach them (34). They neither receive intermittent preventive therapy against malaria (IPT-SP) nor will there be the high index of suspicion recommended by the WHO triad for effective management of malaria in pregnancy (32). Special interventions should be devised to target these groups if maternal and infant mortality from malaria is to be reduced in malaria endemic regions.

Parity

Of the fifteen studies included in the review that investigated the influence of parity on malaria in pregnancy, nine (7-10,12,13,19,20,24) demonstrated a positive relationship between parity and malaria. Overall, the studies indicate that the risk of malaria in pregnancy decreases with increasing gravidity. Prevalence and susceptibility to severe malaria are more common in primigravidae compared to multigravidae. The acquisition of immunity with subsequent pregnancies has been proffered as an explanation for this. In a study in Western Kenya, Fried et al (35) showed that anti-adhesion antibodies are produced by multigravid women against malaria parasites which tend to sequester on the syncytiotrophoblast of the human placenta. Production of these antibodies requires immunological memory from a previous pregnancy (35). The produced antibodies prevent Plasmodium falciparum parasites from binding to chondroitin sulphate A (CSA) molecules on the placenta (35). As a result, multigravidae clear malaria parasites better than primigravidae. The implication of this is that immunity against malaria improves with subsequent pregnancies and the anti-cytoadherance antibodies produced by the body starts after the first pregnancy (35). It is possible that this phenomenon could serve as the basis for production of vaccines against malaria for global use.

It was interesting that Elghazali et al (22), Saute et al (24) and Adam et al (25,26) did not demonstrate statistically significant association between malaria parasitemia and parity. In interpreting results on association of parity and malaria, it is germane to recognize the strong colinearity between age and parity that may make it difficult to completely extricate the overlapping influence of each in a regression model. Secondly, there is also the distorting effect of a high HIV infection rate in the study area; HIV infection is known to distort the parity pattern of malaria infection in pregnancy (36). The studies in Eastern Sudan (25,26) characterize the expectation of malaria patterns in an area of unstable malaria transmission (37). Here, there was no difference in the malaria parasitemia based on parity level.

Gestational stage of pregnancy

Pregnancy is a state of altered immunity resulting from immune modulation from cellular responses to humoral immunity (38). Acquired immunity from malaria wanes during pregnancy (37) especially during the first pregnancies as noted earlier. Consequently, a pregnant woman becomes as vulnerable to malaria as a non-immune child (39). Susceptibility to malaria is thought to start as early as the twelfth week of pregnancy. Before this time, the incidence or at least the clearance of malaria parasite is similar to what is observed in the non pregnant female (39). Two of six studies demonstrated higher susceptibility in the 1st and 3rd trimester, while one (24) indicated greater risk in the second semester. The latter finding is in harmony with findings of the review by Desai et al (2), which indicated that the second trimester remains the most vulnerable period for malaria infection in all mothers. Yet, some others have reported that the last trimester (37) and first trimester (40) may be equally risky. Based on their work in Eastern Sudan, Elghazali et al (22) found that the peak incidence of malaria was the third trimester. They however attributed this finding to the fact that most of the patients presented for prenatal services towards the end of the second semester.

In his analysis of malaria in pregnancy in Africa, Brabin (41) likened the situation of malaria in pregnancy to one in which an infant or child acquires immunity to malaria over a couple of years. The pregnant woman on the other hand, first loses this immunity, and then reacquires it over a period of nine months. Thus, the effectiveness with which she reacquires this immunity may vary in accordance with the initial level of immunity (3) and the competence of her immune system, which in turn, is predetermined by a host of other factors including her nutritional status. Most studies illustrate that the peak in malaria susceptibility is the second trimester but the truth lies possibly somewhere between the second and third trimesters for each individual. Clearly, adequate provision for prevention of malaria needs to target the entire duration of the pregnancy.

Seasonality

Van Eijk et al (9) found a lack of difference in the risk of malaria by season of the year in their study despite perennial transmission of malaria. The reason for this has not been fully elucidated. In an area of unstable malaria, Adam et al. also found no disparity in transmission by season even at the submicroscopic level (26). Dicko et al's (10) findings were consistent with that of other investigators who found a significantly increased risk for malaria parasitemia during the rainy season, OR=4.85 (95% CI = 2.42-9.75). There is a higher rate of inoculation by insects during the rainy season compared to the dry season (40). Mosquito breeding increases during the rainy season as water tends to collect in clear, still, sun-exposed receptacles such as ponds, wells, water tanks, paddy fields and indiscriminately disposed bottles, tins and coconut shells (42). The warm temperatures and humidity also promote mosquito longevity and parasite sporogeny. Pregnant women are also at risk of mosquito bites as the rainy season is also associated with increased involvement in agricultural activities. It has been shown that mosquitoes have a higher predilection for pregnant women compared to non-pregnant women (43).

Geographical site (Urban/rural residence)

Disparities in the prevalence of malaria and the susceptibility patterns of populations are seen in urban and rural areas. Brentlinger et al (18) found a higher prevalence of malaria parasitemia in women from rural areas (48.1%) compared to those from an urban clinic (8.8%) where there was an indoor residual spraying campaign. This difference was persistent despite the inclusion of women who had recently taken preventive Sulphadoxine-pyrimethamine (SP) in the rural site and notwithstanding the higher seroprevalence of HIV in the urban site. This finding was consistent with those from another study conducted in Bandiagara, Mali (10), which found that residence in the rural area was associated with a 2.5-fold increase in the odds of malaria parasitemia OR = 2.49 (95% CI = 0.99-6.27).

Residents of urban areas tend to be more affluent and take steps to prevent contact with parasites. Disease control programs in these places are frequently better managed. Availability of different brands of insecticides with varying price ranges means residents are able to choose from available brands. Disparity in the distribution of health infrastructure and services between rural and urban areas also means that bednets and large scale insecticide use favor urban residents. As noted earlier, availability of programs to reduce malarial parasitemia e.g., in women who use bednets and malarial prophylaxis is significantly associated with lower incidence of malaria (2).

Another factor that may alter the risk to malaria in urban population is the spraying of houses with insecticides especially in the urban areas (44). The higher incidence of HIV in the urban setting may however alter the overall picture. Thus the actual effect of the urban-rural differential may be masked by the unknown HIV serostatus of the rural dwellers and the known status of the urban dwellers (18). Poor nutrition and seasonal changes in nutritional level of rural dwellers may also impact on their immunity response to malaria (2). In developing countries such as Malawi and Nigeria, those who live in rural areas are also more likely to be in the low socioeconomic strata. A large proportion of these groups are outside the delivery loop of the orthodox health care system (45). Even if they have access, poor literacy level predicts their tendency to self-treat, delay presentation to the clinic and hence they suffer the consequences of delayed therapy (46). Thus, any program designed to reduce malaria in these populations must look holistically at predisposing factors, such as poverty, and presence of chronic infections (e.g., helminthiasis) which increase their susceptibility to malaria and accentuate the effect of hemolysis from acute malaria (47). Comparative studies have shown that residents of urban areas expend a larger proportion of their income in procuring insecticide sprays and mosquito screening than those in the urban areas (44).

Ethnicity/region

Only one Kenyan study examined the significance of ethnicity as a determinant of malaria in pregnancy (21). In this study, being of Luo ethnicity was a risk factor for malaria at delivery (RR= 1.74, 95% CI = 1.35-2.24). However, when gravidity and use of Sulphodoxine-Pyrimethamine were excluded, the risk ratio reduced (ARR=1.43, 95% CI= 1.10-1.85). Dicko et al (10) did not find any association between ethnicity and malaria in pregnancy in Bandiagara, Mali. Further studies need to be conducted to compare this observed role of ethnicity in other ethnic groups inhabiting the same area in order to exclude potential confounders. Though none of the studies explored the role of Duffy antigens in modulating P vivax malaria, studies have demonstrated that being of West African origin confers protection from P vivax as a result of the absence of Duffy antigens on the red blood cells. It is therefore not surprising that maternal malaria from P vivax is less prevalent in this area compared to other areas. Besides, P. vivax is not associated with the type of placental cytoadherance observed with P falciparum. In other regions of the world such as South and East Asia, Western Pacific, Eastern Mediterranean, and South America, P vivax malaria is responsible for severe malaria among pregnant women (48). Studies using P vivax Duffy Binding Proteins (PvDBP) suggest the possibility of using PvDBP for the development of a vaccine against P. vivax malaria (49).

Socio economic status

Malaria disproportionately affects 58% of the world's poorest 20% (50). In a study of maternal malaria and socioeconomic status that used absence of electricity as an indicator, the authors found an associated increased risk of malaria in pregnancy (21). One would argue that in many rural and peri-urban regions in low income countries, electricity is a publicly financed infrastructure which may not be a valid indicator of socioeconomic status at the individual and household levels. Brentlinger et al (18) working in central Mozambique, independently arrived at the same conclusion regarding the relationship between socioeconomic status and malaria prevalence. They found that the unavailability of electricity, absence of running pipe-borne water and dirt-floor housing were predictors of malaria parasitemia among pregnant women. In most African countries, women have limited economic power. When they are ill, they rely on the husband to provide resources to initiate therapy. The funds for this may not be readily provided, thus leading to a delay in seeking care (25). This delay is compounded by poor knowledge about signs and symptoms that may be indistinguishable from those witnessed in early pregnancy (44). Though no study has explored the effect of malnutrition on malaria susceptibility, like malaria, maternal nutrition shows the same seasonality as malaria (40) with more cases of malaria occurring during the rainy season when the previous farming season's crops have been exhausted (51).

Brentlinger et al (18) in their study in Mozambique, demonstrated a significant association between lack of education among pregnant women and malaria parasitemia, OR=1.38 (95% CI=1.15-1.66). As would be expected, mothers who with higher levels of education were likely to be of higher socioeconomic status compared to those without formal education. They were likely to eschew activities that would potentially increase their susceptibility to malaria (52) and were more likely to attend prenatal care services (53). This study lends credence to earlier studies that associate higher rates of bednet use among individuals with superior educational exposure (51). Pregnant women with formal education tend to be better informed and are likely to participate in community efforts to control the vector e.g., proper refuse disposal and even community organized insecticide spraying.

HIV infection

The burden of malaria in pregnancy is exacerbated by co-infection with HIV. Because of an altered state of the immune system, HIV positive patients are more vulnerable to the malaria parasite (23). There is a higher prevalence of malaria in HIV+ pregnant women compared to HIV- women (RR=1.7, CI= 1.52-1.90, P<001) (21); there is also an increase in the density of parasites in blood (P=0.0005) (15). These observations are responsible for the higher prevalence of febrile episodes, and chronic parasitemia in pregnant women living with HIV/AIDS (27). HIV infection also reduces the protective effect of higher gravidity on malaria (23). Van Eijk (21) found that HIV-positive young multigravidae had a two-fold increased probability and young HIV-seropositive primigravidae had more than three-fold increased probability of parasitemia. HIV infected mothers also demonstrate less benefit from intermittent preventive therapy with SP to prevent malaria compared to HIV seronegative women (54).

Conclusions

It is possible that there are a plethora of socio-demographic factors other than the ones discussed in this study that influence malaria among pregnant women. Our review focused on the 19 studies that were judged to be of good enough quality to permit rational evidence-based conclusions. Overall, the key message of this review is that while it is known that all pregnant women in malaria endemic regions are predisposed to the dangers of malaria, some are at greater risks than others as a result of their varying exposures to different socio-demographic factors. We hope that with a holistic view of these determinants, program planners can prioritize the deployment of resources to reduce the impact of malaria among pregnant women and device new strategies for reaching those at the greatest risk, particularly primigravidae, adolescents and young adults, the poor and rural dwellers. For them, WHO's recommended triad of insecticide treated bednets, intermittent preventive therapy and decisive case management of malaria in pregnancy is still a fantasy reserved only for the few that traditionally have unfettered access to prenatal services.

References

[1] Centers for Disease Control and prevention (CDC). The history of malaria, an ancient disease. http://www.cdc.gov/malaria/history/index.htm

[2] Desai M, Ter Kuile F, Nosten F, et al. Epidemiology and burden of malaria in pregnancy. Lancet Infect Dis 2007;7:93-104.

[3] World Health Organization. Roll back Malaria. Malaria in pregnancy [http://www.rbm.who.int/cmc_upload/0/ 000/015/369/RBMInfosheet_4.htm Accessed 2008 Nov 01.

[4] Guyatt HL, Snow RW. Impact of malaria during pregnancy on low birth weight in sub-Saharan Africa. Clin Microbiol Rev 2004;17(4):760-9.

[5] Higgins J, Green S. Cochrane Handbook for Systematic Reviews of Interventions 4.2.5. May 2005; http://www.cochrane.org/resources/handbook/hbook.htm. Accessed 2008 Oct 11.

[6] Schulz K, Chalmers I, Hayes R, Altman D. Empirical evidence of bias. Dimensions of methodological quality associated with estimates of treatment effects in controlled trials. JAMA 1995;273(5):408-12.

[7] Okwa O. The status of malaria among pregnant women: a study in Lagos, Nigeria. Afr J Reprod Health 2003;7(3):77-83.

[8] Nnaji G, Okafor C, Ikechebelu J. An evaluation of the effect of parity and age on malaria parasitaemia in pregnancy. J Obstet Gynaecol 2006;26:755-8.

[9] van Eijk A, Ayisi J, ter Kuile F, et al. Risk factors for malaria in pregnancy in an urban and peri-urban population in western Kenya. Trans R Soc Trop Med Hyg 2002;96(6):586-92.

[10] Dicko A, Mantel C, Thera M, et al. Risk factors for malaria infection and anemia for pregnant women in the Sahel area of Bandiagara, Mali. Acta Tropica 2003;89:17-23.

[11] Adam I, Khamis A, Elbashir M. Prevalence and risk factors for Plasmodium falciparum malaria in pregnant women of Eastern Sudan. Malaria J 2005;4(18):1-4.

[12] Singh N, Shukla M, Sharma V. Epidemiology of malaria in pregnancy in central India. Bull World Health Org 1999;77:567-72.

[13] Kochar D, Thanvi I, Joshi A, Subhakaran AS, Kumawat BL. Falciparum malaria and pregnancy. Indian J Malariol 1998;35:123-30.

[14] Marchant T, Schellenberg J, Edgar T, et al. Socially marketed insecticide-treated nets improve malaria and anemia in pregnancy in southern Tanzania. Trop Med Int Health 2002;7(2):149-58.

[15] Ladner J, Leroy V, Simonon A, et al. Pregnancy and HIV Study Group (EGE). HIV infection, malaria, and pregnancy: a prospective cohort study in Kigali, Rwanda. Am J Trop Med Hyg 2002;66(4):56-60.

[16] Barcus M, Basri H, Picarima H, et al. Demographic risk factors for severe and fatal vivax and falciparum malaria among hospital admissions in northeastern Indonesian Papua. Am J Trop Med Hyg 2007;77:984-991.
[17] Adam I, Elbasit E, Salih I, ElBashir M. Submicroscopic Plasmodium falciparum infections during pregnancy in an area of Sudan with a low intensity of malaria transmission. Ann Trop MedParasitol 2005b;99:339-44.
[18] Brentlinger P, Montoya P, Rojas A, et al. Prevalence and predictors of maternal peripheral malaria parasitemia in central Mozambique. Am J Trop Med Hyg 2007;77:228-34.
[19] Walker-Abbey A, Djokam R, Eno A, et al. Malaria in pregnant Cameroonian women: the effect of age and gravidity on submicroscopic and mixed-species infections and multiple parasite genotypes. Am J Trop Med Hyg 2005;72(3):229-35.
[20] Tako E, Zhou A, Lohoue J, Leke R, Taylor D, Leke R. Risk factors for placental malaria and its effect on pregnancy outcome in Yaoundé, Cameroon. Am J Trop Med Hyg 2005;72(3):236-42.
[21] van Eijk A, Ayisi J, ter Kuile F, et al. HIV increases the risk of malaria in women of all gravidities in Kisumu, Kenya. AIDS 2002;17(4):595-603.
[22] Elghazali G, Adam I, Hamad A, El-Bashir M. Plasmodium falciparum infection during pregnancy in an unstable transmission area in Eastern Sudan. East Mediterr Health J 2003;9:570-580.
[23] Ayisi J, Branch O, Rafi-Janajreh A, et al. Does infection with Human Immunodeficiency Virus affect the antibody responses to Plasmodium falciparum antigenic determinants in asymptomatic pregnant women? . J Infect 2003;46:164-72.
[24] Saute F, Menendez C, Mayor A, et al. Malaria in pregnancy in rural Mozambique: the role of parity, submicroscopic and multiple Plasmodium falciparum infections. Trop Med Int Health 2002;7:19-28.
[25] Adam I, Khamis A, Elbashir M. Prevalence and risk factors for Plasmodium falciparum malaria in pregnant women of eastern Sudan. Malaria J 2005;4(18):1-4.
[26] Adam I, Elbasit E, Salih I, ElBashir M. Submicroscopic Plasmodium falciparum infections during pregnancy in an area of Sudan with a low intensity of malaria transmission. Ann Trop Med Parasitol 2005;99:339-44.
[27] Verhoeff F, Brabin B, Hart C, Chimsuku L, Kazembe P, Broadhead R. Increased prevalence of malaria in HIV-infected pregnant women and its implications for malaria control. Trop Med Int Health 1999;4(1):5-12.
[28] Subramanian S, Subramanyam M, Selvaraj S, Kawachi I. Are self-reports of health and morbidities in developing countries misleading? Evidence from India. Soc Sci Med 2008, Epub ahead of print.
[29] Hassan E. Recall bias can be a threat to retrospective and prospective research designs. Internet J Epidemiol 2006;3(2).
[30] Adams S, Matthews C, Ebbeling C, et al. The effect of social desirability and social approval on self-reports of physical activity. Am J Epidemiol 2005;161(4):389-98.
[31] Runsewe-Abiodun I, Ogunfowora O, Fetuga B. Neonatal malaria in Nigeria - a 2-year review. BMC Pediatr 2006;6:19.
[32] World Health Organization. Lives at risk: malaria in pregnancy. http://www.who.int/features/2003/04b/en/ Accessed 2008 Oct 11.
[33] Fomulu N, Nana P, Wiysonge S, Kouam L, Doh A. Adverse perinatal outcomes of adolescent pregnancies in Cameroon. Matern Child Health J 2008;2:149-52.
[34] David GL, Peju O, Piero O. Malaria in adolescence: burden of disease, consequences, and opportunities for intervention. Lancet Infect Dis 2006;6(2):780-93.
[35] Fried M, Nosten F, Brockman A, Brabin B, Duffy P. Maternal antibodies block malaria. Nature 1998;395:851-2.
[36] Ter Kuile F, Parise M, Verhoeff F, et al. The burden of co-infection with human immunodeficiency virus type 1 and malaria in pregnant women in sub-Saharan Africa. Am J Trop Med Hyg 2004;71(2):41-54.
[37] CDC. Human Host and Malaria. http://www.cdc.gov/malaria/biology/humanhost/ Accessed 2008 Oct 12.
[38] Stirrat G. Pregnancy and immunity. BMJ 1994;308 (6947):1385.
[39] Brabin B. Epidemiology of infection n pregnancy. Rev Infect Dis 1985;7:579-603.

[40] Rogerson S, Mwapasa V, Meshnick S. Malaria in pregnancy: Linking immunity and pathogenesis to prevention. Am J Trop Med Hyg 2007;77(6):14-22.

[41] Brabin B. An analysis of malaria in pregnancy in Africa. Bull World Health Org 1983;61:1005-16.

[42] Kakkilaya BS. Anopheles Mosquito. Malaria Site [June, 05, 2007; http://www.malariasite.com/MALARIA/ AnophelesMosquito.htm Accessed 2008 Oct 13.

[43] Himeidan Y, Elbashir M, Adam I. Attractiveness of pregnant women to the malaria vector, Anopheles arabiensis, in Sudan. Ann Trop Med Parasitol 2004;98:631-3.

[44] Worrall E, Basu S, Hanson K. Is malaria a disease of poverty? A review of the literature. Trop Med Int Health 2005;10(10):1047-59.

[45] Uzochukwu B, Onwujekwe F, Onoka C, Ughasoro M. Rural-Urban differences in maternal responses to childhood fever in South East Nigeria. Plos One 2008;12:1788.

[46] Fawole O, Onadeko M. Knowledge and home management of malaria fever by mothers and care givers of under five children. West Afr J Med 2001;20:152-7.

[47] Brooker S, Akhwale W, Pullan R, et al. Epidemiology of plasmodium-helminth co-infection in Africa: populations at risk, potential impact on anemia, and prospects for combining control. Am J Trop Med Hyg 2007;77:88-9.

[48] Langhi DJ, Bordin J. Duffy blood group and malaria. Heamatology. 2006;11:389-98.

[49] Grimberg B, Udomsangpetch R, Xainli J, et al. Plasmodium vivax invasion of human erythrocytes inhibited by antibodies directed against the Duffy binding protein. Plos Medicine 2007;4(12):337.

[50] Lawrence M, Barat NP, Suprotik B, Eve W, Kara H, Anne M. Do malaria control interventions reach the poor? A look through the equity lens. Am J Trop Med Hyg 2004;71:174-8.

[51] Noor A, Omunbo J, Amin A, Zurovac D, Snow R. Wealth, mother's education and physical access as determinants of retail sector net use in rural Kenya. Malaria J 2006;26:5.

[52] Sharma A, Bhasin S, Chaturvedi S. Predictors of knowledge about malaria in India. J Vector Borne Dis 2007;44:189-97.

[53] Fekede BG, Mariam A. Antenatal care services utilization and factors associated in Jimma Town (South west Ethiopia). Ethiop Med J 2007;45:123-33.

[54] Parise M, Ayisi J, Nahlen B. Efficacy of sulfadoxine pyrimethamine for prevention of placental malaria in an area of Kenya with high prevalence of malaria and human immunodeficiency virus infection. Am J Trop Med Hyg 1998;59(5):813-22.

Submitted: November 15, 2008.
Revised: December 27, 2008.
Accepted: January 07, 2009.

In: Public Health Yearbook 2009
Editor: Joav Merrick
ISBN: 978-1-61668-911-7

Chapter 3

THE EFFECT OF DEVELOPMENT OF PROBLEM-SOLVING SKILLS ON THE DEPRESSIVE SYMPTOMS IN WOMEN IN A PRIMARY CARE SETTING IN TURKEY

Meral Kelleci**, RN, PhD and Sevim Buzlu, RN, PhD

Department of Nursing, Cumhuriyet University Health of Science of Faculty, Sivas and Istanbul University Florence Nightingale School of Nursing, Istanbul, Turkey

Abstract

The aim of this study was to investigate the effect of developing problem-solving abilities on depressive symptoms of women in primary care settings. Study subjects consisted of women with complaints of physical health problems not caused by a well-defined medical disease. The study was performed on 76 women randomized into the study group ($n = 38$) and controls ($n = 38$). The data of the research were obtained by using the interview form, Beck Depression Inventory and Problem-Solving Inventory at baseline and three and six months later. The study group and controls were comparable with regard to demographic data ($p > 0.05$). Depression and problem-solving scores of the study group and controls were comparable at baseline ($p > 0.05$). Overall, depression and problem-solving scores of the study group were significantly lower than those of the controls ($p < 0.05$). In the study group, depression and problem-solving scores at month 6 were significantly lower than those at baseline and month 3 ($p < 0.05$) and depression and problem-solving scores at month three were significantly lower than those at baseline ($p < 0.05$). In the control group, there were no significantly differences in depression and problem-solving scores measured at baseline and three and six months later ($p > 0.05$). The findings of our study demonstrated that with increase in problem-solving abilities of women, the depressive symptoms decreased. In primary care settings, there is need to implement programs to increase problem-solving skills of women, who have physical symptoms such as gastrointestinal, reproductive and neurologic symptoms in order to decrease depressive symptoms.

* Correspondence: Meral Kelleci, PhD, Cumhuriyet University Science of Health of Faculty, Psychiatric Nursing Department, 58140 Sivas, Turkey. Tel: +346 2191260; Fax: +346 2191261; E-mail: meralkelleci@yahoo.com

Keywords: Depression, problem solving abilities, women, nursing, primary care settings.

Introduction

Depression is the most common mental health problem. It has been reported that prevalence of depressive symptoms in the society is between 13-20% (1-3). The cost of depression to society is considerably due to lost ability to work, participate in society and increased frequency of visits to physicians and high-cost medical-diagnostic testing (4,5). Women are two to three times as likely as men to be depressed regardless of race, income, or education (4,6). Furthermore, women have twice the risk for unreported and unacknowledged depression (6,7).

A number of explanations have been forthcoming, as for example, that marriage has a less protective effect for women than for men. Such factors as the absence of relationships or partnership supporting women, the presence of little children for them to look after, and the lack of work or something to occupy them outside the home make them inclined towards depression (4,6-9). Also important is the assumption that female hormones lead to depression biologically. The changes that appear in the hormones in the menstruation cycle in particular leads to such feelings as tension, touchiness and restlessness. This state, in turn, increases the inclination towards depression (6).

The existence of depressive symptoms significantly affect quality of life (10-13). By making these individuals with depressive symptoms deal with problem solving skills, one may improve coping skills, thus leading to a decrease in depressive symptoms, thus impacting their life in a positive manner (12-14).

Effective skills for solving interpersonal and social problems encountered in everyday life are considered vital to personnel well-being. Studies have revealed that the problem-solving abilities in individuals with depression are destroyed or deteriorated (15-22). Some authors have defined the problem as a difficult situation in which the individual does not have the necessary performance abilities or as a situation in which he or she is not ready for an answer, while others have defined it as the absence of an open way to a purpose or as an obstacle or by-road. It is supposed that a problem arises when there is a difference between the real and ideal states of the events and when the individual fails to adapt himself or herself to a state quickly and to meet a requirement. The solution is reaching the target or fulfilling the purpose through a series of actions (20,22-24). The individuals in depression determine the fields of problems, but have difficulty in solving these problems (20,22).

Problem solving training can be implemented as a preventive measure and integrated into everyday life. In a study by Dowrick et al (16) problem-solving abilities of the group with depression were found 17% lower than those in the control group and following a one-year education and follow-up, no significant differences was found with another group given anti-depressants. In a study done by Katon et al (5) to prevent the relapses of depression in primary care, it was determined that relapses of depression were fewer in the group, where problem-solving therapy was applied (5). Meade et al (1) stressed that the problem-solving approach along with anti-depressant treatment in primary care made a great contribution to the individuals organizing their lives (1). Ludman et al (25) showed that depression could be prevented by using the methods of improving the decision-making abilities and cognitive-behavior methods and found that 62% of these patients dis not need any drug treatment (25).

It is a known fact that women tend to go to primary care setting more often than men with the explanation that their physical complaints often are due to their repression and personalization of their own feelings and thoughts (9,26,27). Because the treatment is directed towards physical problems, depression is often overlooked or under-diagnosed (7,9,26). However, depressive symptoms may be reduced and a better life standard secured, if nursing practices are implemented to enhance problem-solving abilities in order to combat hopelessness, helplessness, reluctance, worthlessness, loss of meaning and significance of life. It has been remarked in several studies that nurses trained to develop problem-solving abilities can apply this treatment to the individuals with emotional disturbances and this approach can be effective in the primary care of depression (21,28,29). It is therefore considered important for the protection and improvement of public and individual health that women with depression should be recognized by nurses in the primary care setting.

The aim of this study was to assess the effect of the problem-solving approach on depressive symptoms in women coming to health centers with complaints of physical health problems not caused by a well-defined medical disease.

Methods

This study used the pre- and post test controlled-group experimental model. The participants consisted of 76 women, whose score was greater than 12 on the Beck Depression Inventory (BDI) (30). All had a risk of depression; but without exhibiting major depression symptoms; none of them were receiving pharmacologic or psychotherapeutic treatment, all were literate and consented to participate in this study.

Procedure

The research was carried out at a primary care setting after the required permission and consent was achieved. The women who applied to this health centre with physical health problems formed the sample for the research. Meeting the criteria of admission to the research by the simple randomized sampling method, the women were determined as the study group and controls. The women who applied to the health centre during a whole day were given numbers according to the order of their treatment; thus, the women with an odd number were included in the study group while the ones with an even number were controls. The sample consisted of 76 women, 38 in the study groups and 38 in the controls on the basis of a 0.05 error level and .85 power value.

Criteria for admission

The women admitted to the research were expected:

- To have a grade between 12 and 45 from Beck Depression Inventory (those with a grade equal to or higher than 25 were asked to be evaluated by a psychiatrist)
- To have no suicidal thoughts and ideas (those with such thoughts were sent directly to see a psychiatrist)
- Not to have a well-defined or diagnosed physical or mental illness
- Not to be pregnant or not to have delivered a baby in recent times
- To have graduated from a primary school at least
- To have no communication disability
- To be between the ages of 18 and 45 years and not to be in the menopause period.

Seeing that each of the women had a different familial environment, a distinct personality and different facilities, it was assumed that the subjects included in the study would be influenced by these conditions in similar ways.

The interviews were carried out at the primary care setting. The interviews were conducted, where the women could feel comfortable and at ease without noise or disturbance. The women who met the required criteria and agreed to participate were randomly sampled as the study group and controls in the order of their visit to the primary care setting. Each woman was interviewed face to face in a session that lasted for about 45 minutes. The women in the study group were given the program of developing problem-solving abilities in ten sessions (450 minutes in sum). They were called back for observations three and six months later (90 minutes in sum). The women in the control group were, however, interviewed in three sessions and each session lasted for 30 minutes (90 minutes in sum). They were also called back for observations three and six months later.

Hypotheses of the research

We formulated the following hypotheses for our research:

- There is a difference between the pre-approach depressive symptom level faced by the women to whom the program of developing problem-solving abilities was applied and their post-approach depressive symptom level.
- There is a difference between the depressive symptom level faced by the women to whom the program of developing problem-solving abilities was applied and the depressive symptom level faced by the women to whom the program of developing problem-solving abilities was not applied.
- There is a difference between the pre-approach problem-solving abilities of the women to whom the program of developing problem-solving abilities was applied and their post-approach problem-solving abilities.
- There is a difference between the problem-solving abilities of the women to whom the program of developing problem-solving abilities was applied and the problem-

solving abilities of the women to whom the program of developing problem-solving abilities was not applied

Intervention

Women in this study group were taught problem solving skills by the nurse researcher. Training was carried out according to the principles of D'Zurilla and Golfield (31). In the initial D'Zurilla and Goldfried formulation, problem solving was characterized by five general stages (31):

- Problem orientation stage (sessions 1-2) to reduce or distract attention from negative emotional states and thoughts (self statements) that disrupt problem-solving and focus instead on the stimulus of these negative responses
- Problem definition and formulation (sessions 2-3) to identify a realistic goal or objective for problem solving
- Generation of alternatives (sessions 3-4) using a brain-storming method, to make available many solution alternatives
- Decision making (sessions 5-8) to evaluate to consequences of available solution alternatives and select the most effective one for short and long term, personnel and social reasons
- Solution implementation and verification (sessions 9-10) to verify the efficacy or outcome of the chosen solution in real life.

Sociodemographic questionnaire

The form prepared by the researcher with reference to literature is composed of the parts formed to determine the demographic qualities of the individuals included in the research, their existing and potential problems, their thoughts and responses about them, their level of awareness, the factors that may affect their problem-solving abilities and the stages of problem solving (22,23,32,33).

Beck Depression Inventory

Beck Depression Inventory (BDI) was developed by Beck and associates in 1961 and translated into Turkish by Tegin (1980). The BDI is a 21 item forced-choice questionnaire. The BDI is commonly used to measure a person's depressive symptoms by surveying several areas including emotional states, relationships with others, physical indices of depression (e.g., loss of appetite, change in amount of sleep needed, change in body weight), performance on daily task, and outlook toward the future. The total score ranges from 0 to 63. Although the BDI is not a diagnostic scale, it has been often used for indicating the level of depression and depression. The BDI has had high internal consistency, with alpha coefficients of 0.86 and 0.81 for psychiatric and nonpsychiatric populations, respectively. Reported split-half reliability for the BDI was 0.74 a Turkish population (30). In this study, split-half reliability coefficient was 0.75.

Problem Solving Inventory

Problem Solving Inventory (PSI) was developed by Heppner and Petersen in 1982 is a tool of determining the stages of problem-solving process and evaluating the individual thoughts about own problem-solving approaches and attitudes. The inventory can be used in determining the way the individual solves or copes with his or her problem in fields of psychological guidance, medicine and education. The inventory is easy to use and score. There is no time limit in answering, but the average time of answering is 15 minutes. The inventory consists of 35 items of 6-point likert type. In the inventory, “1” means “I completely agree.” while “6” means “I completely disagree.” A low score is indicative of efficiency in problem-solving and behavior and attitudes towards success in problem-solving. A high point, however, is tantamount to the failure to find effective solutions to problems. The adaptation of the inventory to Turkish and studies on its reliability and validity were carried out by Taylan (1990). The results obtained from the versions of the inventory in both languages have shown that both forms are quite equivalent (30). That the reliability score obtained in the present research is .99 shows that the inventory is a reliable tool for the study.

Statistical analysis

Data were presented as mean ± SD and number (percentage). Demographic data were analyzed with chi-square test. Depression and problem-solving scores were compared with repeated measures ANOVA followed by post hoc Tukey test. A p value of <0.05 was considered as statistically significant.

Results

Table 1 presents age groups, marital status, education level, profession, economic status, marriage type, marriage duration, husband’s education, family structure, and child number. The study group and controls were comparable with regard to demographic data ($p > 0.05$).

Figures 1 and 2 show depression and problem-solving scores measured at baseline and three and six months later of the study group and controls. Depression and problem-solving scores of the study group and controls were comparable at baseline ($p > 0.05$). Overall, depression and problem-solving scores of the study group were significantly lower than those of the controls ($p < 0.05$). In the study group, depression and problem-solving scores at month 6 were significantly lower than those at baseline and month 3 ($p < 0.05$) and depression and problem-solving scores at month 3 were significantly lower than those at baseline ($p < 0.05$). In the control group, there were no significantly differences in depression and problem-solving scores measured at baseline and months 3 and 6 ($p > 0.05$).

Discussion

To the authors' knowledge, this study is the first nursing intervention study to reduce the prevalence of depressive symptoms for women in Turkey. Our results indicate the importance of receiving nursing training for depressive symptoms. The finding of the study supported our hypothesis that problem solving training decreased depressive symptoms. Depression is widely and frequently seen in societies and leads to a considerable loss of ability, pain and suffering to the family and society. Nevertheless, it is underdiagnosed and women visit the primary care setting more frequently than men do but they tend to attribute their complaints to physical symptoms. However, when a group of women who visit the primary care setting with such complaints as ache, vomiting and nausea though without any physical health problem are examined in details, it appears that they are unable to solve their problems and have difficulty expressing their feelings. Moreover, there is some sort of prejudice against the use of anti-depressants in the society, since people are of the opinion that such drugs will lead to addiction.

Table 1. Demographic data

	Study group n (%)	Controls n (%)	P[a]
Age groups (y)			
18-26	9 (23.6)	9 (23.6)	p>0.05
27-35	12 (31.5)	15 (39.5)	
36-45	17 (44.9)	14 (36.7)	
Marital status			
Married	20 (52.6)	19 (50)	p>0.05
Single	9 (23.7)	10 (26.3)	
Widow/Divorced	9 (23.7)	9 (23.7)	
Education level			
Primary	15 (39.5)	17 (44.7)	p>0.05
Secondary	14 (36.8)	13 (34.2	
University	9 (23.7)	8 (21.1)	
Profession			
House wife	12 (31.6)	13 (34.2)	p>0.05
Cleaning service	6 (15.8)	5 (13.2)	
Children care	5 (13.2)	5 (13.2)	
Clothing industry	8 (21.1)	7 (18.4)	
State official	7 (18.4)	8 (21.1)	
Economic status			
Low	22 (57.9)	22 (57.9)	p>0.05
Medium	11 (28.9)	10 (26.3)	
Good	5 (13.2)	6 (15.8)	
Duration of marriage			
1-5 years	4 (20)	5 (26.3)	p>0.05
6-11 years	6 (30)	6 (31.6)	
12-17 years	10 (50)	8 (42.1)	

[a]Chi-square test.

Therefore, it seems essential that women be strengthened with another method than drugs and enabled to cope with depression. It is thought that developing women's problem-solving abilities will enhance their power of coping with the problems and thus prevent depression from becoming chronic (16,17).

In our study, women were chosen with the random sampling method. The women in the study group and controls were similar with regard to demographic data. The study group and controls were comparable at baseline with regard to the depression and problem-solving scores. Overall, depression and problem-solving scores of the study group were lower compared to the controls. In the study group, the depression and problem-solving scores at month six were lower than those at baseline and month three. In the controls, the depression and problem-solving scores were similar measured at baseline and three and six months later.

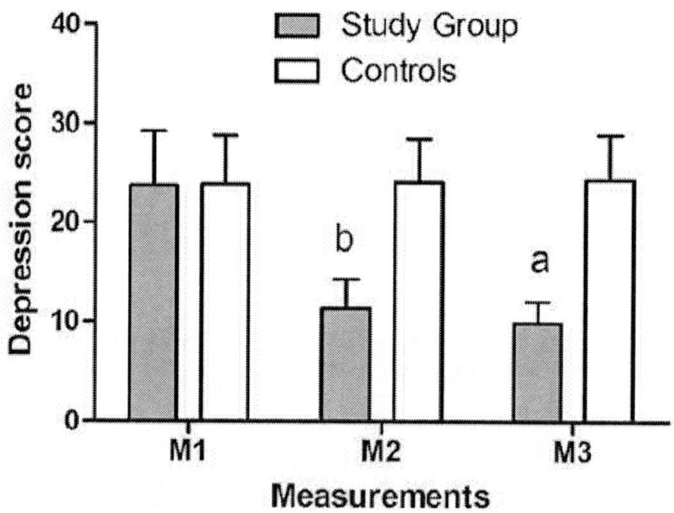

[a]P < 0.05 vs. M1 and M2.
[b]P < 0.05 vs. M1.

Figure 1. Depression scores measured at baseline and months 3 and 6 of study group and controls. M1, baseline; M2, at month 3; and M3, at month 6.

These findings demonstrated that as problem-solving score increased, depression scores decreased. However, there was no change in the problem-solving and depression scores in the control group.

Cannon and Millar (15), who applied the problem-solving program to 15 patients with depression, reported that the BDI score, which was between 27.6 and 31.5 before the program, decreased considerably after the program and the women who had had suicidal ideas got rid of such thoughts. Wallis et al (34) reported that treatment of developing problem-solving abilities was as effective as anti-depressants, more effective than placebo and more accepted by the patients. In their study on 91 randomly chosen patients, they found a significant difference between the patients to whom treatment of developing problem-solving abilities was applied and those who were given placebo as regarding their depression scores, whereas there was no significant difference between the patients to whom treatment of developing problem-solving abilities was applied and those who were given amitriptyline. As a result of the program of developing problem-solving abilities for 3,5 hours over 12 weeks totally, the patients expressed their satisfaction with the program and applications (34).

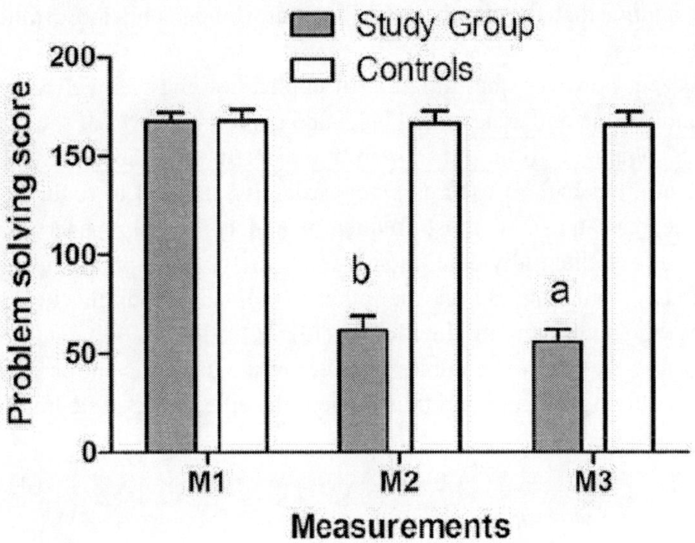

[a]P < 0.05 vs. M1 and M2.
[b]P < 0.05 vs. M1.

Figure 2. Problem solving scores measured at baseline and months 3 and 6 of study group and controls. M1, baseline; M2, at month 3; and M3, at month 6.

Walling (22) stressed that depressive disorders were a significant cause of morbidity and satisfactory results can be obtained in a primary care setting and prevent the illness becoming chronic. It is reported that treatment is usually done with drugs in the primary care of depression, but patients' adaptation to the drugs is not satisfactory. It is also stated that 41% of the patients stop using the drugs within two weeks after they are given the drugs and 68% within four weeks (22). Researchers, therefore, emphasize that alternative different methods ought to take the place of drug-treatment. It is remarked that especially in the program of developing problem-solving abilities, they have learned to cope with their existing problems effectively by using their own abilities and they feel safe about the way they will solve any problem they may face in the future (16,20,34).

In their randomized control study Munos et al (35) applied the program of problem solving to 150 primary-care patients with a low socio-economic level from rural areas and found that depression level decreased to a large extent. Dowrick et al (16) carried out a multi-center randomized control study to determine the acceptability of group psycho-training and program of problem solving for depression and the effect of these applications on their diseases and lives. In this study, 452 subjects were chosen as the sampling group; 128 of them were given problem-solving program and 108 were trained on preventing depression; 189 were, however, included in the control group.

The scores taken six months later from BDI by the patient group to whom problem-solving program was applied were seen to have decreased significantly and problem-solving program was more acceptable and effective than the other programs. Mischoulan et al (33) carried out a study on 40 patients, 36 female and 4 male, with a BDI score higher than 16 by using BDI and PSI and found that level of depression had decreased following the three-month-long treatment.

Researchers (20,21,28) also stress the significance that problem-solving program is short and acceptable, adding that the other applications are longer and more time-consuming as well as more expensive.

It is emphasized, however, that duration of application may as well vary, depending on such factors as motivation and educational level and depression level of the group treated.

The findings obtained from our research indicated that the program of developing problem-solving abilities can be used as a very effective method in reducing the depressive symptoms. As depression is the most frequently and commonly observed disease in the society and costs a lot to the individual, family and society, it is a public health problem to be dealt with seriously. Nursing is, on the other hand, an important health discipline in improving the health and preventing the illnesses (32,34).

It is thought that especially the nurses working in the units for public health can develop women's problem-solving abilities and thus prevent the emergence of depressive symptoms.

Conclusions

The findings of our study suggested that if the problem-solving abilities of women are developed, their depressive symptoms will be decreased. In primary care settings, there was need to conduct programs to increase problem-solving skills of women who have physical symptoms such as gastrointestinal, reproductive, and neurologic symptoms and who have depressive symptoms.

Acknowledgments

This study was supported by a grant from the Istanbul University Research Fund. This article was based on the doctoral thesis of the first author under the supervision of the second author.

References

[1] Meade N, Bower P, Gask L. Emotional problems in primary care: What is the potential for increasing the role of nurses? J Adv Nurs 1997;26(5):876-90.

[2] Cetin I, Bilici M, Bekaroglu M. Saglik ocaklarina basvuran hastalarda depresyon yayginligi ve sosyo-demografik degiskenlerle iliskisi. Ulusal Psikiyatri Kongresi ve Uluslar arasi Kros Kültürel Psikiyatri Uydu Sempozyumu Özet Kitabi, Trabzon, 1999. [Turkish]

[3] Donmez L, Dedeoglu N, Özcan E. Saglik ocaklarina basvuranlarda ruhsal bozukluklar. Türk psikiyatri Dergisi 2000;11(3):198-203. [Turkish]

[4] Hammer CH, Martsolf DS, Zeller RA. Depression and codependency in women, Arch Psychiatr Nurs 1998;12(6):326-34.

[5] Katon W, Rutter C, Ludman EJ. A randomized trial of prevention of depression in primary care. Arch Gen Psychiatry 2001;58(3);241-7.

[6] Kirli S. Kadin ve depresyon. Sürekli Tip Egitimi Dergisi 1999;8(3):104-6. [Turkish]

[7] Beeber LS, Charlee ML. Depressive symptom reversal for women in a primary care setting: A pilot study. Arch Psychiatr Nurs 1998;7(12):247-54.

[8] Gordon V, Gordon E. Short-term group treatment of depressed women: A replication study in Great Britain. Arch Psychiatr Nurs 1987;2:111-24.

[9] Schreiber R. Understanding and helping depressed women. Arch Psychiatr Nurs 1996;10(3):165-75.

[10] Askin R. Depresyon El Kitabi (Depression handbook), Vol 2. Istanbul. Baski Roche Mustahzarlari San. AS, 1999. [Turkish].

[11] Blacker CVR, Clare AW. Depressive disorder in primary care. Br J Psychiatry 1987;150:737-52.

[12] Heppner PP, Krauskopf CJ. An information-processing approach to personal problem solving. Couns Psychol 1987;15:371-447.

[13] Nezu AM, Perri MG. Social problem solving therapy for unipolar depression: an initial dismantling investigation. J Cons Clin Psychol 1989; 57:408-13.

[14] Beck AT, Rush AJ, Shaw BF, Emery G. Cognitive therapy of depression. New York: Guilford, 1987.

[15] Cannon B, Millar R Dysfunctional attitudes and poor problem solving skills predict hopelessness in major depression. J Affect Disord 1999;55(1):45-9.

[16] Dowrick C, Dunn G, Ayuso-Mateos JL. Problem solving treatment and group psycho-education for depression: Multi-centre randomized controlled trial. BMJ 2000;9(321):1450-4.

[17] Garland A, Harrington J, House R, Scott JA. Pilot study of the relationship between problem-solving skills outcome in major depressive disorder. Br J Med Psychol 2000;73:303-9.

[18] Zausznievski SA. Health-seeking resources and adaptive functions in depressed and non-depressed adults. Arch Psychiatr Nurs 1994;8(3):159-68.

[19] Fossati P, Ergis AM, Allilaire JF. Problem solving abilities in unipolar depressed patients. Psychiatric Res 2001;104(2):145-56.

[20] Haverkamp R, Arean P, Hegel MT, Unitzer J. Problem-solving treatment for complicated depression in late life: A case study in primary care. Perspect Psychiatr Care 2004;40(2):45-54.

[21] Thornet A, Mynors-Wallis L.Credibility of problem solving therapy and medication for the treatment of depression among primary care patients. Psychiatry Res 2001;104(2):145-56.

[22] Walling AD. Problem solving sessions in patients with depression. Br J Psychiatry 2000;61(10):125-31.

[23] Benson BA. Problem solving skills training. Habil Ment Healthcare Newsletter 1995;14(1).

[24] Haines J, Williams CL. Coping and problem solving of self-mutilators. J Clin Psychol 1997;53(2):177-86.

[25] Ludman E, Von KM, Katon W. The design, implementation and acceptance of a primary care-based intervention to prevent depression relapse. Int J Psychiatr Med 2000;30(3):229-45.

[26] Birsoz S.Türkiye'de depresyonlarin sosyokültürel özellikleri. Depresyon Dergisi 1997;2(1):3-8. [Turkish]

[27] Jimenez AL, Alagria M, Pena M, Vera M. Mental health utilization in women with symptoms of depression Women Health 1997; 25(2):1-21.

[28] Beech BF. The strengths and weaknesses of cognitive behavioral approaches to treating depression and their potential for wider utilization by mental health nurses. J Psychiatr Ment Health Nurs 2000;7:343-54.

[29] Kelleci M. Depresyonu olan bireylerin sorun cozme becerilerinin gelistirilmesi, Hemsirelik Forumu 2004;(3):14-21. [Turkish]

[30] Savasir I, Sahin N. Bilissel Davranisçi Terapilerde Degerlendirme.: Sik Kullanilan Ölçekler. Ankara: Türk Psikologlar Dernegi Yayinlari, 1997. [Turkish]

[31] D'Zurilla TJ, Goldfried MR. Problem solving and behavior modification. J Abnorm Psychol 1971;78:107-26.

[32] Badger TA, Mishel MH, Biocca LJ. Depression assessment and management: Evaluating a community-based mental health training program for nurses. Public Health Nurs 1992;8(3):170-6.

[33] Mischoulon D, Howarth S, Vuolo RM. Management of depression in the primary care setting. Psychother Psychosomat 2001;3:23-8.

[34] Wallis ML, Davies I, Gray AA. Randomized controlled trial and cost analysis of problem solving treatment for emotional disorders given by community nurses in primary care. Br J Psychiatry 1997;170:113-9.

[35] Munoz RF, Ying YW, Bernal G. Prevention of depression with primary care patients: A randomized controlled trial. Am J Community Psychol 1995;23(2):199-222.

Submitted: December 01, 2008.
Revised: January 01, 2009.
Accepted: January 06, 2009.

In: Public Health Yearbook 2009
Editor: Joav Merrick
ISBN: 978-1-61668-911-7

Chapter 4

How well do parents in the United States report heights and weights for children?

Marilyn S. Townsend*, PhD, RD[1], Hugo Melgar-Quinonez, MD, PhD[2], Mark Hudes, PhD[3] and Patricia B. Crawford, DrPH, RD[4]

[1]Nutrition Department, University of California, Davis, California
[2]Department of Human Nutrition, College of Education and Human Ecology, Ohio State University, Columbus, Ohio
[3]Nutritional Sciences and Toxicology, University of California, Berkeley
[4]Center for Weight and Health, University of California, Berkeley, California, United States of America

Abstract

Parent-reported values for children's heights and weights are routinely collected in national, state, and school surveys in the United States. Our purpose was to examine the accuracy of those values for children 2–11 years old. Z scores, means and standard errors, paired t-tests and Spearman rank order correlations were calculated for three age and three ethnic groups to estimate reliability and validity of values. Few parents accurately reported their child's height, weight, and calculated BMI (15.0%, 13.7%, and 5.6%, respectively). Many parents responded 'Don't know' to questions about their children's weight (25%) and height (53%). The typical parent of 2-5 years olds under-reported height by about 4.6 cm. The magnitude and direction of the BMI bias or error for 2-5 years olds was +2.3 BMI units. The decreasing relative bias for height and BMI indicated increasing accuracy as children age. Height and BMI bias was greatest for children in the 2-5 year group; here, the sex-specific bias for non-

* Correspondence: Marilyn S Townsend, PhD, RD, Nutrition Department, University of California, Davis, One Shields Ave, Davis, CA 95616-8669 United States. Tel: (530) 754-9222; Fax: (530) 752-7588; E-mail: mstownsend@ucdavis.edu

Hispanic black and Mexican-American boys and girls exceeded the bias for non-Hispanic white preschoolers ($p = 0.05$). Regarding random error, the coefficients were smaller for height compared to weight indicating that height was a greater source of this error. For clinical and public health environments, use of parent reports introduced random and systematic errors to reported heights and weights particularly height and calculated BMI. The magnitude and direction of the errors varied by child's age and ethnicity.

Keywords: Height, weight, BMI, overweight, children.

Introduction

Reported values of height and weight for children are often collected from parents or caregivers as part of national, state and school surveys in the United States, where time, money, and/or expertise are not available to measure these variables (1). In our search of the literature, only two validation studies of parent or caregiver reports of heights and weights for children were found (2,3). One study reported on the accuracy of parent reported values for Mexican-American 6 mo-11 year old children (3). The second study included 150 parent reports of weight for their obese children (6-11 years), who were participating in a weight control/reduction program (2). With extensive collection of reported values to monitor population trends in weight (and particularly BMI), to monitor individual children by public schools, and in using BMI in chronic disease related studies, it is important to determine the accuracy of this method of estimating children's actual heights and weights.

To our knowledge, this report is the first large-scale analysis of the accuracy with which parents and caregivers in the United States reported their children's height and weight. We examined the relationships of reported and measured heights, weights, and the corresponding calculated BMI using a nationally representative sample of children [n = 7,316]. We assessed both the prevalence of parents or caregivers reporting children's heights and weights accurately as well as the magnitude and direction to which population estimates are biased for sub-groups of children (ie, validity) and the parameters' variance (ie, reliability). Subsequent references to parents in this paper refer to both parent and caregiver respondents.

Methods

The Nutrition and Health Examination Survey (NHANES) III dataset (1989–94) was selected, because this survey collected both reported and measured height and weight for children and was designed to obtain a nationally representative sample of the US civilian population by employing a complex, stratified, multistage, probability cluster sampling design of partial probability samples of households in 48 contiguous states (4). Procedures were reviewed and approved by the University of California, Davis, Institutional Review Board.

During interviews conducted in their homes, parents and caregivers were asked to estimate their children's height and weight (reported height and weight); BMI was calculated based upon these reports. Approximately 99% of the children subsequently were measured (measured height, weight, and calculated BMI) in the Mobile Examination Center (MEC) (5).

Variables

Ten age-years, two sex categories and three ethnic groups in the original analyses generated 60 permutations for weight and 60 for height. A sample size of 30 per cell was estimated to adequately detect correlations and 40 per cell to adequately compare means for each of the 120 age-sex-ethnic groups. To have sufficient sample size, NHANES III datasets from the years 1989-1991 (phase 1) and 1991-1994 (phase 2) were combined.

Reported height and weight. Parents reported values for height and weight for their children during the household interview.

Measured height and weight. Trained health technicians measured children at the MEC using procedures described elsewhere (4,5).

Body mass index (BMI, kg/m^2). The term measured BMI refers to the body mass index calculated from children's measured height and weight. The term reported BMI is calculated from parent-reported values for children's height and weight.

Age, gender and race/ethnicity. Children were originally grouped into ten 12-month age categories and then collapsed into three for the reader's convenience. Data from three ethnic/racial (non-Hispanic white, non-Hispanic black, Mexican-American) and two gender groups were examined.

Statistical analysis

Using Stata (6), sample weights accounted for the unequal probabilities of selection, oversampling, and non-response (5). Using the CDC growth charts, Z scores were calculated for weight-for-age and height-for-age (7). Outliers were defined as ± 4 SDs for height- and weight-for-age Z scores, and removed to correct biological infeasibility, recording error, or coding error. For parent-reported values, extreme values were not removed from analyses.

Using each child's birth date, date of the MEC visit, and date of the interview, age in months for the interview and for the MEC was determined (5).

As there was no established guideline to follow, acceptable accuracy of reported values was defined as ±2% of the corresponding measured values. For example, a reported height for an arbitrary 3-year old child measured at 102 cm. would be considered accurate within a range of 100 to 104 cm. Accuracy (ie, validity) of the reported values (8,9) was estimated from the mean of the differences between measured values for the population (also called the bias or systematic error) for height, weight, and calculated BMI. The bias of sub-groups were compared to determine if the direction of the bias varied between the groups. The differences between reported and measured values relative to the corresponding measured value [(reported–measured)/measured x 100] was termed "relative bias". Analyses of mean relative bias were used to assess which component of BMI (weight, height, or both) was responsible for the observed pattern in the subgroup analyses. Paired t-tests were used to evaluate the significance, if any, of the bias (8,9).

Reliability of reported values was assessed by the Spearman rank-order correlation coefficients (9). Group differences in random error were assessed by comparing the variances of the bias between groups, while the differences in bias (ie, indicating differences in validity) were assessed by testing for statistically significant differences in magnitude of mean errors between groups using t-tests and a weighted analysis of variance. Test statistics associated with chance probabilities of 0.05 or less for Type I errors were considered statistically significant.

Results

When asked, parents had a 53% probability of responding "Don't know" for height and a 25% probability for weight. One of the reported height or weight variables was missing for 55% of the children (n = 4,023). Consequently, children with reported height and weight values to calculate BMI numbered 3,293 (see table 1). The mean age of the 4,023 children for whom BMI pairs were unavailable was younger in comparison to the mean age of the 3,293 children with available BMI pairs (mean age = 5.4 years and 5.8 years, p = 0.001) (data not shown). Children without available BMI pairs were more likely to live in households with lower incomes (68%) compared to children with available BMI pairs (50% low income households) (p = 0.04) (data not shown). The mean measured weight of the 3,293 children in the final sample was 27.7 kg (SE .29) and statistically different from the measured weight of 24.9 kg (SE .29) for the 4,023 children lost to exclusion criteria (p < .0001) (data not shown). The mean measured height of the 3,293 children in the final sample was 123.5 cm (SE .58) and statistically different from the measured height 118.7 cm (SE .64) of children who did not meet exclusion criteria (p < .0001).

Prevalence of accurately reported values

Of the parents of 5,457 children with measured weights in the original sample, 20.1% reported their child's weight within ±2% of the measured weight (see table 2). Of the 3,410 parents reporting heights (47%) in the original sample, 29.5% reported their child's height within ± 2% of the measured height. Including those reporting "Don't know," only 13.7% (1,005/7,316) accurately reported weight and 15.0% (1,095/7,316) accurately reported height. Of these 7,316 children, 5.6% (n = 409) had an accurately estimated BMI based on reported values (see table 2).

Bias in reported values

The direction (ie, negative sign) of the computed bias for height and weight for each of the three age categories indicated under-reporting of the measured values (see table 3). For example, the typical parent of 2-5 years olds under-reported height by about 4.6 cm and weight by about 0.2 kg. Relative to the measured value, the relative bias for weight was small (0.5% of measured weight) while the relative bias for height was large (4.6% of measured height). The bias in reporting for children's height tended to be larger for younger compared to older children.

Table 1. Inclusion and exclusion criteria and sample size for the combined sample of children, 2-11y, in NHANES III Phase 1 (1989-1991) and Phase 2 (1991-1994)

Description	Lost (n)	Sample remaining (N)
Initial sample size, age 2-11 y † Other ethnic/racial group	540	7,981 7,441
Measured weight-for-age outliers ‡	15	7,426
Measured height-for-age outliers ‡	3	7,423
Both measured height and weight available	107	7,316
Reported height and weight Weight pairs (5,457) Height pairs (3,410)	4,023	3,293
Measured and reported values for BMI (4 values available) ††		3,293
FINAL SAMPLE		3,293‡‡

† All subjects with reported ethnicity. Children, other than non-Hispanic white, non-Hispanic black and Mexican-American, where excluded.

‡ Based on ±4 SDs of the measured value. Reported and measured value is available. Figure transferred to Table 2.

†† Measured height and weight, and reported height and weight available in same child for BMI calculations.

‡‡ Includes 1,831 2-5 y olds, 620 6-8 y olds, and 842 9-11 y olds with 1628 boys and 1665 girls.

Table 2. Prevalence (%) of parents/caregivers reporting accurately the heights, weights, and BMI for children, 2-11 y.[a]

	Accurately reported values prevalence (%)					
	Reports of "Don't know" excluded			Reports of "Don't know" included n=7,316		
Age	Height n= 3410	Weight n= 5457	BMI n= 3293	Height	Weight	BMI
2-5y	24.8	20.0	11.5	11.1	15.3	5.0
6-8y	29.2	18.9	10.7	12.5	13.1	4.4
9-11y	39.6	21.1	15.8	22.0	15.8	8.4
All	29.5	20.1	12.4	13.7[b]	15.0[c]	5.6[d]

[a] Accuracy is defined as ±2% of the measured value. Accuracy rate = percent (%) of parents/caregivers reporting within ± 2% of the measured value.

[b] [1,005 children with reported height ±2% of measured height] divided by [3,410 children with reported height + 3,906 children with reported "Don't know"]

[c] [1,095 children with reported weight ±2% of measured weight] divided by [5,457 children with reported weight + 1,859 children with reported "Don't know")]

[d] [409 children with reported BMI ±2% of measured BMI] divided by (3,293 children with reported BMI + 4,023 children with reported "Don't know"]

Table 3. Measured (M) and reported (R) values, mean errors (bias), absolute value of the error for height, weight, and BMI by age category using data from NHANES III, 1988 – 1994[†‡]

			Height n = 3,410			
Age (y)	Mean (cm)		Error mean (±SE)			
	M	R	Bias	Relative bias (%)	Mean absolute error	Mean relative absolute error (%)
2-5	102.32	97.67	-4.64 (0.30) **, [a]	-4.60 (0.29) [a]	7.21 (0.26) [a]	7.07 (0.25) [a]
6-8	125.89	121.69	-4.21 (0.49) **, [a]	-3.33 (0.39) [b]	7.17 (0.43) [a]	5.73 (.35) [b]
9-11	144.59	141.65	-2.94 (0.46) **, [b]	-2.07 (0.33) [c]	5.71 (0.32) [b]	4.01 (.23) [c]
	Weight (kg) N =5,457					
Age (y)	Mean (kg)		Error mean (±SE)			
	M	R	Bias	Relative bias (%)	Mean absolute error	Relative absolute mean error (%)
2-5	16.80	16.65	-0.15 (0.05) *, [a]	-0.54 (0.32) [a]	1.23 (.04) [a]	7.35 (.24) [a]
6-8	26.84	26.10	-0.74 (0.16) **, [b]	-2.16 (0.51) [b]	2.25 (0.14) [b]	8.21, (.43) [b]
9-11	39.60	38.19	-1.41 (0.22) **, [c]	-2.75 (0.47) [b]	2.88 (0.18) [c]	7.13, (.37) [a]
	BMI (kg/m²) n = 3,293					
			Error mean (±SE)			
Age (y)	Mean (kg/m²)		Bias	Relative bias	Mean absolute error	Relative absolute mean error
	M	R		(%)		(%)
2-5	15.98	18.28	2.30 (0.19) **, [a]	14.47 (1.17) [a]	3.32 (0.19) [a]	20.73, (1.12) [a]
6-8	16.64	17.75	1.11 (0.23) **, [b]	7.23 (1.29) [b]	2.63 (0.19) [b]	15.54, (1.07) [b]
9-11	19.04	19.41	0.37 (0.14) *, [c]	3.08 (0.75) [c]	2.10 (0.16) [c]	11.20, (0.80) [c]

† Parent reported for child. Mean bias = mean of reported value minus measured value (reported – measured) for all children in the group and represents the strength and direction of the population mean. Relative mean bias = (bias ÷ measured value) x 100. Mean total error = absolute value of reported height, weight or BMI minus measured value calculated for each individual and then averaged for the population and represents the mean of the absolute bias for each individual. Relative total error = (error ÷ measured value) x 100.

‡ Paired t-test to determine if mean bias (reported minus measured value) is significantly different from zero. Sample weights accounted for the unequal probabilities of selection, oversampling, and non-response.

*$p \leq 0.01$; ** $p \leq 0.001$ [a, b, c] Groups sharing common superscript are not significantly different from each other ($p \leq 0.05$).

As a result, relative bias for BMI was larger for the youngest age categories. The BMI bias for 2-5 year olds was +2.3 BMI units or 14.5% of BMI based on measured values. Unlike the negative bias for height and weight, BMI bias was positive. For each age category, the relative bias for BMI was larger than that for weight and for height (see table 3). The decreasing relative bias for height and BMI indicated increasing accuracy as children age; ie, as children approach puberty, parents are more likely to estimate heights and resultant BMI with more accuracy. The relative bias for BMI was largely explained by height bias as height is squared in the denominator of the BMI calculations.

Height and BMI bias was greatest for children in the 2-5 year group (see table 4); here, the sex-specific bias for non-Hispanic black and Mexican-American boys and girls exceeded the bias for non-Hispanic white preschoolers (p = 0.05). Weight bias (not shown) was relatively small compared to height and BMI bias for each age, sex, and ethnic category.

Extreme bias. Extreme bias in reporting was defined as ± 4 SD of the reported value. Numerous parents made extreme errors in reporting their children's height while only a small number made extreme errors in reporting their children's weight. Specifically, about 16% of parents (531 of 3,410 with reported height available) reported extreme values for height for their children while 1% (57 of 5,457 with reported weight available) reported extreme values for weight.

Table 4. Comparison by race/ethnicity and gender for 3 age categories for height and BMI bias for reported values using NHANES III, 1988 – 1994[†] [‡]

Height bias (cm) (mean ±SE) n = 3,410						
Age	Non-Hispanic White		Non-Hispanic Black		Mexican -American	
	Boys	Girls	Boys	Girls	Boys	Girls
2-5 y	-3.5 (0.6) [a]	-3.6 (0.5) [a]	-8.5 (0.9) [b]	-7.6 (1.1) [b]	-8.4 (0.8) [b]	-9.3 (0.8) [b]
6-8 y	-3.7 (0.8) [a]	-3.8 (0.7) [a]	-4.9 (2.0) [a]	-6.6 (2.2) [a]	-6.6 (1.3) [a]	-5.7 (1.6) [a]
9-11 y	-1.9 (0.7) [a]	-2.5 (0.7) [a]	-1.4 (1.5) [a]	-4.8 (1.2) [a, b]	-6.2 (1.0) [b]	-7.1 (1.0) [b]
BMI bias (kg/m^2) (mean ±SE) n = 3,293						
Age	Non-Hispanic White		Non-Hispanic Black		Mexican –American	
	Boys	Girls	Boys	Girls	Boys	Girls
2-5 y	1.8 (0.3) [a]	1.6 (0.3) [a]	4.5 (0.6) [b]	4.2 (0.9) [b]	4.7 (0.6) [b]	4.9 (0.5) [b]
6-8 y	0.8 (0.4) [a]	0.8 (0.3) [a]	2.4 (0.9) [a, b]	2.6 (0.9) [b]	2.9 (0.7) [b]	1.8 (0.7) [a, b]
9-11 y	0.4 (0.2) [a]	0.0 (0.3) [a]	0.5 (0.6) [a, b]	0.2 (0.5) [a]	1.4 (0.4) [b]	1.1 (0.5) [a]

[†] Mean (±SE.) Bias is defined as the mean difference between measured and reported values for all children in the group.

[‡] Sample weights accounted for the unequal probabilities of selection, oversampling, and non-response.

[a, b, c] Groups were compared across rows with groups sharing a common superscript not significantly different from each other using Tukey's Studentized Range Test at a 5% procedure-wise error rate.

Random error in reported values

As another indicator of accuracy, we calculated the Spearman correlation coefficient (ie, reliability coefficient) for reported and measured values for height, weight, and BMI derived from those reports or measurements. The coefficients were consistently smaller for younger children (2-5 year olds: r = 0.66 height, 0.84 weight, 0.30 BMI) indicating less reliability and more random error in the reported heights and weights compared to older children (6-8 y olds: r = 0.50 height, 0.83 weight, 0.41 BMI; and 9-11 year olds: r = 0.73 height, 0.90 weight, 0.61 BMI). This result implies that randomness of the error is age-dependent.

In addition, the coefficients were smaller for height compared to weight indicating that height was a greater source of random error than weight. Correlation coefficients for BMI were consistently smaller compared to weight and height coefficients for the corresponding age categories. This would be expected given that height was squared in the denominator of the BMI calculation and the coefficients indicated that height was a larger source of random error than weight. These values indicate considerable deviation between reported and measured values for many children. Using the criterion, r = 0.90, for acceptable reliability, parents for this child population generally did not report with acceptable reliability.

Discussion

Although reported heights and weight for children are frequently collected in clinical and public health environments, their validity and reliability have rarely been studied. The present work examined the quality of parent reported heights and weights for boys and girls 2-11 year for three ethnic groups. National surveys such as the Continuing Survey of Food Intakes for Individuals (CSFII) (10), the 1998 CSFII Child Supplement (10), the National Health Interview Survey (11), the Child Development Supplement to the Panel Study of Income Dynamics (PSID) (12), Medical Expenditure Panel Survey (MEPS) (13), and many state surveys rely on reported heights and weights for children. Because reported heights and weights are easily obtained compared to measured values requiring a trained technician, they will continue to be used (14). Consequently, knowledge of the magnitude, direction and variance of this reporting bias (ie, systematic error) is useful in planning and interpreting survey results. It is essential for users of these kinds of surveys to be well-informed about the limitations of using this kind of data. Statistical handling cannot compensate for erroneously reported values.

Prevalence of accurately reported values

About 55% of parents and caregivers in this sample were not able to estimate either their child's height or weight, marking "Don't know" to the question while 24% did not provide estimates for both height and weight. It is reasonable to expect that those responding "Don't know" would report with even less accuracy than those who reported heights and weights. Using the entire sample in the denominator therefore represents 'the most probable' case that can be made for reported values. Including "Don't know" responses as inaccurate estimates of height, 86% of parents did not report their children's height with accuracy. For weight, 85% did not report accurately. For BMI derived from these reports, 94% were classified as inaccurate.

Using the entire sample, only 6% of parents or caregivers reported values within a ± 2% level of accuracy. A large percentage of parents said they did not know their children's heights (53%) and weights (25%). Using the sub-sample of children with reported and measured values, the magnitude and direction of error varied by age, ethnicity, and sex.

Bias in reported values

Our analyses demonstrated that the child's age and ethnic/racial group are important factors when considering the use of parent-reported height and weight for children. Mexican-American and non-Hispanic black children 2-11 years had greater height and BMI errors than non-Hispanic white children. Generally, we observed substantial under-reporting of height for the three age categories with less under-reporting for non-Hispanic white and black boys, 9-11 years. The result of underreported height is larger calculated BMI values. Bias for height and BMI is greater for younger children (see table 2). For example, the mean overestimate of BMI is 14.5% for 2-5 y olds compared with a bias of 3.1% for 9-11 year olds.

Given that heights and weights in the final sample differed from those lost to exclusion criteria, care must be taken with interpretation of results. Those lost to the analysis for bias were younger, and thus in the age category where errors tended to be larger relative to body size.

Comparison to adult studies. The consistent under-reporting of height seen for children is different from the findings for adults who tend to over-report height (1,8,9,14). As height is squared in the denominator of the child's BMI calculation, the bias for BMI is dramatic.

Random errors in reported values

Reported weight reflects well the relative ranking of measured weight, as indicated by the large reliability coefficients. The use of reported weights as continuous variables in multivariate analyses probably would result in only small errors in the values of the coefficient for weight. However, the smaller coefficients for reported height and BMI suggest that these reported data could be problematic as continuous variables in multivariate analyses.

Comparison with similar study. Our results compare favorably with those of Davis who studied Mexican American mothers' reports for their children with the exception of height for 2-5 year olds (3). Our coefficient of 0.66 for height contrasted with Davis' 0.41 value. It should be noted, however, that the cut points for age categories differ between the two studies.

Comparison with adult studies

Compared to studies for adults, our findings with children reveal smaller reliability coefficients. Charney et al (15) reported a correlation of 0.96 between measured and reported weight for 50 adults (20-30 years of age). Jeffrey (16) found weight correlations of 0.99 for both male and female employees at 32 worksites in Minneapolis-St. Paul and Kuczmarski (17) found reliability coefficients of 0.89 to 0.97 for BMI for his nationally representative sample of US adults. We found considerably smaller coefficients for children ranging from .30 to .61 for BMI and .83 to .90 for weight.

The finding that parents of Mexican-American children were less likely to accurately report heights and weights of their young children is of particular interest. The standard unit of measurement for heights and weights is metric in Mexico. Although respondents were given a choice of metric or English units, Mexican-American immigrants may have felt the need to report using English units. Their reports in inches were consistently underestimated. We would expect a larger variability in reported values among lower socioeconomic families where measurement devices may be less likely to be present and the children may make fewer visits to medical offices. In fact, we did observe this to be true in an analysis of household income and BMI errors (not shown).

Limitations

Although the measurement and interview processes used for NHANES were subject to rigorous standardization and quality control procedures, some factors may have influenced our findings and consequently their interpretation. The time lapse between the interview in the home with its reported responses and the examination with its measured weights and heights at the MEC was 2-6 weeks. Some children in the sample may have had a slight growth in stature and body weight during this period. Thus, part of the underreporting could, in fact, be due to actual changes in the two variables. Unlike height, daily fluctuations in the child's weight could account for some of the difference between reported and measured weight. Knowing their children would eventually be measured for weight and height at the MEC, could have influenced parental reporting.

Conclusions

We conclude that reported weight and heights for children are subject to substantial bias and random error. Our results suggest that users of datasets from school, state, and national surveys and clinicians relying on reported values should consider four main issues. First, the majority of parents in this representative sample marked "Don't know" when asked for estimates. Second, of those willing to estimate values, total errors were substantial particularly for height and, consequently, for calculated BMI. Third, calculated BMI was consistently overestimated. Fourth, errors for BMI were particularly high for non-Hispanic black children and young Mexican-American children.

For analyses of public health survey data where height, weight, or calculated BMI is the outcome variable, a case cannot be made for using reported values with the possible exception of weight. For monitoring population trends in BMI and evaluating the effects of relative body weight on health status, the differences between measured and reported heights and calculated BMI are significant. These errors would alter results. Our findings suggest that children's BMI derived from reported weight and height differ significantly from the corresponding measured value and that the deviation differs by age, sex and ethnic/racial groups further confounding conclusions of public health studies. Use of children's BMI values calculated from reported values is misleading at best and completely erroneous at worst.

Acknowledgments

Funding from the Economic Research Service, US Department of Agriculture, supported this study. The authors wish to thank Katherine Flegal, PhD, for her insightful comments, and Janet Peerson, MA, for her guidance with planning the statistical analyses.

References

[1] Rowland ML. Reporting bias in height and weight data. Statistical Bull 1989;2.

[2] Wing RR, Epstein LH, Neff D. Accuracy of parents' reports of height and weight. J Behav Assess 1980;2:105-10.

[3] Davis H, Gergen PJ. Mexican-American mothers' reports of the weights and heights of children 6 months through 11 years. J Am Diet Assoc 1994;94:512-6.

[4] National Center for Health Statistics. Plan and operation of the third National Health and Nutrition Examination Survey:1988-94. Hyattsville, MD: Natl Center Health Stat, Vital Health Stat 1994;1:32.

[5] National Center for Health Statistics. Analytic and Reporting Guidelines: the Third National Health and Nutrition Examination Survey, NHANES III (1988-1994). NHANES III reference manuals and reports on CD-ROM. Hyattsville, MD: CDC, 1996.

[6] Stata, Release 6.0, 1999. Stata Corp. College Station, TX.

[7] Kuczmarski RJ, Ogden CL, Grummer-Strawn LM et al. Advance data from vital and health statistics. Hyattsville, MD: Natl Center Health Stat, 2000;314(314):1-28 Available at http://www.cdc.gov/growthcharts. Accessed 2008 Nov 15.

[8] Stewart AL. The reliability and validity of reported weight and height. J Chron Dis 1982;35:295-309.

[9] Rowland M.L. Reported weight and height. Am J Clin Nutr 1990;52:1125-33.

[10] Tippett KS, Cypel YS. Design and operation: The continuing survey of food intakes by individuals and the diet and health knowledge survey, 1994-96. USDA/ARS Nationwide Food Surveys Report No. 96-1. Riverdale MD: USDA, Food Survey Res Group, 1997.

[11] Benson V, Marano M. Current estimates from the National Health Interview Survey, 1995. Hyattsville, MD: Natl Center Health Stat. Vital Health Stat 1998;10:199.

[12] Modi M. Panel study of income dynamics, child development supplement. Surveys measuring well-being. Available at: http://www.wws.princeton.edu/?kling/surveys /PSID.html. Accessed 2008 Nov 01.

[13] US Department of Health and Human Services, Agency for Health Care Policy and Research. Design and methods of the medical expenditure panel survey household component: Methodology report 1,1997 . http://www.meps.ahrq.gov/mepsweb/data_files/publications/mr1/mr1.pdf. Accessed 2008 Nov 08.

[14] Pirie P, Jacobs D, Jeffery RW, Hannan P. Distortion in reported height and weight data. J Am Diet Assoc 1981;78:601-6.

[15] Charney E, Goodman HC, McBride M, Lyon B, Pratt R. Childhood antecedents of adult obesity: Do chubby infants become obese adults? N Engl J Med 1976;295:6-9.

[16] Jeffrey RW. Bias in reported body weight as a function of education, occupation, health and weight concern. Addict Behav 1996;21:217-22.

[17] Kuczmarski MF, Kuczmarski RJ, Najjar M. Effects of age on validity of reported height, weight, and body mass index: Findings from the third National Health and Nutrition Examination Survey, 1988-1994. J Am Diet Assoc 2001;101:28-34.

Submitted: December 05, 2008.
Revised: December 29, 2008.
Accepted: January 06, 2009.

In: Public Health Yearbook 2009
Editor: Joav Merrick
ISBN: 978-1-61668-911-7

Chapter 5

THE BURDEN OF CHRONIC FATIGUE SYNDROME (CFS) IN CANADA

Frank Mo, MD, PhD*[*1,2], Heidi Liepold[1], Michelle Bishop[1], Lianne Vardy[1] and Howard Morrison[1]

[1]Division for Chronic Disease Management, Centre for Chronic Disease Prevention and Control, Public Health Agency of Canada

[2]The R Samuel McLaughlin Centre, Institute of Population Health, University of Ottawa, Ottawa, Canada

Abstract

Chronic fatigue syndrome (CFS) poses many socioeconomic, psychosocial, disability and quality of life difficulties for people with CFS in Canada. The self-reported prevalence of CFS was 0.78%, 1.22% and about 201,900, 331,500 Canadians have reported having CFS in 2000 and 2005 respectively. Canadians aged 40-64 years old (57.87% in 2000, and 58.59% in 2005) were the most frequently infected. More female Canadians (71.41% in 2000, and 68.44% in 2005) were affected than males (28.59% and 31.56%). Both physical and mental fatigue caused by CFS cost the Canadian economy an estimated $3.5 billion per year, and the annual lost productivity in Canada is estimated at $2.5 billion in 2003. However, the capacity in Canada for prevention and management of CFS is limited. Currently, there are only few medical doctors using the Clinical Working Case Definition, diagnostic and treatment protocols. Therefore, we need more research in the surveillance, diagnosis, treatment, and evaluation of CFS management in Canada.

Keywords: Chronic fatigue syndrome, lifestyle, socioeconomic status, burden, disability, CCHS, Canada.

* Correspondence: Frank Mo, MD, PhD, Medical Research Scientist, Chronic Disease Management Division, Centre for Chronic Disease Prevention and Control, Health Promotion and Chronic Disease Prevention Branch, Public Health Agency of Canada, 785 Carling Avenue, Ottawa, Ontario K1A 0K9, Canada. Tel: 613-946-2616; Fax: 613-954-8631; E-mail: frank_mo@phac-aspc.gc.ca

Introduction

Chronic fatigue syndrome (CFS) is an illness, which is characterized by long term debilitating fatigue that lasts for more than six months. Patients experience a substantial reduction in their ability to participate in occupational, socially or physically demanding activities. Patients with CFS do not recover from their fatigue with rest (1). CFS is prevalent in the Canadian community and it is costly to the health care system. Without treatment, the symptom of CFS worsens with time. Its causes are not fully understood; however, multiple risk factors have been suggested to influence the occurrence, some of the factors include over 40 years of age, being female, having a sedentary or unhealthy lifestyle. The capacity in Canada to accurately monitor and forecast trends or evaluate the effects of interventions is evidently limited (2). At present Canada does not have a CFS surveillance system. For this reason, this nation is not able to accurately measure the potential associations of this syndrome's prevalence, incidence, hospitalization, disability, mortality and economic burden.

Many individuals who suffer from CFS experience financial hardship and psychosocial problems, which reduces their quality of life. The self-reported prevalence of CFS in Canada increased from 0.78% in 2000 (201,940), to 1.22% in 2005 (331,530 cases) (3). Canadians aged 40 years and over were the most frequently affected with CFS compared to other age groups. More females reported having CFS than males. A recent study from the United Kingdom estimated the cost of CFS at 3.46 billion pounds per year. To crudely convert to Canadian dollars and adjust for size of this nation's economy (just under half of the British one) and currency exchange (just over double), the physical and mental fatigue caused by CFS cost the Canadian economy would be about $3.5 billion per year, and the annual lost productivity in Canada due to CFS is estimated at $2.5 billion in 2003 (4). The second study was done through the Center for Disease Control and Prevention in the US. It focuses on calculation of the loss of productivity of just over $20,000 US dollars per CFS patient each year, and there is in total a productivity loss of $9.1 billion US, which has been converted to the Canadian context (adjusting for GDP and exchange rates). This would be about $1 billion in Canadian economic loss (5). However, the capacity in Canada to prevent and manage CFS is limited. Currently, there are few medical doctors working on the clinical case definition, diagnostic and treatment protocols, and research. Furthermore, there is no gold standard laboratory or a specific diagnostic test available in Canada. Presently, there is no consensus among Canadian doctors as to the clinical definition of CFS. Medical training program related to the syndrome do not exist. Furthermore, there is no financial support for research projects relating to CFS (6). Therefore, we need more research in the surveillance, diagnosis, treatment, and evaluation of CFS management in Canada.

Risk factors and diagnosis

The causes of CFS remain unknown. Clinicians have proposed one or more risk factors, which might trigger the occurrence of CFS. These may include viral infection, injury, psychological depression, profound stress or exposure to toxins (7). While a single cause for CFS may yet be identified, another possibility is that CFS represents a common endpoint of disease resulting from multiple precipitating causes (8). In Canada and worldwide, researchers continue to explore possible causes, risk factors and triggering factors for the condition. However, many questions still remain about diagnosis since there is no treatment guideline or CFS case definition. The idea that CFS is an illness that primarily affects white, middle-class, well-educated, professional women still needs to be verified (2).

Methods

The Canadian Community Health Survey (CCHS) (9) is a collaborative effort between Statistics Canada, Health Canada, Public Health Agency of Canada and the Canadian Institute for Health Information. This national household cross-sectional survey was created to gather national health-related data to provide timely estimates of Canadians demographic information, lifestyle, risk factors, and socioeconomic status. The CCHS began collecting its first cycle of data in September of 2000, and subsequent data collection is based on a two-year collection cycle. Data from CCHS Cycle 1.1 (2000) to 3.1 (2005) were used in this analysis. The survey excluded individuals living on crown or reserve land, in institutions, members of the Canadian Armed Forces, and in certain remote areas of the country; but it still represents ~98% of the Canadian population over 12 years of age (10). A multistage stratified cluster design combined with random sampling methods was used to select the sample (10).

Sampling

The CCHS is scheduled to collect data every month from that point forward. Each two-year collection cycle comprises two distinct surveys: a health region-level survey in the first year with a total sample of 130,000, and a provincial-level survey in the second year with a total sample of 30,000. Sample sizes in any particular month or year can increase from provincial or health region-level buy-ins. Both computer-assisted personal and telephone interviews are planned (9). There was one randomly selected respondent per household. Eligibility for the first collection cycle were limited to only those 12 years of age and over; although it is expected that in future cycles, child-specific content will be included.

Definition of covariates

The self-reported covariates in the analysis are age, gender, living area (province/territories, urban/rural) lifestyle (smoking status, frequency of alcohol use, and physical activity) and socioeconomic status (education, income, immigration status). The level of education achieved by all members of the household was grouped into three categories (less than secondary, secondary, postsecondary school or more). Family income was classified on the basis of total household annual income and the number of household members into low (<$30,000 CAD) or middle (>=$30,000 to $59,999 CAD) and high ($60,000 CAD and over) level. Immigration status includes participants that were either born in Canada or were born elsewhere. Other variables were included in the analysis: physical activities were categorized as active, moderate, and inactive, based on kilo-calories per kilogram of body weight per day expended (KKD). Physically active is defined as an energy expenditure of at least 3 KKD; moderately active corresponds to energy expenditure between 1.5 and 3 KKD; physically inactive is defined as less than 1.5 KKD. The highest level of physical activity can be achieved by playing team sports for an hour or a half an hour of running, combined with an accumulated hour of walking throughout the day (11,12). Cigarette smoking was evaluated by three different methods: 1) patients were asked if they had ever smoked a whole cigarette (yes, no)? 2) if they were a 'current smoker' (daily, occasionally, not at all); 3) or a 'former smoker' (stopped smoke meanwhile survey was started). Patients were asked on a questionnaire how often they drank alcohol. They were asked to categorize their drinking habits as being "a regular drinker", "a former regular drinker(one who used to drink regularly, but no longer does)", or "a non-drinker" (a person who does not drink alcohol). The occurrence of CFS related to risk factors or socioeconomic status were calculated for total population and compared in proportions in people with or without CFS, where statistical significance was conducted by Odds Ratio and P values.

Data analysis

A descriptive model has been used to examine demographics, lifestyle, and socio-economic factors that could influence the occurrence of CFS. Multivariate logistic regression was then employed to determine independent factors associated with CFS, with Odds Ratio (OR) and P values calculated for each model. The logistic regression models were bootstrapped to take the design effects of the CCHS into account. Data was analysed using the SAS version 9.1 (SAS Institute, Cary, NC) (13).

Results

The adjusted prevalence of CFS increased from 0.78% to 1.22% from 2000 to 2005 in Canada. Individuals aged 40-64 years were more likely to report having CFS compared to other age groups in both 2000 (OR, 1.51; $P<0.005$) and in 2005 (OR, 2.67; $P<0.001$). Females made up more than two-thirds of reported cases in both 2000 and 2005 (see table 1). There are no significant statistical differences between current smoking and former smoking (OR from 0.51 to 0.86, $P>0.05$). However, the differences for CFS patients with less than secondary school education level (OR, 1.24 in 2000 and OR, 1.25 in 2005, $P<0.01$), and secondary school level (OR, 1.14 in 2000 and OR, 1.08 in 2005, $P<0.05$) are significant in comparison to post-secondary school educated individuals. Regular alcohol users (OR, 1.11, $P<0.05$ in 2000 and OR, 1.27, $P<0.01$ in 2005) have higher occurrences than non-alcohol users, but former regular alcohol users (OR from 0.66 to 0.96, $P>0.05$ in 2000 and in 2005) had no significant differences compared to non-drinking individuals. Moreover, non-immigrant Canadians (OR from 0.83 to 0.89, $P>0.05$) who live in the urban area (OR from 1.21 to 1.28, $P<0.01$), who have low family income level (OR,1.37, $P<0.01$ in 2000 and OR,1.18, $P<0.05$ in 2005), middle family income (OR, 2.48, $P<0.001$ in 2000, OR,1.06, $P>0.05$ in 2005), those who were physical inactive (OR from 1.33, $P<0.01$ to 1.55, $P<0.005$) were exposed to more risk of CFS than others.

The prevalence of CFS is higher in Nunavut (1.09%), Nova Scotia (0.90%), Quebec (0.90%), Alberta (0.80%), and Ontario (0.79%) in 2000; however, this prevalence in Nova Scotia (1.47%), Quebec (1.38%), and Ontario (1.29%) in 2005 is higher than Canadian nation level (1.22%) (see table 1).

Table 1. Adjusted self-reported prevalence of Chronic Fatigue Syndrome (CFS) by age, sex, lifestyle, socioeconomic status and geographic in the CCHS, Canada, 2000-2005

Chronic Fatigue Syndrome	2000		2005	
	Cases of CFS	Prevalence (%)	Cases of CFS	Prevalence (%)
Cases of CFS	201,938	0.78	331,526	1.22
Non-CFS	25,597,000	99.17	27,057,000	98.48
Missing cases	12,131	0.05	82,510	0.30
Total	25,811,069	100.00	27,471,036	100.00
Provinces & Territories				
Newfoundland & Labrador	1,636	0.36	3,197	0.71
PEI	469	0.40	445	0.38
Nova Scotia	7,067	0.90	11,711	1.47
New Brunswick	4,815	0.76	5,838	0.91
Quebec	55,898	0.90	89,317	1.38
Ontario	78,206	0.79	136,457	1.29
Manitoba	3,780	0.42	7,521	0.81
Saskatchewan	4,330	0.54	6,554	0.83
Alberta	19,896	0.80	31,194	1.16
British Columbia	25,502	0.75	38,900	1.08
YUKON	39	0.16	173	0.64
NWT	86	0.27	205	0.59
NUNAVUT	212	1.09	10	0.07
Total	201,938	0.78	331,526	1.22
12-19	8,303	4.11	6,586	1.99
20-39	51,226	25.37	63,731	19.22
40-64	116,864	57.87	194,235	58.59
65 & over	25,544	12.65	66,974	20.20
Total	201,937	100.00	331,526	100.00
Sex				
Males	57,736	28.59	104,639	31.56
Females	144,402	71.41	226,886	68.44
Total	201,938	100.00	331,526	100.00
Smoking status				
Non-smoker	55,180	27.40	86,142	26.00

Table 1. (Continued)

	Cases of CFS	Prevalence (%)	Cases of CFS	Prevalence (%)
Chronic Fatigue Syndrome	2000		2005	
Current smoker	65,792	32.68	112,439	33.93
Former smoker	80,381	39.92	132,760	40.07
Total	201,353	100.00	331,341	100.00
Education levels				
Less than secondary school	30,941	15.77	34,624	11.70
Secondary school	27,969	14.26	29,808	10.07
Post-secondary school	137,248	69.97	231,577	78.23
Total	196,159	100.00	296,009	100.00
Alcohol drinker				
Regularly drinker	137,659	68.34	228,633	70.00
Former drinker	43,954	21.82	79,040	24.20
Non-drinker	19,823	9.84	18,957	5.80
Total	201,436	100.00	326,630	100.00
Living area				
Urban	170,171	84.27	278,304	83.95
Rural	31,767	15.73	53,221	16.05
Total	201,938	100.00	331,526	100.00
Immigrant status				
Immigrant	38,874	19.36	72,108	22.40
Non immigrant	161,959	80.64	249,789	77.60
Total	200,833	100.00	321,897	100.00
Total yearly family income				
Less than $29,999	48,595	25.99	99,505	36.47
$30,000 - $59,999	108,969	58.28	88,992	32.62
$60,000 & over	29,421	15.73	84,322	30.91
Total	186,985	100.00	272,818	100.00
Physical activity				
Active	29,641	16.14	54,614	17.16
Moderate	31,178	16.98	70,092	22.02
Inactive	122,818	66.88	193,619	60.82
Total	183,637	100.00	318,325	100.00

Discussion

Chronic fatigue syndrome (CFS) is one of a group of illnesses which have unexplained and unknown causes; others include fibromyalgia, diffuse pain and irritable bowel syndrome (14). However, these do not necessary have the same causes and symptoms. For example, patients may sleep poorly and thus develop fatigue, whereas people who have disturbed sleep and inactivity may have different conditions (15). The exact risk factors and causes of CFS have not been identified yet. Researches have theorized that this syndrome may be related to infectious and immunologic, psychiatric, behaivioral, socioeconomic and environmental factors (16).

Studies have found that there is a high economic and disability burden associated with CFS, for the families and society as a whole. A conservative estimate of the direct economic impact of CFS and the huge health care expenditure in Canada is about $3.5 billion per year. The cost to governments in Canada is about $2.2 billion per year in 2002 (4). At a personal level, economic losses caused by absenteeism can have a substantial long-term impact on CFS patients' quality of life. With high unemployment rates among individuals with CFS, there is a surcharged cost of medical services that could become even more problematic to CFS patients and their families, due to a loss of health insurance benefits, and thus, increases in out-of-pocket medical expenses (17). Bombardier and Buchwald (18) estimated an average annual medical expenditure of $1,031 CAD per CFS patient. Lloyd and Pender (19) and McCrone et al (20) also used samples from Australia and the United Kingdom respectively, to estimate the same situation.

Table 2. Adjusted Odds Ratio and 95% confidence interval between age, gender, lifestyle, and socioeconomic status for CFS in the CCHS, Canada, 2000-2005

Chronic Fatigue Syndrome	2000		2005	
	Percent(%)	Odds Ratio (OR) and P-Value	Percent(%)	Odds Ratio (OR) and P-Value
[a] Age (year)				
<40 and 65+	42.13	*1.00*	41.41	*1.00*
40 – 64	57.87	1.51; P<0.005	58.59	2.67; P<0.001
[b] Gender				
Males	28.59	*1.00*	31.56	*1.00*
Females	71.41	2.49; P<0.001	68.44	2.46; P<0.001
[c] Risk factors and socioeconomic status				
Smoking status				
Non-smoker	27.40	*1.00*	26.00	*1.00*
Current smoker	32.68	0.51; P>0.05	33.93	0.58; P>0.05
Former smoker	39.92	0.71; P>0.05	40.07	0.86; P>0.05
Education levels				
Post-secondary school	69.97	*1.00*	78.23	*1.00*
Less than secondary school	15.77	1.24; P<0.01	11.70	1.25; P<0.01
Secondary school	14.26	1.14; P<0.05	10.07	1.08; P>0.05

Table 2. (Continued)

Chronic Fatigue Syndrome	2000		2005	
	Percent(%)	Odds Ratio (OR) and P-Value	Percent(%)	Odds Ratio (OR) and P-Value
Alcohol drinker				
Non-drinker	9.84	*1.00*	5.80	*1.00*
Regularly drinker	68.34	1.11; P<0.05	70.00	1.27; P<0.01
Former drinker	21.82	0.66; P>0.05	24.20	0.96; P>0.05
Living area				
Rural	15.73	*1.00*	16.05	*1.00*
Urban	84.27	1.28; P<0.01	83.95	1.21; P<0.01
Immigrant status				
Immigrant	19.36	*1.00*	22.40	*1.00*
Non immigrant	80.64	0.89; P>0.05	77.60	0.83; P>0.05
$60,000 & over	15.73	*1.00*	30.91	*1.00*
Less than $29,999	25.99	1.37; P<0.01	36.47	1.18; P<0.05
$30,000 - $59,999	58.28	2.48; P<0.001	32.62	1.06; P>0.05
Physical activity				
Active	16.14	*1.00*	17.16	*1.00*
Moderate	16.98	0.88; P>0.05	22.02	1.01; P>0.05
Inactive	66.88	1.33; P<0.01	60.82	1.55; P<0.005

a. Adjusted Odds Ratio were controlled by gender, risk factors and socioeconomic status.
b. Adjusted Odds Ratio were controlled by age, risk factors and socioeconomic status.
c. Adjusted Odds Ratio were controlled by age and gender.

The study results in table 1-2 revealed that CFS aflicts people in the age group (40-64 years) at twice the rate of other age groups. The occurrence of CFS in females is also more common than in males. Regular alcohol use, people have a low education level (less than secondary schooling), being a non-immigrant status, being a Canadian living in an urban area, physical inactivity, and having lower annual family income (less than $29,999 CAD) have a higher prevalence and burden.

Conclusions

CFS is a chronic, severely disabling medical disorder. It is problematic to the patients socioeconomic and psychosocial status.It can be more accurately diagnosed and treated symptomatically with improved surveillance, research, and management. Further developing funded knowledge exchange, health education, and research may reduce the burden and result in better outcomes for CFS patient treatment and management.

References

[1] US Department of Health and Human Services Centers for Disease Control and Prevention 2008. URL: http://www.cdc.gov/cfs.

[2] Carruthers BM. Definitions and aetiology of myalgic encephalomyelitis (ME): How the Canadian consensus clinical definition of ME works. J Clin Pathol 2007;60(2):117-9.

[3] Statistics Canada. Canadian Community Health Survey (CCHS), 2000-2005.

[4] The economic impact of ME/CFS. Sheffield Hallam University on behalf of Action for ME, a UK charity. 2003 May 12. http://www.shu.ac.uk/cgi-bin/news_full.pl?id_num= PR405anddb=03.

[5] Reynolds KJ, Vernon SD, Bouchery E, Reeves WC. The economic impact of chronic fatigue syndrome. Cost Eff Resour Alloc 2004; 2(1):4.

[6] Logan AC, Bested AC, Lowe R, Logan A, Howe R. Hope and help for chronic fatigue syndrome and fibromyalgia. Nasville, TN: Cumberland House Publ, 2008.

[7] Chronic fatigue syndrome. Connecticut Centre for Health 2008. http://www. connecticutcenterforhealth.com/chronic-fatigue-syndrome.html.

[8] Fact sheet. Chronic fatigue syndrome. Pamphlet by: National Institute of Allergy and Infectious Diseases, Health Care Industry, 2000.

[9] Statistics Canada. Canadian Community Health Survey (CCHS). 2001-2005. http://www.statcan.ca/english/survey/other/canforgen.htm.

[10] Beland Y. Canadian community health survey—methodological overview. Health Rep 2002;13(3):9-14.

[11] Statistics Canada. National population health survey, 1996-7. Ottawa, ON: Health Stat Div, Public Use Microdata Files, 1997.

[12] Canadian Fitness and Lifestyle Research Institute. Physical activity monitor survey, 1997.

[13] SAS Institute. Statistical Application System (SAS), version 9.1.3. 2005.

[14] Aaron LA, Buchwald D. A review of the evidence for overlap among unexplained clinical conditions. Ann Intern Med 2001; 134:868-81.

[15] Moldofsky H, Scarisbrick P. Induction of neurasthenic musculoskeletal pain syndrome by selective sleep stage deprivation. Psychosom Med 1976;38:35-44.

[16] Natelson BH, Lange G. A status report on chronic fatigue syndrome. Environ Health Perspect 2002;110(Suppl 4).

[17] Jason LA, Benton MC, Valentine L, Johnson A, Torres-Harding S. The economic impact of ME/CFS: Individual and societal costs. Dyn Med 2008;7:6.

[18] Bombardier CH, Buchwald D. Chronic fatigue, chronic fatigue syndrome, and fibromyalgia: Disability and health Care use. Medical Care 1996, 34:924-930.

[19] Lloyd AR, Pender H: The economic impact of chronic fatigue syndrome. Med J Austr 1992;157:599-601.

[20] McCrone P, Darbishire L, Ridsdale L, Seed P. The economic cost of chronic fatigue and chronic fatigue syndrome in UK primary care. Psychol Med 2003;33:253-61.

Submitted: December 05, 2008.
Revised: Decemner 30, 2008.
Accepted: January 07, 2009.

In: Public Health Yearbook 2009
Editor: Joav Merrick
ISBN: 978-1-61668-911-7

Chapter 6

ADOLESCENT TOBACCO USE IN HIMACHAL PRADESH, INDIA

Jayakaran S Job, MD, DrPH [1,2]***, Adamson S Muula****[*]***, MPH, MBBS***[3]***, Seter Siziya PhD*** [4] ***and Emmanuel Rudatsikira, DrPH, MD***

[1]Department of Global Health, School of Public Health, Loma Linda University, Loma Linda, California, United States of America,

[2]Department of Epidemiology and Biostatistics, Loma Linda University, Loma Linda, United States of America,

[3]Department of Public Health, Division of Community Health, College of Medicine, University of Malawi, Blantyre, Malawi and

[4]Department of Community Medicine, School of Medicine, University of Zambia, Lusaka, Zambia

Abstract

To estimate the prevalence and associated factors of tobacco use among school-going adolescents in Himachal Pradesh, India. Data from the Global Youth Tobacco Survey (GYTS) 2004 was used to determine tobacco use prevalence, determinants, attitudes, and exposure to tobacco advertisements among adolescents. Frequencies and their 95% confidence intervals (CI) were calculated. Odds ratios (unadjusted (OR) and adjusted (AOR)) and their 95% CI were obtained using logistic regression analysis. Of the 1,976 respondents for whom gender was recorded, 6.4% males and 3.9% females reported current tobacco use (p = 0.021). After controlling for age, gender, parental tobacco use status, and perception of risks of tobacco use, 'having some friends who were tobacco users' was associated with tobacco use (AOR = 4.65; 95% CI [2.85, 7.58], the association being stronger if all their friends were tobacco users AOR=11.78; 95% CI [4.84, 28.63]. Participants reported high exposure to tobacco advertisements on billboards (71.0%), and television (53.3%). Nearly one in seven respondents (14.7%) reported possessing an item with a tobacco brand on it. The proportion of males who felt that tobacco use was harmful was higher than that for females (p=0.002). Findings from this study emphasize the

[*] *Correspondence:* Adamson S Muula, MPH, MBBS, Department of Public Health, Division of Community Health, College of Medicine, University of Malawi, Private Bag 360, Chichiri, Blantyre 3, Malawi. E-mail: adamsonmuula@yahoo.com

critical role of friends, and the media in influencing adolescent tobacco use behaviours and the need for considering social and domestic environments in planning gender-specific interventions for this vulnerable population subgroup.

Keywords: Tobacco, cigarettes, smoking, adolescents, India

Introduction

Tobacco use is a leading cause of non-communicable diseases such as chronic obstructive pulmonary disease, cardiovascular conditions and a range of cancers (1). There is growing evidence that while tobacco use has stabilised or is in decline in industrialised nations, there is increased prevalence of use in resource-limited settings and emerging economies (2). A list of reasons why this situation has arisen include: aggressive marketing by tobacco firms, limited public health interventions; and a pre-occupation with communicable diseases that has overstretched public heath efforts (3-6). Furthermore, the global proliferation of various mass media, may also have contributed to the "globalisation" of tobacco use (7,8).

While data on tobacco use, especially data on cigarette smoking and associated factors among adolescents in many states in India has been reported, data from some areas are limited. Data is also currently available on the factors that are associated with tobacco use among adolescents in other international settings (9-12). Public health program planners are likely to benefit from data generated from their own geographical areas when considering options to determine the most efficient allocation of often scarce public intervention resources for example, by targeting factors that are strongly associated with tobacco use based on the effect measures. Furthermore, in the absence of published data, it may be difficult to raise the social profile and concerns associated with tobacco use among researchers and policy makers. Finally, meta-analysis of data on the factors that are associated with tobacco use can only be carried out using available published information.

A recent publication by Sinha et al (13) aimed at linking tobacco control policies and data on tobacco use in India considered the prevalence of the following attributes among 13 to 15 year olds in India: smoking, cessation experience, exposure to second-hand smoke, access to, and availability of tobacco; and exposure to advertisements. Not only is this study population restricted to ages 13 to 15 years, as is the focus of the GYTS (Global Youth Tobacco Survey), but only prevalence estimates and not an assessment of the associations between tobacco use and those explanatory variables were reported. It is not clear whether those exposures are in fact associated with tobacco use. Furthermore, Sinha et al (13) aggregated data from all states in the country and average India estimates were obtained and no individual state estimates were reported.

The India Tobacco Control Act (ITCA) was signed into law in 2003 with the goal to reduce tobacco consumption and protect citizens from exposure to secondhand smoke (SHS). In 2005, the Indian government ratified the World Health Organization Framework Convention on Tobacco Control (WHO FCTC). Among the many provisions of the ITCA are sections prohibiting smoking in public places, prohibiting direct or indirect advertisement of cigarettes and other tobacco products on billboards and in all media excluding point of sale, and prohibiting the sale of tobacco products to persons less than 18 years of age that is the focus of the GYTS. Data used in this article were collected in 2004, possibly before the ITCA had enough time to effect meaningful changes regarding tobacco use practices among adolescents in India.

In this paper we attempt to estimate the prevalence and associated factors of tobacco use among in-school adolescents in Himachal Pradesh, India. Previous studies from this setting have not reported on factors that may be associated with tobacco smoking and therefore important in the prevention of smoking.

Methods

The present study was a secondary analysis of publicly available data from the Centers for Disease Control and Prevention (CDC) on the 2004 Global Health Survey for the State of Himachal Pradesh, India. The survey was conducted according to the Global Tobacco Surveillance System (GTSS) as has been described elsewhere (14). The GYTS used a standard survey questionnaire with core questions (the same in all geographical settings) and country-specific questions that countries can add to cover research questions considered pertinent by country cooperating partners as critical for that particular setting.

The GYTS recruits in-school adolescents in classes with the majority of its students being between the ages 13 and 15 years. A two-stage cluster sampling survey approach is used in which the primary sampling units (PSUs) are schools with students in the eligible age group (13-15 years). At the second stage of sampling, eligible classes (classes with the majority of students of ages 13 to 15 years) within the selected schools are randomly selected. All the students within the selected classes are eligible to participate in the study, regardless of their actual ages. Only students who are present on the day the survey is administered in a particular school are surveyed and no replacement of absent students is attempted. While all students eligible and present are invited to participate, the students are informed that they are free to elect not to participate and also free not to answer any question with which they feel uncomfortable. Surveys using the same methodology have been conducted in other settings (13).

The GYTS questionnaire is administered and anonymously self-completed within a single class period. Information collected include the following variables: age, sex, current smoking status, parental smoking, having friends who smoked, perception that smoking is harmful to health, exposure to tobacco advertisements, and approval of smoking among boys and girls.

Data analysis

Data were obtained from the CDC and analyzed using SUDAAN software 9.0 (Research Triangle Institute, Research Triangle Park, North Carolina, United States). Frequencies and 95% confidence intervals (CI) of relevant variables such as demographics, approval of smoking among boys and girls, and exposure to tobacco advertisements were generated and are reported. To assess the associations between a selected list of variables identified from the literature as possibly associated with current cigarette smoking, logistic regression analysis was conducted both at bivariate and multivariate level. These explanatory variables were: sex; age; smoking by the best friend, and parental smoking.

The bivariate logistic regression analysis was conducted to obtain unadjusted odds ratios (OR) with current tobacco use (Yes or No) as the outcome of interest. Tobacco use was defined as having used tobacco in any form (smoking, chewing or applying tobacco) during the past 30 days.

Each of the following variables was considered as explanatory variables: age; sex; peer smoking; parental smoking; and perception that smoking is harmful. Further multivariable models were also fitted to obtain adjusted odds ratios (AOR).

Results

Of the 1,976 students for whom gender was reported, 41.8% were females. The median age for the sample was 15 (Q_1= 16-17, Q_3=14) years. The prevalence of current tobacco use was 6.4% (95% CI [5.1, 8.0]) among males and 3.9% (95% CI [2.8, 5.5]) among females.

Table 1 indicates that in bivariate analysis, males were more likely to use tobacco than females (OR=1.66; 95% CI [1.08, 2.56]). Compared to participants whose parents did not use tobacco, those with parents who were tobacco users were more likely to use tobacco (OR=1.85; 95% CI [1.23, 2.79]). Those with most or all friends who used tobacco were 14 times more likely to use tobacco than those who had no friends who used tobacco (OR=14.36; 95% CI [6.77, 30.46]). Participants who perceived that tobacco use was harmful were less likely to use tobacco than those who did not perceive tobacco as harmful to health (OR=0.56; 95% CI [0.37, 1.00]).

Table 1 also indicates that in multivariate analysis, having close friends who used tobacco was very strongly associated with tobacco use after controlling for age, gender, parental tobacco use, and perception of hazards caused by tobacco use. Those who had most or all friends who used tobacco were more than 11 times likely to use tobacco than those who had no friends who used tobacco (OR=11.71; 95% CI [4.79, 28.64]). Those who had some friends who used tobacco were more than four times likely to use tobacco than those who had no friends who used tobacco (OR=4.65; 95% CI [2.85, 7.58]).

Table 2 indicates that participants were exposed to tobacco advertisements through billboards (71.0%), and television (53.3%). More than one in ten respondents (14.7%) reported possessing an item with a tobacco brand logo on it. There was no gender difference in rates of those who reported having an item with a tobacco brand logo (p =0.851) nor on prevalence of exposure to tobacco advertisements on hoardings (p=0.149) and television (p=0.474).

Table 3 indicates that the majority (84.8%) of respondents felt that tobacco use was harmful to health. The proportion of males (87.1%) who felt that tobacco use was harmful was significantly higher (p=0.002) than that for females (81.6%). All participants thought that male smokers had more friends compared to 12.5% who felt that females who used tobacco had more friends. About 1 in 4 respondents thought that males and females who used tobacco were attractive (26.7% and 24.7% respectively).

Table 1. Factors associated with current tobacco use in Himachal Pradesh, India

Characteristic	Percentage of smokers	Unadjusted Odds ratio (95% Confidence Interval)	Adjusted Odds ratio (95% Confidence Interval)
Age (years)			
11–12	3.8	1.00	1.00
13	6.4	1.71 [0.71, 4.08]	1.29 [0.49, 3.34]
14	3.9	1.03 [0.44, 2.45]	0.87 [0.34, 2.21]
15	4.8	1.27 [0.55, 2.94]	0.98 [0.39, 2.47]
16–17	7.1	1.93 [0.86, 4.31]	1.15 [0.46, 2.84]
Gender			
Female	3.9	1.00	1.00
Male	6.4	1.66 [1.08, 2.56]	1.21 [0.73, 1.99]
Parental tobacco use			
None	4.1	1.00	1.00
One or both parents smokers	7.3	1.85 [1.23, 2.79]	1.30 [0.81, 2.07]
Best friends tobacco users			
None	3.1	1.00	1.00
Some	12.7	4.63 [2.99, 7.16]	4.65 [2.85, 7.58]
Most or all	31.2	14.36 [6.77, 30.46]	11.71 [4.79, 28.64]
Perception that tobacco use is harmful			
No	7.2	1.00	1.00
Yes	4.7	0.56 [0.37, 1.00]	0.87 [0.46, 1.63]
Family member discussed harmful effects of tobacco use			
No	5.9	1.00	1.00
Yes	4.9	0.84 [0.56, 1.28]	0.84 [0.51, 1.39]

Table 2. Exposure to tobacco advertisements distributed by gender among adolescents in Himachal Pradesh, India

Characteristics	Number of participants	% of total and 95% CI [p value]*
		[P=0.474]
Seen tobacco brand name on TV in past 30 days	1973	53.3 [51.0,55.5]
Males	1140	54.0 [51.1, 56.9]
Females	833	52.2 [48.7, 55.6]
		[P=0.851]
Has item with tobacco brand logo	1969	14.7 [13.2, 16.4]
Males	1136	14.8 [12.8, 17.1]
Females	833	14.6 [12.3, 17.1]
		[P=0.149]
Seen tobacco adverts on hoardings in past 30 days	1973	71.0 [68.9, 73.0]
Males	1140	72.3 [69.6, 74.9]
Females	833	69.1 [65.8, 72.2]

* p value comparing levels of exposure between males and females

Table 3. Attitudes towards tobacco use distributed by gender among adolescents in Himachal Pradesh, India

Characteristic	Number of participants	% of total and 95% CI [p value]*
Felt that boys who use tobacco have more friends	1701	100
Males	1000	100
Females	701	100
		[P<0.001]
Felt like girls who use tobacco have more friends	1647	12.5 [10.9, 14.3]
Males	959	15.5 [13.3, 18.0]
Females	688	8.3 [6.4, 10.6]
		[P=0.673]
Felt that boys who use tobacco are attractive	1337	26.7 [24.3, 29.1]
Males	789	27.9 [24.8, 21.2]
Females	548	24.9 [21.5, 28.7]
		[P=0.002]
Felt that girls who use tobacco are attractive	1675	24.7 [22.7, 26.9]
Males	978	27.7 [24.9, 30.6]
Females	697	20.5 [16.7, 23.7]
		[P=0.002]
Felt that tobacco use is harmful to health	1772	84.8 [83.0, 86.4]
Males	1028	87.1 [84.8, 89.0]
Females	744	81.6 [78.6, 84.3]

* p value comparing levels of exposure between males and females

Discussion

We report an overall current tobacco use of 6.4% (95% CI [5.1, 8.0]) among males and 3.9% (95% CI [2.8, 5.5]) among females (p = 0.021). We did not find male predominance of tobacco use after adjusting for possible confounders. The male predominance has been reported with regard to cigarette smoking in other settings (16-18). However, this finding is not universal. For instance, in the United States of America, cigarette smoking rates are similar among male and female adolescents (19), while in other countries like Turkey, the gender gap is closing (20). We suggest that the acceptability of smoking among males compared to females may be responsible for the higher rates found in males in Himachal Pradesh. We found in the current study that tobacco use among boys was perceived as more favourable compared to use in females.

As also reported in other studies, we found that the likelihood of being a tobacco user were higher among adolescents whose friends used tobacco, and among those who had parents who used tobacco, and among males (in univariate analysis only). Although there was higher reported tobacco use among adolescents 16-17 years old (7.1%) compared to those 11-12 years (3.8%), the difference was not statistically significant. When designing specific anti-tobacco intervention programs, these study findings suggest the importance of focusing efforts directed at friends who use tobacco.

In a cross sectional study, and when data on the temporal sequence of events are not available, it is not possible to determine if a factor is causally associated with the outcome (tobacco use) (21,22). In the context of this study analysis, it is not possible to assess whether befriending a smoker is a cause of tobacco use or if tobacco users themselves are more likely to befriend other tobacco users. Perhaps, both mechanisms may be at work. Another explanation for this observation may be that tobacco users are more likely to influence others to initiate and continue this behaviour.

We did not find that adolescents who believed that tobacco is harmful to health were less or more likely to use tobacco. While we posit that adolescent education about the effects of education is a worthwhile exercise, it may not necessarily result in significant behavioural change. This is not surprising as knowledge alone has been found to be insufficient to effect positive behavioural change (24).

We report in the present study levels of exposure to tobacco advertisement in various forms of media. We consider the study results as baseline findings to assess the potential future impact of the India Tobacco Control Act (which was signed into law the same year of the survey) and the WHO FCTC efforts to prevent tobacco advertisement in India.

Despite the inherent strengths of this study (such as, obtaining a cross state sample and using a standardized questionnaire), the present study has several limitations. First, as data were collected by a cross sectional survey, the effect measures reported (odds ratios) are only indicative of associations between the variables. Hence, one cannot ascribe causation. Second, self-reported data is based on the subject's memory and honesty. To the extent that study participants intentionally misreported or failed to recall any of the variables, our results may be biased. Third, no attempt was done to verify or validate current tobacco use with tobacco metabolites laboratory analysis of specimens such as saliva or urine (25). Finally, the data were collected from adolescents attending school and available on the day their school was visited by the data collection team. If out of school adolescents and students who were absent differed from other students in their tobacco use, our results may not be representative of all adolescents in Himachal Pradesh.

Conclusions

Using data from the 2003 Himachal Global Youth Tobacco Survey, we report a prevalence of all forms of tobacco use at 6.4% among males and 3.9% in females. Adolescent tobacco use was associated with tobacco use among friends. The proportion of males who felt that tobacco use was harmful was significantly higher than that for females. These findings call for consideration of the adolescents' social and domestic environments in the design, implementation and evaluation of gender-specific interventions to prevent tobacco use.

Acknowledgments

The authors declare that they have no financial disclosures or competing interests. We are grateful to the Centers for Disease Control and Prevention (CDC), Atlanta, Georgia, United States, for making the data available for our analysis. The CDC however did not influence the decision to analyse the data or submission of manuscript for publication. We also thank the students who participated in the Himachal Pradesh GYTS conducted in 2004.

References

[1] Mathers CD, Loncar D. Projections of global mortality and burden of disease from 2002 to 2030. PLoS Med 2006;3:e442.

[2] Lopez AD, Mathers CD. Measuring the global burden of disease and epidemiological transitions: 2002-2030. Ann Trop Med Parasitol 2006;100:481-99

[3] Haddock CK, Hoffman K, Taylor JE, Schwab L, Poston WS, Lando HA. An analysis of messages about tobacco in the Military Times magazines. Nicotine Tob Res 2008;10:1191-7.

[4] Suzuki S, Itano D, Yamamoto LG. Prime-time television exposure to high priority school-aged social-developmental issues. Hawaii Med J 2008;67:74-5, 83.

[5] Belstock SA, Connolly GN, Carpenter CM, Tucker L. Using alcohol to sell cigarettes to young adults: a content analysis of cigarette advertisements. J Am Coll Health 2008;56:383-9.

[6] Braun S, Mejia R, Ling PM, Pérez-Stable EJ. Tobacco industry targeting youth in Argentina. Tob Control 2008;17:111-7.

[7] Yach D, Bettcher D. Globalisation of tobacco industry influence and new global responses. Tob Control 2000;9:206-16.

[8] Beaglehole R, Yach D. Globalisation and the prevention and control of non-communicable disease: the neglected chronic diseases of adults. Lancet 2003;362:903-8.

[9] Rudatsikira E, Muula AS, Siziya S, Mataya RH. Correlates of cigarette smoking among school-going adolescents in Thailand: findings from the Thai global youth tobacco survey 2005. Int Arch Med 2008;1:8.

[10] Rudatsikira E, Dondog J, Siziya S, Muula AS. Prevalence and determinants of adolescent cigarette smoking in Mongolia. Singapore Med J 2008;49:57-62.

[11] Unger JB, Palmer PH, Dent CW, Rohrbach LA, Johnson CA. Ethnic differences in adolescent smoking prevalence in California: are multi-ethnic youth at higher risk? Tob Control 2000;9(Suppl 2):II9-14.

[12] Alexander C, Piazza M, Mekos D, Valente T. Peers, schools, and adolescent cigarette smoking. J Adolesc Health 2001;29:22-30

[13] Sinha DN, Gupta PC, Reddy KS, Prasad VM, Rahman K, et al. Linking Global Youth Tobacco Survey 2003 and 2006 data to tobacco control policy in India. J Sch Health. 2008;78:368-73.

[14] The Global Tobacco Surveillance System Collaborating Group. The global tobacco surveillance system (GTSS): purpose, production and potential. J Sch Health 2005;75:15-24.

[15] Warren CW, Jones NR, Peruga A, Chauvin J, Baptiste JP, et al. Centers for Disease Control and Prevention (CDC).Global youth tobacco surveillance, 2000-2007. MMWR Surveill Summ 2008;57:1-28.

[16] Siziya S, Rudatsikira E, Muula AS. Antismoking messages and current cigarette smoking status in Somaliland: results from the Global Youth Tobacco Survey 2004. Confl Health 2008;2:6.

[17] Centers for Disease Control and Prevention (CDC).Tobacco use among students aged 13-15 years--Sri Lanka, 1999-2007. MMWR Morb Mortal Wkly Rep 2008;57:545-9.

[18] Gururaj G, Girish N. Tobacco use amongst children in Karnataka. Indian J Pediatr 2007;74:1095-8.

[19] Centers for Disease Control and Prevention (CDC). Cigarette use among high school students--United States, 1991-2007. MMWR Morb Mortal Wkly Rep 2008;57: 686-8.

[20] Erguder T, Soydal T, Uğurlu M, Cakir B, Warren CW. Tobacco use among youth and related characteristics, Turkey. Soz Praventivmed 2006;51:91-8.

[21] Kaufman JS, Poole C. Looking back on "causal thinking in the health sciences". Annu Rev Public Health 2000;21:101-19.

[22] Rothman KJ, Greenland S. Causation and causal inference in epidemiology. Am J Public Health 2005;95(Suppl 1):S144-50.

[23] Glanz K, Lewis FM, Rimer BK. Health behavior and health education: Theory, research and practice, 3rd ed. San Francisco: Jossey-Bass, 2002.

[24] Lubin JH, Caporaso N, Hatsukami DK, Joseph AM, Hecht SS. The association of a tobacco-specific biomarker and cigarette consumption and its dependence on host characteristics. Cancer Epidemiol Biomarkers Prev 2007;16:1852-7.

Submitted: December 03, 2008.
Revised: January 01, 2009.
Accepted: January 07, 2009.

In: Public Health Yearbook 2009
Editor: Joav Merrick
ISBN: 978-1-61668-911-7

Chapter 7

Design, Implementation and Assessment of an Innovative Anti-Smoking Preventive Program in Greek Preschool Children

*Stylianos M. Piperakis, BSc, PhD, Angeliki Thanou, BSc, PhD, Fotini Garagouni-Areou, BSc, PhD, Konstantinos A Kouziokas, BSc and Maria Zafiropoulou, BSc, PhD**

Department of Preschool Education, University of Thessaly, Volos, Greece

Abstract

Child focused anti-smoking programs are almost non-existent in preschool education, despite the fact that a large number of young children are being brought up in environments, which are not tobacco free. The main purpose of the present study was first to record the perceptions, attitudes and familiarization of 4 to 6 year-olds about smoking and, second, to design, implement and assess the effectiveness of an innovative psycho-educational preventative program, focusing on smoking and its effects on health. Fifty-four preschool children attending state-run kindergarten schools in Central Greece participated in the study. Their perceptions, attitudes and familiarization with smoking were first assessed using an especially designed questionnaire. Approximately half of the children (experimental group) participated in a series of especially designed psycho-educational activities regarding smoking, immediately after the above assessment. All children were once again assessed with the same questionnaire after the psyco-educational activities were completed. The implementation and assessment of the program showed that it was suitably and effectively designed for preschoolers. Our results indicated that preventative programs could change young children's ideas regarding tobacco use and Environmental Tobacco Smoke and could, potentially, contribute to the formation of anti-smoking attitudes.

* Correspondence: Professor Maria Zafiropoulou, PhD Department of Pre-School Education, University of Thessaly, Argonafton and Filellinon Street, Volos 38221, Greece. Tel/Fax: +30 2108075978; E-mail address: mzafirop@ece.uth.gr

Keywords: Anti-smoking education, prevention program, preschool education, health education.

Introduction

Smoking is one of the most serious causes of death worldwide. According to Price et al (1) experimentation with smoking usually begins at an early age. More precisely, those who become regular smokers usually begin to smoke before the age of 18 years (2). Research suggests that adult smoking in Greece is the highest in Europe and the 3rd highest in the world (3,4). Adolescent smoking in Greece is also estimated to occur at a high rate (5).

Apart from tobacco use and its immediate effects on smokers, another issue that must be taken into consideration is the exposure of children to Environmental Tobacco Smoke (ETS). More precisely, ETS could cause respiratory diseases, asthma, sudden infant death syndrome (SIDS), cancer, or DNA damage (6-11). According to the World Health Organization (8) 90% of children in the Balkans are exposed to ETS. In Greece children are exposed to high levels of ETS (12). In their study with preschoolers and their parents, Vardavas et al (13) found that 63% of households had at least one current smoker.

Research supports the notion that children's attitude towards smoking is a reliable predictor of their future smoking behavior (14,15). These attitudes are correlated with a series of factors such as the socioeconomic status of the child's family (16,17), parent's attitudes towards smoking (18-21), smoking habits of the child's social environment (parents and friends) (22-25) and school environment (26,27). It appears that antismoking preventive interventions should be implemented early in the life of children, so that they adopt negative smoking attitudes from an early age.

Preventive Health Education intervention programs have been developed worldwide during the past several decades (28-31). These programs concern actions taken during the early education stages and which engage students, teachers, parents and even the wider society. In their research paper, Ariza et al (32) describe the effects of a Spanish smoking prevention program, conducted in the context of a European project on regular smoking, in a sample of Barcelona adolescents. The intervention included a school based program, reinforcement of a smoke-free school policy, smoking cessation for teachers, brochures for parents and other community-based activities involving youth clubs and tobacco sales. According to their results, after 12 and after 36 months fewer individuals in the experimental group became smokers in relation to those of the control group. In general, research review supports that school based prevention programs usually have short-term positive effects on children's smoking behavior, but there are limited evidence regarding long-term effects of those interventions (31).

On the other hand, there is controversy regarding some anti-smoking interventions. Some feel that educating children in issues that deal with smoking and the use of other dangerous substances often results in encouraging them to experiment with the substances concerned (33). Research evidence regarding the smoking behavior of school age children in Britain showed that they begin to experiment and try the first cigarette approximately at the age of 10-11 years (34). The same phenomenon appears in Greece, according to the studies conducted by the Childs' Health Institute (35). Experts, therefore, support that education on these issues should be delayed until children reach the appropriate age level. It is interesting to note that similar positions are also held about sex education. More precisely, some feel that sex education encourages children to try casual sex. These same people feel that sexuality education should be delayed (36). However, there is always the risk that the appropriate health education messages reach the children too late, when they would have already formulated wrong perceptions and attitudes.

Taking all these into account, a preventive psycho-educational program about tobacco use and ETS in young children was designed and implemented. With the help of a fairy-tale scenario and the use of a number of creative methods and techniques the program aimed at conveying to preschool children the appropriate knowledge and perceptions that would potentially help them formulate a critical attitude towards smoking, smokers and ETS.

Purpose of the study

The objective of the study was to design, implement and assess an innovative health education preventive program on smoking and its effects in health, addressed to preschool children. The design of the program was based: a) on the developmental capabilities of preschool aged children, and b) on the Greek Kindergarten Curriculum (37). The study aimed at helping preschool children:

1. Familiarize themselves with the serious impact of smoking on human health.
2. Learn and engage in basic hygiene and protective habits.
3. Develop the right attitudes and behaviors towards smoking.

The content of the program should provide the children with:

- Knowledge about the origin and history of tobacco and smoking.
- Skills for decoding symbols relative to smoking (e.g. the non-smoking sign).
- Knowledge about the effects of active and passive smoking on human health.
- Anti-smoking perceptions and attitudes.
- Decision making skills.
- Enhanced self-esteem and assertiveness so as to be able to fight for their rights.
- Ability to convey the knowledge and experience acquired during the intervention program to members of their close social environment.

Methods

Fifty-four (N=54) randomly selected preschoolers attending Greek state kindergarten schools participated in the study (N=25 boys and N=29 girls). Children originated from both urban and rural areas of Central Greece (Magnesia prefecture) and were of middle socio-economic background. The children in the study were 4.2 to 5.9 years of age.

After primary assessment, children were divided in two groups: Twenty- eight (N=28) children formed the Experimental Group and 26 children formed a Control Group. Children in the control group matched those of the experimental in age, gender and socioeconomic status.

Instruments

For the purpose of the present research study the following methodological tools were designed:

1. The Smoking Perceptions–Attitudes Test (SPAT): It was designed by two of the writers (MZ and AT). The SPAT is a developmentally appropriate instrument with open-ended and closed questions. It is addressed to pre-school children aged 4-6 years, and is administered during a structured interview. This is divided in ten subjects (see Appendix) and is accompanied by three pictures (a, b and c) and two posters (I and II) relevant to content of the questionnaire. Picture a, which accompanies subject 1, presents a number of adults, of whom some are smokers and some are not. Each child is asked to point to the researcher, which person smokes and which doesn't. Picture b, which accompanies subject 8, depicts a number of people holding their noses. Picture c, which accompanies subject 10, depicts a monkey, which smokes a cigarette, and children are asked to state what they would say to the monkey had they met. Poster I accompanies subject 7 and depicts a race track with two persons about to start racing - one of the runners is a smoker. The child is asked to answer, if those two persons raced, which one would terminate first and why. Poster II accompanies subject 9 and depicts a train and two passengers (a smoker and a non-smoker). Children are asked to say where they would seat the smoker and where the non-smoker in the train. More precisely:

- The first 3 items seek information about children's familiarity with smoking (e.g. "Point to me which person is a smoker and which is a nonsmoker in these pictures") and their experience regarding smoking environment (familial and social) (e.g. "Is there anybody at home who is a smoker?", "Have you ever been to a place where people smoked?").
- The following 4 items investigate children's perceptions about smoking (e.g. "Why do you think those people smoked?"), and about the effects of smoking on man (e.g. the child is shown a poster depicting a race track with 2 persons about to start racing – one of the runners is a smoker) and he/she is asked to answer the following question "If those two persons raced, which one would finish first and why?", or do you mean and after being shown the poster with the a train and two persons (a smoker and a non-smoker) children were asked "Where would you seat the smoker and where the non-smoker in the train,?".).
- The last 3 items aim at exploring children's attitudes towards smokers and smoking environment (e.g. "How do you react when you are annoyed by smoking?" or after been shown a picture of a monkey smoking the child is asked "What would you say to the monkey had you met?").

2. Educational activities: A total of nine psycho-educational antismoking preventive sessions were specially designed and adapted to the program of the Greek state pre-school education system. The experts, involved in the design of the psycho-educational sessions were highly experienced preschool educators, psychologists and one biologist.

The content of the sessions was designed on the basis of:

- The information extracted by SPAT pre-test results.
- The Greek Pre-school Education Curriculum, as referred in the Cross-Thematic Curriculum Framework for Nursery School (Official Gazette, issue B, nr 1366/18–10– 2001).
- The Health Action Model, which, according to Athanasiou (38) aims at reinforcing the individual's self-esteem, as this is believed to be a very important issue in both education and health promotion. The essence of the model is based on the notion that individuals with high self-esteem are more efficient in taking responsibility of their own health (38,39).
- The Creative Learning Model, which promotes the child's critical thinking and creativity (40). According to this model, by using creative teaching methods i.e. brainstorming, concept mapping, role playing games, etc, children's creative learning process is activated, leading to knowledge acquisition (40).

Techniques and methods employed in the program were methods of creativity with allegorical, metaphorical and symbolic content based on active learning e.g. brainstorming, story writing and dramatization, role playing games, theatrical play, peer tutoring, and experiential learning e.g. story narration, art, drama, doll animation, etc. Furthermore, visual aids (pictures and slides projection), conversation and work sheets were also used.

The psycho-educational program titled "Cowslip and Tobacco" was based on a fairy-tale scenario in which "Cowslip", the insect and "Tobacco", the plant, were the central heroes.

The story begins with Cowslip flying gaily in the countryside, when she decides to get some rest on Tobacco's leaf. While resting, Cowslip bites a little bit of the Tobacco leaf and complains about its bitter taste and heavy smell. It is then, when Tobacco decides to tell his story (origin, ways of cultivation, use etc) to Cowslip.

The two heroes, Cowslip and Tobacco, are, then, acting as animators engaging children in various playful activities that aimed at achieving the objectives of the study. In general, the content of sessions concerned:

- Children's acquaintance with the heroes of the story and the origin of tobacco through the fairy-tale scenario.
- Narration of the story of tobacco with the use of technology (e.g. slides regarding the processing of tobacco).
- Getting children in contact with anti-smoking messages through reading and artistic learning activities.
- Creating and communicating anti-smoking messages.
- Manifestation of anti-smoking attitude through a "contract of honor" that the children composed and signed, with the help of Cowslip.
- Children's familiarization with passive smoking and the non-smokers' prerogatives and rights.
- Creation of a book titled "The tobacco that became Jimmy".

Contents, implementation methods and techniques of both SPAT and the psycho-educational antismoking activities were finalized after a pilot study conducted on eight kindergartners. During the pilot study the internal validity of the SPAT was tested (Cronbach's a = 0.87). All the necessary corrections were conducted based on the information collected during the pilot study.

Procedure

Before the implementation of the program, the second author (AT) visited the participating kindergartens for a whole week so that the children got familiar with her and her presence in class during lessons.

The research procedure lasted 11 weeks. The 1st and the 11th week the children were individually assessed with the use of the Smoking Perceptions – Attitudes Test (SPAT) (pre and post test respectively). This took place in a quiet room of the school and each testing was videotaped.

During the first assessment, each child was asked for his/her consent to participate in the program, which was described to it as a game. It should be noticed, here, that preschoolers are extremely willing when they get informed on the kind of collaboration they are asked to take part and are freely and easily engaged when their participation is presented to them as a game (41).

The psycho-educational preventive sessions were conducted by the second author (AT), once a week, on a regular day and time basis, and in a specially designed area inside the school. Sessions lasted 30-45 minutes and took place in the presence of the class teacher.

Statistical analysis

Thematic analysis was performed on children's answers to SPAT, which was undertaken by two researchers. Namely, all interviews were transcribed verbatim creating a numbered interview protocol for each participant. The analysis and coding of responses began with reading the transcriptions several times. Meanings seemed to cluster together and formed some patterns permitting the grouping of information. This grouping, based on the techniques of 'the categorization of meanings' proposed by Kvale led to subsequent study of the categories to obtain the context of what had been said and its meaning (42). At this stage, five transcripts were also coded by a second outside coder to enhance credibility of coding. Agreement of 93% was obtained for the two researchers' coding, based on manual calculations of percentage of agreement for the presence of the coded theme (43).

Descriptive statistics on the categorized children's answers were performed using SPSS 15.0. Furthermore, x2 test was performed and a level of at least 0.05 was used to determine significance.

Results

Pre- and post-test frequencies and percentages of Smoking Perceptions–Attitudes Test (SPAT) for both experimental and control groups are presented below. The contents of the interviews are organized into the above three categories.

Familiarity and experience regarding smoking

Our results revealed that all children are aware of the smoking habit (100%). Of the 54 children, 49 (90.5%) experience ETS exposure in their close environment (family), while 77.8% stated that they have been exposed to ETS while being in a place where other people smoked. All children exposed to ETS stated that they are annoyed by this experience.

Children's perceptions about smoking

Table 1 presents children's answers (before and after intervention) to the question "why they thought some people smoked". Content analysis revealed five categories:

- "Pleasure" (e.g. "they smoke because they like it" or "to get a rest")
- "Addiction" (e.g. "because they can't stand without smoking" or "so they are not agitated")
- "Age" (e.g. "because they are old" or "because he is a daddy")
- "Image" (e.g. "to be good looking")
- "Ignorance" (e.g. "don't know").

As it can be observed (see table 1), after intervention, children's answers in the experimental group were differentiated. That is, no child in the experimental group stated ignorance and, most importantly, more than half of the children recognized "addiction" as a reason for smoking ($p<0.05$). On the contrary, no differences were found in the control group answers, before and after intervention.

Table 1. Preschoolers answers in the question *"Why do you think some people smoke?"*

"Why do you think some people smoke?"	Experimental Group (N = 28)		Control Group (N = 26)	
	Pre-test N (%)	Post-test N (%)	Pre-test N (%)	Post-test N (%)
Pleasure	12 (42.9%)	12 (42.9%)	9 (34.6%)	10 (38.5%)
Addiction	0 (0%)	15 (53.6%)	1 (3.8%)	1 (3.8%)
Age	6 (21.4%)	1 (3.6%)	4 (15.4%)	5 (19.2%)
Image	0 (0%)	0 (0%)	1 (3.8%)	1 (3.8%)
Ignorance	10 (35.7%)	0 (0%)	9 (34.6%)	8 (30.8%)
Total	28 (100%)	28 (100%)	26 (100%)	26 (100%)

Table 2a. Preschoolers' answers in the question "If those two persons (the smoker or the non –smoker) raced, which one would terminate first?"

"If those two persons (the smoker or the non –smoker) raced, which one would terminate first?''	Experimental Group (N = 28)		Control Group (N = 26)	
	Pre-test N (%)	Post-test N (%)	Pre-test N (%)	Post-test N (%)
The non-smoker	20 (71.4%)	27 (96.4%)	20 (76.9%)	20 (76.9%)
The smoker	6 (21.4%)	1 (3.6%)	6 (23.1%)	6 (23.1%)
No one	2 (7.1%)	0 (0%)	0 (0%)	0 (0%)
Total	28 (100%)	28 (100%)	26 (100%)	26 (100%)

Table 2b. Preschoolers' justification of their answer to the question "If those two persons (the smoker or the non –smoker) raced, which one would terminate first and why?"

"Why the smoker (or the non –smoker) would terminate first?"	Experimental Group (N = 28)		Control Group (N = 26)	
	Pre-test N (%)	Post-test N (%)	Pre-test N (%)	Post-test N (%)
Strength – Health	4 (14.3%)	23 (82.1%)	8 (30.8%)	9 (34.6%)
Functionality	9 (32.1%)	2 (7.1%)	11 (42.3%)	11 (42.3%)
Ignorance	13 (46.4%)	3 (10.7%)	7 (26.9%)	6 (23.1%)
No answer	2 (7.1%)	0 (0%)	0 (0%)	0 (0%)
Total	28 (100%)	28 (100%)	26 (100%)	26 (100%)

At pre-test and after children were shown the racing track poster with the two runners and asked to indicate "which one would terminate first", the majority of them in both experimental and control groups opted for "the non-smoker" (see table 2a). At the post-test, the percentage of children in the experimental group raised up to 96.4% for the "non-smoker" while no differences were found in the control group.

Children were then asked to justify the answer given in the previous question. The ways in which they rationalized their answers were very interesting. Content analysis revealed three justification categories (see table 2b):

- "Strength – Health" (e.g. "because he is stronger" or "because he is not coughing", when suggesting that the non-smoker would win)
- "Functionality" (e.g. "the smoker will be delayed because he holds the cigarette package and the other person will overtake him" or "the smoker will stop to shake the cigarette's ash and the other person will run ahead")
- "Ignorance" (e.g. "don't know")
- "No answer".

As presented in table 2b, after the intervention the majority of preschoolers in the experimental group were able to associate the racer's performance with his/her smoking habit ($p<0.05$). Such changes were not found in the control group.

Children's attitudes and behaviors towards smoking

To explore their attitudes and behaviors towards smoking, children were asked to state, "what they did when they were in a place where people smoke". The answers given were divided in four categories, as presented below (see table 3):

- "Passivity" (e.g. "I do nothing" or "what can I do, they don' t listen to me")
- "Activation" (e.g. "I shout to make them stop" or "I leave and go to the other room and close the door behind me")
- "Exhibition of physical reactions" (e.g. "I cough" or "my eyes tingle")
- "Ignorance" (e.g. "don't know").

Table 3 shows that after the intervention, most children in the experimental group appeared more active regarding ETS exposure, showing that they were willing to take action to protect themselves from ETS exposure ($p<0.05$). No differences were observed in the control group.

In the question with the picture of a little monkey smoking a cigarette where children were asked to state "What they would say to the monkey, had they met", children's answers were divided into four categories according to their content (see table 4):

- "Annoyance" (e.g. "get out of here, you smell bad" or "you smell of smoke!")
- "Advise" (e.g. " animals don't smoke" or "if you smoke, you will get sick" or "take the cigarette out of your mouth")
- "Ignorance" (e.g. "don't know")
- "No answer".

According to post-test results, the great majority of the children in the experimental group would act as advisors, so as to help the monkey to quit smoking while at pre-test assessment less than half were interested in acting as advisors ($p<0.05$). Regarding children in the control group, although more than half of them reported that they would act as advisors, no important changes were found in their post-test results, as presented in the table 4 below.

In the question about where they would seat a smoker and where a non-smoker in the train, all children (100%) placed the smoker away from the non-smoker. When asked to justify why they placed the smoker away from the non-smoker, they gave various explanations, which were divided in four categories (see table 5):

- "Protection" (e.g. "so that the other person will not get sick" or "so that he/she will not rub his/her eyes")
- "Annoyance" (e.g. "he/she will bother" or "he/she will smell bad" or "he/she will smell of smoke")
- "Hazardousness" (e.g. "if he/she sits close to the engine, the train will blaze up")
- "Ignorance" (e.g. "don't know").

After implementation of the program, the percentage of preschoolers in the experimental group that appeared to care about the non-smokers' health rose more than 50%, showing that they became more sensitive to matters relating to ETS exposure ($p<0.05$). On the contrary no noticeable differences were observed in the control group (see table 5).

Table 3. Preschoolers' answers in the question *"What do you do when you are in a place where people smoke?"*

"What do you do when you are in a place where people smoke?"	Experimental Group (N = 28)		Control Group (N = 26)	
	Pre-test N (%)	Post-test N (%)	Pre-test N (%)	Post-test N (%)
Passivity	10 (35.7%)	1 (3.6%)	5 (19.2%)	5 (19.2%)
Activation	14 (50.0%)	22 (78.6%)	17 (65.4%)	17 (65.4%)
Exhibition of physical reactions	4 (14.3%)	5 (17.9%)	3 (11.6%)	4 (15.4%)
Ignorance	0 (0%)	0 (0%)	1 (3.8%)	0 (0%)
Total	28 (100%)	28 (100%)	26 (100%)	26 (100%)

Table 4. Preschoolers' answers in the question *"What would you say to the monkey had you met?"*

"What would you say to the monkey, had you met?"	Experimental Group (N = 28)		Control Group (N = 26)	
	Pre-test N (%)	Post-test N (%)	Pre-test N (%)	Post-test N (%)
Annoyance	9 (32.1%)	3 (10.7%)	6 (23.1%)	6 (23.1%)
Advise	13 (46.4%)	25 (89.3%)	17 (65.4%)	18 (69.2%)
Ignorance	4 (14.3%)	0 (0%)	2 (7.7%)	1 (3.8%)
No answer	2 (7.1%)	0 (0%)	1 (3.8%)	1 (3.8%)
Total	28 (100%)	28 (100%)	26 (100%)	26 (100%)

Table 5. Preschoolers' answers in the question *"Where would you seat the smoker and where the non-smoker in the train?"*

"Where would you seat the smoker and where the non-smoker in the train?"	Experimental Group (N = 28)		Control Group (N = 26)	
	Pre-test N (%)	Post-test N (%)	Pre-test N (%)	Post-test N (%)
Protection	2 (7.1%)	17 (60.7%)	5 (19.2%)	6 (23.1%)
Annoyance	14 (50.0%)	10 (35.7%)	11 (42.3%)	12 (46.2%)
Hazardousness	3 (10.7%)	1 (3.6%)	4 (15.4%)	5 (19.2%)
Ignorance	9 (32.1%)	0 (0%)	6 (23.1%)	5 (19.2%)
Total	28 (100%)	28 (100%)	26 (100%)	26 (100%)

Discussion

There is an ancient Greek saying which states "prevention is better than cure". Nowadays, the demand for prevention and health promotion actions appears to be vital due to the variety of diseases that people are faced with in their lifespan.

The objective of the present study was the design, implementation and evaluation of an anti-smoking preventative psycho-educational program addressed to preschool children.

Although, there are programs implemented in primary and secondary schools (3,31, 32,44-47), the implementation of anti-smoking prevention programs in preschool children is extremely limited. In the mid-80's, Parcel, Bruhn and Murray (48) found that preschool children who were taught the Preschool Health Education Curriculum expressed significantly less intention to smoke in the future. In another study, Philips, Longoria, Parcel and Ebeling (49) found that, after the implementation of their program in preschoolers, twice the number of children expressed their intention to take action in order to protect themselves from passive smoking.

According to our findings, and in agreement with other studies (50) preschoolers were familiar with the habit of smoking. Moreover, the majority of the children who participated in our study (90.5%) were exposed to ETS. In another study conducted in Greece, it was found that 73% of children aged up to 14 years old were exposed to ETS (51). All children exposed to ETS in this study stated that this was a nuisance to them. Similarly, Woods, Sprigett, Porcellato and Dudill (52) found that 90% of the children 4-7 years old were annoyed when they were in a smoky area. Porcellato, Dugdill and Springett (53) have also revealed that young children (4 to 7 year-olds) express a negative disposition towards smoking.

Post-test assessments revealed considerable changes in the children's perceptions, attitudes and behaviors towards smoking. More precisely, after the implementation of the program, most preschoolers in the experimental group were able to recognize that smoking is a form of addiction that causes serious health problems. Likewise, Porcellato et al (53) found that children of this age can refer to the negative effects of smoking. After the implementation of our program, children in the experimental group appeared to be more sensitive regarding ETS and more willing to take action to face the problem. This is in concordance with Philips et al (49), who found that after their prevention program the children were more likely to protect themselves from ETS.

As regards children's behavior towards smokers, after the end of the program, preschoolers in the experimental group declared that they would prefer acting as advisors towards a smoker.

This strengthens the finding that children in the experimental group were able to perceive smoking as an addictive behavior, thus, non-smokers should counsel smokers on the hazards of this habit, rather than be just being negative and hostile.

Research has revealed that even very young children have their views about smoking, and, therefore, such intervention programs should be suitable in the preschool education level (50,52,54). Woods et al (52) found that as elementary school children grow older, they express more positive ideas towards smoking than younger ones, and, thus, children under 6-7 years old would be more receptive to information about the negative aspects of smoking. According to Greenlund et al (55) health behaviors are established at an early developmental stage and are difficult to change, once they are adopted. Therefore anti-smoking programs should be implemented as early as possible. The results obtained in this study suggest that health educators and early education experts should begin implementing smoking prevention programs at nursery school level, in an attempt to help children develop the necessary skills and adopt negative attitudes towards smoking. This has been suggested by other experts as well (56,57).

To summarize our results, it seems that children, as young as preschool-aged, are capable of receiving anti-smoking preventive interventions, in order to be 'inoculated' with negative attitudes towards smoking. However, these programs should be designed specially for preschool children, since they are a very sensitive age group with certain developmental capabilities and educational needs.

Finally, the limitation of the study described is the small number of participating children in both experimental and control groups. This fact is evidently affecting the generalizability of the study. In an attempt to come up with more reliable results regarding the effectiveness of the program, a further project has already been designed which will involve the implementation of the program in larger numbers of pre-school children, together with a four-year follow-up study.

Conclusions

The evaluation of our preventive psycho-educational program revealed that it is an effective antismoking program to be used with kindergartners. It is essential, however, that others carry out similar research to support our findings. In addition, longitudinal randomized control trials are also necessary to determine the best methods of promoting antismoking attitudes and behaviors in young children.

Acknowledgments

The authors wish to thank the preschool educators Heleni Poulakopoulou, Stella Petraki, Irini Antoniou and Eftixia Moutselou, who cooperated with the research team during the intervention program. This research project was partially funded by the Research Committee of the University of Thessaly, Greece.

Appendix: The Smoking Perceptions – Attitudes Test (S.P.A.T.)

Name

....
....

Place of testing

....
....

Address

....
....

	Day	Month	Year
Date of testing			
Date of birth			

1st Subject	Distinguishing smokers from non-smokers[1]		R / W /NA[2]
Perceptions	Q[3]	Point out to me which person is a smoker and which is a non-smoker in these pictures	
	A[4]		

2nd Subject	Familial environment		NA
Perceptions	Q	Is there anybody at home who is a smoker? (If Yes, we ask Who?)	
	A		

If the child's answer to the above is No, then we move on to the third subject otherwise we move on to the 4th subject.

3rd Subject	Broader Social Environment		NA
Perceptions	Q	Have you ever been to a place where people smoked?	
	A		

4th Subject	Personal Judgment		NA
Perceptions	Q	"Why do you think some people smoke?	
	A		

5th Subject	Myself and Smoking		NA
Attitudes	Q	Is there anything, which annoys you when people smoke? If Yes, What is it that annoys you?	
	A		

---

1 Picture a accompanies the question.
2 R=Right, W=Wrong, NA=No Answer
3 Q=Question
4 A=Answer

If the child's answer to the above is No, then we move on to the 7th subject

6th Subject	Myself and Smokers		NA
Intentions / Attitudes	Q	What do you do when you are in a place where people smoke?	
	A		

7th Subject	Endurance[5]		NA
Perceptions	Q	If those two persons raced, (the smoker or the non –smoker) which one would terminate first and why?	
	A		

8th Subject	Aesthetics[6]		NA
Perceptions	Q	Why do you think these people are holding their noses?	
	A		

9th Subject	My own assessment[7]		NA
Perceptions/ Attitudes	Q	Where would you seat the smoker and where the non-smoker in the train?	
	A		
10th Subject	I express my own position[8]		NA
Intentions / Attitudes	Q	What would you say to the monkey had you met?	
	A		

Remarks

....

....

[5] We show to the child poster 1 which accompanies the test.
[6] Picture b accompanies the question.
[7] We show children Poster II.
[8] Picture c accompanies the question.

References

[1] Price J, Beach P, Everett S, Telljohann SK, Lewis L. Evaluation of a three-year urban elementary school tobacco prevention program. J Sch Health 1998;68(1):26-31.

[2] Tingle LR, DeSimone M, Covington B. A meta-evaluation of 11 school-based smoking prevention programs. J Sch Health 2003;73(2):64-70.

[3] Koumi I, Tsiantis J. Smoking trends in adolescence: report on a Greek school-based, peer-led intervention aimed at prevention. Health Promot Int 2001;16(1):65-72.

[4] Huisman M, Kunst AE, Mackenbach JP. Educational inequalities in smoking among men and women aged 16 years and older in 11 European countries. Tobac Contr 2005;14(2):106-13.

[5] Kyrlesi A, Soteriades ES, Warren CW, Kremastinou J, Papastergiou P, Jones NR, Hadjichristodoulou C. Tobacco use among students aged 13–15 years in Greece: the GYTS project. BMC Publ Health 2007;7(1):3.

[6] Nuhoglu C, Gurul M, Nuhoglu Y, Karatoprak N, Sonmez EO, S. Yavrucu S, Özgüner A. Effects of passive smoking on lung function in children. Pediatr Int 2003;45:426-8.

[7] Zalata A, Yahia S, El-Bakary A, Elsheikha HM. Increased DNA damage in children caused by passive smoking as assessed by comet assay and oxidate stress. Mutat Res 2007;629:140-7.

[8] World Health Organization Regional. Exposure of children to environmental smoking. Fact sheet 3.4. Copenhagen: WHO; 2007. Accessed 2008 Jul 10. URL: http://www.euro.who.int

[9] Chatzimicael A, Tsalkidis A, Cassimos D, Gardikis S, Spathopoulos D, Tripsianis GA, Kambouri K, Aivazis V, Vaos G, Bouros D. Effect of passive smoking on lung function and respiratory infection. Indian J Pediatr 2008;75(4):335-40.

[10] Dostál M, Milcová A, Binková B, Kotesovec F, Nozicka J, Topinka J, Srám RJ. Environmental tobacco smoke exposure in children in tow districts of the Czech Republic. Int J Hyg Environ Health 2008;211:318-25.

[11] Hendreson AJ. The effects of tobacco smoke exposure on respiratory health in school-aged children. Paediatr Respir Rev 2008;9:21-8.

[12] Vardavas CI, Tzatzarakis MN, Tsatsakis AM, Athanasopoulos D, Balomenaki E, Linardakis MK, Kafatos AG. Biomarkers of passive smoking among Greek preschool children. Eur J Pediatr 2006;165:891-6.

[13] Vardavas CI, Athanasopoulos D, Balomenaki E, Niaounaki D, Linardakis MK, Kafatos AG. Smoking habits of Greek preschool children's parents. BMC Publ Health 2007;7:112.

[14] Higgins A, Conner M. Understanding adolescent smoking: The role of the theory of planned behaviour and implementation intentions. Psych Health Med 2003;8(2):173-86.

[15] Trafimow D, Brown J, Grace K, Thompson LA, Sheeran P. The relative influence of attitudes and subjective norms from childhood to adolescence: Between-participant and within-participant analyses. Am J Psychol 2002;115(3):395-414.

[16] Tyas S, Pederson L. Psychosocial factors related to adolescent smoking: a critical review of the literature. Tobac Contr 1998;7(4):409-20.

[17] Droomers M, Schrijvers C, Casswell S, Mackenbach JP. Father's occupational group and daily smoking during adolescence: Patterns and predictors. Am J Public Health 2005;95(4):681-8.

[18] Newman IM, Ward JM. The influence of parental attitude and behavior on early adolescent cigarette smoking. J Sch Health 1998;59(4):150-2.

[19] Dusenbury L, Kerner J, Baker E. Predictors of smoking prevalence among New York Latino youth. Am J Public Health1992;82(1):55-8.

[20] Adamczyk-Robinette A, Fletcher A, Wright K. Understanding the authoritative parenting-early adolescent tobacco use link: the mediating role of peer tobacco use. J Youth Adolesc 2002; 31(4):311-8.

[21] Hill KG, Hawkins JD, Catalano RF, Abbott RD, Guo J. Family influences on the risk of daily smoking initiation. J Adolesc Health 2005;37:202–10.

[22] Wang MQ, Fitzhugh E, Westerfield RC, Eddy JM. Family and peer influences on smoking behavior among American adolescents: an age trend. J Adolesc Health 1995;16:200-3.

[23] Kurtz M, Kurtz JC, Johnson S, Beverly EE. Exposure to environmental tobacco smoke – Perceptions of African American children and adolescents. Prev Med 1996;25:286-92.

[24] Jackson C, Henriksen L, Dickinson D, Levine DW. The early use of alcohol and tobacco: its relation to children's competence and parents' behavior. Am J Public Health1997;87(3):359-64.

[25] Pinilla J, Gonzalez B, Barber P, Santana Y. Smoking in young adolescents: and approach with multilevel discrete choice models. J Epidemiol Community Health 2002;56:227-32.

[26] Kumar R, O'Malley PM, Johnston LD. School tobacco control policies related to students' smoking and attitudes toward smoking: National Survey Results, 1999-2000. Health Educ Behav 2005;32(6):780-94.

[27] Leatherdale ST, Manske S. The relationship between student smoking in the school environment and smoking onset in the elementary school setting. Cancer Epidemiol Biomarkers Prev 2005;14(7):1762-5.

[28] Kalantzi-Azizi A. Applied Clinical Psychology in the school, 5th Edition. Athens: Ellinika Grammata,1999. [Greek]

[29] Kalantzi-Azizi A, Zafiropoulou M. School adjustment: Prevention and intervention in difficulties. Athens: Ellinika Grammata, 2005. [Greek]

[30] Zafiropoulou M, Thanou A. Laying the foundations of well being: A creative Psycho – Educational Program for young children. Psychol Rep 2007;100:136-46.

[31] Thomas RE, Perera R. School-based programmes for preventing smoking. Cochrane Database Syst Rev 2008;4.

[32] Ariza C, Nebot M, Tomas Z, Gimenez E, Valmayor S, Tarilonte V, De Vries H.. Longitudinal effects of the European smoking prevention framework approach (ESFA) project in Spanish adolescents. Eur J Public Health 2008;18(5):491-7.

[33] Downie RS, Fyfe C. Health education in schools. In: Doxiadis S (ed.) Ethics in health education. Chichester: John Wiley, 1990.

[34] Goddard E, Ikin C. Smoking among secondary schoolchildren in 1986. London: OPCS, HMSO, 1987.

[35] Davou M, Perdiki M, Megalooikonomou, T. Habits, knowledge and attitudes of adolescents towards smoking. Psycho-social factors. Iatriki 1991;59(5):472-81 [Greek]

[36] Grunseit A, Kippax S, Aggleton P, Baldo M, et al. Sexuality education and young people's sexual behavior: a review of studies. J Adolesc Res 1997;12(4):421-53.

[37] Greek Pedagogical Institute. Cross-Thematic Curriculum Framework for Nursery School: Greece, 2003. Accessed 2008 Jun 02. URL: http://www.pi-schools.gr

[38] Athanasiou K. Health Education. Athens: Grigoris Publications, 2007.[Greek]

[39] Tones, K, Tilford, S. Health promotion: Effectiveness, efficiency and equity. London: Nelson Thornes, 2001.

[40] Xanthakou Y, Kaila M. The creative problem solving. Athens: Atrapos, 2002. [Greek]

[41] Mellon R. Psycho-diagnostic methods. Athens: Ellinika Grammata, 1998. [Greek]

[42] Kvale S. Interviews: An introduction to qualitative research interview. London: Sage, 1996.

[43] Voyatzis RE. Transforming qualitative information: Thematic analysis and code development. Newbury Park, CA: Sage, 1998.

[44] Skara S, Sussman S. A review of 25 long-term adolescent tobacco and other drug use prevention program evaluations. Prev Med 2003;37:451–74.

[45] La Torre G, Chiaradia G, Ricciardi G. School-based smoking prevention in children and adolescents: review of the scientific literature. J Publ Health 2005;13:285-90.

[46] Côté F, Godin G, Gagné, C. Efficiency of an evidence-based intervention to promote and reinforce tobacco abstinence among elementary schoolchildren in a school transition period. Health Educ Behav 2006;33(6):747-59.

[47] Baan B. Prevention of smoking in young children in Holland: Education and changing attitudes. Lung 1990; 168(1):320-6.

[48] Parcel GS, Bruhn JG, Murray JL. Effects of a Health Education curriculum on the smoking intentions of pre-school children. Health Educ Behav 1984;11(1):49-56.

[49] Philips BU, Longoria JM, Parcel GS, Ebeling EW. Expectations of preschool children to protect themselves from cigarette smoke: results of a smoking prevention program for preschool children. J Canc Educ 1990;5(1):27-32.

[50] Dalton MA, Bernhardt AM, Gibson JJ, Sargent JD, Beacj ML, Adachi-Mejia AM, Titus-Ernstoff LT, Heatherton T. Use of cigarettes and alcohol by preschoolers while role-playing as adults. "Honey, have some smokes". Arch Pediatr Adolesc Med 2005;159: 854-9.

[51] Bakoula CG, Kafritsa YJ, Kavadias GD, Haley NJ, Matsaniotis NS. Factors modifying exposure to environmental tobacco smoke in children (Athens, Greece). Canc Causes Contr 1997;8:76.

[52] Woods SE, Sprigett J, Porcellato L, Dugdill L. "Stop it, it's bad for me": Experiences of and views on passive smoking among primary-school children in Liverpool. Health Educ Res 2005;20(6), 645-55.

[53] Porcellato L, Dugdill L, Springett J. A longitudinal study exploring Liverpool primary schoolchildren's perspectives on smoking. Childhood 2005;12(4):425-43.

[54] Porcellato L, Dugdill L, Springett J, Sanderson FH. Primary schoolchildren's perceptions of smoking: implications for health education. Health Educ Res 1999;14(1):71-83.

[55] Greenlund KJ, Johnson CC, Webber LS, Berenson GS. Cigarette smoking attitudes and first use among third- through sixth-grade students: The Bogalusa Heart study. Am J Public Health 1997;87(8):1345-8.

[56] Melissa-Halikiopoulou C, Natsiopoulou T. Health education in Greek preschool settings. The importance of reading children's books on health promotion. ICUS Nurs Web J 2005;24. Accessed 2008 Nov 02. URL: http://www.nursing.gr

[57] Damianaki A, Kaklamani S., Tsirakis S., Clarke R, Tzanakis N, Makris D. Risk factors for smoking among school adolescents in Greece. Child Care Health Dev 2008; 34(3):310-5.

Submitted: November 28, 2008.
Revised: December 30, 2008.
Accepted: January 07, 2009.

In: Public Health Yearbook 2009
Editor: Joav Merrick
ISBN: 978-1-61668-911-7

Chapter 8

NATIONAL SURVEY 2002 ON MEDICAL SERVICES FOR PERSONS WITH INTELLECTUAL DISABILITY IN RESIDENTIAL CARE IN ISRAEL

Joav Merrick, MD, MMedSc, DMSc*[*1,2], Isack Kandel, MA, PhD[1,3], Efrat Kenig-Merrick, MD[1] and Mohammed Morad, MD[1,4]

[1]National Institute of Child Health and Human Development, Office of the Medical Director, Division for Mental Retardation, Ministry of Social Affairs, Jerusalem
[2]Kentucky Children's Hospital, University of Kentucky, Lexington, United States of America
[3]Faculty of Social Sciences, Department of Behavioral Sciences, Ariel University Center of Samaria, Ariel, Israel
[4]Department of Family Medicine, Faculty of Health Sciences, Ben Gurion University of the Negev, Beer-Sheva, Israel

Abstract

In Israel, the Office of the Medical Director of the Ministry of Social Affairs is responsible for the medical service in residential-care centers for persons with intellectual disability (ID). During 1997-1998 a standard annual questionnaire was developed and the first national survey study conducted in 1998. This present paper presents the findings of the fifth national survey in 2002, for which the following information was gathered via questionnaires: information on the age, gender, and level of intellectual disability of persons served at the residential care center in question, status of the population served, profile, nursing, medical, and allied professional staff, number of annual examinations, preventive medicine aspects, medications, number of annual cases of infectious disease, annual unintentional injury, number of deaths, number of hospitalizations, internal residential center hospitalization, ambulatory out-patient use, use of outside laboratory examinations and dental care. In

* Correspondence: Professor Joav Merrick, MD, MMedSci, DMSc, Medical Director, Division for Mental Retardation, Ministry of Social Affairs, BOX 1260, IL-91012 Jerusalem, Israel. E-mail: jmerrick@zahav.net.il

2002, 6,352 persons were served in nine government, 36 private and 12 public centers. The average number of persons per center was 111.44 (range 16 to 398). Of the patient population, 78.4% were between 20 and 60 years old, 50.4% had severe or profound intellectual disability, and 41.9% moderate disability. 25% were nursing patients, 18.7% were confined to a wheelchair, 28.9% suffered from epilepsy. Of the total population, 80.3% were receiving medication daily for chronic illness and 50.8% received psychotropic medication.

Keywords: Intellectual disability, developmental disability, mental retardation, residential care, long term care, nursing, Israel.

Introduction

In 1997 it was decided to develop an instrument to monitor the health service for people with intellectual disability living in residential care centers in Israel and conduct annual surveys (1-4). We want to continue to improve our service to this population and the data provided each year will guide us in our work. This paper describes the findings from the fifth annual survey in 2002.

Methods

The questionnaire developed for the residential care centers have the following sections: age, gender and level of ID of persons served at the care center in question; the status of the population served (educational, treatment, rehabilitation; nursing, challenging behavior); profile (various aspects of the nursing load like number of persons with gastric tubes, catheters, gastrostomy, dialysis, oncology, epilepsy, diabetes, hypertension, blindness etc); nursing, medical and allied professional staff; number of annual examinations; preventive medicine aspects; medications; number of annual cases of infectious disease; annual unintentional injury; number of deaths; number of hospitalizations; internal residential center hospitalization; ambulatory out-patient utilization, utilization of outside laboratory examinations, and dental care (1). The questionnaire was sent to each residential care center in Israel with a medical clinic to survey the activity of the clinic for the 12-month period of 2002.

Results

Questionnaires were received from all 55 residential care centers (100% response rate). In the year 2002 there were nine government, 36 private and 12 public (not-for-profit) centers serving a total of 6,352 persons (see table 1). The average number of persons per center was 111.44 (range 16 to 398). The level of ID or mental retardation (MR) in the population of persons with ID in residential care centers is shown in table 2. Mild ID: IQ 55-70; moderate: IQ 35-54; severe IQ 20-34; and profound: IQ < 20. Other refers to 21 persons who were placed for other reasons.

Table 1. The population of persons with intellectual disability in 55 residential care centers in Israel, 2002

Age (yrs)	Males	Females	Total	Percent
0-9	100	69	1697	2.66
10-19	475	372	847	13.33
20-39	1,589	1,078	2,667	41.99
40-49	721	691	1,412	22.23
50-59	463	436	899	14.15
> 60	1667	192	358	5.64
TOTAL	3,514	2,838	6,352	100.00

Table 2. The level of intellectual disability in persons in 55 residential care centers in Israel, 2002

Age (yrs)	Mild	Moderate	Severe	Profound	Other Total		Percent
0-9	3	11	98	57	0	169	2.66
10-19	42	302	354	146	3	847	13.33
20-39	169	1,009	1,017	466	6	2,667	41.99
40-49	132	680	456	136	3	1,407	22.23
50-59	95	458	256	85	4	898	14.15
> 60	28	200	92	39	5	364	5.64
TOTAL	469	2,660	2,273	929	21	6,352	100.00
Percent	7.38	41.88	35.78	14.63	0.33	100.00	

In table 3 is shown the profile of the population. There were 1,392 nursing patients and 207 intensive nursing care patients. Educational category is the term for persons with a level of self care, social skills, and ability to work.

Table 3. Profile of the population in residential care 2002 according to educational, treatment, rehabilitation, nursing and challenging behavior

Profile	Numbers	Percent
Educational	675	10.63
Treatment	1,456	22.92
Rehabilitation	372	5.86
Nursing	1,392	21.91
Intensive nursing	207	3.26
Challenging behavior	2,250	35.42
TOTAL	6,352	100.00

Treatment category is a person with normal-to-moderate self-care functions and social skills, able to accomplish simple tasks and skills in a limited number of activities. Rehabilitation category is for a person with poor adaptive skills, in need of support, instruction, and assistance. Challenging behavior means persons that are hyperactive and in need of constant supervision. The total population in residential care centers is very much in need of nursing care, and the medical profile or medical/nursing problems can be seen in table 4.

Table 4. Nursing profile of the population in residential care, 2002 (N=6,352)

Profile	Numbers	Percent
Gastric tube feeding	19	0.30
Urinary catheter	18	0.28
Gastrostomy	135	2.13
Pressure sore (decubitus)	59	0.93
Dialysis	9	0.14
Oncology treatment	41	0.65
Down syndrome	581	9.15
Fragile X	68	1.07
Epilepsy	1,836	28.90
Diabetes mellitus	253	3.98
Hypertension	329	5.18
Asthma	131	2.06
Phenylketonuria (PKU)	19	0.30
Self injurious behavior (SIB)	216	3.40
Blindness	292	4.60
Wheelchair users	1,187	18.69

In residential care centers there is a need for a multidisciplinary staff, which will provide medical, nursing, and allied health professional service to this population, and the number of full-time equivalent positions is shown in table 5.

Table 5. Medical and allied professional staff in 55 residential care centers, 2002

Profession	Number of equivalent full-time positions
Physicians	36.50
Chief nurse	25.75
Other nurses	243.56
Psychiatrist	14.05
Other medical specialist	4.53
Pharmacist	3.24
Physiotherapist	43.16
Communication and speech therapist	14.67
Nutritionist	9.32
Medical secretary	4.25
Occupational therapist	20.83

In each residential care center, a regular clinic is held daily, providing not only treatment to patients with complaints or problems during the previous night in need of examination, but also routine health surveillance. Table 6 shows the number of examinations for the year 2002. Blood is also drawn in the residential care center, but sent out to laboratories run by the local area health maintenance organizations (HMOs).

Table 6. Number of examinations at the 55 residential care centers in 2002

Examination/ treatment by	Total 2002	Exams/person with ID/y
Physician	104,532	16.46
Psychiatrist	20,216	3.18
Other physician	5,515	0.87
Physiotherapist	94,260	14.84
Blood test, urine, stool, other	23,412	3.69

Preventive medicine is an important aspect of the practical work in residential care centers with some shown in table 7.

Table 7. Preventive medical aspects in 55 residential care centers, 2002 (N=6,352,2,838 females)

Measure	Number	Percent of population
Influenza vaccination	5,423	85.37
Hepatitis B vaccination	305	4.80
Hepatitis A vaccination	24	0.38
Breast examination (females)	823	29.00
Gynecological examination (females)	1,013	34.37

In this population, 80% were in need of daily medication (see table 8), 31% received anti-epileptic drugs, and 51% psychotropic medication. Daily medication is usually given three times per day, but for acute situations (usually challenging behavior) extra medication is given (SOS).

Infectious disease is often seen in this population. Some statistics can be seen in table 9 for 2002.

The medical clinics in the residential care centers are usually staffed with nurses (most are still practical nurses) 24 hours every day. The physician makes visits during the day, but is not on call and therefore, the medical clinic at the residential care center may send the resident to the emergency room or for hospitalization, whereas several residential care centers have a small number of beds for observation (called internal institutional hospitalization in table 10). Emergency and hospital utilization in 2002 is shown in table 10.

Table 8. Medication for persons with intellectual disability in residential care, 2002 (N=6,352)

Type of medication	Number	Percent
Chronic medication	5,098	80.26
AED (for epilepsy)	1,967	30.97
Psychotropic	3,225	50.77
Oral contraception	88	3.10 (female population)
Depo-Provera	320	11.28 (female population)
SOS	6,814	

Table 9. Infectious diseases in 2002

Disease	Number of cases
Septicemia	3
Salmonellosis	2
Shigellosis	3
Scabies	785
Lice	112
Other	56

Table 10. Emergency room visits and hospitalizations in 55 residential care centers in 2002 (6,352 persons)

Activity	Number	Days	Rate per 1,000
Emergency room	1,569	0	247.01
Internal medicine	535	3,206	84.23
Pediatrics	140	955	22.04
Surgery	163	887	25.66
Other	152	822	23.93
Total somatic hospitalization	990	5,870	155.86
Psychiatric hospitalization	31	452	4.88
Total hospitalization	1,021	6,322	160.74
Internal institutional Hospitalization	145	3,679	22.83
Total external and internal hospitalization	1,166	10,001	183.56

The physician in each residential care center is usually a family physician or a physician without specialization for the adult population and a pediatrician for the pediatric population. The number of specialist referrals outside the residential care center in 2002 is shown in table 11, and the number of special examinations in laboratories or clinics outside the residential care center is shown in table 12. It should be noted here that ECG is also done in the centers, where they have the equipment available. The nursing staff will often have to be involved to explain to and calm the resident and sometimes to follow and participate with the resident at the out-patient clinic, dental visit, or during hospitalization. Another aspect of the medical is dental surveillance and treatment.

Table 11. Use of ambulatory services outside residential 55 residential care centers in 2002 (6,352 persons). Numbers and rate per 1,000 study population

Type of service	Visits in 2001	Rate/1,000
Surgery	740	116.5
Internal medicine	78	12.3
Eye	1,274	200.6
Optometrist	250	39.4
Dermatology	849	133.7
Orthopedics	841	132.4
Gynecology (females)	721	254.1
Neurology	531	83.6
Oncology	88	13.9
ENT	546	86.0
Diabetes	223	35.1
Cardiology	188	29.6
Endocrinology	258	40.6
Pulmonology	117	18.4
Child development	12	1.9
Urology	499	78.6
Gastroenterology	228	35.9
Auditory	84	13.2
Proctology	39	6.1
Rehabilitation	82	12.9
Vascular	62	9.8
Hematology	94	14.8
Physiotherapy	101	15.9
Plastic surgery	100	15.7
Oral surgery	206	32.4
Hemodialysis	594	93.5
Psychiatrist	64	10.1
Other	140	22.0
TOTAL	9,009	1,418.29

The number of dental visits for 2002 is shown in table 13. People with intellectual disability or challenging behavior who live in residential are prone to injuries. Each injury (intentional, unintentional, or a case of death) must be reported to the medical director.

Table 12. Use of ambulatory laboratory services outside 55 residential care centers in 2002 (6,352 persons). Number of examinations and rate per 1,000 study population

Type of laboratory	No. exams	Rate/1,000
Chest X ray	468	73.7
Other X ray	692	108.9
Ultrasound	675	106.3
ECG	381	60.0
EEG	252	39.7
Mammography	273	42.98
ECHO	117	18.4
CT	197	31.0
MRI	17	2.7
Other	64	10.1
TOTAL	3,136	497.9

Table 13. Dental treatment (examination, hygienist and general anaesthesia) for all persons in 55 residential care centers in 2002 (N = 6,352)

Examination	Numbers	Percent
Dental examination	7,043	110.88
Dental hygienist	6,298	99.15
Treatment under GA	234	3.68

Discussion

The Office of the Medical Director (OMD) of the Division for Mental Retardation at the Ministry of Social Affairs (MSA) provides medical services for persons with intellectual disability (ID) in residential care centers in Israel. The OMD sets the standard of care, and a medical/allied professional health team carries out inspections and supervision to staff at the local institutional level.

This situation is different from that in many other countries, where large institutions have been closed and supervision de-centralized. Israel has never had large institutions like those in the United States, but rather smaller centers having an average of 111 persons per center. Only about 27% of the total registered population of persons with ID (in 2002 the total registered population was 23,340 persons) reside in this manner, whereas the majority remain at home, but receive services from the Division for Mental Retardation.

Table 14. Reported cases of injuries from 55 residential care centers in 2002 (N=6,352)

Injury	Numbers	Percent of population
Death (unintentional injury)	17	0.27
Burns	40	0.63
Fractures	116	1.83
Wounds	825	12.99
Runaway	205	0.31
Care staff injured resident	3	0.05
Resident injured other resident	127	2.00
Abuse of resident	2	0.03
Drowning	1	0.02
Other	181	2.85
TOTAL	1,332	20.97

Table 15. Cause of death for 85 cases in 55 residential care centers in 2002

ICD Classification	Numbers
1. Infectious	12
2. Neoplasms	5
3. Endocrine	0
4. Blood	0
6. Nervous system	4
7. Circulatory	31
8. Respiratory	18
9. Digestive	0
10. Genitourinary	2
14. Congenital	0
16. Ill-defined	9
17. Injury	4
TOTAL	85

The present survey is the fifth on a national basis in Israel conducted to obtain a picture of the population served and to analyze trends in service provision. The survey in 2002 showed that 78.4% of the population with ID in residential care in Israel was between 20 and 60 years old, 50.4% with severe or profound ID, 41.9% with moderate and 7.4% with mild ID. This distribution, because the persons with ID who can be served outside of the residential care framwork will be served in the community. Twenty-five percent were nursing patients, with a high workload for the care staff, and 18.7% confined to a wheelchair. The present survey showed 28.9% with epilepsy, which is much higher than the usual 0.5% to 1% in the general population (5) but has been reported in other studies (6,7), where the prevalence of epilepsy in residential care was around 32%. For community studies with persons with ID, the prevalence was lower—around 16% (6,7).

This population of persons with ID in residential care has many associated medical problems and therefore a higher prevalence of daily medication. In this survey, 80.3% were found to be receiving medication daily for chronic illness, and 50.8% received psychotropic medication for psychiatric illness. Ambulant (out-patient clinics) or specialist service in this survey showed that the sub-specialties of ophthalmology, dermatology, orthopedics, surgery and gynecology were the most requested specialist visits. Dental care and hygiene are very important in this population. Most of this population was examined by a dentist and over time, we have seen an increase to 99% that are now treated by dental hygienist.

Conclusions

This paper is a report on the fifth national survey on medical care for persons with intellectual disability in residential care centers in Israel. We have observed over time that the information gathered has been very helpful for the planning and development of services. The questionnaire has resulted in a uniform data collection that is important for not only the Office of the Medical Director, but also for the clinic itself, the local administration of the specific residential care center, and the Division for Mental Retardation in particular.

Acknowledgments

We thank the medical and nursing care staff of all residential-care centers for their time and efforts to fill out the questionnaire and collect the data.

References

[1] Merrick J. National survey 1998 on medical services for persons with intellectual disability in residential care in Israel. Int J Disabil Hum Dev 2005;4(2):139-46.
[2] Merrick J. National survey 1999 on medical services for persons with intellectual disability in residential care in Israel. Int J Disabil Hum Dev 2006;5(3):303-8.
[3] Merrick J. National survey 2000 on medical services for persons with intellectual disability in residential care in Israel. Int J Disabil Hum Dev 2007;6(1):91-6.
[4] Morad M, Kandel I, Merrick J. National survey 2001 on medical services for persons with intellectual disability in residential care in Israel. Int J Disabil Hum Dev 2007;6(3):317-22.
[5] Kerr M. Improving the general health of people with learning disabilities. Adv Psychiatr Treat 2004; 10: 200-6.
[6] Mariani E, Ferini-Strambi L, Sala M et al. Epilepsy in institutionalized patients with encepha-lopathy. Clinical aspects and nosological consider-ations. Am J Ment Retard 1993;98:27-33.
[7] Morgan CL, Baxter H, Kerr MP. Prevalence of epilepsy and associated health service utilisation and mortality among patients with intellectual disability. Am J Ment Retard 2003;108:293-300.

Submitted: December 15, 2008.
Revised: January 01, 2009.
Accepted: January 02, 2009.

In: Public Health Yearbook 2009
Editor: Joav Merrick
ISBN: 978-1-61668-911-7

Chapter 9

BLACK MARKET MEDICINE: AN ETHICAL DILEMMA IN ISRAEL

Isack Kandel, MA, PhD[*1,2]
and Joav Merrick, MD, MMedSci, DMSc[2,3]

[1]Faculty of Social Sciences, Department of Behavioral Sciences, Ariel University Center, Samaria, Ariel, Israel; [2]National Institute of Child Health and Human Development, Jerusalem, Office of the Medical Director, Division for Mental Retardation, Ministry of Social Affairs, Jerusalem, Israel
[3]Kentucky Children's Hospital, University of Kentucky, Lexington, United States

Abstract

Black market medicine contradicts the ethical and moral codes obligating every physician to act ethically and not accept bribery for care provided or to accept compensation for a service that should be provided equally and without charge. The phenomenon is not new and has been described by various professionals working within the health and medical system in Israel. This paper is a short overview of black market medicine. We believe that if physicians are made aware of the issue of black market medicine and its immorality, emphasizing the harm that it causes them and the entire population due to its avaricious portrayal, perhaps in the future this practice will be reduced and more easily eliminated.

Keywords: Public health, medical ethics, professional ethics, Hippocratic oath.

[*] Correspondence: Senior lecturer Isack Kandel, MA, PhD, Faculty of Social Sciences, Maaleh Shomron, IL-44852 Lev Shomron, Israel. Tel 972-9-7929180; Fax: 972-9-7920316; E-mail: kandelii@zahav.net.il

Introduction

The prevalence of black market medicine in Israel is extensive. This practice is in contradiction with the Patient's Rights Act from 1996, chapter C, clause 3-4, which states that "every person in need is entitled to receive medical care in accordance with all laws and regulations and the conditions and arrangements reigning at any given time in the Israeli health care system" and "no medical facility or clinician shall discriminate between patients on grounds of religion, race, sex, nationality, country of birth, or other such grounds."

The existence of black market medicine is troublesome for the Israel Ministry of Health and a black stain on the white gown of the medical profession. Black market medicine contradicts the ethical and moral codes obligating every physician to act ethically and not accept bribery for care provided or to accept compensation for a service that should be provided equally and without charge.

The phenomenon is not new and has been described by nurses working at the largest hospital in Israel (1), who called it immoral medicine. They described (1) that nurses have been exposed to many instances of immoral medicine in hospitals, where they have observed demands for money from patients who are waiting for surgical intervention and physicians accepting bribes or financial compensation in return for their services.

We have decided to review this subject, since we also have encountered this phenomenon of physicians, who are financially compensated by patients for health care services for which they are already paying as members of the HMOs. This practice is prevalent in almost all hospital departments and expressed by the concept of the "department fund" – insinuating to the patient, "that should you wish to receive prompt treatment or to expedite surgery, or should you wish to order the services of a specific surgeon, you are expected to deposit money in the fund". Black market medicine in the hospitals is also expressed by donations, including gifts to the staff, patients who organize staff outings, purchasing equipment for the wards, etc. This issue is very significant and it has a great deal of influence on the nature of medical care. For this reason we should be aware of it, discuss it, and examine why it is surrounded by a conspiracy of silence.

What is black market medicine?

The definition provided by the Knesset (the Israel Parliament) in the bill prohibiting black market medicine as an amendment to the Health Care Act (prohibiting the acceptance of payments, clause 10B): "A public health care worker or institution may not request or accept, whether directly or indirectly, any payment in return for the provision of health care or any service that are part of the worker's duties, unless this payment is made through a public health care institution or with its consent. Said payment includes money, money equivalent, services, or any other benefit".

In the legal directory black market medicine is defined as a white-collar crime. This term includes various types of illegal and nonviolent behavior performed by groups or individuals and including theft, fraud, and other violations of trust, which are performed during the rendition of the offender's professional activities (for example: fraud, bribery, violations of anti-monopoly laws, price adjustment, manipulation of the capital market, inside trading) (2).

Further legal explanation can be given as using special resources (positions, assets, and political influence) to generate illegal profits by means of disguise and deception and while preventing exposure by controlling sources of information. At the same time, the legal definitions of these prohibitions create a conspicuous obscurity that makes it difficult to differentiate between a criminal act and an act that carries only civil liability.

In an investigation by the State Comptroller on the role and efficiency of the Israeli medical system black market medicine was defined as: "Medical services provided under the auspices of a public institution involving any display of preference that does not stem from medical considerations and not in the required transparent and formal manner – in return for financial or other gain provided by the patient to the physician treating him as part of his responsibilities in a public hospital."

From an economic point of view black market medicine and black market economy has been described as a state of imbalance (3). The law determines the level of services in economic terms, but since the present level is poor a state of imbalance exists. The market must achieve a state of balance by searching for alternative products, such as private and "black market" medicine. Physicians receive significant financial compensation for providing alternative services and this complements their lack of satisfaction with the compensation received from the system, leading to illegal conduct (4). From a sociological point of view white-collar criminals do not perceive themselves, and often are not perceived by society, as criminals and deviants, but rather as honest citizens.

We see black market medicine as an extensive field related to immoral and unethical medicine, including all medical compensation expressing the relationship between caregiver and patient in a manner unrecognized by the establishment, such as department compensation or organized department fund (issuing receipts), handing the physician money in an envelope before or after an operation or after performing a certain procedure, selecting a private surgeon by paying him, reserving beds on surgical wards, private consultations at the hospital.

Perceptions of black-market medicine

The Legislature Service Commission in Israel decided to formulate a bill defining black market medicine as a criminal offense. This is an additional attempt to fight this reality, against which all administrative means of supervision used in the last few years within healthcare institutions have been exposed as inefficient. Government service regulations concerning private employment state that physicians in government service may not accept payment from a patient in a hospital for surgery or consultation. This is also forbidden according to the labor constitution of Union (Histadrut) workers and according to the procedures of the various health care providers in Israel (HMOs).

In the public debate around this issue and the work of the commission there were recognition that a law cannot solve the problem of black market medicine and that it could cause damage to the health care system. For all intents and purposes, black market medicine is already considered bribery in criminal law (5).

The medical profession itself can also be seen as ambivalent to this issue. Both for personal reasons related to the fact of being a physician, the presence or absence of compensation (promotion, studies, research), structural causes related to the type of workplace (surgical or internal ward or other) or the physician's ability to support himself by practicing private medicine and supplement his low pay in public hospital service. So from the chair of the Israel Medical Association it was claimed that a bill prohibiting black market medicine would be a callous violation of the basic constitutional foundations of the democratic state, since "it is inconceivable that a modern state would apply a unique discriminatory penal code to a specific group of workers", while the representative of the HMOs felt that "private and public medicine should not merge within a public institution. Such a combination causes discrimination between affluent and less prosperous patients, while providing personal benefits to selected physicians."

Within the economic system black market medicine relates to the economic perspective, dividing it into a number of aspects and levels (6), where the first level is the health care budget as part of the total budget of society and level two the manner in which the medical budget is divided between various medical objectives. In his article, Benjamin Mozes (6) quoted renowned jurist Guido Calabresi, who dealt with alternative ways of distributing resources, which are on the one hand significantly limited and on the other hand related to very important matters. Calabresi offers four approaches to the question of resource allocation:

- Pure market: Resources are distributed according to a free market (each medical procedure has a price) and consumers compete with each other. People of means will always receive better care. This approach is immoral, since there are "poor people", who will not receive any care as they lack the resources to pay for it.
- Political: The state decides how resources will be divided, based on considerations, such as military service. This is similar to a democracy. The will of the people, expressed by chosen representatives for public matters, decides which treatments should receive medical priority.
- Fortuitous: The division of medical care will be decided by lottery, the moral question is whether human life should be decided by lottery.
- Customary practice: According to this approach, society decides not to decide tragic matters, i.e. nature is permitted to take its course. Social powers, pressures, coincidence, different behavior when visiting physicians, form a distribution of the limited resources. The disadvantage of this approach is that the moment a person understands it he objects to it when it is not in his favor.

In order to regulate and have exceptions medical services is now provided as part of a complementary insurance policy and special medical services that are not included in the basket of health care services can be paid for on condition that the compensation is paid directly to the hospital management. This service will be a more efficient use of existing infrastructure, such as operating rooms and cardiac catheterization rooms and will cause more senior and professional physicians to remain at the hospitals and thus be available to care for patients (5). This AMS (Additional Medical Service) has so far only been implemented in a few hospitals.

Legal struggle

The low level of exposure and punishment in regard to black market medicine is not surprising. In the current state of the medical system, black market medicine is a social need offense (an offense contrary to the economic situation), similar to violations of the alcohol prohibition in the "dry years" of the United States. As such it satisfies needs of both the offender and the "victim" and thus both sides possess a vested interest in preventing exposure. In the few cases in which the practice was exposed, additional factors were at play, such as poor objective outcomes of the treatment, together with a sense of medical malpractice or an intention to harm to the victim. The current deterring punishment should be a prison term.

Since the offense is basically financial, another possible deterrent would be heavy fines, which would neutralize profits. However the value of such fines would also be limited due to the low level of exposure. We must also remember that punishing a black market medicine offender does not end with the penalty imposed by the criminal system. There are supplemental penalties that hold serious implications, such as the possibility of revoking or suspending the physician's license to practice medicine in cases of criminal conviction, administrative removal from senior positions (head of department, assistant head of department, senior physician) and even dismissal with slim chances of being employed by other public employers. A primary fact regarding "social need offenses" is that they cannot be stopped by administrative or legal means. These offenses are not the main problem, rather only symptoms of another, more deeper illness, and until it is treated no real remedy is possible.

The Ministry of Health support the organized implementation of the AMS system, since there is a demand for this service and the public wishes to determine the identity of the surgeons operating on them. It is time to stop ignoring the obvious, to acknowledge changing needs and to prepare for them accordingly in order to determine uniform rules and prevent distortions.

Operating an additional medical service will enable more efficient utilization of expensive equipment and installations, increase the availability of physicians and staff for the public system in the evening and night hours as well, and enable final elimination of the need for corrupt black market medicine (5). The argument against is that it is wrong to use an installation funded by the public in order to provide physicians with the opportunity to generate additional personal gain. In all modern states there is a separation of private medicine from public medicine (5).

Conclusions

From a professional point of view, members of the medical staff provide a unique service and must maintain neutrality and work according to codes acquired during their training. The State of Israel strives to grant equal care to all its citizens according to the welfare model. The authority invested in the physicians comprises power, a great deal of professional knowledge, and professional judgment.

In light of these conclusions, we would like to recommend a number of ways in which hospitals should handle the issue of black market medicine:

- The provision of directives and conducting of seminars for caregiving staff and physicians in all departments, emphasizing the negative implications of this practice.
- Increasing patients' awareness of the issues relating to black market medicine by publicizing the prohibition on large signs throughout the hospitals.
- Abolishing hospital "department funds" and establishing a general donation funds managed by an external element, so that only those interested in contributing will approach this fund of their own initiative.
- Another solution suggested (2) was structural changes in the health care system, such as the establishment of a public health system, that would create a balance in regard to the interests of the public, on the one hand enabling them to receive better medical treatment and on the other providing a solution to the practice of black market medicine.

We believe that if physicians are made aware of the issue of black market medicine and its immorality, emphasizing the harm that it causes them and the entire population due to its avaricious portrayal, perhaps in the future this practice will be reduced and more easily eliminated.

References

[1] Carmon P, Tabak N. Immoral behavior in medicine. Nurs Ethics 1997;4(2):115-22.
[2] Wafner L. MPs actions in the Knesset. Michtav Lehaver 1996;6:10-3. [Hebrew]
[3] Berglas E, Tzedakah E. Economic analysis of the health system. Tel Aviv: Pinchas Sapir Dev Center, 1988;10. [Hebrew]
[4] Lachman R, Noy S. Black market medicine in Israel: Perceptions, circumstances, and implications. Tel Aviv: Tel-Aviv Univ, 1992. [Hebrew]
[5] Sofer R. The operation succeeded and the patient paid. Michtav Lehaver 1977;59(1):31-2. [Hebrew]
[6] Mozes B. [Rationing health care: ethical, medical and economic aspects]. Harefuah 1993;124(10): 625-8. [Hebrew]

Submitted: August 20, 2008.
Revised: January 01, 2009.
Accepted: January 18, 2009.

Section two
Can we make a difference?

In: Public Health Yearbook 2009
Editor: Joav Merrick

ISBN: 978-1-61668-911-7

Chapter 10

EOSINOPHIL CATIONIC PROTEIN IN PEDIATRIC ASTHMA

Eugenia Panagiotopoulou, MD[1], Michael B. Anthracopoulos, MD, PhD, FAAP[*1] and Kostas N. Priftis, MD, PhD[2]

[1]Respiratory Unit, Department of Pediatrics, University Hospital of Patras, Rio-Patras
[2]Department of Allergy-Pneumonology, Penteli Children's Hospital, P Penteli, Athens, Greece

Abstract

Eosinophil granulocytes (eosinophils) are white blood cells that develop from bone marrow precursor cells. Their major morphological characteristic is eosinophilic granules within the cytoplasm, which are divided into specific and small granules. Four cationic proteins have been recognized within the eosinophil specific granules that include eosinophil cationic protein (ECP). It displays a variety of biological activities, most notably cytotoxicity that is due to its ability to make pores in cell membranes. ECP exerts this action on parasites, viruses, bacteria, tumor cells, and even respiratory epithelial cells. Other biological functions include stimulation of mucus production in the airway, interaction with the coagulation and complement systems, and immunomodulation. The role of ECP as a marker of eosinophil activity has been investigated in a variety of body fluids and diseases, particularly in wheezing children. The role of ECP has been investigated in acute viral bronchiolitis of infants and preschool wheezing in reference to both pathogenesis and prognosis of the disease. There is evidence that ECP can be used in asthma to evaluate severity, patient compliance to anti-asthma treatment, and to step-down inhaled corticosteroid dosage in stabilized patients. Further studies are required in order to elucidate its role as a diagnostic and prognostic tool in pediatric asthma.

[*] Correspondence: Michael Anthracopoulos MD, PhD, FAAP, Department of Pediatrics, University of Patras School of Medicine, Rio 265 04, Greece. Tel: +30-2610-999544; Fax: +30-2610-994533; E-mail: manthra@otenet.gr

Keywords: Eosinophil cationic protein, asthma, bronchiolitis, children, wheezing.

Introduction

Eosinophil granulocytes (eosinophils) are white blood cells that develop from bone marrow precursor cells and differentiate under the control of various growth and colony-stimulating factors. After a five day maturation period, eosinophils circulate in the peripheral blood. Only a small fraction of eosinophils remains in the bloodstream, while most mature cells immigrate to the tissues, preferably those exposed to the external environment such as the respiratory and gastrointestinal tract. Numerous studies suggest that they play a significant role in the proinflammatory process in various diseases, particularly those of allergic origin such as asthma.

Their major morphological characteristic is the presence of eosinophilic granules within the cytoplasm, which are divided into two main types: specific and small granules (1,2). The specific granules are arginine-rich and stain reddish-brown with basic aniline dyes such as eosin. Various inflammatory mediators and particularly active proteins are stored in these granules. Among them, four cationic proteins are recognized: a) eosinophil peroxidase (EPO), b) major basic protein (MBP), c) eosinophil-derived neurotoxin or protein X (EDN or EPX) and d) eosinophil cationic protein (ECP); these proteins are held responsible for the eosinophil biologic actions (3). The small granules are mainly seen in the mature eosinophil and contain acid phosphatase and arylsulphatase B (1).

The present article discusses the biochemical characteristics of ECP, its biological functions, its role in the inflammatory process and its clinical significance in pediatric asthma.

Biochemical and biological aspects

ECP was first purified in 1971 from the granules of myeloid cells taken from patients with chronic myeloid leukemia (4). At that time it was presumed to be a component of the family of neutrophilic basic proteins, but in 1975 ECP was aggregated among the products of eosinophilic origin (5), however similarly to EDN, it has also been isolated in neutrophils (6,7).

ECP is a single-chain, zinc-containing protein. Its molecular weight ranges from 16 to 22 kDa due to differences in glycosylation of the three available sites in its amino acid sequence. The molecule is characterized by a content of 2.5 mol of zinc per mole, and a relatively high isoelectric point of 10.8 that is the result of its 20 arginine residues.

When compared, ECP and EDN show a 67% sequence homology, with 37 identical residues from a total of 55 (8). Despite their similarity, ECP has a 100-fold weaker ribonuclease activity as compared to EDN. Conversely, ECP demonstrates great toxicity against various cells (bacteria, parasites, viruses, several mammalian cell lines) whereas EDN lacks such cytotoxic properties [9].

ECP demonstrates a variety of cytotoxic and non-toxic activities that are summarized in table 1. The most important among its recognized functions appears to be its cytotoxic activity against parasites, bacteria and viruses that has been reported in numerous of studies (10).

Secretion from the eosinophil and measurements in body fluids

A wide variety of stimuli is implicated in the activation and degranulation processes of eosinophils at the site of inflammation. Among these, the role of cytokines –such as IL-5, and IL-3– and that of immunoglobulins –such as IgE, IgG and IgA– is deemed fundamental (10,11). Other stimuli that induce eosinophil degranulation include eosinophil-chemotactic cytokines: regulated upon activation, normal T- expressed and secreted cytokine (RANTES) and macrophage inflammatory protein-1 alpha (MIP-1a), the complement fragments C5a and C3a, the lipid mediator platelet activating factor (PAF) (12), even the eosinophil derived proteins per se can cause eosinophil degranulation (13).

Table 1. Major biologic functions of ECP

Cytotoxic effects	Non-toxic effects
• Parasites	• Stimulates airway mucus secretion
○ *Schistosoma mansoni*	• Induces TGF-β1 release
○ *Trypanosoma cruzi*	• Induces proteoglycan production by fibroblasts
○ *Trichinella spiralis*	• Stimulates histamine and tryptase release from mast cells
○ *Brugia malayi*	• Stimulates histamine release from basophils
○ *Brugia pahangi*	• Inhibits T-cell proliferation
• Bacteria	• Inhibits immunoglobulin synthesis by B-cells
• Viruses	• Increases coagulation time at high doses
• Tumor cells	• Activates urokinase-induced plasminogen
• Respiratory epithelial cells	• Inhibits anticoagulant action of heparin
• Neurotoxic activity	• Induces ICAM-1 and IGF-1 expression

ECP can be measured in various body fluids such as sputum, saliva, nasal lavage fluid, BALF, serum, plasma and urine. A sensitive radioimmunosorbent assay for quantitative measurement of ECP was developed by Venge et al (14). Circadian variation in serum ECP levels has been reported, with high concentrations noted during the night and peak levels at 06.00 hours (15). ECP levels in various body fluids of normal and asthmatic subjects are summarized in table 2.

Table 2. Levels of ECP in normal and asthmatic subjects in various body fluids

Body fluid	Healthy controls (μg/ml)	Asthmatic patients (μg/ml)
Serum	2-20	>20
Sputum	20-1280	76,8-32,000
Saliva	250-450	450-850
Bronchoalveolar lavage	1-3	5-100

In order to obtain ECP sputum measurements sputum induction is often required via inhalation of hypertonic saline as described by Pin et al (16). Using this method ECP was studied in healthy and asthmatic subjects; the results showed a wide range of ECP levels that partially overlap in the two groups (17,18). Sputum levels have been associated with asthma severity, and shown to reflect inhaled corticosteroid (ICS) treatment (19).

Furthermore, higher ECP levels have been observed in selected portions of induced sputum as compared to the entire expectorate (20); therefore, standardization of sputum acquisition and processing is crucial in order to achieve meaningful results.

ECP has also been measured in BALF. Due to dilution differences among procedures, BALF ECP is best expressed as micrograms per liter recovered fluid. Bousquet et al have demonstrated that levels of ECP in BALF samples from asthmatic patients correlate positively with asthma severity (21). Increased levels of ECP have been detected in BALF of infants with recurrent wheezing episodes even during the intermittent asymptomatic periods, thus suggesting a chronic inflammatory process of the airways (22). Surprisingly, in the same study ECP levels did not correlate with the absolute number of eosinophils in BALF, but rather with the neutrophil count. In addition, increased levels of ECP in BALF have been reported in idiopathic pulmonary fibrosis (23), eosinophilic pneumonia (24,25) and in patients after lung transplantation (26,27). However, researchers failed to demonstrate a relationship between elevated levels of BALF ECP and acute rejection (28). Serious drawbacks still exist in the use of BALF ECP in routine clinical practice as bronchoalveolar lavage constitutes an invasive technique and standardization of methodology is critical in order to obtain reproducible measurements.

The role of ECP in inflammation

Eosinophils contain numerous proinflammatory mediators that include granule proteins, cytokines and lipid mediators. Accumulation and degranulation of eosinophils are thought to participate in the pathogenesis of various disorders such as asthma, allergic rhinitis, inflammatory bowel, and rheumatoid disease via release of their toxic products, including ECP (29). This phenomenon may lead to tissue destruction and remodeling.

In an effort to describe airway inflammation patterns in asthma, Gibson et al (30) compared sputum ECP concentrations in two groups of asthmatic children: one group with eosinophilic invasion and the other with combined neutrophilic and eosinophilic invasion. The median value of ECP levels was higher in the second group suggesting greater eosinophil degranulation in children with eosinophil-neutrophil exacerbation, thus implying a supportive role –via ECP activity– of neutrophils in asthma exacerbations. Elevated serum ECP levels represent eosinophilic activation and are considered to be a sign of airway inflammation in asthma (31).

Elevated ECP levels were also found in tracheal aspirates of neonates who subsequently developed bronchopulmonary dysplasia, thus proposing an important role of eosinophils and their products in lung inflammation and injury (32).

With regard to bronchiolitis, ECP may contribute to its pathogenesis by damaging the respiratory epithelium (33) and by inducing mucus secretion (34). There are in vitro studies of the effect of ECP release by eosinophils on human lung type II alveolar epithelial cell cultures infected by respiratory syncytial virus (RSV) (35-37). The results of these studies highlight the fact that RSV per se or non infected epithelial cells alone cannot provoke eosinophil degranulation. Conversely, epithelial cells, when infected with RSV, are capable of releasing a significant amount of ECP. These findings support the hypothesis that infected cells release mediators that activate adjacent eosinophils, which in turn release their toxic products that affect both healthy and abnormal cells, thus causing tissue injury.

ECP in pediatric asthma

Episodic airway obstruction, not an uncommon finding during childhood, is apparently the final common pathway of different disease processes. Our understanding of the epidemiology of childhood wheezing has been greatly advanced over the past twenty years and a number of cohort studies in children have shown that wheezing, especially during infancy and preschool age, is a heterogeneous condition with different predominant characteristics at different ages; the old paediatric motto "All that wheezes is not asthma" appears today more true than ever (38-42). After the first two months of life the incidence of wheezing increases markedly with a peak occurrence between two and five months of age, then decreases after the sixth month, and remains low until the third year (43). Three common phenotypes of recurrent wheezing have been identified, i.e. transient early wheeze, non-atopic persistent wheeze, and atopic wheeze, but there is considerable overlap among them (38-42). Timing of initiation of wheezing is important, but both atopic and non-atopic wheeze can be of early or late onset, while the presence or absence of atopy is the critical factor that determines pathogenesis and long-term prognosis. Finally, it is worth mentioning that there is a small group of infants and young children with unusual causes of wheezing who present with atypical wheeze. This group is of great clinical importance and includes children with foreign body aspiration, cystic fibrosis, primary ciliary dyskinesia, gastroesophageal reflux, immune deficiency, and congenital pulmonary or cardiac anomalies. The characteristics of the three common wheezing phenotypes are briefly described below:

- Transient early wheeze (about 60% of wheezers <3 years) is characterized by risk factors such as: smoking during pregnancy [44], decreased level of lung function shortly after birth (before the occurrence of any respiratory symptoms) (45), early day care attendance or living with older siblings (39), male sex, young age of mother and low birth weight, and bottle feeding (41).
- Non-atopic persistent wheeze (about 20% of wheezers <3 years) occurs during viral infections and is characterized by a different set of risk factors that include: beginning at age ≤1 year, history of RSV lower respiratory tract infection (LRI), and prematurity (39, 40). It has been speculated that dysregulation of airway tone is responsible for the decrease in lung function and the increase in prevalence of bronchial hyperresponsiveness (BHR) in these children [46]. Genetic predisposition, damage due to RSV-LRI, or both may determine the alterations of airway tone of viral wheezers. On the other hand, altered autonomous regulation and/or disruption of the development of the lung may be responsible in prematurely born children.

Non-atopic wheezers do not respond to ICS, but their wheezing appears to be responsive to bronchodilators (47). Wheezing and BHR decrease with age (39,40). It should be noted that non-atopic wheeze apparently constitutes a much larger portion of wheezing disorders in developing as compared to developed societies and its long-term prognosis may not be as favourable (47).

- Atopic asthma can start at any age; however, most cases present clinically in the first 6 years of life. Atopic wheeze (about 20% of wheezers <3 years) usually starts later than non-atopic wheeze, usually in the second and third years of life. Symptoms are generally more severe and may occur with or without colds. This group is also characterized by a positive family history of asthma (x4 the risk of other groups in this age range) and a history of atopic dermatitis (x2-3 the risk). Although these infants eventually become sensitized to local aeroallergens, only few exhibit positive skin-prick tests at the time of their initial symptoms. Detection of specific serum IgE against aeroallergens (in the few infants that exhibit such a finding) has a high positive predictive value for wheezing at a later age. Sensitization to both aeroallergens and food allergens increases further the risk of persistent wheezing, but sensitization to food allergens alone is of no predictive value (48). An association also exists with total serum IgE (38). In addition, atopic wheeze is associated with eosinophilia (≥4%) and an increased eosinophilic response is observed during virally induced wheezing episodes (39,40). This group is characterized by normal initial lung function (before the inception of wheezing), increased BHR that appears to be the result (not the cause) of the disease, and a progressive decline in lung function (38-40). Young atopic wheezers usually respond –albeit often only partially– to ICS and bronchodilators.

The need to target long-term anti-inflammatory prophylactic treatment to those that have a better chance of a favourable response and to address the parents' pressing question "Will my child outgrow his/her asthma?" has driven researchers to identify markers of asthmatic inflammation. ECP has been studied extensively in this context.

ECP in acute bronchiolitis

The role of ECP has been investigated in acute viral bronchiolitis of infants in reference to both pathogenesis and prognosis of the disease. The ECP concentration in nasopharyngeal secretions was found to be significantly higher among patients with bronchiolitis as compared to those with other respiratory tract infections; a positive correlation with disease severity was also established (49).

It is well recognized that degranulation of eosinophils occurs in the respiratory epithelium of infants with bronchiolitis caused by RSV, suggesting a potential role of eosinophil-derived proteins in the progress of virus induced airway obstruction (50). Moreover, nasopharyngeal ECP levels greater than 50 ng/ml were found to be predictive of the development of bronchiolitis at the time of RSV infection (50) and increased nasopharyngeal and serum ECP has been observed in RSV induced bronchiolitis (51,52). Interestingly, girls have been found to have almost twice as high ECP levels when compared to boys, suggesting that constitutional factors may influence the response of the infant (51). Elevated levels of ECP in nasal washings were found in wheezing children with either RSV or rhinovirus infection and levels exceeding 200 ng/ml were associated with the highest risk for wheezing (53).

In an attempt to study the value of serum ECP in predicting subsequent wheezing in RSV bronchiolitis, Pifferi et al (54) measured serum ECP levels in forty-eight infants with RSV acute bronchiolitis; they reported significantly higher levels of serum ECP in these infants as compared to healthy controls. Furthermore, higher levels of ECP during acute disease correlated with persistence of wheezing during a five year follow-up period; conversely, peripheral eosinophil count and total serum IgE were unable to predict outcome. However, high serum ECP was not predictive of the development of allergic sensitization in the same study, although serum ECP levels above 8mg/ml were associated with a tenfold higher risk of developing subsequent wheezing.

It should be noted that not all studies support the role of ECP in predicting post-bronchiolitic wheeze. Counil et al (55) reported no difference in the pharyngeal levels of ECP between RSV positive and RSV negative wheezy infants. However, they did show an increase in histamine levels in the RSV positive group; this finding suggests mast cell induced rather than eosinophilic inflammation. In accordance to these results, Priftis et al (56) found that serum ECP levels did not differ between RSV positive and RSV negative bronchiolitic infants; surprisingly, in this study it was the RSV positive group that demonstrated decreased levels of serum ECP.

The discrepancies among the aforementioned studies may be due to differences in the study populations and/or variations in sampling and measurement procedures that have not been standardized as yet. Careful recruitment of subjects and design of studies is crucial if comparable results are to be obtained.

ECP and diagnosis of asthma

The identification of a marker or constellation of markers –preferably non invasive– continues to the present day to represent the "search for the holy grail" in the understanding of the natural history of pediatric wheezy illness. ECP has been extensively studied as a potential marker that may differentiate among the various "asthma phenotypes" particularly in infancy and preschool age. It has been measured in serum, nasal, and other body fluid samples in wheezy children and attempts have been made to correlate its levels with other atopic markers. In one of the earlier studies, Ingram et al (57) measured ECP levels in serum and nasal fluids of wheezing children and asymptomatic controls. Serum levels of ECP were found to be significantly higher in the first group, correlated positively with total blood eosinophil count, and showed a tendency to increase with age; however, there was no relationship between ECP serum measurements and RAST results. In addition, ECP concentrations in nasal wash specimens were significantly elevated in the wheezing group as compared to controls and on many occasions outnumbered the serum levels, thus suggesting that assessment of eosinophilic products in peripheral blood may underestimate the degree of inflammation at the site of interest.

There is an overwhelming body of literature that has reported similar findings. In a prospective study by Frischer et al (58), nasal ECP levels were found to be significantly higher in those infants that subsequently developed "wheezy bronchitis". In addition to the ability of such measurements to predict the development of later episodes of recurrent wheezing, it has also been demonstrated that high levels of ECP in nasopharyngeal secretions in children with acute bronchiolitis can predict subsequent hospitalization and physician-diagnosed bronchial obstruction (59), while the use of anti-inflammatory therapy with budesonide or nebulized cromolyn sodium appears to be effective in decreasing the number of physician-diagnosed bronchial obstruction episodes in children with elevated naso-pharyngeal ECP (59). When sputum ECP was compared among groups of children with asthma, recurrent wheeze, and first time wheeze, significantly higher levels were found in the asthmatic patients' group versus first-time or recurrent wheezers (60). However, no correlation was established between sputum ECP levels and the presence of RSV antigen (60).

As already mentioned, the identification of those infants that will eventually develop persistent wheezing after their first episode continues to pose a major challenge to practitioners and researchers alike. Various inflammatory mediators have been studied in order to predict short- and long-term outcome, while ECP has been measured in body fluids of wheezy infants in an attempt to support its potential role in the prediction of subsequent persistence of wheezing and airway inflammation (61). Villa et al (62) found that an ECP serum threshold of over 20 μg/ml can differentiate infants with an increased risk of persistent wheeze from transient wheezers two years after the measurement; these findings imply that an inflammatory process mediated by eosinophils is responsible for the persistence of symptoms, whereas a problem in airway geometry appears more likely among transient wheezers. Similar results have been reported by other investigators suggesting that eosinophil degranulation markers such as ECP may in fact help to predict childhood asthma (63). Reijonen et al (64) determined that a threshold limit of at least 16 μg/ml of serum ECP could predict wheezing within 16 weeks after acute bronchiolitis; this cut-off level was highly specific but had poor sensitivity. In a later study, they showed that risk factors for developing asthma after initial hospitalization for wheezing included elevated serum ECP, age over 12 months, history of prior wheezing episode, atopy, and family history of atopy (65).

In their attempt to investigate the same question, Øymar et al (66) came to different conclusions in their retrospective study of first-time wheezers. Serum concentration of ECP was determined and subsequent development of asthma was assessed by questionnaire after a three year period. Surprisingly, serum ECP failed to predict those destined to develop asthma; furthermore, children that had higher levels of ECP during the wheezing episode did not develop asthma. These findings were supported by those of Sigurs et al (67). These researchers, by using ECP/albumin ratios in nasal secretions, also failed to predict subsequent development of asthma during a two year follow up period of children with RSV bron-chiolitis. Disappointing results were also reported among children with cough-variant asthma with regard to the use of ECP level as a predictive marker of subsequent development of classic asthma (68).

ECP and asthma severity

There are controversial findings with regard to ECP levels and airway inflammation. The role of ECP in both asthma and infant wheeze and its relation to disease severity were assessed by Marguet et al (69) in BALF samples of asthmatic children and viral wheezers and were compared to those of children with no airway pathology. ECP levels did not differ in the three groups, while positive correlations of ECP levels were found with the eosinophil count in the asthma group and with the neutrophil count in the infant wheezers group. The investigators failed to show any relation between ECP levels and disease severity, even though they established a 20 ng/ml threshold for persistence of symptoms. In another study of chronic asthmatics, serum ECP did not differ between symptomatic and asymptomatic children, thus failing to indicate disease activity (70). Finally, increased levels of serum ECP were found by Vanto et al (71) in children recently diagnosed with atopic asthma as compared to non-atopics; however, they did not correlate with disease severity.

Other studies have come to different conclusions. In an attempt to assess airway inflammation in the different clinical patterns (phenotypes) of asthma, Gibson et al (72) compared induced sputum samples from children with diagnosed asthma that were divided into three groups: infrequent asthma symptoms, frequent episodic asthma, and persistent asthma; healthy subjects were also studied. They noticed that ECP levels and eosinophil numbers were significantly increased in those with persistent or frequent episodes of asthma as compared to healthy controls; moreover, increasing levels of sputum ECP were noted with increasing asthma severity. Conversely, children with infrequent asthma symptoms and controls had similar levels of sputum eosinophils and ECP. Interestingly, symptomatic children showed significantly increased ECP levels and eosinophil counts as compared to asymptomatic asthmatics, regardless of asthma category. These results suggest that as the clinical pattern of asthma worsens regarding its frequency and severity, a concomitant increase in airway inflammation is detected, as reflected by ECP.

Moreover, Zubovic et al (73) showed an association between serum ECP and asthma severity. In other studies, ECP levels in BALF of asthmatic patients also correlated with disease severity (21), were found to be increased among asthmatic children (74,75) and corresponded well to symptoms or atopy (76,77). Similar observations were reported for ECP levels in serum (78,79), urine, and nasal lavage fluid; in these studies, the levels of ECP were also found to be higher in asthmatic children as compared to healthy controls. In asymptomatic children with a history of wheeze, ECP was found to be raised only in the subgroup of atopic asthmatics, in contrast to the findings in subjects with viral associated wheeze, non-atopic asthmatics, and healthy controls (80). These findings imply persistence of eosinophilic activation and degranulation, even during the asymptomatic periods of atopic asthma.

Carlsen et al (81) demonstrated that serum ECP was significantly higher in children with persistent as compared to episodic asthma, among those with atopic as compared to non-atopic asthma, and in those with active atopic eczema. Thus attention should be paid to the presence of atopy and active eczema when interpreting serum ECP measurements in the evaluation of asthma severity.

The results from studies on the relation of serum ECP and bronchial hyper-responsiveness (BHR) are controversial. A positive correlation of BHR to histamine and serum ECP has been demonstrated in asthmatic children (82), whereas no relationship was found in another study between serum ECP and BHR to histamine and cold air challenge (83). In addition, an increase in serum ECP was associated with BHR after bronchial challenge with hypertonic saline (84) or adenosine-5'-monophosphate (85), but not after challenge with metacholine (85).

ECP and monitoring asthma treatment

The fact that reductions in ECP concentration in fluid samples have been noted during withdrawal of anti-inflammatory therapy in asthmatic children (86) is of significant clinical interest. With regard to the role of ECP in assessing effectiveness of asthma therapy, the results of a small patient sample showed significant reduction of ECP levels in asthmatics, who received a five month course of inhaled budesonide, but not in the group that received sodium cromoglycate; however, no correlation with disease severity or pulmonary function was established (87). Furthermore, ECP concentrations in induced sputum decreased in asthmatic children following clinical improvement after treatment with ICS (88). The compliance to corticosteroid therapy, oral and inhaled, has also been monitored by ECP concentrations as has been demonstrated by several studies (89-91).

Supporting evidence of the usefulness of ECP in directing clinical decisions concerning asthma therapy also comes from a pilot study by Prehn et al (92). In this study, ECP serum levels were used in order to assess the initial ICS dose needed by 21 asthmatic children, and to step down the anti-inflammatory therapy during the follow up period. Thus, children with ECP levels over 30 μg/L received budesonide 400 μg twice daily, and those with ECP levels between 15 and 30 μg/L were given budesonide 200 μg twice daily. During the study period, the anti-inflammatory therapy changed according to ECP serum concentrations. When ECP levels decreased below 15 μg/L, ICS were substituted by 10 mg of sodium cromoglycate twice daily. The researchers demonstrated a decrease in both symptoms and serum ECP levels with ICS, but not with sodium cromoglycate. Furthermore, the children enrolled in the study did not require any emergency room treatment, hospital admission or oral steroid bursts during the study period. An increase in ECP levels was observed in non compliant patients. These findings support the use of ECP in the selection of the initial dosage of anti-inflammatory drugs and subsequent evaluation of asthma therapy. Other anti-inflammatory drugs also affect ECP levels. ECP from nasal washings decreased after treatment with montelukast, a leukotriene receptor antagonist with proven anti-inflammatory activity (93).

Other researchers, however, have failed to demonstrate a decrease in markers of inflammation such as ECP during treatment with ICS in children with moderate asthma, despite clinical and pulmonary function improvement (94).

Conclusions

Eosinophil cationic protein has been studied in various inflammatory diseases and particularly in childhood wheezing illness, including asthma. ECP measurements in various body fluids have been shown in many studies to correlate with disease severity and fluctuations of ECP levels may reflect the inflammatory process in asthmatic airways. There is evidence that ECP may prove to be a useful marker in guiding anti-inflammatory therapy and assessing patient compliance. Perhaps more importantly, the measurement of ECP in infants presenting with their first episode of wheezing may potentially assist in prognosing the development of asthma, and thus help to identify those infants that could benefit from early anti-inflammatory treatment. In addition, the role of eosinophil granule proteins, including ECP, in airway injury and inflammation is of great research interest in the quest for elucidating the pathogenesis of asthma (95).

To date, however, despite a large body of information, the exact role of ECP in clinical practice remains elusive. Sampling methods and measurements should be carefully standardized in order to obtain comparable results and larger patient samples need to be studied. Undoubtedly, more concrete evidence should be sought regarding the role of ECP in airway inflamation not only as a marker of disease severity and a guide to therapeutic decision making, but also as a potential target for anti-inflammatory treatment.

References

[1] Kroegel C, Virchow Jr JC, Luttmann W, Walker C, Warner JA. Pulmonary immune cells in health and disease: the eosinophil leucocyte (Part I). Eur Respir J 1994;7:519-43.

[2] Kroegel C, Warner JA, Virchow Jr JC, Matthys H. Pulmonary immune cells in health and disease: the eosinophil leucocyte (Part II). Eur Respir J 1994;7:743-60.

[3] Gleich GJ, Adolphson CR. The eosinophil leukocyte: structure and function. Adv Immunol 1986;39:177-253.

[4] Olsson I, Venge P. Cationic proteins of human granulocytes. I. Isolation of the cationic proteins of the granules of leukaemia myeloid cells. Blood 1974;44:235-46.

[5] Olsson I, Venge P, Spitznagel JK, Lehrer RI. Arginine-rich cationic proteins of human eosinophil granules. Comparison of the constituents of eosinophilic and neutrophilic leukocytes. Lab Invest 1997;36:493-500.

[6] Sur S, Glitz DG, Kita H, Kujawa SM, Peterson EA, Weiler DA, et al. Localization of eosinophil-derived neurotoxin and eosinophil cationic protein in neutrophilic leukocytes. J Leukoc Biol 1998;63:715-22.

[7] Monteseirín J, Vega A, Chacón P, Camacho MJ, El Bekay R, Asturias JA, et al. Neutrophils as a novel source of eosinophil cationic protein in IgE-mediated processes. J Immunol 2007;179:2634-41.

[8] Gleich GJ, Loegering DA, Bell MP, Checkel JL, Ackerman SJ, McKean DJ. Biochemical and functional similarities between human eosinophil-derived neurotoxin and eosinophil cationic protein: homology with ribonuclease. Proc Natl Acad Sci USA 1986;83:3146-50.

[9] Rosenberg HF, Domachowske JB. Eosinophils eosinophil ribonucleases and their role in host defense against respiratory virus pathogens. J Leukoc Biol 2001;70:691-8.

[10] Venge P, Bystrom J, Carlson M, Hakansson L, Karawacjzyk M, Peterson C, et al. Eosinophil cationic protein (ECP): molecular and biological properties and the use of ECP as a marker of eosinophil activation in disease. Clin Exp Allergy 1999;29:1172-86.

[11] Gleich GJ. Mechanisms of eosinophil-associated inflammation. J Allergy Clin Immunol 2000;105:651-63.

[12] Rot A, Krieger M, Brunner T, Bischoff SC, Schall TJ, Dahinden CA. RANTES and macrophage inflammatory protein 1 alpha induce the migration and activation of normal human eosinophil granulocytes. J Exp Med 1992;176:1489-95.

[13] Kita H, Abu-Ghazaleh RI, Sur S, Gleich GJ. Eosinophil major basic protein induces degranulation and IL-8 production by human eosinophils. J Immunol 1995;154:4749-58.

[14] Venge P, Roxin LE, Olsson I. Radioimmunoassay of human eosinophil cationic protein. Br J Haematol 1977;37:331-5.

[15] Wolthers OD, Heuck C. Circadian variations in serum eosinophil cationic protein and serum and urine eosinophil protein X. Pediatr Allergy Immunol 2003;14:130-3.

[16] Pin I, Gibson PG, Kolendowicz R, Girgis-Gabardo A, Denburg JA, Hargreave FE, et al. Use of induced sputum cell counts to investigate airway inflammation in asthma. Thorax 1992;47:25-9.

[17] Ronchi MC, Piragino C, Rosi E, Stendardi L, Tanini A, Galli G, et al. Do sputum eosinophils and ECP relate to the severity of asthma? Eur Respir J 1997;10:1809-13.

[18] Pizzichini E, Pizzichini MM, Efthimiadis A, Evans S, Morris MM, Squillace D, et al. Indices of airway inflammation in induced sputum: reproducibility and validity of cell and fluid-phase measurements. Am J Respir Crit Care Med 1996;154:308-17.

[19] Bacci E, Cianchetti S, Ruocco L, Bartoli ML, Carnevali S, Dente FL, et al. Comparison between eosinophilic markers in induced sputum and blood in asthmatic patients. Clin Exp Allergy 1998;28:1237-43.

[20] Spanevello A, Beghe B, Bianchi A, Migliori GB, Ambrosetti M, Neri M, et al. Comparison of two methods of processing induced sputum: selected versus entire sputum. Am J Respir Crit Care Med 1998;157:665-8.

[21] Bousquet J, Chanez P, Lacoste JY, Barnéon G, Ghavanian N, Enander I, et al. Eosinophilic inflammation in asthma. N Engl J Med 1990;323:1033-9.

[22] Azevedo I, de Blic J, Vargaftig BB, Bachelet M, Scheinmann P. Increased eosinophil cationic protein levels in bronchoalveolar lavage from wheezy infants. Pediatr Allergy Immunol 2001;12:65-72.

[23] Hällgren R, Bjermer L, Lundgren R, Venge P. The eosinophil component of the alveolitis in idiopathic pulmonary fibrosis. Signs of eosinophil activation in the lung are related to impaired lung function. Am Rev Respir Dis 1989;139:373-7.

[24] Janin A, Torpier G, Courtin P, Capron M, Prin L, Tonnel AB, et al. Segregation of eosinophil proteins in alveolar macrophage compartments in chronic eosinophilic pneumonia. Thorax 1993;48:57-62.

[25] Boomars KA, van Velzen-Blad H, Mulder PG, Koenderman L, Lammers JW, van den Bosch JM. Eosinophil cationic protein and immunoglobulin levels in bronchoalveolar lavage fluid obtained from patients with chronic eosinophilic pneumonia. Eur Respir J 1996;9:2488-93.

[26] Riise GC, Scherstén H, Nilsson F, Ryd W, Andersson BA. Activation of eosinophils and fibroblasts assessed by eosinophil cationic protein and hyaluronan in BAL. Association with acute rejection in lung transplant recipients. Chest 1996;110:89-96.

[27] Dosanjh AK, Elashoff D, Kawalek A, Moss RB, Esrig S. Activation of eosinophils in the airways of lung transplantation patients. Chest 1997;112:1180-3.

[28] Riise GC, Kjellström C, Ryd W, Scherstén H, Nilsson F, Mårtensson G, et al. Inflammatory cells and activation markers in BAL during acute rejection and infection in lung transplant recipients: a prospective longitudinal study. Eur Respir J 1997;10:1742-6.

[29] Walsh GM. Eosinophil granule proteins and their role in disease. Curr Opin Hematol 2001;8:28-33.

[30] Gibson PG, Norzila MZ, Fakes K, Simpson J, Henry RL. Pattern of airway inflammation and its determinants in children with acute severe asthma. Pediatr Pulmonol 1999;28:261-70.

[31] Venge P. Soluble markers of allergic inflammation. Allergy 1994;49:1-8.

[32] Raghavender B, Smith JB. Eosinophil cationic protein in tracheal aspirates of preterm infants with bronchopulmonary dysplasia. J Pediatrics 1997;130:944-7.

[33] Motojima S, Frigas E, Loegering DA, Gleich GJ. Toxicity of eosinophil cationic proteins for guinea pig tracheal epithelium in vitro. Am Rev Respir Dis 1989;139:801-5.

[34] Lundgren JD, Davey RT Jr, Lundgren B, Mullol J, Marom Z, Logun C, et al. Eosinophil cationic protein stimulates and major basic protein inhibits airway mucus secretion. J Allergy Clin Immunol 1991;87:689-98.

[35] Olszewska-Pazdrak B, Pazdrak K, Ogra PL, Garofalo RP. Respiratory syncytial virus-infected pulmonary epithelial cells induce eosinophil degranulation by a CD18-mediated mechanism. J Immunol 1998;160:4889-95.

[36] Kimpen JL, Garofalo R, Welliver RC, Ogra PL. Activation of human eosinophils in vitro by respiratory syncytial virus. Pediatr Res 1992;32:160-4.

[37] Kimpen JL, Garofalo R, Welliver RC, Fujihara K, Ogra PL. An ultrastructural study of the interaction of human eosinophils with respiratory syncytial virus. Pediatr Allergy Immunol 1996;7:48-53.

[38] Martinez FD, Wright AL, Taussig LM, Holberg CJ, Halonen M, Morgan WJ. Asthma and wheezing in the first years of life. N Engl J Med 1995;332:133-8.

[39] Taussig LM, Wright AL, Holberg CJ, Halonen M, Morgan WJ, Martinez FD. Tucson children's respiratory study: 1980 to present. J Allergy Clin Immunol 2003;111:661-75.

[40] Stein RT, Martinez FD. Asthma phenotypes in childhood: lessons from an epidemiological approach. Paediatr Respir Rev 2004;5:155-61.

[41] Rusconi F, Galassi C, Corbo GM, Forastiere F, Biggeri A, Ciccone G, et al. Risk factors for early persistent and late-onset wheezing in young children. Am J Respir Crit Care Med 1999;160:1617-22.

[42] Young S, Arnott J, O'Keeffe PT, LeSouëf PN, Landau LI. The association between early lung function and wheezing during the first 2 yrs of life. Eur Respir J 2000;15:151-7.

[43] Holberg CJ, Wright AL, Martinez FD, Ray CG, Taussig LM, Lebowitz MD. Risk factors for respiratory syncytial virus-associated lower respiratory tract illnesses in the first year of life. Am J Epidemiol 1991;133:1135-51.

[44] Strachan DP, Cook DG. Health effects of passive smoking. 1. Parental smoking and lower respiratory illness in infancy and early childhood. Thorax 1997;52:905-14.

[45] Martinez FD, Morgan WJ, Wright AL, Holberg CJ, Taussig LM. Diminished lung function as a predisposing factor for wheezing respiratory illness in infants. N Engl J Med 1988;319:1112-7.

[46] Palmer LJ, Rye PJ, Gibson NA, Burton PR, Landau LI, LeSouëf PN. Airway responsiveness in early infancy predicts asthma lung function and respiratory symptoms by school age. Am J Respir Crit Care Med 2001;163:37-42.

[47] Martinez F, Godfrey S. Wheezing disorders in the preschool child. Pathophysiology and management. London: Martin Dunitz-Taylor Francis, 2003

[48] Illi S, von Mutius E, Lau S, Nickel R, Niggemann B, Sommerfeld C, et al. The pattern of atopic sensitization is associated with the development of asthma in childhood. J Allergy Clin Immunol 2001;108:709-14.

[49] Garofalo R, Dorris A, Ahlstedt S, Welliver RC. Peripheral blood eosinophil counts and eosinophil cationic protein content of respiratory secretions in bronchiolitis: relationship to severity of disease. Pediatr Allergy Immunol 1994;5:111-7.

[50] Garofalo R, Kimpen JL, Welliver RC, Ogra PL. Eosinophil degranulation in the respiratory tract during naturally acquired respiratory syncytial virus infection. J Pediatrics 1992;120:28-32.

[51] Colocho Zelaya EA, Orvell C, Strannegård O. Eosinophil cationic protein in nasopharyngeal secretions and serum of infants infected with respiratory syncytial virus. Pediatr Allergy Immunol 1994;5:100-6.

[52] Sung RY, Hui SH, Wong CK, Lam CW, Yin J. A comparison of cytokine responses in respiratory syncytial virus and influenza A infections in infants. Eur J Pediatr 2001;160:117-22.

[53] Rakes GP, Arruda E, Ingram JM, Hoover GE, Zambrano JC, Hayden FG, et al. Rhinovirus and respiratory syncytial virus in wheezing children requiring emergency care. IgE and eosinophil analyses. Am J Respir Crit Care Med 1999;159:785-90.

[54] Pifferi M, Ragazzo V, Caramella D, Baldini G. Eosinophil cationic protein in infants with respiratory syncytial virus bronchiolitis: predictive value for subsequent development of persistent wheezing. Pediatr Pulmonol 2001;31:419-24.

[55] Counil FP, Lebel B, Segondy M, Peterson C, Voisin M, Bousquet J, et al. Cells and mediators from pharyngeal secretions in infants with acute wheezing episodes. Eur Respir J 1997;10:2591-5.

[56] Priftis KN, Papadopoulou A, Liatsis E, Katsikas D, Nicolaidou P, Kanariou M. Serum eosinophil cationic protein and CD23 in acute RSV bronchiolitis. Med Sci Monit 2005;11:CR493-7.

[57] Ingram JM, Rakes GP, Hoover GE, Platts-Mills TA, Heymann PW. Eosinophil cationic protein in serum and nasal washes from wheezing infants and children. J Pediatrics 1995;127:558-64.

[58] Frischer T, Halmerbauer G, Gartner C, Rath R, Tauber E, Schierl M, et al. Eosinophil-derived proteins in nasal lavage fluid of neonates of allergic parents and the development of respiratory symptoms during the first 6 months of life. Collaborative SPACE team. Study on the Prevention of Allergy in Children in Europe. Allergy 2000;55:773-7.

[59] Reijonen TM, Korppi M, Kleemola M, Savolainen K, Kuikka L, Mononen I, et al. Nasopharyngeal eosinophil cationic protein in bronchiolitis: relation to viral findings and subsequent wheezing. Pediatr Pulmonol 1997;24:35-41.

[60] Nagayama Y, Tsubaki T, Toba T, Nakayama S, Kiyofumi O. Analysis of sputum taken from wheezy and asthmatic infants and children with special reference to respiratory infections. Pediatr Allergy Immunol 2001;12:318-26.

[61] Shields MD, Brown V, Stevenson EC, Fitch PS, Schock BC, Turner G, et al. Serum eosinophilic cationic protein and blood eosinophil counts for the prediction of the presence of airways inflammation in children with wheezing. Clin Exp Allergy 1999;29:1382-9.

[62] Villa JR, García G, Rueda S, Nogales A. Serum eosinophilic cationic protein may predict clinical course of wheezing in young children. Arch Dis Child 1998;78:448-52.

[63] Koller DY, Wojnarowski C, Herkner KR, Weinländer G, Raderer M, Eichler I, et al. High levels of eosinophil cationic protein in wheezing infants predict the development of asthma. J Allergy Clin Immunol 1997;99:752-6.

[64] Reijonen TM, Korppi M, Kuikka L, Savolainen K, Kleemola M, Mononen I, et al. Serum eosinophil cationic protein as a predictor of wheezing after bronchiolitis. Pediatr Pulmonol 1997;23:397-403.

[65] Reijonen TM, Korppi M. One-year follow-up of young children hospitalized for wheezing: the influence of early anti-inflammatory therapy and risk factors for subsequent wheezing and asthma. Pediatr Pulmonol 1998;26:113-9.

[66] Øymar K, Bjerknes R. Is serum eosinophil cationic protein in bronchiolitis a predictor of asthma? Pediatr Allergy Immunol 1998;9:204-7.

[67] Sigurs N, Bjarnason R, Sigurbergsson F. Eosinophil cationic protein in nasal secretion and in serum and myeloperoxidase in serum in respiratory syncytial virus bronchiolitis: relation to asthma and atopy. Acta Paediatr 1994;83:1151-5.

[68] Kim CK, Kim JT, Kang H, Yoo Y, Koh YY. Sputum eosinophilia in cough-variant asthma as a predictor of the subsequent development of classic asthma. Clin Exp Allergy 2003;33:1409-14.

[69] Marguet C, Dean TP, Basuyau JP, Warner JO. Eosinophil cationic protein and interleukin-8 levels in bronchial lavage fluid from children with asthma and infantile wheeze. Pediatr Allergy Immunol 2001;12:27-33.

[70] Ferguson AC, Vaughan R, Brown H, Curtis C. Evaluation of serum eosinophilic cationic protein as a marker of disease activity in chronic asthma. J Allergy Clin Immunol 1995;95:23-8.

[71] Vanto T, Koskinen P. Serum eosinophil cationic protein in the evaluation of asthma severity in children. Allergy 1998;53:415-9.

[72] Gibson PG, Simpson JL, Hankin R, Powell H, Henry RL. Relationship between induced sputum eosinophils and the clinical pattern of childhood asthma. Thorax 2003;58:116-21.

[73] Zubovic I, Rozmanic V, Ahel V, Banac S. Manifold significance of serum eosinophil cationic protein in asthmatic children. Acta Med Croatica 2002;56:53-6.

[74] Carlson M, Håkansson L, Peterson C, Stålenheim G, Venge P. Secretion of granule proteins from eosinophils and neutrophils is increased in asthma. J Allergy Clin Immunol 1991;87:27-33.

[75] Durham SR, Loegering DA, Dunnette S, Gleich GJ, Kay AB. Blood eosinophils and eosinophil-derived proteins in allergic asthma. J Allergy Clin Immunol 1989;84:931-6.

[76] Zimmerman B, Enander I, Zimmerman R, Ahlstedt S. Asthma in children less than 5 years of age: eosinophils and serum levels of the eosinophil proteins ECP and EPX in relation to atopy and symptoms. Clin Exp Allergy 1994;24:149-55.

[77] Zimmerman B, Lanner A, Enander I, Zimmerman RS, Peterson CG, Ahlstedt S. Total blood eosinophils serum eosinophil cationic protein and eosinophil protein X in childhood asthma: relation to disease status and therapy. Clin Exp Allergy 1993;23:564-70.

[78] Koller DY, Halmerbauer G, Frischer T, Roithner B. Assessment of eosinophil granule proteins in various body fluids: is there a relation to clinical variables in childhood asthma? Clin Exp Allergy 1999;29:786-93.

[79] Hoekstra MO, Hovenga H, Gerritsen J, Kauffman HF. Eosinophils and eosinophil-derived proteins in children with moderate asthma. Eur Respir J 1996;9:2231-5.

[80] Ennis M, Turner G, Schock BC, Stevenson EC, Brown V, Fitch PS, et al. Inflammatory mediators in bronchoalveolar lavage samples from children with and without asthma. Clin Exp Allergy 1999;29:362-6.

[81] Carlsen KH, Halvorsen R, Pettersen M, Carlsen KC. Inflammation markers and symptom activity in children with bronchial asthma. Influence of atopy and eczema. Pediatr Allergy Immunol 1997;8:112-20.

[82] Krug N, Napp U, Enander I, Eklund E, Rieger CH, Schauer U. Intracellular expression and serum levels of eosinophil peroxidase (EPO) and eosinophil cationic protein in asthmatic children. Clin Exp Allergy 1999;29:1507-15.

[83] Gruber W, Eber E, Pfleger A, Modl M, Meister I, Weinhandl E, et al. Serum eosinophil cationic protein and bronchial responsiveness in pediatric and adolescent asthma patients. Chest 1999;116:301-5.

[84] de Meer G, Postma DS, Janssen NA, de Jongste JC, Brunekreef B. Bronchial hyper-responsiveness to hypertonic saline and blood eosinophilic markers in 8-13-year-old schoolchildren. Clin Exp Allergy 2004;34:1226-31.

[85] Choi SH, Kim DK, Yu J, Yoo Y, Koh YY. Bronchial responsiveness to methacholine and adenosine 5'-monophosphate in young children with asthma: their relationship with blood eosinophils and serum eosinophil cationic protein. Allergy 2007;62:1119-24.

[86] Lönnkvist K, Hellman C, Lundahl J, Halldén G, Hedlin G. Eosinophil markers in blood serum and urine for monitoring the clinical course in childhood asthma: impact of budesonide treatment and withdrawal. J Allergy Clin Immunol 2001;107:812-7.

[87] Juntunen-Backman K, Järvinen P, Sorva R. Serum eosinophil cationic protein during treatment of asthma in children. J Allergy Clin Immunol 1993;92:34-8.

[88] Sorva R, Metso T, Turpeinen M, Juntunen-Backman K, Björksten F, Haahtela T. Eosinophil cationic protein in induced sputum as a marker of inflammation in asthmatic children. Pediatr Allergy Immunol 1997;8:45-50.

[89] Prehn A, Seger RA, Faber J, Torresani T, Molinari L, Gerber A, et al. The relationship of serum eosinophil cationic protein and eosinophil count to disease activity in children with bronchial asthma. Pediatr Allergy Immunol 1998;9:197-203.

[90] Wolthers OD, Heuck C. Impact of age and administration regimens on the suppressive effect of inhaled glucocorticoids on eosinophil markers in children with asthma. Pediatr Asthma Allergy Immunol 2004;17:45-51.

[91] Lönnkvist K, Anderson M, Hedlin G, Svartengren M. Exhaled NO and eosinophil markers in blood nasal lavage and sputum in children with asthma after withdrawal of budesonide. Pediatr Allergy Immunol 2004;15:351-8.

[92] Prehn A, Seger RA, Torresani T, Molinari L, Gerber A, Sennhauser FH. Evaluation of a clinical algorithm involving serum eosinophil cationic protein for guiding the anti-inflammatory treatment of bronchial asthma in childhood. Pediatr Allergy Immunol 2000;11:87-94.
[93] Volovitz B, Tabachnik E, Nussinovitch M, Shtaif B, Blau H, Gil-Ad I, et al. Montelukast a leukotriene receptor antagonist reduces the concentration of leukotrienes in the respiratory tract of children with persistent asthma. J Allergy Clin Immunol 1999;104:1162-7.
[94] Hoekstra MO, Grol MH, Hovenga H, Bouman K, Stijnen T, Koëter GH, et al. Eosinophil and mast cell parameters in children with stable moderate asthma. Pediatr Allergy Immunol 1998;9:143-9.
[95] Castro M, Ramirez MI, Gern JE, Cutting G, Redding G, Hagood JS, et al. Strategic plan for pediatric respiratory diseases research: an NHLBI working group report. Pediatr Pulmonol 2009;44:2-13.

Submitted: December 29, 2008.
Revised: February 05, 2009.
Accepted: February 17, 2009.

In: Public Health Yearbook 2009
Editor: Joav Merrick
ISBN: 978-1-61668-911-7

Chapter 11

ARE WHO/EURO SYSTEM FRAMEWORK FUNCTIONS APPLICABLE TO PUBLIC HEALTH SERVICES?

Itamar Grotto, MD, MPH, PhD*[1,2] and Alex Leventhal, MD, MPH, MPA[3,4]

[1]Public Health Services, Ministry of Health, Jerusalem, Israel
[2]Ben-Gurion University of the Negev, Beer-Sheva, Israel
[3]Department of International Relations, Ministry of Health, Jerusalem, Israel
[4]Braun School of Public Health, Hebrew University, Jerusalem, Israel

Abstract

In the World Health Report of 2000 a new concept was introduced, which gained acceptance among health policy scientists and the various World Health Organization agencies. This concept has been called the Four Health System Framework Functions: resource generation, financing, stewardship and service provision. These functions are interlinked and suppose to determine the way inputs are transformed to outcomes in health systems and have become the working language of policy makers and scholars, while they are not common for public health professionals. In this paper we deal with the applicability of the Four Health System Framework Functions for assessing and reforming Public Health Services (PHS). We suggest a model for this application in order to allow a discussion, which could provide a practical frame for systematic PHS assessment and planning of specific goals, objectives and interventions for efficient use of outputs and reform interventions at the public health level.

Keywords: Public health, health systems.

* Correspondence: Itamar Grotto MD, MPH, PhD, Israel Ministry of Health PO Box 1176, Jerusalem 91010, Israel. Tel: 972 2 6247850; Fax: 972 2 6233058; E-mail: itamar.grotto@moh.health.gov.il

Introduction

The World Health Report of 2000 (1) devoted entirely to health systems introduced a new concept that gained acceptance among health policy scientists and various World Health Organization (WHO) regional offices. This new concept was called the Four Health System Framework Functions, which are interlinked and supposed to determine the way inputs are transformed to outcomes in health systems. The Function of "service provision" is listed with the three other Functions of: resource generation, financing, and stewardship. The integration of these Four Health System Framework Functions is needed for developing human, material and conceptual resources – required for the system to work. It enables mobilizing and channeling financing, and ensures that the individuals and organizations that compose the health system act as good stewards of the resources and trust given to the health services provided by them,

Application to Public Health Services (PHS)

The above mentioned terms of the World Health Report 2000 has become the working language of policy makers and scholars, while they are not common concepts/language for public health professionals. For instance the European Region of WHO has incorporated these functions into its working environment over the past few years and in 2008 the European ministerial conference of the WHO/Euro on "health systems, health and wealth" also mentioned these functions and they became the core of "The Tallinn Charter" (2) accepted by all member states.

In this paper we deal with the applicability of the Four Health System Framework Functions for assessing and reforming PHS. Since we are of the opinion that public health academics and professionals should consider to apply these functions to the public health vocabulary and thinking, we suggest a modified or applied model as described in figure 1.

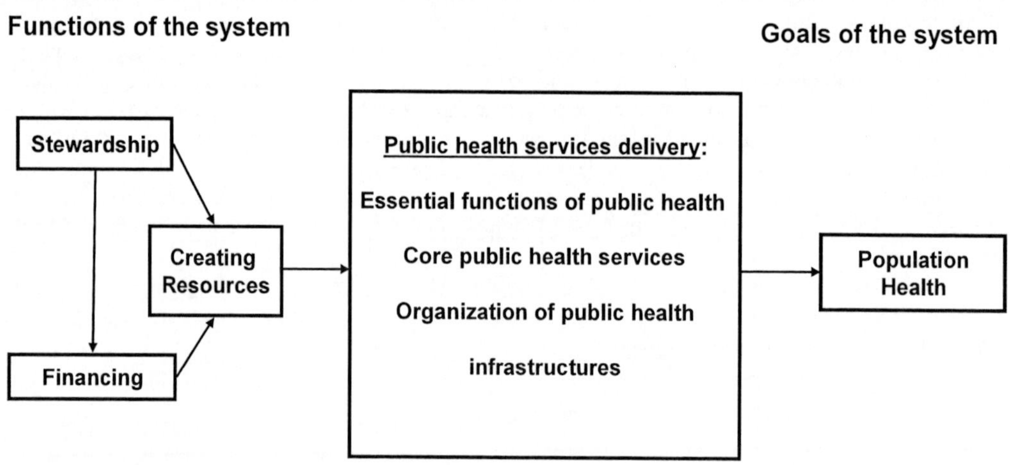

Figure 1. The health system framework functions in public health.

The "service delivery function" is the core of PHS delivery and has been intensely discussed previously and includes the "essential public health operations" and the "core public health services", which determine the organizational infrastructure of PHS. However, the public health arena involves not only delivery of services, but requires also a high-quality performance of the three other functions: stewardship, resource generation and financing.

This paper will focus on the application of these three other functions to PHS in order to allow a discussion that could provide a practical frame for systematic PHS assessment and planning of specific goals, objectives and interventions. We will also consider the efficient use of outputs and reform interventions at the public health functions level.

Stewardship in public health

Stewardship has recently been defined as a “function of a government responsible for the welfare of the population and concerned about the trust and legitimacy with which its activities are viewed by the citizenry"(1,3). Although other sectors play a part in promoting the health of the population, the government has the most important stewardship role in public health. The government as a whole and the Ministry of Health as its "health agency" are defining strategic health policy directions, which is a central public health duty. The government has the responsibility for the legislative and regulatory framework for public health (4) and the tools for implementing it e.g. adequate and modern health information system (5). It will enable the PHS to monitor the health system performance in order to ensure accountability and transparency. This stewardship role is essential to make possible the attainment of each health system goal and improving health of the public, which is the legitimate expectation of the population. The roles of government as a steward in public health include:

- Development of public health policies and plans that promote and protect population health.
- Health protection: advancement of legislation, control and enforcement of laws and regulations in public health.
- Supervision of delivery of PHS.
- Creation of partnership (coalitions) for encouraging public health knowledge and practice, synchronization and efficient resource allocation.
- Support research in public health.

Creating resources in public health

The resource function is dealing in general with the resources required for the operation of the health system. It includes human, material, technological and conceptual resources that are essential not only to deliver services, but also having an important role in the other two basic functions of the health system – financing and stewardship.

In the application of "creating resources" for public health one should note that public health requires more than ever before both personnel and infrastructure in order to cope with the new challenges imposed on its workforce in the last decade. The resources that are needed for public health include:

- Development and education of the human resources in public health.
- Development and maintenance of laboratory resources.
- Production and/or purchasing of public health supplies such as childhood and adult vaccines, chemo-prophylactic agents, iron, vitamins and food supplementation and screening tests for early detection of diseases.
- Applying information technology resources.

Financing in public health

The purpose of health financing as one of the functions is to make funding available, as well as to set the right financial incentives for providers, to ensure that all individuals have access to effective public health and personal health care. Applying "financing" to public health should be based on the following principles:

- Social solidarity, equity and financial protection as core values (6).
- Universal coverage, equity in access and distribution of public health services and benefits according to need.
- Regulation and dissemination of information to the public health services providers and the public (transparency).
- Sources include domestic public funds, domestic private funds, external public funds and external private funds.

The "financing" function in the World Health Report 2000 included three interrelated sub-functions: revenue collection, pooling of resources, and purchasing of interventions. The following is their application to public health:

- Revenue collection is the process by which the public health system raises and secures sufficient funds. Regulation and legislation should secure that appropriate financial resources are allocated for public health to cover specified public health services and to regulate proportion of the health budget that should be allocated to public health. This is done by setting up a budget that is separated from the overall health budget – the "ring fence" mechanism (7) and secure differential funding for public health services according to its cost.
- Pooling is the accumulation and management of revenues in such a way as to ensure that the risk of having to pay for public health services is borne by all the members of the pool and not by each contributor individually. The pooling of the resources designated for public health services will allow the application of the following principles of public health: 1) Social solidarity and equity, 2) Contribution according to ability to make a payment and 3) Universal coverage, equity in access and distribution of services and benefits according to need. A large-scale governmental pool will allow the policymakers to prioritize public health interventions at the

national level. Insurance-based pooling will allow health-care providers to provide high-cost individual preventive health services to the entire population.

- Strategic purchasing where purchasing is the process by which pooled funds are paid to providers in order to deliver various public health interventions to maximize population health outcomes (strategic purchasing) as well as setting up provider payment systems that offer them incentives to perform better.

The Challenge

We believe it is important that public health professionals start to deal with the World Health Report 2000. The leadership of the European Region of WHO has adapted this new vocabulary of the four functions in its documents and strategic planning. On an initial glance these functions seemed remote from the public health culture and thinking, because of the stress on the economic part, as is expressed in the terms of stewardship, resource generation and financing. But as we have worked on these terms in order to try and fit them into an upgrading and reforming PHS, it has become clear to us that these functions makes sense. However, in public health we are talking about "essential public health functions" (8) that are different from the Four Health System Framework Functions and we argue that two of them can fit in a modular way, as we have elaborated in this article. In order not to mix between these two sets of functions maybe the suggestion would be to call them "essential public health operations" . In this paper we would like to challenge it and to put it forward for discussion and debate.

References

[1] The World Health Report 2000. Health systems: improving performance. Geneva: World Health Organization, 2000.

[2] The Tallinn Charter. Health system for health and wealth, 2008 Jun 27. http://www.euro.who.int/document/e91438.pdf. accessed on 2008 Dec 30.

[3] World report on knowledge for better health. Strengthening health systems. Geneva: World Health Organization, 2004.

[4] Beaglehole R, Bonita R, Horton R, Adams O, McKee M. Public health in the new era: improving health through collective action. Lancet 2004;363:2084-6.

[5] AbouZahr C, Boerma T. Health information system: the foundation of public health. Bull World Health Organ 2005;83:578-83.

[6] The Ljubljana Charter on reforming health care. Ljubljana, 1996.

[7] Durham G, Kill B. Public health funding mechanisms in New Zealand. Aust Health Rev 1999;22:100-12.

[8] WHO Regional office for the Western Pacific. Essential public health functions: The role of Ministries of Health. Kyoto, Japan: Regional Comm WPR/RC53/10, 2002.

Submitted: January 01, 2009.
Revised: February 15, 2009.
Accepted: February 19, 2009.

In: Public Health Yearbook 2009
Editor: Joav Merrick
ISBN: 978-1-61668-911-7

Chapter 12

ADVANCING YOUTH TOBACCO USE CESSATION IN DEVELOPING COUNTRIES: PRACTICAL CONSIDERATIONS

Steve Sussman, PhD* and David S. Black, MPH
Institute for Health Promotion and Disease Prevention Research, Departments of Preventive Medicine and Psychology, University of Southern California, Alhambra, California, United States of America

Abstract

Tobacco use is a major public health concern among youth in developing countries, and it is a leading cause of behavior-related morbidity and mortality. Although youth tobacco use cessation efforts appear to almost double quit rates among youth, and have increased in the United States and some European countries, few cessation efforts have been initiated in developing countries. This paper provides general guidelines for initiating and advancing teen tobacco use cessation research and practice in developing countries. Initially, countries' larger social climate needs to be prepared for youth tobacco use cessation efforts, which requires recognition that tobacco use cessation programming is needed, and adequate resources such as funding and training. Subsequently, effective cessation programming targeting tobacco-using youth needs to be developed, implemented, evaluated, and institutionalized. Guidance and examples are provided for each step.

Keywords: Tobacco cessation, international, smoking, developing countries, adolescents.

* Correspondence: Steve Sussman, PhD, FAAHB, FAPA, Professor of Preventive Medicine and Psychology, Institute for Health Promotion and Disease Prevention Research, University of Southern California, 1000 S Fremont Avenue, Unit 8, Alhambra, CA 91803, United States. E-mail: ssussma@usc.edu

Introduction

Tobacco use is the most prevalent behavioral cause of death in the world (1). Tobacco use mortality includes deaths resulting from cancers of the lungs, oral cavity, nasal cavity, pancreas, stomach, and liver, bronchitis, cardiovascular disease, pneumonia, emphysema, and other diseases (1). In high-income countries such as the United States, tobacco use prevalence is on the decline, but in many low-to-middle income countries, tobacco use prevalence is rising (2). The burdens of tobacco use are disproportionately exacted on developing countries where 84% of the 1.3 billion current smokers reside (3). Worldwide, WHO attributes about five million deaths per year to tobacco use, and this figure is expected to double to about ten million deaths in just over a decade, with seven million of these deaths occurring in developing countries (4). Current tobacco use cessation programming appears to almost double cessation among youth compared to persons not exposed to cessation programming (5). These efforts will need to be a priority in developing countries if substantial reductions in tobacco-related morbidity and mortality are to be achieved.

Based on the Global Youth Tobacco Survey (GYTS) (6), which assesses 13-to-15 year old youths in school settings around the world, just under 10% of youths are current cigarette smokers, and over 10% currently use tobacco products other than cigarettes. These cigarette alternatives include cigar and tobacco pipes, kreteks (clove cigarettes), chuttas (handmade filtered cigars smoked by placing the lit end inside the mouth), water pipes (e.g., hookahs), bidis (tobacco in hand-rolled dried leaves), and smokeless tobacco (tobacco that is consumed orally or nasally) (7). Beyond prevalence estimates, and consequences of long-term use, the need for tobacco use cessation efforts among youth in developing countries is evident for at least three other reasons. First, there is a relatively steep daily smoking inflexion curve evident during the teen years (see http://www.globaltreatmentpartnership.org/treatment_case.html) (8). This inflexion curve suggests that the adolescent years are a critical period for implementation of tobacco use cessation programming, before the tobacco use habit becomes much more firmly embedded in memory. Second, internationally, a large proportion of young tobacco users (60-85%) are likely to have made at least one quit attempt and failed (9-13). Most youth appear unable to quit on willpower alone (14); this suggests a need for formalized cessation programming.

Finally, the tobacco industry has made recent attempts to capitalize on the physiological vulnerabilities of youth through promoting tobacco uptake in developing countries with marketing and advertisement campaigns (15). Tobacco industry documents indicate a desire for global penetration in markets throughout Europe, Asia and Africa (16). From 1993 to 1996, exports of tobacco products increased by 42% coupled by a 5% increase in international consumption (17). Partly in response to the expansion of the World Trade Organization's Global Agreement on Tariffs and Trade (GATT) to agricultural products in 1994, which opened international trade as a non-discriminatory enterprise, tobacco industries now are operating as transnational organizations that have been able to provide tobacco products at relatively lower prices, team up with local growers, provide incentives to local storeowners, and market themes of sophistication, wealth, or attractiveness that compose a global cosmopolitan cultural demand for tobacco products (17,18). Moreover, trade liberalization has been associated with increased cigarette smoking, particularly in low to middle-income countries (19). Thus, tobacco industry efforts are likely to increase tobacco use prevalence and need for cessation programming among youth in developing countries. There are few documented youth tobacco use cessation efforts in developing countries; this lack of programming is discussed in the next section.

International youth tobacco use cessation efforts

Evidence from a recent empirical review of teen tobacco use cessation, which examined an exhaustive sample of 64 evaluated youth cessation trials with comparison groups (11), published in the English language, highlight the dearth of cessation programming efforts in developing countries. The review found only 17 studies completed outside of the US (four from Australia, three from Canada, one from China, one from Finland, two from New Zealand, one from Singapore, one from Switzerland, and four from the UK). Results of cessation programming failed to vary systematically by whether or not data were obtained from samples in the US. However, these eight countries all were of high per capita income, aside from China. One recent study documented implementation of tobacco use cessation programs in nine Southeast Asian developing countries (20). Cessation treatment was mostly available only in hospitals and primary care settings, and appeared to be targeted primarily at adults.

International organizations have developed guidelines that may assist in initiating youth tobacco use cessation efforts. In particular, in 2003, member countries of the World Health Organization (WHO) adopted the Framework Convention on Tobacco Control (FCTC). The FCTC is an international-based agreement that commits countries to adopt strong tobacco control policies. To become binding agreements, countries must ratify the agreement. The FCTC officially entered into force in 2005, and as of January 2009, a total of 168 WHO member states have signed the treaty, and 161 of those signatories have become parties to the treaty (21). The FCTC adopts an institutional mechanism of public monitoring of compliance, and has raised the profile of tobacco control internationally to a high level of visibility.

The FCTC contains 38 articles, which lay out the treaty provisions (see www.fctc.org). Some key articles developed from the FCTC include taxation, large warning labels, no smoking policies, restrictions on advertisements, restrictions on selling tobacco to youth, and tobacco education, cessation, and activism efforts (18).

Articles directly mentioning tobacco cessation efforts include Articles 4, 12, and 14. Article 14 provides the most input on cessation efforts; FCTC recommendations are provided in table 1.

Although tobacco cessation efforts do not explicitly refer to youth within the FCTC articles, many of these regulations may help decrease youth tobacco use (11, 22). Many developing countries have been involved in the World No Tobacco Day (the 2008 campaign focused on the multi-billion dollar efforts of tobacco companies to attract young people to its addictive products through marketing) and the 'Quit and Win Campaign' (an international smoking cessation competition to motivate primarily adult smokers to quit). These events could influence tobacco cessation through increasing motivation to quit, quit attempts, and use of cessation social support (23). However, since only a few isolated programs have targeted youth in developing countries, we suggest that several steps should be taken to initiate and maintain use of this type of programming.

The following sections outline a protocol to be considered when creating teen tobacco use cessation work in developing countries. It is beyond the scope of this paper to detail all efforts required for effective youth tobacco cessation programming; however, six general steps for tobacco use cessation endeavors are provided (see Appendix for further details on the six steps).

Table 1. Article 14 Cessation Efforts of the FCTC

(a)	Design and implement effective programmes aimed at promoting the cessation of tobacco use, in such locations as educational institutions, health care facilities, workplaces and sporting environments
(b)	Include diagnosis and treatment of tobacco dependence and counseling services on cessation of tobacco use in national health and education programmes, plans and strategies, with the participation of health workers, community workers and social workers as appropriate
(c)	Establish in health care facilities and rehabilitation centres programmes for diagnosing, counseling, preventing and treating tobacco dependence
(d)	Collaborate with other Parties to facilitate accessibility and affordability for treatment of tobacco dependence including pharmaceutical products pursuant to Article 22. Such products and their constituents may include medicines, products used to administer medicines and diagnostics when appropriate

Preparing the social climate for teen cessation

Initially, the social environment in a country needs to be prepared to support youth tobacco use cessation programming. National and local governments in developing countries may not recognize the extent of the problem of tobacco use among youth in their country. Creating awareness of the public health problem of youth tobacco use can be accomplished through the collection and provision of data from developing countries that demonstrates the prevalence of teen smoking, and youths' desire to quit. The World Health Organization (WHO) and Centers for Disease Control and Prevention's (CDC) Office on Smoking and Health developed the Global Youth Tobacco Survey (GYTS) as a surveillance tool to track tobacco use among young people across countries using a common methodology and core questionnaire. The GYTS is now the largest global surveillance system for any major public health risk, is operational in over 150 international locations and has completed questionnaires on over one million young people between the ages of 13 and 15 years in randomly selected schools (6,24). Through assessments such as the GYTS, several countries have established that there exists a problem with youth tobacco use (cigarettes, smokeless tobacco, bidis, clove cigarettes) within their country, and that a large percentage of young smokers have tried to quit and have failed (e.g., Barbados, China, Costa Rica, Fiji, Jordan, India, Kenya, Nepal, South Africa, Sri Lanka, Tanzania, Thailand, Venezuela, Zambia, Zimbabwe; 9,13,25-29).

Another aspect of preparing the large social environment is to achieve an understanding of the difficulties youth may face when trying to quit. Measures might include the cultural/social context of tobacco use, and using/quitting motives and barriers. Some of these data have been collected with the GYTS. These data indicate that 10% to 50% of youth use tobacco at their home or the home of a friend (13). Depending on the country, 20% to 60% of teen tobacco users purchase their tobacco (illegally) themselves at a store. A majority have been exposed repeatedly to tobacco advertisements and promotional events, and many perceive smokers as being more socially popular among peers (13,26). It appears that, in general, adults tend to ignore youth tobacco use. Interestingly, these social-based reasons for tobacco use appear to be universal (30). Teen quit attempts in developing countries appear to be related to having anti-tobacco use attitudes, lower levels of tobacco use, relatively high tobacco cessation self-efficacy, less pocket money, and a relatively more supportive non-smoking social environment; these are also apparently universal reasons for quitting (13,26,27,30).

Still, country-specific reasons for youth tobacco use or quitting should be considered. For example, tobacco may be used as a reflection of ritual, such as in ceremonies or as gifts, as a way to cope with hunger, and as an expression of male prowess, which may vary in importance by specific country or group (e.g., many American Indian nations view tobacco as sacred and use it in ceremonies) (31). Rebellion against male control may lead females to engage in smoking as an unhealthy expression of liberation, which can be capitalized on by the tobacco industry (13,32). Youth may be more motivated to quit if, as examples, commercial tobacco use is differentiated from ritual-based tobacco use (the latter which may not have to be smoked) (31), or if personal liberation was contrasted directly with nicotine dependence (an alternative expression of lack of freedom) .

Anti-tobacco activist activity is essential to get key messages publicized and change attitudes in the large social environment, which may subsequently facilitate teen tobacco use cessation activities. For example, Essential Action is an international anti-tobacco use activism organization that facilitates global partnerships for tobacco control (www.essential action.org). Key activist messages include confronting tobacco industry tactics, emphasizing dangers of tobacco use and international consensus on the FCTC, discussing the difficulties of breaking a nicotine addiction (and relying more on assistance and less on ignoring use or punishing teen use), and emphasizing the importance of quitting tobacco use while one is young (32).

Resource acquisition

A second step involves a consideration of the need each country has for resources to develop youth cessation programming (see Appendix). These resources include informational, financial, and technical assistance. Health care providers in developing countries often lack the knowledge and skills to delivers tobacco cessation interventions, and tobacco cessation education is often lacking from medical school curricula, even directed at adults (33). Some tobacco cessation and treatment information tailored for adults is contained on the Web (www.fctc.org), and this information may possibly be adapted for youth. Moreover, reliable tobacco cessation information for youths may be found on the Youth Tobacco Cessation Collaborative (YTCC) website (http://www.youthtobaccocessation.org/).

Developing countries often lack the financial power to develop an effective social and public health infrastructure, which can provide youth with wide-reaching tobacco cessation programming. Proven but expensive programs such as mass media campaigns, telephone quit lines, and insurance or government subsidized coverage for treatment and pharmaceutical medication (medications currently are not indicated for teens) (11) may be especially difficult to implement in low income countries (34). However, several funding mechanisms currently exist that may support work on youth tobacco use cessation, dependence, and cessation including the World Health Organization (WHO), Centers for Disease Control and Prevention (CDC), United Nations, World Bank, Non-Governmental Organizations (NGOs), and Save the Children Foundation. Moreover, international efforts of various countries (e.g., US [NIH-Fogarty, USAID], Netherlands, Canada), national efforts, and grassroots efforts (donations, activism) may provide resources for youth tobacco use cessation efforts.

Policy makers, health care workers and cessation programmers in developing countries require education and training to acquire resources such as grant money and program implementation and evaluation skills. One option to consider is the National Institutes of Health Fogarty Center program (NIHFC). The NIHFC is a granting agency that provides assistance to reduce the burden of tobacco use in low to middle income countries. The program is designed to promote international collaboration between investigators in high-income nations pursuing research programs on tobacco control, and scientists and institutions in low-to-middle income nations.

Moreover, program developers in low-to-middle income countries may contact youth tobacco use cessation program developers directly through e-mail and through program websites. Communication of this type may lead to research, technical assistance, and training or otherwise facilitate utilization of evidence-based programming. Program developers may also want to consult the evidence based tobacco use programming features located on the National Cancer Institute (NCI) or Substance Abuse and Mental Health Services (SAMHSA) websites (http://www.cancer.gov/cancertopics/smoking; http://www.modelprograms.samhsa.gov/). Moreover, identifying cessation programs implemented locally that better reflect countries' own cultures may result in a more expedient uptake of cessation programming; however, empirical validation of such programming is imperative.

Health care providers including physicians, pharmacists, nurses, therapists and healers in developing countries are a vital resource often not utilized for youth tobacco cessation efforts. However, they must be convinced that youth tobacco use is a problem and informed of treatment options. Helping providers understand that tobacco use is an addictive disease and that treatment options are available is the first step to engaging them in treatment. Also, educating students about tobacco use addiction and treatment in medical or public health schools will help mainstream cessation treatment. Studies have indicated that even simple advice to quit smoking from a reliable source may be effective in reducing tobacco use (1), and minimal interventions are relatively easy to teach to healthcare workers. Integration of tobacco use cessation into other healthcare programs such as HIV/AIDS, cancer treatment, family planning has been postulated relatively feasible and cost effective (34).

Youth tobacco cessation program development

A third step involves the use of appropriate youth tobacco cessation program development strategies. When planning a program, the developer needs to carefully consider the settings in which programming might be delivered (schools, homes, mass media, sports clubs, health centers). For example, important information regarding tobacco cessation can be transmitted through media channels such as television, radio, and newspapers. However, the limitations of each type of communication channel should be understood by the program developer such as the lack of active involvement of the viewer, as well as the current evidence base (11). As other examples, while delivery in urban areas may involve health educator visits to schools, or youth visits to local health clinics, program delivery in some rural areas may be more difficult. Transportation resources such as roving vans may be needed to travel from village to village. In some countries, involvement of village elders, tribal/village leaders, or traditional healers may be needed before programming can be delivered.

The participants for which programming will be directed needs to be specified prior to implementing an intervention since different youth may have different needs, and since programs are likely to be more effective if they are tailored to specific youth groups. For example, cessation programming for street youth (who tend to exhibit high smoking rates compared to youth residing in homes) will tend to be different from programming for general groups of adolescent smokers. For street youth, basic necessities may need to be offered for attendance at cessation clinics, as well as opportunities to help them transition into mainstream society (e.g., school enrollment, residential or community housing), whereas these more intensive treatments may not be needed with general groups of smokers.

Selecting a pre-existing evidence-based youth tobacco use cessation program may be the most efficient route for program translation. Tailoring these programs to the cultural lives of participants can be accomplished by conducting discussion groups with local teens. Focus groups of this type offer an opportunity to assess the perceived efficacy of a youth cessation program. Moreover, youth can provide helpful feedback regarding program components that are likely to fail when used with a specific cultural group. In addition, a cessation program may be implemented on a small-scale basis to assess its receptivity among youth in a given country (29,35).

The program developed internally or selected from elsewhere for translation should consist of empirically validated contents; that is, include motivation-enhancement plus cognitive behavioral strategies provided in a format engaging to youth (e.g., including local games) with at least five sessions (5,11). Support for the feasibility of these structural characteristics with youth has been documented in diverse samples in South Africa and the United Kingdom (27,36). Cessation program developers may adapt interventions to a developing country in minor but important ways. For example, names of characters depicted in program curriculum and materials may be refined to match appropriate cultural milieu. In addition, policy or other knowledge-based information (e.g., cost of obtaining tobacco, prevalence of use) should be localized (35).

Some tobacco prevention and youth cessation programs being translated to countries such as India and China are being delivered very similarly to the way they were in their country of origin (generally, the US), with intermediate results indicating high receptivity (29,35,37). These results may be due to the apparent universality of major tobacco use acquisition variables. Alternatively, a country may develop a very different type of program which retains some principles of evidence-based programming but which involves new types of strategies. For example, some attempts at youth tobacco use prevention have involved appeals to Buddhism, and have been provided by monks, in some areas of Thailand (Jeremiah Mock, personal communication, May 1, 2007) (18). However, much more work is needed to establish whether program translation in developing countries requires little rather than substantial change of original program content.

Youth tobacco cessation program implementation

A fourth step involves youth tobacco use cessation program implementation. The most complete international statement regarding tobacco prevention and control program implementation for youth was made subsequent to a conference in Singapore in September of 1999. The conference was titled, "International Consultation on Tobacco and Youth: What in the World Works?" The UN Convention on the Rights of the Child was mentioned, which frames tobacco promotion as an unethical antagonist to the child's right to attain the highest standards of health. Moreover, the creation of new policies (larger warning labels, bans on tobacco promotion, taxation, limits on youth access), anti-tobacco use marketing, coordinating mechanisms with community and international organizations, and technical expertise were mentioned as being needed components to implement (40). While the importance of youth cessation was stated in this report, and use of the mass media, youth empowerment, counteracting tobacco industry promotion, stress management, weight gain concerns, nicotine dependence issues, and tailoring cessation approaches to youth also were mentioned, the report did not provide any specific examples of evidence-based youth cessation program that might be implemented. Examples of successful implementation are needed to develop scientific understanding of the tobacco cessation program implementation process in developing countries.

The present state of the research suggests that youth tobacco cessation programming might best be delivered in a school-based context (e.g., 11); schools have served as a main modality for tobacco use intervention. Interestingly, according to the GYTS, more than half of students (57.6%) reported having been taught in school about the dangers of tobacco during the preceding school year (6). However, there remain many barriers to delivering health programming in a school context internationally, including lack of understanding of the importance of school health programs, inadequate coordination and lack of a sense of responsibility for student health among school staff, and lack of resources for complete implementation (8). Key areas to consider include the logistics of cost, time, and human resources required for the implementation of the intervention.

Regarding non-school based programs, there is an ongoing single group study by Chan and colleagues (38) in Hong Kong, which indicates notable cessation rates among teens that receive telephone counseling (17.5 mean intent-to-treat quit rate at 6-month follow-up among 12-to-25 year olds; no control group). Moreover, a recent cell phone text messaging intervention in New Zealand showed that this communication modality might serve as a future promising youth tobacco cessation intervention (nearly doubling quit rates compared to a control group at 3-months post-program, though effects deteriorated by 6-months post-program) (39).

Youth tobacco cessation program evaluation

A fifth step involves program evaluation. It is important that programs are evaluated based on scientific methods to assess the actual change in tobacco use behavior due to an intervention. Ideally, change in tobacco use should be assessed from baseline, immediately prior to providing cessation material, immediately after the program, and at multiple follow-up periods (e.g., 3, 6, 12 months). Several indicators of smoking cessation and reduction should be measured during these data collection points. For example, point-prevalence of tobacco use cessation (e.g., use in last 7-days; use in last 30-days), continual tobacco use cessation (cessation assessed across multiple time-points), reduction in tobacco use, and intention to quit tobacco use in the near future should be measured. Previously tested and valid measures similar to these are provided by Health Canada and can be found on the on the Youth Tobacco Cessation Collaborative (YTCC) website (http://www.youthtobaccocessation.org/). Cessation evaluation questionnaires may also be obtained by contacting youth cessation program developers (e.g., Project EX pretest-posttest questionnaires can be found on http://tnd.usc.edu/ex/index.php?sub_flag=7).

Institutionalizing youth cessation programming

The sixth step involves institutionalization of youth tobacco use cessation programs in a developing country. A country should enact policy that provides support for youth smoking cessation efforts, a safe setting for youth to go to quit their tobacco use, and enforcement of the existence of such settings. Policy implementation and enforcement generally involves cooperation among several groups including anti-tobacco activists, NGOs, public health professionals, and government officials. Monitoring of decision makers may be needed to ensure that votes are not biased due to influences from business interests such as the tobacco industry (32). Information on how countries have been institutionalizing the FCTC regulations might serve as a good model.

Conclusions

In 2004, the US Department of Health and Human Services published the first guide for making informed decisions regarding teen cigarette smoking cessation (http://www.cdc.gov /tobacco/quit_smoking/cessation/youth_tobacco_cessation/). The recommendations provide practitioners with information on how to select a cessation program, what contents to include, how to implement a program, and how to evaluate it. The applicability of these guidelines to developing countries has yet to be established. Yet, effective youth tobacco cessation efforts are needed soon to reduce rates of preventable morbidity and mortality. Concern is great for youth in developing countries since tobacco prices are low and tobacco industry campaign efforts have been targeted at the regions. This paper highlighted the need to further youth cessation programming research and practice in developing countries. In addition it provided general guidelines for advancing youth cessation program efforts and offered several current resources that are publicly available. The "big question" for consideration is whether cessation programming in developing countries can be implemented on a large scale in a way that will be acceptable by policy makers and the general public, sustainable and cost-effective. Researchers will be able to better examine effect sizes among the theories and modalities, and other variables, when there are a greater number of studies to represent the experiences of developing countries.

Acknowledgments

This paper was supported by grants from the National Institute on Drug Abuse (#sDA13814, DA016090, DA020138 and P50 DA16094).

Appendix: Six Steps to Consider When Trying to Establish Teen Tobacco Use Cessation in Developing Countries

Preparing the Large Social Environmental Climate	Consider why tobacco is being used in the country (e.g., cultural gift, deal with hunger, male prowess, advertisements and other social influences). Emphasize dangers of tobacco use. Emphasize the difficulties of breaking a nicotine addiction. Emphasize the importance of quitting tobacco use while one is young. Emphasize the international consensus on the FCTC. Through assessments such as the Global Youth Tobacco Survey (GYTS), establish that there is a problem with youth tobacco use in the country. Emphasize the importance of providing cessation programming rather than punishment. Create policy favorable to teen tobacco use cessation in the country.
Resources	NIH-Fogarty, USAID, WHO (GYTS), CDC (GYTS), UN, WB, NGOs, Save the Children Foundation, international efforts of various countries (e.g., U.S., Netherlands, Canada), national efforts, grassroots efforts (donations, activism). The provision of funding and technical assistance. Tobacco cessation & treatment information is contained on www.fctc.org and on http://www.youthtobaccocessation.org/, and the latter site contains the consensus report as well as other information.
Program Development	Consider the settings in which programming can be delivered (schools, home, mass media, sports clubs, health centers). Consider type of programming (self-help, 1:1 counseling, or groups). Locate evidence-based programs for possible translation. Assess perceived efficacy of program in discussion groups of teens. Select program for translation (probably motivation plus cognitive behavioral, at least 5 sessions). Adapt program to country, or retain some principles of program but develop new program.
Program Implementation	Consider implementation setting (urban/rural). Maximize reach, recruitment, and retention.
Program Evaluation	Assess change in tobacco use from baseline, just prior to the provision of cessation material, immediately after the program, and at follow-up (e.g., 3, 6, 12 months).
Program Institutionalization	After ratifying the FCTC, enact a policy that provides support for teen smoking cessation efforts, a safe setting for youth to go to quit tobacco use, and enforce the existence of such settings.

Note. All web sites were last accessed on January 1, 2009.

References

[1] Fiore MC, Bailey WC, Cohen SJ, Dorfman SF, Goldstein MG, Gritz ER, et al. Treating tobacco use and dependence. Clinical practice guideline. Rockville, MD: US Dept Health Hum Serv, Public Health Serv, 2000;23:73-7.

[2] Lopez AD, Collishaw NE, Piha T. A descriptive model of the cigarette epidemic in developed countries. Tob Control 1994;3(3):242.

[3] Jha P, Chaloupka FJ, eds. Tobacco control in developing countries. Oxford: Oxford Univ Press, 2000.

[4] CDC. Smoking and tobacco use. Accessed 2009 Jan 01. URL: www.cdc.gov/tobacco/media_communications/calendar/2009/may_pressrelease.htm

[5] Sussman S, Sun P, Dent CW. A meta-analysis of teen cigarette smoking cessation. Health Psychol 2006;25(5):549-57.

[6] CDC. Global Youth Tobacco Surveillance, 2000-2007. MMWR 2008;57(SS01):1-21.

[7] Prokhorov AV, Winickoff JP, Ahluwalia JS, Ossip-Klein D, Tanski S, Lando HA, et al. Youth tobacco use: A global perspective for child health care clinicians. Pediatrics 2006;118(3):e890.

[8] The Global School Health Initiative and Health and Human Development Programs. Improving health through schools: National and international strategies. Geneva, Switzerland, WHO, 1999.

[9] Sirichotiratana N, Techatraisakdi C, Sujirarat D, Rahman K, Warren CW, Jones NR, et al. Linking Global Youth Tobacco Survey (GYTS) data to the WHO Framework Convention on Tobacco Control: The case for Thailand. Bangkok, Thailand: WHO-Southeast Asia Regional Office, 2005.

[10] Sithole EGV. Global school-based health survey Zimbabwe 2003. Harare, Zimbabwe: Min Health Child Welfare, 2003.

[11] Sussman S, Sun P. Youth tobacco use cessation: 2008 update. Tob Induc Dis, in press.

[12] Swart D, Reddy P, Pitt B, Panday S. The prevalence and determinants of tobacco-use among Grade 8-10 learners in South Africa. Cape Town, South Africa: Natl Health Promot Res Dev Group Med Res Council, 2001.

[13] Warren CW, Riley L, Asma S, Eriksen MP, Green L, Blanton C, et al. Tobacco use by youth: A surveillance report from the Global Youth Tobacco Survey Project. Bull World Health Organ 2000;78(7):868-76.

[14] Mermelstein R. Teen smoking cessation. Tob Control 2003;12(1):i25-34.

[15] Wen CP, Chen T, Tsai YY, Tsai SP, Chung WS, Cheng TY, et al. Are marketing campaigns in Taiwan by foreign tobacco companies targeting young smokers? Tob Control 2005;14:i38.

[16] Yach D, Bettcher D. Globalisation of tobacco industry influence and new global responses. Tob Control 2000;9(2):206-16.

[17] Chaloupka FJ, Nair R. International issues in the supply of tobacco: Recent changes and implications for alcohol. Addiction 2000;95(4):S477-89.

[18] Sussman S, Pokhrel P, Black D, Kohrman M, Hamann S, Vateesatokit P, et al. Tobacco control in developing countries: Tanzania, Nepal, China, and Thailand as examples. Nicotine Tob Res 2007;9:S447-57.

[19] Taylor A, Chaloupka FJ, Guindon E, Corbett M. The impact of trade liberalization on tobacco consumption. In: Jha P, Cahloupka FJ, eds. Tobacco control in developing countries. Oxford: Oxford Univ Press, 2000:343-64.

[20] Sirichotiratana N, Sovann S, Aditama TY, Krishnan M, Kyaing NN, Miguel-Baquilod M, et al. Linking data to tobacco control program action among students aged 13-15 in Association of South East Asian Nations (ASEAN) member states, 2000-2006. Tob Control 2008;17(6):372-8.

[21] WHO. WHO Framework Convention on Tobacco Control (WHO FCTC). Accessed 2008 Dec 12. URL: http://www.who.int/fctc/en/

[22] Tauras JA, Chaloupka FJ. Determinants of smoking cessation: An analysis of young adult men and women. Working paper 7262. Cambridge, MA: Natl Bureau Econ Res, 1999.

[23] Hey K, Perera R. Quit and win contests for smoking cessation. Cochrane Database Syst Rev 2005(2):1465-858.

[24] Strong K, Bonita R. The SuRF Report 1. Surveillance of risk factors related to noncommunicable diseases: Current status of global data. Geneva, Switzerland: WHO, 2003.

[25] Astrøm AN, Ogwell EA. Use of tobacco in Kenya: Sources of information, beliefs and attitudes toward tobacco control measures among primary school students. J Adolesc Health 2004;35(3):234.
[26] Gururaj G, Girish N. Tobacco use amongst children in Karnataka. Indian J Pediatr 2007;74:1095-8.
[27] Panday S, Reddy SP, Ruiter RA, Bergstrom E, de Vries H. Determinants of smoking cessation among adolescents in South Africa. Health Educ Res 2005;20(5):586-99.
[28] Siziya S, Rudatsikira E, Muula AS. (2007). Cigarette smoking among school-going adolescents in Katue, Zambia. Malawi Med J 19:75-78.
[29] Stigler MH, Perry CL, Arora M, Shrivastav R, Mathur C, Reddy KS. Intermediate outcomes from project MYTRI: Mobilizing Youth for Tobacco-Related Initiatives in India. Cancer Epidemiol Biomarkers Prev 2007;16(6):1050-6.
[30] Sussman S, Dent CW, Burton D, Stacy AW, Flay BR. Developing school-based tobacco use prevention and cessation programs. Thousand Oaks, CA: Sage, 1995.
[31] Unger JB, Soto C, Thomas N. Translation of health programs for American Indians in the United States. Eval Health Prof 2008;31(2):124-44.
[32] Sussman S, Gufranova U, Demin A. Speculation about options for teen tobacco use cessation in the Russian Federation. Tob Induc Dis, 2007;3:1-15.
[33] Richmond R, Larcos D, Debono D. A worldwide survey of teaching about tobacco in medical schools. Educating Medical Students About Tobacco Planning and implementation. Paris, France: Int Union Against Tuberculosis Lung Dis, 1996:281-96.
[34] Jha P, Paccaud F, Nguyen S. Tobacco control in developing countries. In: Jha P, Chaloupka F. New York: Oxford Univ Press, 2000
[35] Zheng H, Sussman S, Chen X, Wang Y, Xia J, Gong J, et al. Project EX: A teen smoking cessation initial study in Wuhan, China. Addict Behav 2004;29(9):1725-33.
[36] Markham WA, Aveyard P, Thomas H, Charlton A, Lopez ML, De Vries H. What determines future smoking intentions of 12-to 13-year-old UK African Caribbean, Indian, Pakistani and white young people? Health Educ Res 2004;19(1):15-28.
[37] Chen HH, Yeh ML. Developing and evaluating a smoking cessation program combined with an internet-assisted instruction program for adolescents with smoking. Patient Educ Couns 2006;61(3):411-8.
[38] Chan SS, Wong DC, Fong DY, Leung AY, Lam DO, Mak YW, et al. The establishment and promotion of the first youth quitline in Hong Kong: Challenges and opportunities. Eval Health Prof 2008;31(3):258-71.
[39] Rodgers A, Corbett T, Bramley D, Riddell T, Wills M, Lin RB, et al. Do u smoke after txt? Results of a randomised trial of smoking cessation using mobile phone text messaging. Tob Control 2005;14(4):255-61.
[40] Bell, B. International Consultation on Tobacco and Youth [ICTY]. What in the world works? 28-30 September 1999, Singapore, final conference report. Geneva, Switzerland, WHO, 1999.

Submitted: December 22, 2008.
Revised: February 16, 2009.
Accepted: February 23, 2009.

In: Public Health Yearbook 2009
Editor: Joav Merrick
ISBN: 978-1-61668-911-7

Chapter 13

Postpartum Depression. Effects on the Mother-Infant Relationship and Child Development

Deana B. Davalos*[*], *PhD, Alana M. Campbell, BS and Amanda L. Pala

Department of Psychology, Colorado State University, Fort Collins, Colorado, United States of America

Abstract

During the last two decades there has been an increase in research focusing on the effects of maternal depression on the developing child. Research in this field has apparently developed out of the recognition of a relatively higher prevalence of postpartum maternal depression than once believed and recurring observations of differences in mother/offspring relationships or child behavior associated with maternal postpartum depression. The offspring behaviors that have been implicated have included slight, transient effects to longer term deficits. Some researchers have argued that even in to young adulthood, individuals who experienced interactions with depressed mothers are at significantly greater risk of experiencing a variety of psychological symptoms, including depression, anxiety, and problems with addiction. Again, this view is controversial and others in the field link these increased risks to alternative factors such as low socioeconomic status or marital discord. While there appears to be consensus among most researchers in recognizing that there are likely effects of maternal postpartum depression on offspring, there is little consensus regarding the specific details of these effects. In our review, we will systematically analyze research focusing on the effects of postpartum depression on the offspring and those variables that are believed to be affected from potential difficulties in this bond.

Keywords: maternal depression, postpartum depression, depression.

[*] Correspondence: Deana B Davalos, PhD, Department of Psychology, Colorado State University, Fort Collins, CO 80523-1876 United States. Tel: 970-491-5548; Fax: 970-491-1032; E-mail: Davalos@ColoState.Edu

Introduction

The mother infant bond has long been recognized as being crucial in multiple areas of infant development. The value that is placed on this relationship is recognized throughout the world and across socioeconomic status (1). The multitudes of variables that are thought to be influenced by the mother infant relationship are impressive, even staggering. Research suggests that, depending on the level of bonding or lack thereof, infants may suffer outcomes such as cognitive deficits, interpersonal difficulties, or the development of long-standing psychopathology (2). Others have argued that the effects are likely much more subtle, but certainly still important. During the last two decades there has been an increase in research focusing on, possibly one of the most prevalent threats to the mother infant bond, maternal depression. Research in this field has apparently developed out of the recognition of a higher prevalence of postpartum maternal depression than once believed and recurring observations of differences in mother/infant relationships or infant behavior resulting from maternal postpartum depression.

Longitudinal data suggest that while some problems appear to resolve relatively quickly, there are select characteristics that endure long after infancy. Specifically, some researchers have argued that children, adolescents, and even young adults who experienced problems bonding with their depressed mothers are at significantly greater risk of experiencing a variety of psychological symptoms, including depression, anxiety, and problems with addiction (3). Again, this view is controversial and others in the field link these increased risks to factors other than maternal depression, such as low socioeconomic status or marital discord. While there appears to be consensus among most researchers in recognizing that there are likely effects of postpartum depression on mother infant bonding that affect early development, there is little consensus regarding the specific details of these effects. In this review, we will systematically analyze research focusing on the effects of postpartum depression on the mother infant bond and those variables which are believed to be affected from potential difficulties in this relationship..

Maternal depression has received increasing attention during the past several years due to interest in the possible implications for both mother and child. However, confounding variables that may also affect children of depressed mothers present a limitation that systematically appears in the maternal depression literature. For example, results from various studies suggest that the following variables may all have an effect on children's well-being, regardless of maternal depression; marital status, socio-economic status, low social support, maternal daily stressors, family adversity, quality of childcare (4). Furthermore, there are difficult issues involved in trying to identify the effects of depression when the onset of symptoms can be vague or difficult to identify. While some mothers with depression only experience depressive symptoms during the postpartum period, there are also mothers who meet diagnostic criteria for depression throughout both the prepartum and postpartum period (5). Given that there are distinct consequences for infants and children exposed to maternal depression during the prenatal period, it is often difficult to ascertain what is a product of postpartum maternal depression instead of maternal depression with an earlier onset during pregnancy.

While a large number of the outcome variables associated with depression during the prenatal period have focused on physiological indices related to prenatal exposure to elevated neurotransmitters and cortisol levels (6,7) the effects of postpartum depression have tended to emphasize the role of compromised bonding between infant and mother and resulting psychological and cognitive outcomes.

To understand the importance of identifying maternal depression and the possible effects on both mother and child, it is critical that one first understands the prevalence of this condition. While it has been argued that perinatal depression is likely grossly underreported, estimates suggest that 8% to 52% of women experience postpartum depression. When one adds those women with children who have experienced depressive symptoms, that estimate consistently jumps to over 50% of women (8). The World Health Organization has posited that for women of child-bearing age, depression is the leading cause of disease burden worldwide (9). And while unfortunate, researchers have argued that mothering young children increases the risk of depression and that, childbirth in particular, is the time when women are most prone to develop psychiatric disturbance. In addition, there appears to be specific risk factors associated with those mothers of young children who endorse the highest rates of depression, including; never being married, achieving less than a high school education, under 25 years of age, specific racial status, and low socioeconomic status. Surveys focusing on women bringing in children for pediatric care have estimated that 15% to 40% of mothers report depressive symptoms (10).

Given that maternal depression borders on epidemic proportion and considering the fact that when we are able to recognize depression and treat it effectively, the duration may be reduced significantly, there is increasing need to understand maternal depression and the outcomes that may result from depression in both mother and child.

The description of maternal depression varies significantly in the literature. Defining maternal depression varies from self-reports, subjective ratings from clinicians or family members, to structured clinical interviews. In addition, women who are included in maternal depression studies vary from individuals who have suffered from severe depressive symptoms for years to others who appear to have more transient mild symptoms of depression. Lastly, it is often unclear whether the symptoms of depression that are reported in the women with depression during the perinatal period are related to their perinatal status or represent long-term depression that simply carries over into the perinatal period. The unifying theme for the studies presented in this chapter is that they reflect a wide range of outcome variables that are thought to result from maternal depression.

Methods

A systematic search was undertaken of the MEDLINE, PsycINFO, and the Social Sciences Citation Index databases from 1950-2008. Search words used were postpartum depression, postnatal depression, perinatal depression and maternal depression. Reference lists of all included articles and review articles were also checked to identify any other relevant studies. Studies were excluded if there appeared to be no method of assessing depression other than maternal complaint or if there were other medical or psychological issues that clearly confounded the effects of maternal depression (e.g. poor physical health of mother, maternal substance use) or if the depressive symptoms appeared to be longstanding in nature rather than associated with the perinatal period.

Results

Maternal depression outcome variables

Physical health and injury

Over the years, researchers have uncovered a number of physical differences which appear to distinguish offspring of depressed mothers compared to those of non-depressed mothers. Many of these characteristics appear as early as infancy. Among these are elevated heart rates associated with sympathetic arousal during interactions with their depressed mothers and lower vagal tone suggestive of lowered parasympathetic activity during interactions (11), both suggesting an elevated degree of stress in these infants with their mothers. While some argue that these characteristics may be inherent in these children from birth, there are compelling findings suggesting that interaction with the depressed mother exacerbates physiological deficits. For example, a number of these physiological indices are not present in infants when they are separated from their mothers and observed with strangers, even when their external observable behavior is unchanged. However, there are other measures which appear to be more chronic, regardless of the presence of the depressed mother during assessment. For example, infants with depressed mothers exhibit elevated cortisol levels across multiple measurement times, suggesting that infants most likely experience chronic stress. Dawson et al (12) furthered the argument that there are likely static physiological conditions in these infants leading to increased stress and chronic negative outcomes. Specifically, the researchers hypothesized that the atypical brain activity that has been observed in infants of depressed mothers may reflect a tendency to experience more frequent and possibly more intense negative affect in addition to a lack of appropriate self-regulatory strategies that are used to modulate negative emotions. Furthermore, the reduced frontal brain activation (EEG) is likely associated not only with cognitive deficits that will be addressed later, but also contribute to difficulties with inhibition and emotional regulation (13). That infants of depressed mothers may be predisposed to experience more frequent and greater negative affect while also lacking sufficient self-regulatory strategies to modulate these negative emotions lends further support to the idea that there may be multiple factors pointing towards chronic stress in infants of depressed mothers.

This perceived relationship between maternal depression and increased stress in their offspring has been of great interest to researchers and has been studied across multiple physical outcome variables. One condition that has been studied in depth is asthma. Given that asthma is considered by many to be a stress-sensitive illness, researchers have questioned the relationship between asthma and psychological distress, specifically focusing on depression (14). The autonomical dysregulation model of asthma (15) suggests that depressive states involve autonomic nervous system dysregulation that may be associated with vagally mediated asthma episodes (16). This model is consistent with past studies which have found a link between high internalizing symptoms and asthma severity and research suggesting higher than average rates of depression in children and those children's mothers who present at hospitals for asthma symptoms. Given these findings, a natural question that arises is whether children of depressed mothers may be at greater risk for developing asthma and/or exhibit greater asthma activity. While it remains controversial whether there is a direct relationship between maternal depression and asthma disease activity, research findings suggests that there is higher prevalence of asthma in children of depressed mothers and that there appears to be an indirect relationship between maternal depression and increased child internalizing symptoms (e.g. depressive and anxiety symptomatology) that result in increased asthma activity (17). Furthermore, there is strong evidence that maternal depression is associated with internalizing disorders, suggesting that maternal depression may play an important role in child asthma as well as a number of other conditions which involve internalizing symptoms.

A different, possibly more controversial, area of research in maternal depression focuses on issues such as the increased prevalence of accidents, injuries, and doctors' appointments in children of depressed mothers. There are numerous studies suggesting overall poorer physical health in children of depressed mothers, greater number of headaches and stomachaches, higher rates of medical problems, and even higher rates of mortality in the offspring of depressed parents in longitudinal studies following participants into middle age. However, there is slightly more controversy surrounding whether children of depressed mothers have more accidents, more physical injuries and greater frequency of doctor's visits.

Lewsinsohn, Olino and Klein (18) found that children of mothers with depression had greater occurrences of treatment for illness. Schwebel and Brezausek (19) found that chronic levels of severe maternal depression were associated with increased risk of injury in infants and toddlers (up to age three). This finding was robust even when the researchers controlled for SES, sex of the child, child temperament, externalizing behavior, and parenting. It should be noted, however, that the risk for injury was not noted when mothers endorsed less severe symptoms of chronic maternal depression. Brown and Davidson (20) also demonstrated a higher rate of accidents in children of depressed mothers as compared with children of nondepressed mothers. However, they point out that other studies noting similar results have introduced the possible role of maternal psychotropic medication use at the time of the child's injury, reporting that 26% of the depressed mothers were receiving prescribed psychotropic medication at the time of injury. Others have argued that a more feasible explanation of increased medical care and increased injuries in children of depressed mothers focuses on the fact that these children may be more likely to have growth failure (both height and weight) due to "failure to thrive". Past studies suggest that low maternal self-esteem and depressive mood are important factors associated with growth failure. These characteristics often viewed as a failure to thrive appear to be related to poor maternal affect and poor child-rearing. However, the relationship between maternal depression and infant growth outcomes is poorly understood with possibilities including; infant growth 'failure' may negatively affect maternal mood, children of mothers with depression may be more likely to be identified with "failure to thrive" due to increased health-seeking behaviors by the mother, difficulty breastfeeding and poor mother-child interaction, or the established relationship between antenatal depression and low infant birth weight (21).

Cognition and language

While many of the physical outcome variables studied in the maternal depression literature are assessed early in development, often at infancy, the outcome measures associated with cognition and language development are often assessed later in development. While there appears to be ample evidence suggesting that children of mothers with depression may exhibit developmental delays and some degree of cognitive and functional impairment, there is quite a bit of variability in the literature. There are clearly certain situations that may lead to different outcomes or select variables that lead to diverse effects. Among these, researchers have identified two main variables that may affect outcome the most: the age of the child at which the onset of maternal depressive symptoms appear and the gender of the child. Some research results suggest that the first two years are the most critical in terms of mother/infant bonding and the potential impairment of cognitive development. Others argue that cognitive impairments are less a function of timing and more likely associated with the gender of the offspring. For example, poor cognitive performance resulting from maternal depression has been found to be selectively limited to sons in some studies, specifically finding that boys of depressed mothers have poorer educational attainment. Others argue that while there are clearly cognitive and linguistic variables that appear to be affected by maternal depression, it is less clear whether this relationship is direct or mediated by another variable. For example, some studies find direct associations between poorer cognitive functioning and maternal depression but others show an association only in the context of family adversity or, as mentioned previously, only for boys.

More general findings have appeared across genders. There are widespread language difficulties and specific cognitive deficits that span early childhood to late adolescence. In terms of language, persistent maternal depression has been associated with delayed language development in children approximately three years of age. Other studies assessing the same age range have noted poor verbal comprehension, poor linguistic functioning, and difficulties with expressive language (22). In addition, there are a number of cognitive outcome measures that may surface later in development, possibly after the mother's depression has resolved. For example, children who have been exposed to maternal depression at age three exhibit deficiency in their reading even at age eight. These difficulties can also persist much later, with studies suggesting that children whose mothers have had persistent depression during childhood are more likely to drop out of high school.

Failure to complete school is not the only education-related variable that has been noted in the literature. Children of depressed mothers tend to show more difficulty with school-readiness (22). From teacher reports, these children are more often described as more aggressive, angry, defiant, and uncooperative than are other children. However, it has been argued that the more external, behavioral problems that have been repeatedly noted by teacher ratings in the literature tend to minimize internalizing symptoms, often reported by family members, such as fear, anxiety, and physical complaints. Instead, given the teachers' instructional role, they are more likely to report these children's behaviors such as aggression, hostility, and hyperactivity, which disrupt classroom routines.

While there are multiple theories about why maternal depression is related to compromised cognitive and linguistic development, it has been suggested that it is likely due to a combination of factors. Many of these include indirect influences that may be more related to the child's environment in the home of a depressed mother (e.g. high stress, limited resources, etc.) while others focus more on the relationship between the mother and child. These mother/child variables range from poor modeling of enriched language and engaged problem solving by the depressed mother to more general issues such as reduced maternal sensitivity to the child's needs and reduced level of engagement with the child (22).

Psychological effects and behavioral correlates

The last facet of development that has arguably received the most attention in the maternal depression literature is the psychological and behavioral correlates of exposure to maternal depression.

While there is definite controversy in the literature regarding the types and the extent of pathology that may be associated with maternal depression, the majority of literature suggests that there are likely at least transient psychological effects and behaviors that result from exposure to maternal depression. For decades, researchers have highlighted the relationship between parental depression and higher rates of depression in their offspring. These rates vary significantly from study to study, 10% to 33% in some studies, 2-6 times greater than in control groups in other studies, with all noting a significant increase in the odds of these children becoming depressed at some point in their life (23). However, the increase in psychopathology is not limited to depression. Children of depressed mothers are also more likely to suffer from other types of clinical disorders including anxiety disorders, attention deficit hyperactivity disorder, conduct disorder and substance abuse, among others. In addition, children of depressed mothers, not only have higher rates of psychopathology, but receive higher levels of treatment for psychiatric disturbance. In longitudinal studies spanning 10-20 years, children of depressed mothers have been found to use more mental health resources during their lifetime and were more likely to report that they had obtained mental health assistance in the past year.

Others who have studied the relationship between maternal depression and pathology in their children agree that there is an increase in psychopathology, however, it appears to vary as a function of exposure and chronicity. When mothers/offspring are assessed at two separate time periods (e.g. spanning months to years), children whose mothers reported depressive symptoms at both ages exhibited significantly elevated rates of hostile behavior problems in the classroom and at home. However, children of mothers who were previously, but not currently, depressed exhibited significantly more anxious and withdrawn behavior at school and at home, while, lastly, children of recently depressed mothers were noted as exhibiting more hyperactivity and demanding behavior.

These higher rates of psychopathology have been noted not only when compared to controls, but also when compared to children of non-depressed mothers or mothers with "medical conditions". Furthermore, these differences appear to persist over time, even decades. In studies spanning 25-32 year follow-ups of adult children of depressed mothers, researchers have found that their risk for specific disorders such as depression, anxiety, social impairment, and substance disorder were significantly increased compared to controls (3). And often, the emergence of pathology did not surface until years following the initial exposure to maternal depression. For example, the period of highest incidence for major depressive disorder was found to be between ages 15 and 20 years. Outcome variables outside the realm of diagnosable mental illness have also been found, specifically in terms of behaviors that appear to be relatively latent until adolescence when children of depressed mothers are described as showing elevated patterns of defiant, rebellious, and withdrawn behavior.

One interesting facet of this area of research is the control groups that have been selected as comparison groups for the mothers with depression. Even when researchers use psychiatric comparison groups, such as mothers with schizophrenia, poor affect regulation and poor affective development continue to appear at greater levels in offspring of mothers with depression. While negative affective outcome variables appear to be greater in children of depressed mothers compared to other psychiatric populations, other studies suggest that the children of depressed parents cannot usually be distinguished from the children of schizophrenic parents on behavioral or attentional measures (24).

These detrimental effects of perceiving one's mother to be depressed have even been witnessed when non-depressed mothers have simply simulated depression. The infants of the mothers with "simulated depression" quickly exhibit high levels of distress. It should be noted that research in "simulated depression" suggests that the distressed behavior observed by the infants was selectively limited to the children of the non-depressed mothers, while the infants of the depressed mothers appeared to be rather unaffected. Results were interpreted as suggesting that infants of depressed mothers may become accustomed to flattened affect and lower activity, decreasing their distress over time (11). What may be one of the least suspected findings in these studies was that the infants of clinically depressed mothers were not only negatively affected by the depressed mood of their mothers, but they also appeared to have a negative effect on the nondepressed mothers participating in the study. Specifically, the nondepressed mothers (blind to the infants' group) appeared to exhibit more depressed symptoms and less optimal interaction with the infants of depressed mothers.

The finding which suggests that infants of depressed mothers actually affected the non-depressed mothers in a negative way is not surprising considering the behaviors that often characterize these offspring. The types of behaviors that have been described in infants and young children of depressed mothers include; disengaged and intrusive interaction styles, withdrawn behavior, looking away, and reduced positive affect. A substantial literature has focused on these variables and how they affect relationships. Specifically, there has been research focusing on the relationship within and outside of the mother/child dyad, with both types of relationships thought to be affected by exposure to maternal depression. Within the dyad, depressed mothers and their infants have been shown to have less positive interaction. Unfortunately, the reduction in positive interaction appears to generalize beyond the interactions between infants with their depressed mothers to others, including non-depressed mothers with whom the infants were not familiar. These findings suggest that the infants' depressed style of interacting with their mothers may generalize to nondepressed adults. There is also evidence that these children have more difficulty in their relationships with their siblings and peers, specifically, children of depressed mothers have been described as exhibiting excessive rivalry with peers and siblings for attention and impatient, deviant, and withdrawn behavior in their interactions.

Other behaviors that have been noted in offspring of mothers with depression that are associated with altered patterns of interactions with others include increased self-regulatory behaviors such as head and gaze aversion which are thought to develop out of a desire to reduce the negative affect that is experienced when mothers are unresponsive.

Research focusing on children of depressed mothers consistently illustrates this widespread difficulty regulating emotions. For example, children whose mothers report chronically high levels of depression have a difficult time learning to control behavior and modulate impulses when upset (25). This poor modulation of emotions is exhibited in increased aggression and acting out. Specifically, Zahn-Waxler et al (25) reported that toddlers of depressed mothers showed increased out-of-control aggression when interacting with peers and were rated higher on externalizing problems at the age of five.

These externalizing behaviors have been noted in multiple studies, often characterized by significantly higher rates of hostile behavior at home and school. These behaviors appear to persist and have been noted in studies focusing on older children also, in which offspring of depressed mothers have been found to have more adjustment problems in early and middle childhood.

In terms of the etiology of these aberrant behaviors, there has been ongoing debate whether psychological symptoms that appear in children of depressed mothers represent genetic contribution, effects of parenting styles of the depressed mother or whether there may be modeling in terms of the child adopting traits and attributes from the depressed mother. Recent research suggests that it is likely that multiple factors contribute to psychological attributes in children of depressed mothers. Lim and colleagues (17) interviewed children and adolescents ages 7-17 and found a direct relationship between maternal depression and increased depressive symptomatology measured using the Children's Depression Inventory and the Child Depression Rating Scale-Revised (CDRS–R) and increased anxiety symptoms, both state and trait, using the State-Trait Anxiety Inventory for Children (STAIC-T; STAIC-S). In addition, maternal depression indirectly affected these psychological variables via negative parenting (e.g. intrusiveness, neglect/distancing, and harsh discipline). Others have also found that in terms of parenting, depressed mothers are less effective than nondepressed mothers in setting limits on their toddlers, and this was reflected in fewer compromise solutions to conflict solutions. Depressed mothers have also been found to be less likely to follow through when they do set limits, leading to less compliance and increased conflict between mother and child. This difficulty with compliance has been noted in a number of studies, with some noting higher rates of "passive noncompliance" associated with less mature expressions of age-appropriate interaction and autonomy. Lastly, mothers with depression may tend to use more guilt in their interactions with the children when they are unable to persuade them to comply via more positive routes. Furthermore, evidence suggests that there are long-standing effects of these guilt-inducing behaviors. Children of well mothers show prototypic expressions of "adaptive guilt" which is thought to involve themes of responsibility and reparation. In contrast, expressions of guilt in children of depressed mothers have been described as aberrant, distorted, and unresolved, indicating that these children may develop different patterns of guilt expression, and likely, may be made to feel guilty for different reasons from the control children (25).

Some have speculated that the lack of consistency in parenting that is often seen in mothers with depression may exacerbate other behaviors that are often observed in this population. Specifically, behavioral problems (such as difficulty being managed, difficulty playing with other children, and having frequent tantrums) may result from both a genetic predisposition and parenting styles that do not foster proper affect regulation.

However, there is evidence that suggests that not all mothers with depression exhibit these deficits in parenting and that the effects of maternal depression on children can be mediated by interventions and specific parenting techniques. For example, research suggests that mothers suffering from depression who engaged in parenting education had children who fared better on certain outcome measures. Specifically, mothers enrolled in parenting education focusing on anticipatory guidance techniques, or techniques which focus on anticipating children's emerging needs at different developmental stages, are believed to have children with fewer behavioral problems during early school-age years than mothers not receiving parent education. These mothers were described as more proactive in their parenting and appeared to exhibit less negative affect, use less guilt in their parental interactions, have more secure attachments, and appeared to be more consistent with their young children (25).

Discussion

During the last decade, there has been increased interest and concern about the prevalence of maternal depression. Researchers and policy-makers alike appear to recognize the importance of this condition and the far-reaching effects that maternal depression has on children and families. While not specific to only maternal depression, the US Surgeon General has pointed out that the impact of maternal mental health on children is vastly under-recognized (26).

It becomes clear when one systematically assesses the literature that there are social and practical limitations that have made research in the area of maternal depression and the effects on offspring difficult. One of the primary barriers for researchers in their quest to understand maternal depression and the prevalence of this condition is the fact that depression, for many, carries a stigma. When one adds the fact that there are additional expectations about motherhood, in terms of mothers themselves believing that the period of time following the birth of their child should be filled with happiness and reward compounded by society placing these same expectations on mothers, the reporting of depression during this period is likely vastly underreported (27). There is a significant amount of literature which reports that even if mothers would discuss their postpartum depression, there are multiple barriers in terms of having them adequately assessed by their physicians. There are a number of reasons that are reported by physicians to explain the lack of screening for depression. Some physicians are not aware of appropriate screening tools. Others worry that adding depression screening to their visits will be both time-consuming and expensive and, in the worst case, they may be put in a position where they have to make decisions about how to treat mothers with depression. Studies have shown that a large number of pediatricians acknowledge concern about addressing depression with new mothers due to possible judgments and stigma that may be associated with maternal depression. Physicians have argued that identification and assessment may be more feasible and desired if they had services to which they could refer these mothers. However, these doctors and other researchers have highlighted the point that even when mothers are successfully identified, they may be hesitant to seek assistance due to perceived judgment (28).

Even in ideal situations, when mothers are successfully identified and willing to seek treatment, new barriers arise in terms of accurately diagnosing and providing the proper treatment. Research suggests that postnatal depression is complex and likely involves a variety of subtypes that should be considered when determining treatment. Watson et al (29) suggest that women with postnatal depression could be classified into as many as six categories with others supporting this argument given the vast etiologies of depression during the postnatal period.

These proposed different categories of postnatal depression have widespread implications in terms of treatment and research alike. In terms of treatment, researchers have argued that, given the different types of depression in this population, personalized client-centered approaches are the most appropriate rather than a blanket approach of drug treatment paired with talk therapy.

In terms of research, different types of depression, levels of pathology, and duration of symptoms have all been found to effect outcome variables in different ways. When one tries to analyze the literature systematically, it quickly becomes apparent that these variables have not been well-assessed across studies and have likely led to much of the disparity in the literature. For example, the aspect of chronicity of symptoms alone is associated with very different outcomes in the mother/child relationship depending on when the symptoms first appear and how long those symptoms persist. Many researchers argue that parenting and bonding appears especially impaired when maternal depression symptoms are chronic; this is compared to women whose symptoms may be equally long in duration but are intermittent with breaks during which depressive symptoms remit (13). Similarly, while some researchers have argued that the first six months of parenting and bonding appear to be selectively involved in poor outcome for children of depressed mothers, others have argued that negative consequences of maternal depression are specifically associated with cases in which symptoms persist beyond the immediate postpartum period, specifically following the first year of life and beyond (30).

There are clearly a number of other limitations that enter the picture that may be even more difficult to extricate from the outcome variables that are associated with maternal depression. Probably the most notable variable is whether mothers who report postpartum depression may have had a predisposition for depression existing before the perinatal period. The question of whether offspring of mothers with postpartum depression may have genetic predisposition for depression remains. Depression in the offspring of depressed parents is generally thought to be due to an interaction between genetic factors and environmental factors, including stressors in the family and the social context. However, approximately 40–50% of the relationship between mothers' and children's depressive symptoms are thought to be due to genetic linkage. If this is so, one has to wonder what the extent of this predisposition may have on bonding or other outcome measures that are independent of their mother's symptomatology during early development or whether this predisposition is specifically exacerbated by their mother's depressive symptoms. The other issue that arises when this "interaction" between genes and environment is addressed involves the difficulty that researchers encounter when they attempt to understand this proposed 50-60% of variance that is not due to genetics. The non-genetic variables that ideally should be assessed in studies focusing on the effects of maternal depression on mother infant bonding are extensive and often difficult to assess. For example, multiple studies suggest that the negative effects of maternal depression on their offspring may be due to what we view as more direct influences, such as responding to mothers' sadness or lack of energy or their difficulty parenting. However, children may also exhibit negative symptoms due to secondary variables that not only affect them negatively but also contribute to their mother's symptoms. These secondary variables range from social disadvantage, economic instability, dysfunctional family dynamics, low social support, maternal daily stressors, or insufficient childcare (4). Last, but not least, is the vastly under-examined role of marital status, level of marital discord, and the father's role in both the depressed mother's life and in the offspring's quality of life. Downey and Coyne (31) once described the spouses of depressed mothers as "shadowy figures." There are multiple studies suggesting that the mates of depressed mothers may, in many cases, contribute to the pathology of the mother and to their offspring. Specifically, research suggests that mothers with depression may select mates with mental illness who contribute to pathology in offspring and who also contribute to marital discord (31). However, there is equal, if not more, empirical support to suggest that "well" fathers may actually provide a buffer between negative effects of maternal depression on the child (32). In addition, there are a wide range of studies suggesting that many of the negative outcomes associated with maternal depression appear to be selectively associated with mother's depression, but not with paternal depression, even when the father had been diagnosed with clinical depression. For example, behavioral problems, physical injury, physical illness, and a variety of other negative outcome variables have been found to be selectively involved in maternal depression but absent in cases of paternal depression (33,34). While this area of research is lacking, there is enough empirical support to suggest that future research focusing on the role of the spouse in both the depressed mother's life and the life of the offspring is warranted.

Conclusions

Maternal depression is a condition that has received increasing attention over the past few decades. What appears consistent in the literature is the fact that more must be done in terms of treatment and research in this population. What also appears clear in the literature is that there are multiple layers of barriers that often stand in the way of achieving research and treatment goals with this population. Multiple studies suggest that fear of stigma and embarrassment related to maternal depression may be two of the greatest barriers to getting assistance to this population. While the ideal solution to these barriers would be to reduce stigma and be accepting of maternal depression, very little progress towards this goal has been achieved over the past few decades. As researchers and policy makers work toward educating the public about maternal depression, the treating clinicians may have to focus on getting mothers to seek help for the benefit of their offspring and for the benefit of their relationship with their children. There is substantial evidence, spanning decades, that suggests that the children of depressed mothers pay a great cost in terms of their physical, cognitive, and psychological development for untreated maternal depression. There is also a wealth of literature suggesting that the maternal/child bond is typically compromised whether acutely or chronically as a result of maternal depression. It becomes quickly apparent that new attempts at intervention are needed to help get mothers and their offspring get the assistance they need. Nylen and colleagues (35) captured the needs of this population when they wrote, "The challenge now is to devote continued attention to process and outcome variables as well as to creative manners of designing and implementing interventions such that the propensity of women and infants in need of help are able to access and receive quality mental health services."

Acknowledgments

This research was partially supported by the National Alliance for Research on Schizophrenia and Depression (NARSAD) Young Investigator Award. This paper is an updated version on research first reported in the following book chapter, Davalos DB, Campbell AM, Pala AL.

The effects of maternal depression on the maternal-child relationship. In: Cuyler E, Ackhart, M, eds. Psychology of relationships. New York: Nova Science, in press.

References

[1] Narayanan I. Early mother–infant interaction: Global perspectives and developing country concerns. J Trop Pediatr 1987;33:120-3.

[2] Gunning M, Conroy S, Valoriani V, Figueiredo B, Kammerer MH, Muzik M, Glatigny-Dallay E, Murray L. Measurement of mother–infant interactions and the home environment in a European setting: Preliminary results from a cross-cultural study. Br J Psychiatry 2004;184:38-4.

[3] Peisah C, Brodaty H, Luscombe G, Anstey K. Children of a cohort of depressed patients 25 years later: Psychopathology and relationships. J Affect Disord 2004;82:385–94.

[4] Belsky J. The determinants of parenting: A process model. Child Dev 1984;55:83-6.

[5] Dietz P, Williams S, Callaghan W, Bachman D, Whitlock E, Hornbrook M. Clinically identified maternal depression before, during, and after pregnancies ending in live births. Am J Psychiatry 2007;164(10):1515-20.

[6] Davis EP, Glynn L M, Schetter C D, Hobel C, Chicz-Demet A, Sandman, C. Prenatal exposure to maternal depression and cortisol influences infant temperament. J Am Acad Child Adolesc Psychiatry 2007;46(6):737-46.

[7] Field T, Diego M, Dieter J, Hernandez-Reif M, Schanberg S, Kuhn C, Yando R, Bendell D. Prenatal depression effects on the fetus and the newborn. Infant Behav Dev 2004;27:216-29.

[8] Baker-Ericzen M J, Mueggenborg M G, Hartigan P, Howard N, Wilke T. Partnership for Women's Health: A new-age collaborative program for addressing maternal depression in the postpartum period. Fam Syst Health 2008;26:30-43.

[9] World Health Organization. A message from the Director General. 2001. Available from: URL: http://www.who.int/whr/2001/ dg_message/en/index.html.

[10] Kahn R, Wise P, Finkelstein J, Bernstein H, Lowe J, Homer C. The scope of unmet maternal health needs in pediatric settings. Pediatrics 1999;103:576-81.

[11] Field T. Early interactions between infants and their postpartum depressed mothers. Infant Behav Dev 1984;7:527-32.

[12] Dawson G, Frey K, Self J, Panagiotides H, Hessl D,Yamada E, Rinaldi J. Frontal brain electrical activity in infants of depressed and nondepressed mothers: Relation to variations in infant behavior. Dev Psychopathol 1999;11:589-605.

[13] Ashman SB, Dawson G, Panagiotides H. Trajectories of maternal depression over 7 years: Relations with child psychophysiology and behavior and role of contextual risks. Dev Psychopathol 2008;20: 55-77.

[14] Shalowitz MU, Berry CA, Quinn KA, Wolf RL. The relationship of life stressors and maternal depression to pediatric asthma morbidity in a subspecialty practice. Ambul Pediatr 2001;1:185-93.

[15] Miller BD, Wood BL. Emotions and family factors in childhood asthma: Psychobiological mechanisms and pathways of effect. In: Brown ES, ed. Social and psychological factors and psychosomatic syndromes. Dallas, TX: Karger, 1984:131-60.

[16] Waxmonsky J, Wood BL, Stern T, Ballow M, Lillis K, Cramer-Benjamin D, Mador J, Miller BD. Association of depressive symptoms and disease activity in children with asthma: Methodological and clinical implications. J Am Acad Child Adolesc Psychiatry 2006;45:945-54.

[17] Lim J, Wood BL, Miller BD. Maternal depression and parenting in relation to child internalizing symptoms and asthma disease activity. J Fam Psychol 2008;22:264-73.

[18] Lewinsohn PM, Olino TM, Klein DN. Psychosocial impairment in offspring of depressed parents. Psychol Med 2005;35:1493-1503.

[19] Schwebel DC, Brezausek CM. Chronic maternal depression and children's injury risk. J Ped Psychol 2008;33(10):1-9.

[20] Brown GW, Davidson S. Social class, psychiatric disorder of mothers and accidents to children. Lancet 1978;1:378-81.

[21] Stewart RC. Maternal depression and infant growth: A review of recent evidence. Matern Child Nutr 2007;3(2):94-107.

[22] NICHD Early Child Care Research Network. Chronicity of maternal depressive symptoms, maternal sensitivity, and child functioning at 36 months. Devel Psychol 1999;35(5):1297-1310.

[23] Lieb R, Isensee B, Hofler M, Pfister H, Wittchen H. Parental major depression and the risk of depression and other mental disorders in offspring: A prospective longitudinal community study. Arch Gen Psychiatry 2002;59:365-74.

[24] Orvaschel H, Weissman MM, Kidd KK. The children of depressed parents; The childhood of depressed patients; Depression in children. J Affect Dis 1980;2:1-16.

[25] Zahn-Waxler C, Kochanska G, Krupnick J, McKnew D. Patterns of guilt in children of depressed and well mothers. Devel Psychol 1990; 26:51-9.

[26] Office of the Surgeon General. Mental health: A report of the Surgeon. Rockville, MD: Office Surgeon Gen, 1999.

[27] O'Reilly A, ed. From motherhood to mothering. Albany, NY: State Univ New York Press, 2004.

[28] Heneghan AM, Morton S, DeLeone NL. Pediatricians' attitudes about discussing maternal depression during a pediatric primary care visit. Child Care Health Dev 2007;33(3):333-9.

[29] Watson JP, Elliott SA, Rugg AJ, Brough DI. Psychiatric disorder in pregnancy and the first postnatal year. Br J Psychiatry 1984;144:453-62.

[30] Horwitz SM, Briggs-Gowan MJ, Storfer-Isser A, Carter AJ. Prevalence, correlates, and persistence of maternal depression. J Women's Health 2007;16(5):678-91.

[31] Downey G, Coyne JC. Children of depressed parents: An integrative review. Psychol Bull 1990;108:50-76.

[32] Tannenbaum L, Forehand R. Maternal depressive mood: The role of the father in preventing adolescent problem behaviours. Behav Res Ther 1994;32:321-5.

[33] Kahn RS, Brandt D, Whitaker RC. Combined effect of mothers' and fathers' mental health symptoms on children's behavioral and emotional well-being. Arch Pediatr Adolesc Med 2004;4(158);721-9.

[34] Peisah C, Brodaty H, Luscombe G, Anstey K. Children of a cohort of depressed patients 25 years later: Identifying those at risk. Aust NZ J Psychiatry 2005;39:907–14.

[35] Nylen KJ, Moran TE, Franklin TL, O'Hara MW. Maternal depression: A review of relevant treatment approaches for mothers and infants. Infant Ment Health J 2006;27(4):327-43.

Submitted: October 16, 2008.
Revised: November 14, 2008.
Accepted: November 15, 2008.

In: Public Health Yearbook 2009
Editor: Joav Merrick
ISBN: 978-1-61668-911-7

Chapter 14

Typical and Atypical Expression of Distress: A Study on Cry

Gianluca Esposito, PhD and Paola Venuti, PhD*
Department of Cognitive Science and Education, University of Trento, Rovereto, Italy

Abstract

Crying, which represents the very first communicative channel infants can use to communicate with their environment, plays an important role in child development. Crying is a biological signal that alerts those in the caregiving environment about the needs and wants of the infant and motivates them to respond. Cries act to release specific and appropriate patterns of caregiving actions, thereby ensuring the infant's survival. The aim of this study was to review research that has investigated expressions of distress, specifically crying, during early stages of development in infancy. We have emphasized on the importance of cry evaluation in specific psychopathology, particularly Autism Spectrum Disorders (ASD). First the neurobiological activation that takes place during an episode of crying, both in the caregiver and the infant brain, is described. A description of the function of crying episodes and their evolution, starting from the fetal stage through childhood, follows. Finally, how anomalies in the expression of cry can bias the caregiver's perception of them, and how parents' reactions to pathological crying can be qualitatively different from their reactions to typical crying of same-aged children, is described. Such differences can confound parental attempts to share feelings and develop inter-subjectivity with their children.

Keywords: Crying, responses to young infant's cries, early communication, developmental disorders.

* Correspondence: Gianluca Esposito, PhD, Department of Cognitive Science and Education, University of Trento, Via Matteo del Ben 5b, 38068 Rovereto (TN) Italy. E-mail: gianluca.esposito@unitn.it

Introduction

Crying represents the very first communicative channel infants can use to express their needs and communicate with their environment. These social behaviors, which are driven by genetically predetermined factors, elicit a series of physiological reactions in adults, such as increases in heart rate (1) and endocrine responses (2). These reactions are greater in parents than in non-parents; for example, while hearing episodes of crying, higher levels of testosterone were found in fathers than non-fathers (2). Such physiological reactions activate those listening to cries to take measures to eliminate the cause of the uneasiness that is shared both by newborn and adult (3,4). Starting from these considerations, the aim of this study was to describe expressions of distress, specifically crying, during early stages of development in infancy. In the next pages we describe:

- Physiology of human crying
- Evolutionary trajectory of crying
- Parental reaction to human cries
- Cries in children with atypical development
- How cries are perceived in children with atypical development: The case of Autism Spectrum Disorder

Physiology of human crying

An episode of crying activates the central nervous system (CNS) of both the infant (the producer) and the caregiver (the listener), and this activation creates a state of reciprocal attention. For this reason crying has been considered a complex behavioral mechanism that regulates the infant-caregiver relationship. This complex behavioral mechanism guarantees the building of a specific tie, and this tie assures infant survival. In particular, infant survival is guaranteed primarily because the caregiver hearing the infant crying is alerted and can attend to the infant's primary needs (5) and affective, social, and cognitive needs as well.

In a typically developing infant, an episode of crying is a response to an external or internal negative stimulus and results from the coordination of several brain regions, such as cranial nerves, brainstem, and limbic system. The limbic system, which is the central core of socio-emotional life, is linked to the lower part of the brainstem, which controls the muscles of the larynx, pharynx, and thorax. From a physiological perspective, infant crying comprises a rhythmic alternation of utterances (the cry sounds) and inspiration. Crying is part of the expiratory phase of respiration with phonation (or sound) produced by the larynx. The larynx contains the vocal cords and the glottis vocalis (or simply glottis) that is the opening between the vocal cords. The larynx is the major source of sound during a crying episode and it generates sound through the rhythmic opening and closing of the vocal folds. The production of sound during an episode of crying is the same as every other vocalization (such as speech or song). In particular, in order to oscillate, the vocal folds are brought near enough together so that air pressure builds up beneath the larynx. The cords are pushed apart by this increased subglottal pressure. The elasticity of the cords brings them back together. Under typical conditions, this oscillation pattern sustains itself. In essence, sound is generated in the larynx by cutting the flow of air into little whiffs. This vibration is the fundamental frequency (f0) and is heard as the pitch of the cry (4). Damage in the vagal cranial nerve complex has been related to atypical patterns of fundamental frequency. Extremely rapid shifts in the fundamental frequency are often related to some degree of instability in the neural control system, especially at the level of the brainstem.

Mainly, three different cry modes, related to different vocal fold vibrations, have been identified. Each modality is related to a different infant need (4,6,7):

- basic cry or phonation, characterized by rhythmic vocalizations with cycles of opening and closing of the vocal cord (approximately 250 to 450 Hz or cycles per second in normal, healthy newborns).
- high pitch cry or hyperphonation (1000–2000 Hz or cycles per second). The high frequencies of this mode express a high level of distress; for this reason it is often refereed to as a pain cry. Typically after an initial high frequency pitch the child tends to hold his breath.
- turbulent cry or dysphonation, characterized by no harmonic vibration of the vocal folds. It is often refereed to as a cry of frustration.

These cry modes are present in all typically developing children, and also children from different cultures (6,8). In a recent study, Esposito and Venuti (9) described the shape of the "narrative structure" of a crying cycle. In typically developing infants, some degree of homogeneity across cultures exists (8). In particular the general shape of such cycles seems stable. The general shape or narrative of each crying cycle is composed of 4 phases: (i) an initial phase, when the fundamental frequency starts to increase from a baseline level (usually silence). Soon after this initial phase there is a second phase, called (ii) plateau, when the fundamental frequency reaches its highest level. The plateau phase is then followed by (iii) the aspiration/expiration phase, during which the cry sound follows the breathing rhythm. The last or final phase (iv) concludes the cycle. During this last phase the fundamental frequency decreases to its baseline level. A crying episode can be composed of several cycles, and the proportion of time spent in each phase can differ from cycle to cycle.

For example pain cry, which usually require an immediate response from caregivers in order to assure the infant's safety (and, in extreme cases, survival), tend to have a higher and longer plateau phase and a shorter initial, aspiration/expiration and final phase than other cries. In this way the perceptual system of the caregiver, which, for neurophisiological reasons, is typically more activated by higher pitch stimuli, will be activated sooner. On the other hand, hunger cry, which do not always require an immediate response from the caregiver (the child will survive if the response is not immediate), tend to have a longer initial and aspiration/expiration phase and shorter plateau and final phases.

Evolutionary trajectory of crying

A cry is a signal available to infants from the very early stages of life. In a recent study, Gingras, Mitchell and Grattan (10) reported that a fetal homologue of crying, lasting about 15 seconds, was observed. One of the most replicated findings about crying in early infancy concerns what is called "the cry curve". Crying increases during the first two months of life, with a peak usually found around the sixth week and a decline during the following months (8,11,12). In general, soon after birth, the cry becomes an automatic reaction to signal biological needs (hunger, pain, visceral colic); typically it also elicits soothing behavior from caregivers (e.g., cuddling or moving the child rhythmically) that are universally utilized across different cultures. These responses are the result of cultural norms (8) and caregiver characteristics (13); infant cry characteristics influence responses to crying as well (14,15). The caregiver's adequate behavioral response, which ideally satisfies the newborn's needs, is a mandatory step for good future relations. Deviations in the signal and/or misunderstanding the message can compromise infant care, parental effectiveness, and undermine the budding relationship (4). Not surprisingly, the needs of an infant do not remain stagnant; on the contrary, the baby's needs generally follow a course of development, as does the expression of crying. Initial cries requesting basic wants soon evolve into solicitations rooted outside of biology. Day by day, the reasons for crying episodes become more social. Whatever the reasons, these bouts typically serve to bring or keep the caregiver in the infant's proximity.

Around the 3rd month, episodes of crying can result from a sudden change in environmental stimulation; for example, when the caregiver goes out of the visual field of the child or when the caregiver stops singing or talking. In these scenarios, restoring the environmental stimulation or distracting the baby with new stimuli often succeeds in stopping the crying. Generally speaking, behaviors that cause distress or offer consolation to the child often match the subtle aspects of crying being expressed at the moment. These different aspects of crying and caregiver responses help define the nature of their relationship (16), and also reflect: (i) the new competence of the child to face the world; (ii) the child's ability to modulate internal stimuli; (iii) and other factors such as parental age and personality (15) and infant age (17).

At 8 months, babies can have a specific relationship with their caregivers and a better understanding of the world around them; on the whole, infants are more aware of their needs and they are also more aware of the implications of their cries than earlier. During this stage, to be aware of the power of their cries means that babies are responsive to the effects that their crying can produce, specifically changes in the behavior of others and especially that of their caregiver. Infants also develop, at about 7 or 8 months, both a stronger attachment to the mother and an increased sense of ''stranger fear'' (11,18). Usually stranger fear is expressed through the ''stranger fear cry,'' a specific modality of crying activated when the caregiver is not in sight and another person is closely approaching the child. At 12 months, the cry is an effective and efficient communicative routine, with a narrative and a turn-tacking structure. In short, crying is a base and a guide for the development of language and will be, for the rest of life, a primary communicative approach to express deep and strong feelings (19).

Parental reaction to human cries

Crying is the very first beahvior with a communictaive valence, and it represents an early signal that the neonate can use to express its needs and wants. For this reason it is important to understand how parents react to this signal. Research during the last several decades has focused on three main aspects: (i) responses of adults to infant crying, (ii) effects of those parental responses on infant crying, (iii) differences between parents and non-parents in their responses to infant crying.

Responses of adults to infant crying

In the last several decades many studies have focused on how the frequency and duration of cyring episodes modulate adult responses. For example researchers have reported that parental responses are the results of cultural norms (8), caregiver characteristics (13), and morphological characteristics of the infant cry (14,15). Cry pitch also can influence caregivers' perception: higher frequency cries are often perceived as more aversive and distressful than lower frequency cries. A particular type of cry, characterized by low frequency and typical of children with Down syndrome, is often perceived as less urgent than the moderate frequency cries usually encountered in typically developing children. On the other hand, cries of pre-term infants (considered a high-risk population) are typically of higher frequency and for that reason are considered more urgent than moderate frequency cries. Another example: the cries of children with visceral colic are characterized by higher frequency and are also perceived as more distressful (1).

These patterns have been confirmed using an experimental procedure in which acoustic parameters (frequency and duration) of crying episodes were modified and then participants where asked to listen and judge the different stimuli. The results confirmed that frequency plays a crucial role in determining the urgency of a person's response. Another important acoustic variable is the duration of the pauses during a crying episode. Zeskind and colleagues (20) modified the length of the expiratory phase and pauses in some crying episodes. Participants who were asked to judge those stimuli regarded shorter pauses as more activating, informative, and also distressful.

Irwin (21) has investigated modality effects on cry perception. In her study, she examined whether perceivers can detect more distress in the acoustic or visual signals within the cry. Perceiver ratings differed for high- and low-distress cries at each infant age on the basis of facial and vocal action, but not bodily movement. Perceivers rated the cry sound as more distressed and the cry face as less distressed with increasing infant age. The author speculated that information about distress is available to perceivers in both the crying infant's face and voice.

Effects of parental responses to infant crying

In a naturalistic study, Bell and Ainsworth (11) showed that the promptness of maternal response to crying was related to children's individual differences in their amount of crying and with more favourable outcomes for children. These same results were also described by Moss (22). Other experimental studies (23,24) have analyzed the effectiveness of different interventions. In general, it seems that maternal warmth and promptness of maternal response to cries are important predictors of outcome. Many studies report that a caregiver's responsiveness to infant cries play an important role in the development of the child's personality, temperament, and cognitive and linguistic skills. Some authors suggest that crying should be interpreted as a biosocial phenomenon that directly reflects the status of the nervous system and indirectly mediates development through parental intervention (4,25). Some support for this interpretation is provide by data gathered in a study of preterm infants in which parents were asked to rate the aversiveness of an infant's cry (26). Infants of mothers who better identified their infant's cry as more aversive or less had higher Bayley mental scores and language scores at 18 months than infants whose mothers misperceived their infant's cry (4,25). It has been speculated that agreement between the cry signal and parent perception optimizes child development (4).

Differences between parents and non-parents in their responses to infant crying

Adult brain activation varies enormously in response to infant vocalization; specifically, it is affected by the sex and parental status of the adult. In a study by Seifritz and colleagues (27), functional magnetic resonance imaging (fMRI) was used to analyze brain response to infant crying and laughing in mothers and fathers of young children and in female and male non-parents. Interestingly, they found that women but not men, independent of their parental status, showed neural deactivation in the anterior cingulate cortex, as indexed by decreased blood oxygenation level– dependent signal, in response to both types of infant vocalization. Different patterns emerged in other brain regions, controlling for the role of parental experience. In the amygdala and in the limbic regions connected, parents showed stronger activation from crying, whereas non-parents showed stronger activation from laughing. These results suggest that sex and experience change the brain response pattern. The authors of this study speculated that a "successful recognition and evaluation of infant vocalizations can be critical for bonding mechanisms and for offspring well-being and survival. Thus, the modulation of responses by experience seems to represent an adaptive mechanism that can be related to reproductive fitness" (27).

A number of studies have investigated the differences between parents and non-parents. Fleming and colleagues (2), analyzing endocrine responses in response to infant cries, made an interesting point. In order to determine the responsiveness of experienced fathers, new fathers and non-fathers toward infant cues, they proposed an experimental procedure for which participants were asked to listen to infant cries and other control stimuli, and affective and endocrine responses were measured prior to and after the cry presentations. In particular, they measured salivary testosterone, cortisol and plasma prolactin concentrations. Their results showed that fathers hearing the cry stimuli felt more alert and sympathetic compared to non-fathers. The baseline level of hormones was predictive of the general affectivity of the men toward the infants and was not influenced by prior experience. More specifically (i) adult males (both fathers and non-fathers) with lower testosterone levels had higher sympathy to infant cries than adult males with higher testosterone levels and (ii) fathers with higher prolactin levels were more alert and more positive in response to the cries then fathers with lower levels of it. Another interesting result of this study was related to the level of increase in hormones. In particular, (i) a greater percentage increase in testosterone was reported for fathers hearing the cry stimuli compared to fathers not hearing the cry stimuli and (ii) a greater percentage increase in prolactin levels was reported for experienced fathers hearing the cries compared to first-time fathers or to non-fathers hearing control stimuli. Finally, after accounting for the variance related to parity and experience, both experience and testosterone continued to contribute to the variance in fathers' affective responses to infant cries. This pattern of results led the authors to conclude that human fathers are more responsive to infant distress signal then non-fathers and that both hormones and caregiving experience play an important role in this pattern.

The two studies just described suggest that both direct experience and biological alterations can affect how adults react to infant cries. Others studies have also noted how parents appear more skilled then non-parents. For example, parents are more able to identify episodes of cry with a higher level of fundamental frequency (hyperphonation), often related to expression of pain (28), than non-parents. This result was also replicated with a Japanese sample, which is interesting because in Japan the expression of crying is often culturally inhibited (29).

Others differences between parents and non-parents are related to the amount of information they need to recognise the cause of the cry: parents need less information, (28). Furthermore parents know more soothing strategies than non-parents (30). A similar finding was described by Gustafson and colleagues (3) after using a simulation experiment in which mothers and non-mothers were asked to sooth a manikin resembling an infant. They found that mothers and non-mothers alike began their response with some combination of five different behaviours: (a) pick up the infant; (b) put the infant to their shoulder; (c) verbal stimulation; (d) tactile stimulation (e.g., patting or stroking), and (e) vestibular stimulation (e.g., rocking or swaying). Moreover mothers were somewhat better at guessing the exact cause of the cries, and they spent a greater proportion of their time engaged in activities that might soothe the infant's distress (3).

Cries in children with atypical development

A number of studies that examined cries of infants with a specific medical conditions related to neurological damage were conducted in the twenty-year period from the 1960 to the 1980. Since the instrumentation of that time was limited by today's standards, those early studies gave a description of crying that included only a limited number of acoustic characteristics. In general, those studies demonstrated an association between crying and neurological status. In particular, they highlighted how the fundamental frequency (f0) was particularly sensitive to neurological insult with both higher levels overall and greater variability resulting. The fundamental frequency seems particularly influenced by neurological damage. Among these studies, some identified brain anomalies associated with a higher level of f0, whereas other anomalies were associated with a lower level of f0. In particular, higher levels of f0, more biphonation (f0 instability), and less duration were associated with brain damage (31,32), Krabbe's disease (33), meningitis (34), and asphyxia (35). On the other hand, lower levels of f0, were described in children with Down syndrome (36), children with hypothyroidism (37), and children with trisomy 13 and 18 (38).

Many of the early researchers also examined cry characteristics in infants at risk for poor outcomes based on potential neurological insult (e.g., prematurity). Overall, groups of infants at-risk showed higher and more heterogeneity of fundamental frequency and fewer utterances but increased short utterances, suggesting increased tension and instability of neural control of the vocal tract and poorer capacity of the respiratory system. More recently cry studies have examined the effects of potential prenatal insult during pregnancy (e.g., drug exposure). These studies suggest that drug-exposed infants also show increased fundamental frequency, shorter utterances, a higher level of dysphonation, hyperphonation, and more dysregulation—all signs that indicating poor neural control of the vocal track and respiration (4). Among groups of at-risk children, premature infants are often studied. For example, Corwin and colleagues, (39) showed short cry utterances and lower developmental outcome (measured at 30 months) in preterm infants. Higher f0 and shorter duration in preterms infants has been described as well (40,41).

A number of studies have emphasized that anomalies in cry characteristics can be related to neurological compromise. These findings suggest that undetected neurological damage may be found by analyzing cries, even when no other symptoms seem to be present. In this view, atypical cries may be considered an early indicator of developmental risk. The kind of cry and its perception could thus aid the identification of neonatal risk. Starting from this point of view, some researchers have begun to analyze episodes of crying in children with Autism Spectrum Disorder (ASD). Considering the tight connection between crying and the functioning of the brainstem and limbic system (both areas highly compromised in ASD children), it seems reasonable to expect some anomalies in the expression of cry in ASD infants. Moreover ASD afflicts individuals by compromising their communicative and social skills and their activity repertoire, and crying can be viewed as both the first communicative system and the first social structure in human development. The analysis of acoustic features of crying episodes has found a number of differences among children with ASD and matched controls. In particular, in ASD children episodes of cry were characterized with shorter duration, less waveform modulation, and more dysphonation (42). In a more recent study (9), the shape of the "narrative structure" of cry cycles in infants with ASD has been described. This specific narrative of a cycle of cry in ASD children has showed some anomalies in the 4 phases, specifically: (i) the initial phase was often shorter than usual; (ii) the plateau phase presented a series of repetitive peaks with high frequency; (iii) the aspiration/expiration phase was usually not present and when present was shorter than expected; and the last phase (iv) was also shorter then for the matching control cases. The authors speculated that these differences can lead to caregivers misinterpreting the child's needs and create problems in the child-caregiver relationship.

How cries are perceived in children with atypical development: The case of autism spectrum disorder

In typical situations, parents understand the level of distress of a crying episode. They pay attention to the sound (in particular evaluating the intensity and the height of the pitch), evaluate the facial expression of the child, and take the environmental situation into account (such as the hour of the day, the time since the previous meal, etc). Furthermore, when a child has a specific, previously diagnosed neurological condition, and if the parent has received appropriate training from a specialist, those parents can correctly interpret the distress signals of their child even though their child's cries are quite atypical. An excellent example of this process of accommodation, where the parent can understand a signal after training, is provided by the Cri-du-Chat syndrome. The Cri-du-Chat syndrome (deletion 5p syndrome) is a rare genetic disorder due to a missing portion of chromosome 5. The condition affects an estimated 1 in 20,000 to 50,000 live births. The disorder is found in people of all ethnic backgrounds and is slightly more common in females by a 3-1 ratio. The peculiarity of this syndrome (form which it gets its name) is the characteristic cry sound, which sounds just like a meowing kitten and is characterized by cries of very high pitch and short duration. Although the meaning of an episode of cry-du-chat is difficult to impossible to understand at first, parents of children with this disorder can, after adequate training, come to understand their child's needs and wants. But what happens when parents cannot adequately understand their children's cries? An instructive example occurs when a parent interacts with a child with neurological deficits, but before those deficits are diagnosed. This situation often happens in the case of children with ASD (9), for whom diagnoses are usually provided only after 24 months of age.

In later interviews with parents whose children have been diagnosed with ASD, the parents often report that they had great difficulty decoding the emotional signals of their children, especially during the first year. They report, in particular, problems with understanding the causes of crying episodes. Such misunderstandings regarding why their infant is crying can initiate a vicious cycle. The caregiver fails to recognize the child's needs, and these results in inadequate feedback to the child.

A number of studies (9,42-44) have investigated how parents perceive crying in children with ASD compared to typical developing children and children with intellectual disabilities. In a first study (42), an interview was administrated to parents of children with ASD and those of typically developing children. Qualitative analysis showed that negative patterns with respect to crying episodes were more often mentioned by parents of ASD children, who often mentioned difficulty understanding those episodes. In a successive study (9), an experimental procedure was designed to test whether the atypical structure of crying episodes typical of children with ASD could bias parents' perception. In particular, a ''Listen-and-Response'' experiment was carried out. Twelve episodes of crying at different ages (13 and 20 months) from retrospective home video of children with ASD and from matching control group children were presented to participants. Participants were asked to listen to the 12 stimuli, randomly presented, and then answer three questions: (a) guess the age of the child who was crying; (b) guess the reasons why the child was crying, (c) and describe what they felt while hearing the cries.

The results of this study showed some specificity of ASD crying episodes. In particular, participants assigned younger ages to ASD cries. Nevertheless, when listening to ASD crying episodes, participants felt more negative states. In contrast, more positive mental states were felt when listening to crying episodes of children in the other two groups. These different patterns may be interpreted as resulting from an incorrect decoding of the acoustic stimulus. In particular, because of the acoustic characteristics (few peaks, small modulation, small rhythm, and absence of turn-taking), the crying episodes of the children with ASD are difficult to interpret and for this reason may evoke mental states of uneasiness (9). This suggestion agrees with Zeskind and Marshall (45) who found that shorter pauses were perceived to be more arousing and aversive.

Some important implications follow from these results. In particular, the authors speculated that the relationship between caregivers and their children with ASD may be prey to a vicious cycle (43,44). This vicious cycle, could start from a series of brain anomalies present in ASD children since birth (and possibly even before). Given these hypothesized brain anomalies, the various acoustic qualities of a crying episode may not be easily understood by the caregiver. Problems in understanding their infant's cries creates distress and can make the caregivers uneasy. The distress leads caregivers to provide their children with inadequate feedback, which is not effective in addressing the cause of specific crying episodes. As a result, caregivers do not receive an adequate response from their children and so start to feel inadequate, not able to provide their children with a sense of well being. Sensing something amiss, caregivers may attempt to modify their parenting skills. For their part, children who cannot adequately communicate with their caregivers may engage in such compensatory behaviors as isolation, stereotyped behavior, hyper or hypocinesia, etc.). Thus something related to a neurological disorder (in this example, crying) becomes a starting point for a problem in interaction and sets the tone for the overall relationship between the caregiver and child with ASD, undermining the development of intersubjectivity processes for the child with ASD.

Conclusions

The aim of this paper was to describe expressions of distress, specifically crying, during early stages of development in infancy. In particular, we wanted to briefly describe the physiology of human crying and its evolutionary trajectory. Then, keeping in mind the communicative valence of crying episodes, our intention was to discuss parental reactions to human cries, focusing on how adults respond to infants crying and how their responses affect infant crying, and also whether or not parents and non-parents differ in their response to crying. Finally, we described some results of studies concerning the cries of children with atypical development and whether or not acoustic anomalies in the cries of children with atypical development can lead to parental misperception of the signal itself.

The core idea of this study was that cries serve as an important signal of distress, but moreover, they play a crucial role in human development, representing both the first communicative and the first social structure in infant development. Before neonates smile or visually fixate on objects, they can communicate with the environment by crying. They can use cries to signal their caregiver and make their primary (5) and affective, social, and cognitive needs known.

This behavior, activating the central nervous system (CNS) of both infant and caregiver, creates a state of reciprocal attention and regulates the infant-caregiver relationship. Moreover, it guarantees the building of a specific tie that assures the survival of the infant. Crying starts early communication between caregiver and infant and, based on the maternal (or paternal) skill to give a meaning to the child's cries, their parents' behavior assures the infant about caregiver proximity, thus the infant acquires a sense of reliance in the external environment. Furthermore the strict connection that exists between the cry expression and the central nervous system, gives to the cry the status of an important early indicator of mental health. The cry behavioral system can be altered in two ways: (i) the child's cries can be atypical or (ii) the caretaker's reactions to cries can be atypical. Both these two possibilities need to be considered in order to assure an infant's ideal development. Moreover, although many studies have focused on the acoustic or social features of children's cries, less emphasis has been given to the ways parents face episodes of cry. Especially during the first months after the birth, pediatricians and other health personnel should dedicate more attention to the difficulty parents may have in understanding and responding to their infant's cries. In general we believe that training programs should start during pregnancy to educate new-parents on the language of cries. With this additional skill, parents could better monitor their children's cries and report to their pediatrician any anomalies that could be related to potential medical problems.

Moreover, cry evaluation could be included in screening tools that assess the neurological activity of the new-born and in order to activate early intervention programs with families. In this view, intervention with families, to help parents understand their children's crying, could help them avoid interactional problems and reduce parental stress and child anxiety.

References

[1] Huffman LC, Bryan YE, del Carmen R, Pedersen FA, Doussard-Roosevelt JA, Porges SW. Infant temperament and cardiac vagal tone: Assessments at twelve weeks of age. Child Dev 1998;69(3):624-35.

[2] Fleming AS, Corter C, Stallings J, Steiner M. Testosterone and prolactin are associated with emotional responses to infant cries in new fathers. Horm Behav 2005;42:399-413.

[3] Gustafson G, Wood R, Green J. Can we hear the causes of infants' crying? In: Barr R, Hopkins B, Green J, eds. Crying as a sign, a signal, and a symptom. London: Mac Keith, 2000:8-22.

[4] LaGasse L, Neal AR, Lester BM. Assessment of Infant Cry: acoustic Cry analysis and parental perception. Ment Retard Dev Disabil 2005;11:83-93.

[5] Murray AD. Infant crying as elicitor of parental behaviour: An examination of two models. Psychol Bull 1979;86:191-215.

[6] Wolff P. The natural history of crying and other vocalizations in early infancy. In: Foss B, ed. Determinants of infant behaviour (vol. 4). London: Mathuen, 1969.

[7] Golub HL. A physioacoustic model of the infant cry. In: Lester MB, Boukydis CFZ, eds. Infant crying: Theoretical and research perspectives. New York: Plenum, 1989:59-82.

[8] Barr RG, Konner M, Bakeman R, Adamson L. Crying in Kung San infants: A test of cultural specificity hypothesis. Dev Med Child Neurol 1991;33:601-10.

[9] Esposito G, Venuti P. Is this a cry? A study on early communication signals in children with Autistic Spectrum disorder (ASD). Proceed Int Cry Workshop, Denmark, 2007.

[10] Gingras JL, Mitchell EA., Grattan KE. Fetal homologue of infant crying. Arch Dis Child Fetal Neonatal Ed 2005;90:415-8.

[11] Bell SM, Ainsworth MDS. Infant crying and maternal responsiveness. Child Dev 1972;43:1171-90.

[12] St James-Roberts I. Persistent crying in infancy. J Child Psychol Psychiatry 1989;30:189–95.

[13] Frodi A. When emphathy fails. Avversative infant crying and child abuse. In: Lester BM, Boukydis CFZ, eds. Infant crying: theoretical and research perspectives. New York: Plenum, 1995:263-77.

[14] Gustafson GE, Green JA. On the importance of fundamental frequency and other acoustic features in cry perception and infant development. Child Dev 1989;60(4):772-80.

[15] Ziefman DM. Predicting adult responses to infant distress: Adult characteristics associated with perceptions, emotional reactions, and timing of intervention. Infant Ment Health J 2003;24:597-612.

[16] Dunn J. Emotional development in early childhood: A social relationship perspective. In: Davidson R, Goldsmith HH, Scherer K, eds. The handbook of affective science. Oxford: Oxford Univ Press, 2002:332-46.

[17] Schuetze P, Zeskind PS, Eiden RD. The perceptions of infant distress signals varying in pitch by cocaine-using mothers. Infancy 2003;4:65-83.

[18] Trevarthen C, Aitken K, Papoudi D, Robarts J. Children with autism: Diagnosis and interventions to meet their needs. London: Jessica Kingsley, 1998.

[19] Rothganger H. Analysis of the sounds of the child in the first year of age and a comparison to the language. Early Hum Dev 2003;75:55-69.
[20] Zeskind PS, Klein L, Marshall TR. Adult's perceptions of experimental modifications of durations of pauses and expiratory sounds in infant crying. Child Dev 1992;59:193-6.
[21] Irwin JR. Parent and non-parent perception of the multimodal infant cry. Infancy 2003;4:503-16.
[22] Moss HA. Communication in mother-infant interaction. In: Krames L, Plin P, Alloway T, eds. Advances in the study of communication and affect. New York: Plenum, 1974:171-91.
[23] Korner AE, Grobstein R. Visual alertness as related to soothing in neonates: Implications for maternal stimulation and early deprivation. Child Dev 1966;37:867-76.
[24] Korner AE, Thoman EB. Visual alertness in neonates as evoked by maternal care. J Exp Child Psychol 1970;10:67-79.
[25] Lester BM. A biosocial model of infant crying. In: Lipsitt L, Rovee-Collier C, eds. Advances in infant research. Norwood, NJ: Ablex, 1984.
[26] Lester BM, Boukydis CF, Garcia Coll CT. Developmental outcome as a function of the goodness of fit between the infant's cry characteristics and the mother's perception of her infant's cry. Pediatrics 1995;95:516-21.
[27] Seifritz E, Esposito F, Neuhoff JG, Luthi A., Mustovic H, Dammann G, et al. Differential sex-independent amygdala response to infant crying and laughing in parents versus nonparents. Biol Psychiatry 2003;12(54):1367-75.
[28] Green JA, Jones LE, Gustafson GE. Perception of cries by parents and non-parents: Relation to cry acoustics. Dev Psychol 1987; 23:370-82.
[29] Adachi T, Murai N, Okada H, Nihei Y. Maternal perception of infant cries. Japanese J Edu Psychol 1985;33:146-51.
[30] Zeskind PS, Lester BM. Analysis of infant crying. In: Singer LT, Zeskind PS, eds. Biobehavioral assessment of the infant. New York: Guilford, 2001:149-66.
[31] Fisichelli, VR, Karelitz, S. Frequency spectra of the cries of normal infants and those with Down's Syndrome. Psychon Sci 1966; 6:195-6.
[32] Sirvio P, Michelsson K. Sound-spectrographic cry analysis of normal and abnormal newborn infants: A review and a recommendation for standardization of the cry characteristics. Folia Phoniatr Logop 1976;28:161-73.
[33] Thoden CJ, Michelsson K. Sound spectrographic cry analysis in Krabbe's Disease. Dev Med Child Neurol 1979;21:400-1.
[34] Michelsson K, Sirvio P, Wasz-Hockert O. Pain cry in full-term asphyxiated newborn infants correlated with late findings. Acta Paediatr Scand 1977;66:611-6.
[35] Michelsson K. Cry analyses of symptomless low birth weight neonates and of asphyxiated newborn infants. Acta Paediatr Scand 1971; 216(Suppl):9-45.
[36] Wasz-Hockert O, Lind J, Vuorenski V, Partanen T, Valanne E. The infant cry: A spectrographic and auditory analysis. Clin Dev Med 1968;29:1-42.
[37] Michelsson K, Sirvio P. Cry analysis in congenital hypothyroidism. Folia Phoniatr Logop 1976;28:40-7.
[38] Michelsson K., Tupperainen N, Aula P. Cry analysis of infant with karyotype abnormality. Neuropediatrics 1980;11:365-76.
[39] Corwin MJ, Lester BM, Sepkoski C, McLaughlin S, Kayne H, Golub HL. Effects of in utero cocaine exposure on newborn acoustical cry characteristics. Pediatrics 1992;89:1199-1203.
[40] Michelsson K, Jarvenpaa AL, Rinne A. Sound spectrographic analysis of pain cry in preterm infants. Early Hum Dev 1983;8:141-9.
[41] Lester BM. Prediction of developmental outcome from acoustic cry analysis in term and preterm infant. Paediatrics 1987;80:529-34.
[42] Venuti P, Esposito G, Giusti Z. A qualitative analysis of crying and vocal distress in children with autism. J Int Dis Res 2004;48(4):338.
[43] Venuti P, Esposito G. Come piangono i bambini con disturbo dello spettro autistico? [How do children with Autism Spectrum Disorder cry?] Psic Clin Svil 2007;12(2):325-44. [Italian]

[44] Esposito G, Venuti P. How is crying perceived in children with Autistic Spectrum Disorder? Res Autism Spectr Disord 2008; 2(2):371-84.

[45] Zeskind PS, Marshall TR. The relation between variations in pitch and maternal perceptions of infant crying. Child Dev 1988; 59(1):193-6.

Submitted: May 08, 2008.
Revised: June 01, 2008.
Accepted: June 06, 2008.

In: Public Health Yearbook 2009
Editor: Joav Merrick

ISBN: 978-1-61668-911-7

Chapter 15

New psychosocial methods in child health care: Can we make a difference under routine conditions?

Dagmar Lagerberg, PhD*[*1], Margaretha Magnusson, MD[1,2] and Claes Sundelin, MD[1,2]

[1]Department of Women's and Children's Health, University of Uppsala, Uppsala University Children's Hospital, Uppsala. Sweden

[2]County Unit for Child Health Care, Uppsala University Children's Hospital, Uppsala, Sweden

Abstract

The study was inspired by general allegations against the preventive child health services of failing to take into account problems faced by modern families, e.g. attachment difficulties and stress. Objective: In order to improve the psychosocial effectiveness of the health services for preschool children, a comprehensive programme was tested. Study group and setting: Mothers of 1,963 children participated. 967 were recruited at 18 months (Cohort I, baseline, no intervention), 996 shortly after birth and followed until 18 months (Cohort II) in two arms: intervention – non-intervention. Thirty-six child health centres within primary care in Uppsala county (experiment) and 36 centres in five other Swedish counties (control) were enrolled. Methods: Quasi-experimental controlled trial under routine conditions. The intervention included screening for postpartum depression, a curriculum for attachment and interaction, book gifts, parent groups, encouragement to participate in network activities, and extended home visits if needed. Main outcome measures: management of postpartum depression, mother-child interaction, child vocabulary, group participation, stress in parents. Results: The programme was not implemented according to the plans. Apart from more invitations to parent groups and higher participation in parent groups, there were no effects attributable to the intervention. The experiences are discussed with a view to general recommendations for intervention research put forward in the

* Correspondence: Associate professor Dagmar Lagerberg, PhD, Department of Women's and Children's Health, Uppsala University Children's Hospital, SE-751 85 Uppsala. Tel. +46-18 611 59 73. Fax +46-18 50 45 11. e-mail: dagmar.lagerberg@kbh.uu.se

literature. Conclusions: Intervention trials in primary care should not be launched without extra resources in terms of financial support, manpower, and monitoring. Recommendations of careful pre-planning and development of interventions in several stages should be followed.

Keywords: Children, experimental research, prevention, psychosocial methods, public health.

Introduction

Since the 1930's, Sweden has been offering preventive health care to children of preschool age. All children are invited to Child Health Centres (CHC) at certain key ages. The services are free of charge and accepted by almost all parents (1).

The present study was inspired by a general criticism of the Child Health Services (CHS) for failing to take into account challenges faced by parents in a modern society, such as attachment difficulties and parental stress. New political and financial trends had resulted in claims of evidence-basing the services (2). According to the final document of a state-of-the-art conference in 1999 (3), non-evidence-based practices were to be removed successively, and the CHS should take particular responsibility for infants below two years of age.

The aim of the present study was to develop a new model for the psychosocial tasks of the CHS. As far as possible, the programme components were to be evidence-based. The programme differed from common international standards in being performed under routine conditions, with no additional financial or manpower contributions.

Methods

The study relied on sources of inspiration retrieved from research literature. The main parts of the intervention addressed postpartum depression, parent-child interaction, language development, social relations, and stress in parents.

Postpartum depression

Postpartum depression affects 8-15 % of all mothers (4) and is a substantial risk factor for suboptimal parent-child attachment, social development (5), and insufficient safety measures for children (6,7). The Edinburgh Postnatal Depression Scale (EPDS) was applied, a screening tool for postpartum depression validated on Swedish-speaking mothers (4,8). Counselling by the nurse has proven effective with moderately depressed infant mothers (9). Four to six counselling sessions were to be offered to mothers scoring 12-16; mothers scoring 17 or more were to be referred to a psychologist. Outcomes: proportion of mothers screened and case management of high scorers.

Parent-child interaction

Associations have been found between attachment security and children's social relationships and social functioning (10). A parent curriculum aimed at improving interaction in everyday situations, implemented in individual and group sessions, was used: International Child Development Programmes (ICDP) (11). The program aims at making parents reflect on eight themes: showing affection; awareness of child's needs; communication about interesting things; encouragement; helping child to pay attention to things and events; describe shared experiences; explain shared experiences; setting limits in a positive way. Outcomes: implementation of the programme; mother's own perception of her capacity to satisfy each theme (1: very little, 5: very much). A mean based on the eight themes was calculated.

Reading and language development

The effectiveness of reading information and book gifts to parents in producing a more advanced language in children has been established (12). Differences in reading frequency with small children have shown associations with SES and number of siblings (13,14). A special brochure was developed and book gifts were to be offered at 10, 12 and 18 months. Outcomes: parent's or other family member's looking in a book with the child (10 or more times/week, 6-9 times, 3-5 times, 1-2 times, never); expressive vocabulary of the child measured from a standardised list of 90 simple words, where the mother was asked to indicate whether the child could understand, or understand and say the word (15).

Social relations

Substantial proportions of parents experience a lack of social support and high stress levels (16). Social support and stress have been found to be related to the quality of parent-child communication (17). Parent groups, supposed to offer opportunities for families of making acquaintances and discussing common problems, have been an integrated part of the CHS since about 30 years. The ”open preschool”, an informal organisation for parents and young children, aims at supporting social networking among parents. Parents were to be invited systematically to groups and encouraged to take part in the activities of the open preschool. Outcomes: invitation rates to parent groups, participation in groups by mothers and fathers, information about the open preschool by the nurse, mother's participation in the open preschool and her appreciation of the services (very valuable, valuable, not very valuable, don't know). Mothers were asked about their overall experience of the CHC (very great benefit, certain benefit, no benefit, don't know).

Parenthood stress

It was hypothesised that social networking through groups and the open preschool would result in lower levels of stress. The Swedish Parenthood Stress Questionnaire (SPSQ) has been validated on a Swedish population (16), and treatment for behaviour problems in children has been found to decrease stress in parents (18). The Swedish version consists of a total scale and five subscales (Socisol: Social isolation, Roler: restriction due to parenting role, Incomp: incompetence in parenting tasks, Spouse: stress in relation to spouse, Health: stress related to health; 1: low stress, 5: high stress). Outcomes: means on total SPSQ and the five subscales.

Home visits

Based on the positive findings reported by Olds from intensive nurse visiting to deprived mothers (19), a home visiting programme was planned. The families were to be selected by the nurse according to her personal knowledge of the family. This was a different approach from the ordinary Swedish programme, where the nurse typically makes one home visit to inform about the services and establish a working relationship. All mothers were to have at least one home visit and those with psychosocial needs substantially more (e.g., in case of mental health problems or risks of neglect). Outcomes: proportion of families visited, number of home visits per family.

Special efforts were to be made to include immigrant and refugee families, defined as families where the mother was born outside Sweden. Interpreters were to be engaged and paid by the project in case of need. Outcome: participation of immigrant and refugee families.

Setting and participants

The CHC:s were to be situated in non-privileged areas, particularly with high proportions of immigrant families. Eighteen CHC:s from Uppsala county constituted the experiment group. Eighteen CHC:s from other counties served as controls (Stockholm, Östergötland, Värmland, Västmanland, and Dalarna). The main reason for not randomising within one county was the risk of "contagion effects" which could have influenced nurses and participants in uncontrollable ways.

At the beginning of the study, a part time university course in child health care and social paediatrics was arranged for the experiment nurses, and a manual for the intervention was developed by the project management in collaboration with the nurses.

Information about the children was obtained from the population register or directly from CHC registers. Baseline children were born September 2000 – August 2001 (cohort I). When these children, who were given "services as usual", came for their 18-month check-up (March 2002 – February 2003), the mothers were asked to complete a questionnaire covering background data, participation in and appreciation of services, child health and behaviour, language, stress, and life situation. The nurse extracted certain data from the children's health records. The intervention started with follow-up infants (cohort II) born April 2003 – March 2004. The children were offered the intervention if they belonged to an experiment centre or moved into the area no later than at one month of age. All children were followed until the youngest had passed their 18-month check-up, i.e., September 2005. Health and intervention data were registered continually by the nurses. The mothers completed the same questionnaire as cohort I (see table 1).

Table 1. Study materials and steps in data retrieval

Material	EXPERIMENT		CONTROL	
	Baseline Cohort I[1]	Follow-up Cohort II[2]	Baseline Cohort I[1]	Follow-up Cohort II[2]
	N	N	N	N
Eligible children	752	758	778	842
External drop-out (moved out before check-up)	91	108	46	56
Remaining for study	661	650	732	786
Declined/refused or nurse did not ask mother	57	116	65	72
Remaining for study after refusal	604	534	667	714
Accepted but questionnaire not returned	147	112	157	140
Questionnaire returned	457	422	510	574
Questionnaire returned, % of those remaining	69.1	64.9	69.7	73.0
Health record from CHC	604	533	667	712

[1] Due for 18-month check-up, born September 2000-August 2001.
[2] Born into study April 2003-March 2004.

The children's age variation at questionnaire delivery was 14-32 months. 72.8 % (1430/1963) were 17-19 months old, and 40.8 % (800/1963) exactly 18 months. There were 50.6 % (993/1963) boys and 49.4 % (970/1963) girls. The questionnaire return rate was 69 % (1963 of 2829 after external dropout), with variations 69.1 % - 73.0 % (see table 1). All 2519 children whose mothers accepted to participate, except three, had a health record completed by the nurse.

The numbers of nurses were 20 experiment and 21 control during baseline and 21 in each arm during follow-up. A fact not intended or noticed in advance was that all nurses in the experiment centres were district nurses working with child health as part of their tasks ("integrated" CHC:s). The control nurses worked exclusively with children ("focused" CHC:s). There was more personnel turnover during the study in experiment than control areas. The study was approved by the Research Ethics Committees of the universities involved (Dnr Ups 01-342).

Statistical methods

The SAS package for personal computers was used (20). Significance was tested by X^2, Fisher's exact test, t-test, and logistic regression analyses with dichotomizations of continuous variables by the means. Effect sizes for means (Cohen's d) and X^2 were calculated (21). As to means, an effect size of about 0.8 is considered large, 0.5 medium and 0.2 small. For effect sizes based on X^2, 0.5 is considered large, 0.3 medium and 0.1 small. Observations with missing values were excluded from the calculations concerned, which resulted in varying N and n values.

Results

The implementation of programme components is shown in table 2. About 90 % of the mothers were screened with the EPDS, however significantly fewer of the immigrant mothers. Of 449 mothers screened, 48 (11 %) had a score of 12 or more (range 12-23). Fourteen of these, six with a score of 12-16 and eight scoring 17 or more, were referred to a psychologist (29.2 %). Five declined because they had already a helping contact. Of the 48 high-scoring mothers, 20 received no counselling, 25 were offered 1-6 counselling sessions (mean: 1.9), and three were already taken care of. Fourteen mothers scoring under 12 received 1-6 counselling sessions, most of them only one.

About 90 % participated in at least one ICDP session, immigrant mothers significantly less. However, fewer than half had two group sessions and/or five individual sessions. About 90 % received three children's books, but a substantial proportion of mothers did not receive the brochure.

Table 2. Implementation of programme components. Percentages of experiment children, cohort II, whose mothers were offered the intervention, total and by maternal ethnicity. Mean number of home visits for those who had at least one visit. Source: nurses' records of programme implementation and maternal questionnaires

Part of programme	Children with nurse records	Children with returned questionnaires (and nurse records)			
	N=533	All N=422	Mother born in Sweden N=345	Mother not born in Sweden N=77	P (country of birth)
EPDS screening, %	84.2	87.2	89.3	77.9	0.007
ICDP at least one session, %	89.3	91.5	92.8	85.7	0.046
ICDP 2 group and/or 5 individual sessions, %	41.7	44.5	45.2	41.6	0.56
Three books, %	90.6	91.9	91.6	93.5	0.58
Three books + brochure, %	57.8	59.7	60.0	58.4	0.80
Parent group at least once, mother and/or father, %	44.7	49.3	54.2	27.3	<0.0001
Parent group at least 5 times, mother and/or father, %	7.7	9.5	10.7	3.9	0.064
Information about open preschool, %	70.2	69.4	68.7	72.7	0.49
At least one home visit, %	84.2	84.1	84.6	81.8	0.54
Number of home visits (if any), mean	1.39	1.42	1.43	1.35	0.38
N	449	355	292	63	
Range	1-5	1-5	1-5	1-5	

Group participation was low, about 50 %, particularly in immigrant families. One-third had not been informed about the open preschool, and a little more than 15 % had no home visit. No child received more than five home visits. (In the total material, including baseline and controls, no mother had more than six home visits, the majority just one).

We divided the programme into six components to evaluate the completeness of implementation: at least two home visits, screening with the EPDS, at least one ICDP session, mother participated in a parent group at least once, information about the open preschool, and three book gifts. 35.5 % (189/533) of the children were reached by 5-6 components, 57.4 % (306/533) by 3-4, 6.8 % (36/533) by 1-2, and 0.4 % (2/533) by none.

No special home visiting programme was developed. Immigrant families were not particularly attended to, and their questionnaire return rate was lower than for Swedish mothers (45.7 %, 523/1144, vs. 72.5 %, 1440/1986, classified by surname).

Effect outcomes

With two exceptions, there were no significant differences in socio-demographic background between cohorts I and II. The proportion of immigrant mothers was larger in experiment cohort I than in experiment cohort II, and the proportion of less educated mothers was larger in control cohort I than in control cohort II. Therefore, significant differences between cohorts I and II were controlled for by logistic regressions yielding adjusted p values (experiment cohorts adjusted for mother born in Sweden – not born in Sweden; control cohorts adjusted for maternal education compulsory or less – higher). In view of the differences in organisation between the experiment and control CHC:s, all comparisons were made within each arm (experiment-experiment and control-control). Potential programme effects were defined as adjusted significant differences between cohorts I and II in the experiment group, without corresponding differences among the controls.

Adjusting for maternal ethnicity, and relating the outcomes to the intensity of the relevant programme components, there were no significant effects on interaction scores or children's frequent "reading" (data not shown). Experiment children's (singletons aged 17-19 months) expressive vocabulary was significantly higher after the intervention than at baseline (32.5 (n=288) vs. 27.9 (n=332), adjusted p=0.03, effect size=0.22). However, vocabulary was not related to the reading programme (number of book gifts, brochure).

The only robust effects were certain increases related to parent groups, with no corresponding differences in the control group. The proportion of experiment children whose mothers had been invited to parent groups, according to maternal questionnaires, was 70.4 % (290/412) at follow-up vs. 58.7 % (262/446) at baseline, adjusted p=0.0015, effect size 0.12. The proportion of experiment children whose mothers had participated in groups, according to the questionnaires, was 47.0 % (193/411) at follow-up vs. 38.1 % (169/444) at baseline, adjusted p=0.029, effect size 0.09. The corresponding figures for experiment fathers were 12.3 % (50/406) and 7.6 % (33/432) (adjusted p=0.032, effect size 0.08).

Fewer mothers found the parent groups very valuable after intervention (11.5 %, 22/191) than at baseline (21.9 %, 37/169, adjusted p=0.0081, effect size –0.14). Mothers' perceived benefit from the CHC was more favourable at follow-up than at baseline, but this was the case also for control mothers. There were no intervention effects whatsoever on participation in the open preschool, evaluation of the preschool, or parenthood stress (data not shown).

Discussion

Our study was explicitly intended to try a new psychosocial model under routine conditions and without extra resources. Our interest lay in trying something that might work in real life (effectiveness, not efficacy). Due to the risk of contagion and also to practical problems and costs associated with a genuine randomisation, the approach was quasi-experimental. This may be considered a methodological weakness, but on the other hand, experiment and control areas were selected in order to be comparable. Assessments of mother-child interaction were collected from maternal questionnaires and not from observations, which would have been preferable but was not feasible. The scales measuring assessments of interaction and maternal stress had good psychometric properties: Cronbach's alpha for the former was 0.92, for the various SPSQ scales 0.67-0.89.

The programme was not implemented as expected. Only a minority were offered the total programme at an intensive enough level. The counselling programme for depressed mothers was not implemented. Frequent home visits to vulnerable mothers were not carried out. The study did not succeed in attracting immigrant mothers. No substantial effects could be observed except somewhat higher proportions of parents invited and participating in groups. Whatever "effects" there may have been on interaction, reading and language, they could not be explained by the intensity of the relevant programme components. In sum, our study must be characterised as something of a failure.

Possible explanations – a comparison with recommended standards

In a recent review, Olds et al (22) summarised a number of items recommended for preventive interventions, with particular stress on the importance of following a series of pre-stages in the process. Epidemiologic research should be used to establish relevant aspects of parenting to address. Theory and empirical findings should be consulted for developing valid strategies, and the intervention should be pre-tested and tried in small-scale RCTs before the larger trial. The shortcomings of the present study can perhaps be explained with a view to this work.

Identification of relevant aspects of parenting. The study addressed postpartum depression, attachment and interaction, language stimulation, social support, and stress. Difficulties in all these respects are enough prevalent to be a matter of concern. Thus the aspects of parenting chosen for the intervention seem to have been relevant.

Valid strategies to influence aspects of parenting. Certain components of the programme must be considered firmly based on empirical research, i.e. counselling sessions against postpartum depression (9), and encouragement of reading to facilitate language development (12). Home visiting by nurses has proven effective with deprived mothers (19). However, this component was modelled upon studies performed in social contexts different from Swedish communities and may have been low in ecological validity. Conclusive studies of the effectiveness of the ICDP are insufficient, particularly for the general public as opposed to vulnerable families, although the programme is widely recommended in Sweden. It can be doubted, on theoretical grounds, whether our method of improving social relationships was in a position to be effective. Parent groups and preschool activities may not be sufficient to strengthen social relationships and reduce stress.

Another aspect of methodological validity is the potential of an intervention not just for change, but for substantial change. Only statistically significant changes will not do; the efforts also have to result in differences of clinical significance. None of our effect sizes exceeded 0.22, and several lay below 0.10. Even in the few successful cases, our effects were small or just a little less than medium.

Pre-tests and small RCT trials

It is recommended by Olds et al. (22) that programme feasibility and acceptability on the part of parents and service providers should be pre-tested in advance. This can be done with the help of theory and research, including qualitative studies and focus groups. No such test was made in our study. A preparatory stage involving the nurses would probably have contributed to a higher programme fidelity. Some nurses expressed doubts in advance about the feasibility of the intervention. They were worried about lack of time and possibilities to implement the programme. Several nurses left their CHC during the study, and those replacing them were not given the total course in social paediatrics but only a short introduction. The practical implementation could not be monitored continuously, i.e. on an almost day-to-day basis which would have been desirable.

Efficacy trials under nearly ideal conditions and small-scale RCT:s are recommended (22) before effectiveness trials are made under real life conditions. This was not carried out in our study.

Apart from certain weaknesses as to the effectiveness of some programme components, the main shortcoming of the present study was its lack of preliminary tests of feasibility and acceptability among service providers (nurses). With hindsight, it can be concluded that our real life approach did not work. However, we think that our study may serve as an instructive example of difficulties to be expected in large field intervention trials. Such trials are seldom undertaken in our country.

Acknowledgment

The study was supported by the Swedish Council for Working Life and Social Research, the County Council of Uppsala, and Allmänna Barnhuset. Sincere thanks are due to all experiment and control nurses for their interest in the study and their generous contribution in time and efforts.

Conflicts of interest: none.

References

[1] Magnusson M. Barnhälsovård: studier av effektivitet och föräldratillfredsställelse [Child health services: Effectiveness and parental satisfaction. In Swedish with English summary.] Comprehensive Summaries of Uppsala Dissertations from the Faculty of Medicine 882. Uppsala: Acta Universitatis Upsaliensis, 1999.

[2] Hall DM, Stewart-Brown S. Screening in child health. Br Med Bull 1998;54:929-43.

[3] Sundelin C, Håkansson A. The importance of the Child Health Services to the health of children: summary of the state-of-the-art document from the Sigtuna conference on Child Health Services with a view to the future. Acta Paediatr Suppl 2000; 89(434):76-9.

[4] Wickberg B, Hwang CP. The Edinburgh Postnatal Depression Scale: validation on a Swedish community sample. Acta Psychiatr Scand 1996;94:181-4.

[5] Luoma I, Tamminen T, Kaukonen P, Laippala P, Puura K, Salmelin R, Almqvist F. Longitudinal study of maternal depressive symptoms and child well-being. J Am Acad Child Adolesc Psychiatry 2001;40:1367-74.

[6] McLennan JD, Kotelchuck M. Parental prevention practices for young children in the context of maternal depression. Pediatrics 2000;105:1090-5.

[7] Leiferman J. The effect of maternal depressive symptomatology on maternal behaviors associated with child health. Health Educ Behav 2002;29:596-607.

[8] Cox JL, Holden JM, Sagovsky R. Detection of postnatal depression: development of the 10-item Edinburgh Postnatal Depression Scale. Br J Psychiatry 1987;150:782-6.

[9] Wickberg B, Hwang CP. Counselling of postnatal depression: a controlled study on a population based Swedish sample. J Affect Disord 1996;39:209-16.

[10] Rydell AM, Bohlin G, Thorell LB. Representations of attachment to parents and shyness as predictors of children's relationships with teachers and peer competence in preschool. Attach Hum Dev 2005;7:187-204.

[11] Hundeide K. Ledet samspill: håndbok til ICDPS sensitiviseringsprogram [Guidance for interaction: a handbook to the sensitivity program of ICDP. In Norwegian.] International Child Development Programs. Nesbru: Vett Viten, 1996.

[12] High PC, LaGasse L, Becker S, Ahlgren I, Gardner A. Literacy promotion in primary care pediatrics: can we make a difference? Pediatrics 2000;105:927-34.

[13] Scarborough HS, Dobrich W. On the efficacy of reading to preschoolers. Dev Rev 1994;14:245-302.

[14] Kuo AA, Franke TM, Regalado M, Halfon N. Parent report of reading to young children. Pediatrics 2004;113:1944-51.

[15] Westerlund M, Berglund E, Eriksson M. Can severely language delayed 3-year-olds be identified at 18 months? Evaluation of a screening version of the MacArthur-Bates Communicative Development Inventories. J Speech Lang Hear Res 2006;49:237-47.

[16] Östberg M. Parenting stress: conceptual and methodological issues. Comprehensive Summaries of Uppsala Dissertations from the Faculty of Social Sciences 83. Uppsala: Acta Universitatis Upsaliensis, 1999.

[17] McCurdy K. The influence of support and stress on maternal attitudes. Child Abuse Negl 2005;29:251-68.

[18] Östberg M, Hagekull B, Lindberg L, Dannaeus M. Can a child-problem focused intervention reduce mothers' stress? Parenting Sci Pract 2005;5:153-74.

[19] Olds DL. Prenatal and infancy home visiting by nurses: from randomized trials to community replication. Prev Sci 2002;3:153-72.

[20] SAS® Introductory Guide. Third Edition. Cary, NC: SAS Institute Inc, 1985.

[21] Hojat M, Xu G. A visitor's guide to effect sizes: statistical significance versus practical (clinical) importance of research findings. Adv Health Sci Educ Theory Pract 2004;9:241-9.

[22] Olds DL, Sadler L, Kitzman H. Programs for parents of infants and toddlers: recent evidence from randomized trials. J Child Psychol Psychiatry 2007;48:355-91.

Submitted: January 08, 2009.
Accepted: February 17, 2009.

In: Public Health Yearbook 2009
Editor: Joav Merrick
ISBN: 978-1-61668-911-7

Chapter 16

WATCHING HEALTH THREATS ON THE NEWS: PREDICTING HEALTH RISK PERCEPTIONS, FEAR AND BEHAVIOR INTENTIONS

Marijke Lemal, MA ***and Jan Van den Bulck, PhD, DSc***
Faculty of Social Sciences, School for Mass Communication Research, Katholieke Universiteit Leuven, Leuven, Belgium

Abstract

The aim of this study was to examine the relationship between watching health content on television news programs and fear of health problems, risk perceptions and health behavior intentions. We explored the possibility that television exposure may not only be directly related to perceptions of risk, but also indirectly trough fear. 923 randomly selected adult respondents completed a Health and Media Interview Survey. Structural Equation Modeling confirmed that fear was an intervening variable between television news exposure and risk perception about health problems. There was a direct link between watching health content on television news and risk perception, but this was only true for rarely experienced health problems. While risk estimates were not related to intended health behavior, both fear of health problems and news exposure directly predicted respondents' intentions to engage in positive health actions.

Keywords: Public health, television news, risk perception, fear, health behavior.

* Correspondence: Marijke Lemal, MA, Faculty of Social Sciences, School for Mass Communication Research, Parkstraat 45 Box 3603, BE-3000 Leuven, Belgium. Tel: +32 16323312; Fax: +32 16323312; E-mail: marijke.lemal@soc.kuleuven.be

Introduction

There is a growing body of research on the role of mass-media exposure in influencing a variety of health beliefs and attitudes. Studies have linked regular exposure to health topics in television entertainment to heightened awareness of health topics (1), beliefs that health outcomes are determined by chance (2) and preventive health behavior (3).The association between television news exposure and health beliefs has received less attention, even though research has shown that television news is an important source of health information. A large scale survey study on health news and the American public by the Kaiser Family Foundation and the Harvard School of Public Health found that four in ten adults followed health news stories closely (4). And research on health communication channels suggests that television is a primary source of health information for less healthy individuals (5).

Television news programs frequently portray health content. According to an analysis of local television news, one in ten news stories dealt with health topics (6). A similar study found that 11% of news airtime was filled with stories about health (7). Berry, Wharf-Higgins and Naylor (8) investigated the construction of health information in the news media. They observed that messages about health problems were frequently discussed in terms of risk. News items about cancer were also likely to focus on personal stories of patients. According to research on narrative persuasion, such personal illness narratives may be vivid, touching and memorable (9), and therefore have the potential to influence health beliefs.

Television news and health risks

Several theories on health behavior view risk perception as a crucial factor in individuals' decisions concerning health promoting behaviors (10). They assume that the greater a person's perceived health risk, (typically defined as beliefs about susceptibility to a disease) the more likely it is he or she will engage in preventive health actions.

Whereas several factors have been identified that can influence the perception of risk, such as cultural differences or risk characteristics (e.g. controllability, dread) (11), none of the available risk perception theories appear to make predictions about the role of mass media in the construction of vulnerability beliefs. One framework which does refer explicitly to television in conjunction with risk perception is Social Amplification Theory (12). This model describes the dissemination and transformation of risk information trough several transmitters such as social organizations, personal networks and the news media. These transmitters are thought to amplify or attenuate risk information so that it spreads or ripples trough society. Mass media are seen as important agents of risk amplification and attenuation because "most of society learns about the parade of risks and risk events trough information systems rather than trough direct personal experience" (12, page 97). There is, however, little empirical evidence to support this theory.

Although not generally referred to as a theory on risk perception, George Gerbner's Cultivation Theory offers a framework for the study of media effects on risk perception. (13). The main assumption of Cultivation theory is that heavy viewers of television, who are repeatedly exposed to the dominant and repetitive patterns of mainstream television content, are more likely to develop a personal view of the world that resembles the TV version of what the world looks like. Evidence can be found for first-order and second-order cultivation effects. First-order cultivation measures typically refer to judgments of probability or occurrence of real-world facts, while second-order cultivation effects involve the construction of value judgments and attitudes. While the theory has been developed in the context of studying entertainment content, watching television news has also been found to cultivate viewers' perceptions of reality (14). From a Cultivation perspective it could be hypothesized that viewers who are frequently exposed to health threats on television news will be more likely to display heightened perceptions of vulnerability for health hazards.

Hypothesis 1: Respondents who are frequently exposed to health content in television news programs will be more likely to give higher personal risk estimates.

The number of studies regarding the first hypothesis is limited and their conclusions are contradictory. Coleman (15) assessed the relationship between exposure to informational mass-media content and societal and personal health risk judgments, including heart disease, AIDS, smoking, and hazards from drinking water, household radon, chemicals in food, household chemicals, and low-level radioactive waste. Respondents who were frequently exposed to these topics in national or local television news and news documentaries were more likely to give higher personal risk estimates. But watching health content was not related to risk judgments at a societal level. Snyder and Rouse (16) studied the differences in the impact of news and entertainment television coverage of AIDS on risk perceptions. Exposure to AIDS content in entertainment television programs was associated with higher estimates of personal risk, whereas exposure to news media stories about AIDS was negatively related to personal risk judgments in one study and unrelated in another. Discussing their results, Snyder and Rouse (16) suggested that only vivid and dramatic television content, such as entertainment TV, has the potential to influence perceptions of personal risk. But a subsequent study by Morton and Duck (17) found no evidence of an association between risk judgments about skin cancer and exposure to skin cancer coverage in either entertainment TV or television news. Contrary to what might be expected from the Cultivation hypothesis some of these studies failed to find a significant direct relationship between exposure to health topics in television news and perceptions of vulnerability. If a link between television exposure and risk perception exists, it is likely to be the result of a more complex causal pathway.

The role of fear

The traditional view in decision making research has been that risk perception is constructed using cognitive shortcuts or heuristics (18). But a growing body of research is recognising the role of affect or specific emotions in the construction of risk estimates. Slovic, Finucane, Peters and MacGregor (19) have proposed the 'affect heuristic' and Loewenstein, Weber, Hsee, and Welch (20) have suggested the 'risk-as-feelings' hypothesis as a framework for the influence of affect on risk perception. Both theories make a distinction between rational, cognitive-based evaluations and affective or feeling-based decision making. They belief that people do not only make risk judgments based on rational and argument-based thinking, but also based on affective or emotional reactions to a health threat. Several studies support this idea. Most researchers have investigated the role of affect or emotions that are induced before exposure to a health message instead of exploring the influence of emotions that are a result of the message content itself. Results suggest that whereas anxious individuals judge their risks to be higher, angry participants are more likely to express more optimistic risk perceptions (21).

Following the affect-approach, we expect that viewers who are confronted with news stories about health problems may not merely adjust their probabilities of experiencing a health threat, but that they may also undergo feelings of fear and anxiety. Those feelings may in turn serve as a cue for risk perceptions. Cultivation research on media-effects (in the context of violent content) has shown that frequent exposure to threats can be related to fear (14). There is, however, little or no evidence on the relationship between television exposure and fear of health hazards. And despite increasing attention on the role of affect in decision making, few studies have included fear as a possible intervening variable between media exposure and risk judgments. The current study therefore aims to explore the role of fear in the construction of risk perceptions from television exposure.

Hypothesis 2: Respondents who are frequently exposed to health content in television news programs will be more likely to be afraid of health problems.

Hypothesis 3: Fear of health threats will serve as an intervening variable between television news exposure and judgments about health risks.

News and health promoting behavior

Whereas cultivation theory has paid scant attention to the association between television exposure and behavior or behavioral intentions. Fear Appeal theories such as the Parallel Process Model (EPPM) (22) have been used widely in health communication to investigate how health risk messages motivate positive health behavior. The EPPM suggests that the depiction of a health hazard produces a perception of vulnerability to the threat. When people perceive they are likely to be at risk for the depicted disease they become motivated to reduce the threat by taking action. Research has found, however, that an increased perceived risk is not a sufficient factor for behavior change. Efficacy, or the perceived ability to cope with the threat, is important in determining which action is taken. Low efficacy beliefs tend to result in denial or avoidance of the threat, whereas high efficacy perceptions are likely to lead to health promoting intentions or actual health promoting behavior.

Because exposure to health threats on television may increase risk perceptions, and because risk perceptions may be related to taking positive health actions, Snyder and Rouse (16) hypothesised that television exposure should be positively related to health promoting behavior. Their results indicated that respondents who reported higher perceived susceptibility to AIDS were more likely to have engaged in AIDS preventing behaviors. But contrary to their hypothesis, television exposure was not directly related to health behavior. A look at content analyses offers an explanation of why they failed to find a significant direct relationship. Berry et al (8) found that health problems on local television news were twice as often discussed in terms of risk than in terms of prevention or treatment. In addition, Wang and Gantz (6) reported that health news stories were generally too short in length to offer follow-up information. A lack of information about treatment options and preventive measures in television news is not likely to increase viewers' efficacy beliefs. Following the EPPM, low efficacy beliefs are likely to lead to avoidance instead of health promoting action. Thus, it can be hypothesised that television exposure will not be related to health promoting behavior directly, but may be related to such behaviours indirectly by increasing risk perceptions, at least in people who score high on efficacy.

Hypothesis 4: Risk perception will be positively related to health promoting behaviors in respondents who report high health efficacy beliefs.

Hypothesis 5: Television exposure will be indirectly related to intentions to engage in positive health behavior by increasing risk perception.

Predicted model

The aim of this study is to explore the relationship between exposure to health content on television news, personal risk perceptions and intentions to engage in health promoting behavior. In particular, this study investigates the possibility that television exposure is not only directly related to perceptions of risk, but also indirectly trough fear. The predicted model (see figure 1) proposes a number of paths, based on our hypotheses.

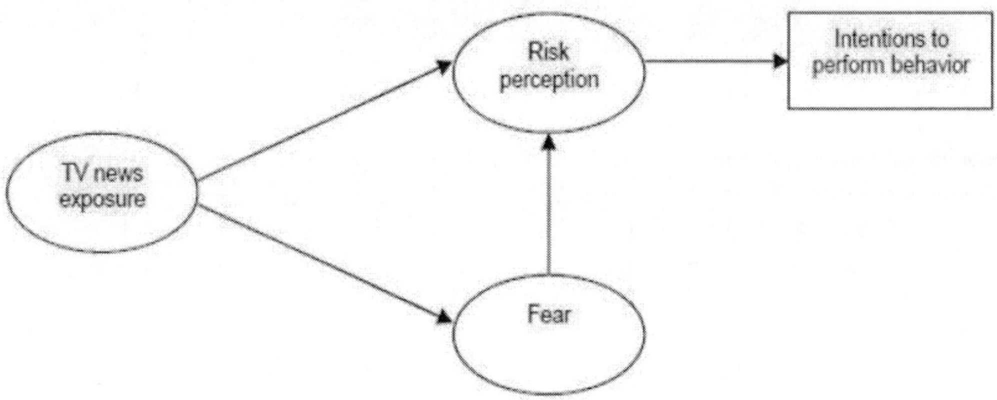

Figure 1. Predicted Model.

Methods

First year undergraduate students enrolled in an introductory communication course received credit for conducting three face-to-face interviews. 308 students agreed to conduct interviews and underwent a standardized interviewer training course. The interviewers received randomly selected interview addresses. At these addresses, the person of the household with the most recent birthday was selected as respondent.

Between October and November 2007, 923 Flemish respondents completed the standardized Health and Media Interview Survey. Of these participants 416 were male

(45.1%) and 502 were female. Ages ranged from 18 to 87 years (Mean age= 44). 41.7% of the respondents were between 18 and 40 years old, 37.6% were 41 to 60 years old and the smallest proportion (20.7%) was 60 years old or older. Among the participants 37.8% completed high school education and 52.4% was still attending or completed some college education or higher.

Measures

Demographics. Standard questions assessed gender, age and level of education.

Risk perception. Personal risk perception was measured by asking the participants: "How likely is it that you will get each of the following health problems in your lifetime?" We offered the respondents a list of six health problems (cancer, heart problems, pulmonary and respiratory problems, serious injury, paralysis and infectious disease). These health threats have been found to receive frequent television news coverage (6-8) Answers were coded on a 7-point scale from 1: this will certainly not happen to 7: this will certainly happen. A similar measure has been used in previous research on risk perception (15) and has been found to be reliable and valid (23).

A Confirmatory Factor Analysis (Amos™ 7.0) was conducted on the six risk perception items. A single factor model did not fit the data well (χ^2= 67.842, p=.000; CFI=0.947; RMSEA= 0.084; χ^2/df=7.538). Modification indices showed three pairs of variables (risk estimates about cancer, heart disease and pulmonary problems) with high correlations among their error terms. A two-factor model was tested with these three items loading on one common factor, and the remaining items on another. The revised model provided a better fit for the data (χ^2= 28.639, p=.000; CFI=0.982; RMSEA= 0.053; χ^2df=3.580). When ranking respondents' answers about their vicarious experience with health threats, the most commonly encountered health problems in friends or family members were cancer, heart disease and pulmonary problems (factor 1). Paralysis, infectious disease and serious injury (factor 2) were encountered less often. The first factor, thus, appears to represent 'risk perception about frequently experienced health problems' and the second factor 'risk perception about rarely experienced health problems'.

Fear of health problems. Participants rated how much they feared being diagnosed with each of the six health problems on a 7-point scale ranging from 1: not afraid at all to 7: very much afraid. We conducted a Confirmatory Factor Analysis on the six items. A one-factor solution did not provide an adequate fit to the data (χ^2= 216.170, p=.000; CFI=0.943; RMSEA= 0.158; χ^2/df=24.019). Similar to the CFA of risk perception, we revised the model according to the modification indices. Again, a two-factor model (factor 1= cancer, heart disease, pulmonary problems) provided a better fit (χ^2= 20.940, p=.002; CFI=0.996; RMSEA= 0.052; χ^2df=3.490).

Perceived health efficacy. Participants completed the Perceived Health Competence Scale (24). This is a measure of the degree to which an individual feels capable of effectively managing his or her health outcomes. The scale asked respondents to rate their agreement with 8 statements (e.g., "I succeed in the projects I undertake to improve my health") on a 7-point scale from 1: totally disagree to 7: totally agree. Item responses were summed to form a composite measure of health efficacy (Cronbach's alpha = .80). A dichotomous variable (low/high efficacy) was created by means of a medium split.

Intentions to engage in health promoting behavior. Participants rated their agreement with seven statements about their intention to perform several positive health behaviors (e.g.: "I intent to exercise regularly", "I intent to go to my physician for a regular check-up). Response categories ranged from 1: disagree strongly to 7: agree strongly. Scores on the seven items were summed to create a measure of health promoting behavior intentions (Cronbach's alpha= .77).

Exposure to health threats in television news programs. Television news exposure was assessed with a measure that has previously been used in studies on television exposure and health risk perceptions (14,15). Respondents were asked to rate how often they had encountered depictions of the selected health threats in television news programs in the month preceding the administration of the survey. Response options ranged from 1: never, 2: rarely, 3: occasionally, 4: frequently to 5: very frequently.

Analysis

The relationship between television news exposure, risk perception, fear and behavioral intent was estimated using structural equation modeling (Amos™ 7.0). The fit of the models was assessed by Chi-Square (χ^2), Comparative Fit Index (CFI) and Root Mean Square Error of Approximation (RMSEA). Because the Chi-Square index is sensitive to variations in data and sample size, models tested with large sample size data will almost always produce a statistical significant χ^2 (25). Therefore, the chi square to degrees of freedom ratio (χ^2/df) was also used as a fit index (cutoff point <3). All non-significant paths ($p>0.05$) were excluded from the final fitted models.

Results

Correlations, means, and standard deviations for the variables in the structural equation model are reported in table 1 and table 2. A predicted model was tested for risk perception and fear about frequently experienced health problems and risk perception and fear about rarely experienced health problems. Demographic measures were included in both models as control variables. In addition, a multiple group analysis was conducted to test for differences between high and low efficacy groups in their intended health behavior.

Model 1: Risk perception and fear about frequently experienced health problems. The proposed model did not fit the data well (χ^2= 586.197, p=.000; CFI=0.851; RMSEA=0.101; χ^2/df=10.468). The model was revised using the Modification Indices provided by the program. The modified model (Figure 2) fitted the data well (χ^2= 136.465, p=.000; CFI=0.976; RMSEA= 0.042; χ^2/df=2.624). The model accounted for 18% of the variance in risk perception about frequently experienced health problems, 10% of the variance in fear of frequently experienced health problems and 16% of the variance in intentions to engage in health promoting behavior.

As suggested by the predicted model, exposure to health content in television news programs was significantly related to fear of health problems (ß=.30, $p<0.01$) and fear of health problems, in turn, predicted risk perception (ß=.35, $p<0.01$). Television news exposure was, however, no significant direct predictor of risk perception (ß=-0.01, ns). The total standardised effect of television exposure on risk perception added up to 0.10.

Although the proposed model predicted a significant association between risk perception and positive health behavior intentions, this could not be confirmed by the data. A multiple group analysis for levels of health efficacy beliefs (χ^2= 194.755, p=.000; CFI=0.973; RMSEA= 0.032; χ^2/df=1.909) indicated that the path from risk perception to behavioral intent was not significant for both the low and high efficacy group (low efficacy: ß=-0.13, ns; high efficacy: ß=0.04 ns). Although unanticipated, the revised overall model suggested a small, but significant, direct path from television news exposure to intended health actions (ß=.09, p<0.05) and a link between fear of health problems and behavioral intent (ß=.11, p<0.01). The total effect of TV exposure on behavior intentions (directly and indirectly trough fear) was 0.12.

Model 2: Risk perception and fear about rarely experienced health problems. The predicted model did not fit the data well (χ^2= 356.464, p=.000; CFI=0.917; RMSEA= 0.074; χ^2/df=6.042). Paths were added or removed according to Modification Indices. Fit indices for the refined model (see figure 3) suggested a closer fit to the data (χ^2=165.799, p=.000; CFI=0.968; RMSEA= 0.048; χ^2/df=3.128). The fitted model accounted for 8% of the variance in fear of health problems, 14% of the variance of risk perception and 15% of the variance in behavioral intent.

Respondents who were exposed to health content in television news programs frequently were more likely to give higher risk estimates about rarely experienced health problems (ß=.13, p<0.01) and to report higher levels of fear (ß=.23, p<0.01). Because there was a significant path between fear of health problems and risk perception (ß=.23, p<0.01), television exposure was also indirectly related to respondents' risk estimates. The total standardised effect of exposure to television content about health problems on risk perception (directly and indirectly trough fear) was 0.18.

Table 1. Means, Standard Deviations and Zero-order Correlations among Variables in Model for Frequently Experienced Health Problems

	1	2	3	4	5
1. Risk perception about frequently experienced health problems	1.00				
2. Fear of frequently experienced health problems	.33**	1.00			
3. Health efficacy	-.32**	-.23**	1.00		
4. Health promoting behavior intentions	-.03	.15**	.24**	1.00	
5. Exposure to frequently experienced health problems on TV news programs	.06	.27**	-.07*	.15**	1.00
Mean	10.62	11.58	64.20	34.25	6.08
SD	2.60	4.47	12.47	8.29	2.35

**p<.01, N=923.

Table 2. Means, Standard Deviations and Zero-order Correlations among Variables in Model for Rarely Experienced Health Problems

	1	2	3	4	5
1. Risk perception about rarely experienced health problems	1.00				
2. Fear of rarely experienced health problems	.27**	1.00			
3. Health efficacy	-.11**	-.09**	1.00		
4. Health promoting behavior intentions	-.02	.12**	.24**	1.00	
5. Exposure to rarely experienced health problems on TV news programs	.15**	.20**	-.01	.09**	1.00
Mean	11.03	12.81	64.20	34.25	5.76
SD	3.19	6.03	12.47	8.29	2.29

**p<.01, N=923.

As in the first model, there was no significant association between risk perception and health promoting behavior intentions (ß=-0.03, ns), even when the path was tested for differences between low (ß=-0.04, ns) and high efficacy (ß=.03, ns) groups (χ^2=225.037, p=.000; CFI=0.965; RMSEA= 0.036; χ^2/df=2.164).

As in the first model respondents who were frequently exposed to health content in television news programs were more likely to take positive health actions, directly (ß=.07, p<0.05) and indirectly trough fear (ß=.10, p<0.01). The total effect of television news exposure on health behavior intentions was 0.09.

Discussion

Content analyses have shown that television news frequently covers stories about health problems. To date there has been little research on the association between television news exposure and the construction of health beliefs or behaviors. The goal of this study was to examine the relationship between exposure to health topics in television news programs, risk perception and intentions to engage in health promoting actions. Because previous research has found that emotional reactions can be important cues for risk perception, we reasoned that television exposure would not only be related to perceptions of health risks directly, but also indirectly through fear responses.

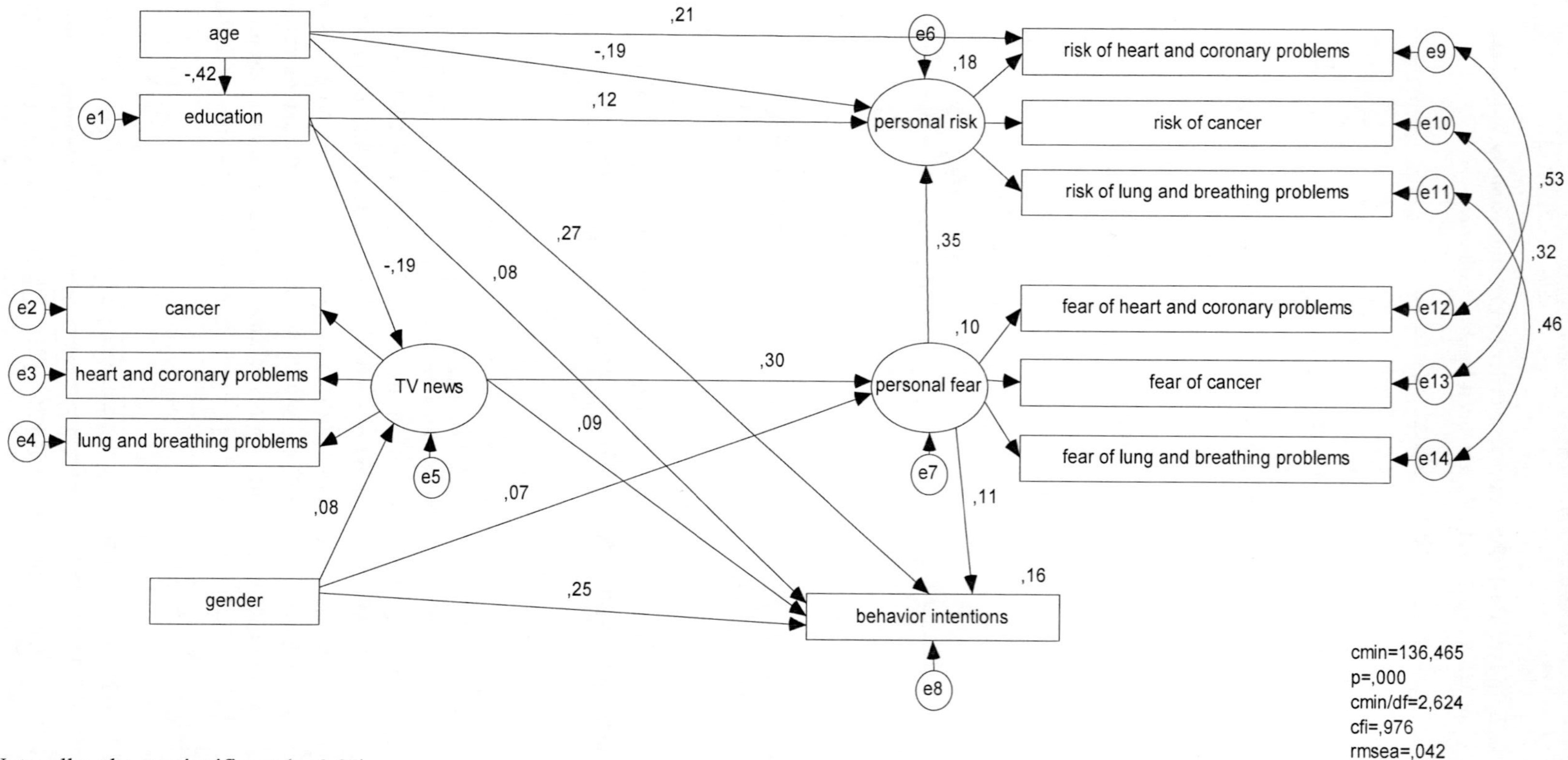

Note: all paths are significant (p<0.05).

Figure 2. Modified Model for Frequently Experienced Health Problems.

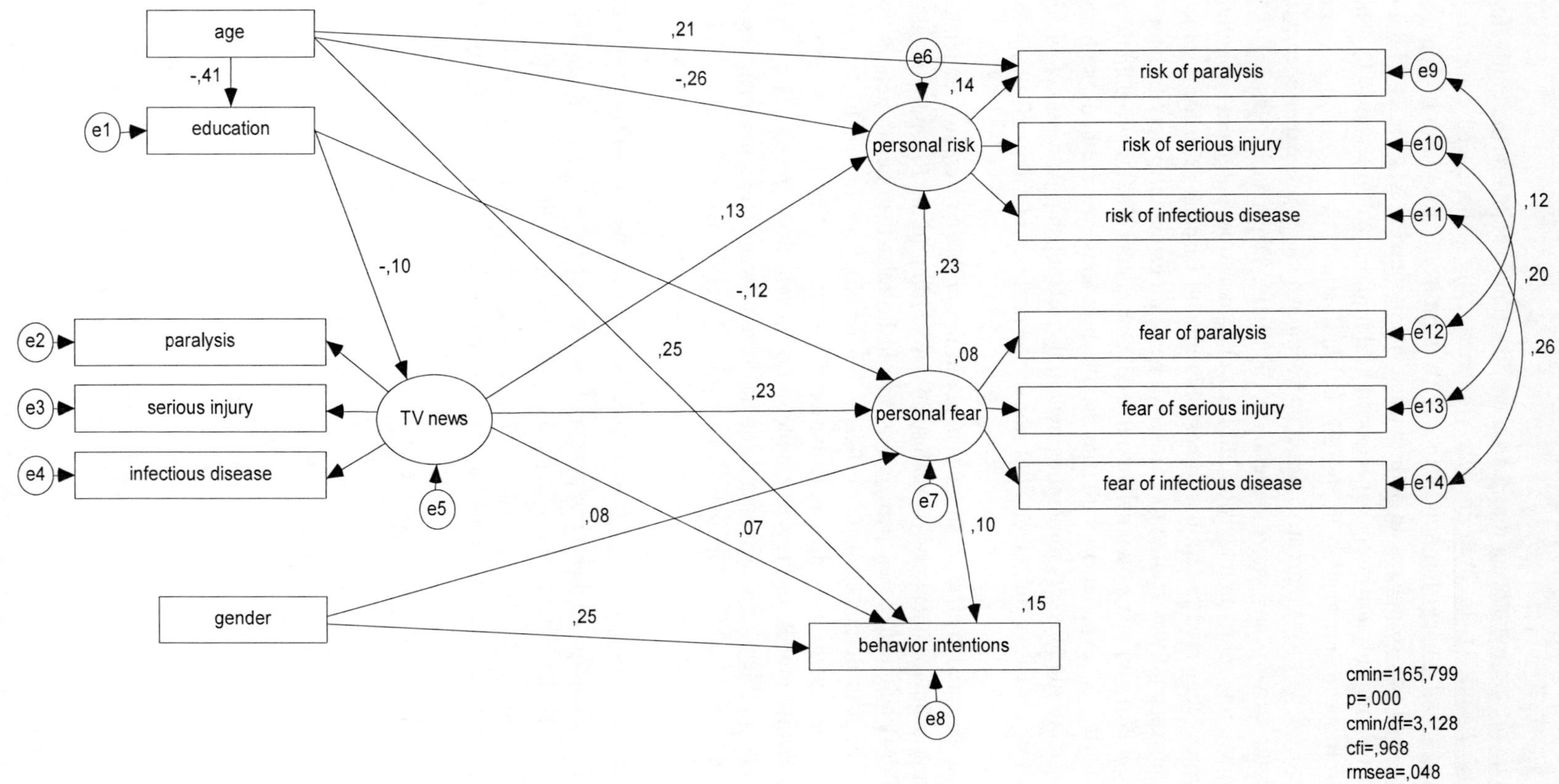

Note: all paths are significant (p<0.05).

Figure 3. Modified Model for Rarely Experienced Health Problems.

Our findings support the hypothesis that fear is an important variable in the cultivation process (hypotheses 2 and 3). In both models (for frequently experienced and rarely experienced health problems) television news exposure was indirectly related to perceptions of risk trough heightened fear responses. In addition, television viewing was directly related to health risk estimates, but only for rarely experienced health problems (hypothesis 1). This seems consistent with the mainstreaming hypothesis of Cultivation (13). According to this view, television exposure will have a greater impact on people who have less experience with the topic, than for those who have more experience. Similarly, Dependency Theory (26) predicts that people will rely more on television information to construct judgments or beliefs about unfamiliar topics (compared to familiar topics). Shrum and Bischak (27), for instance, found that television exposure was related to crime risk perceptions about society but not to risk perceptions about crime in one's own neighbourhood. Our results did, however, indicate that whereas familiarity or experience with the health problems we studied predicted television impact on risk estimates (cognitive judgments), the relationship between television news exposure and fear (affective judgments) did not vary with level of familiarity with the topic.

Contrary to what was predicted, risk estimates about health problems were not associated with health promoting behavior intentions (hypothesis 4). According to the Extended Parallel Process Model (EPPM) heightened risk perceptions should be related to health actions for individuals who are high in perceived health efficacy, but results from our multiple group analyses did not indicate a significant difference between the efficacy groups. Although not hypothesised in the initial model, the revised models did contain a significant association between fear of health problems and behavioral intent. Several researchers have suggested that there may be a causal relationship between emotional reactions and behavior (28). According to these theorists, each emotion is associated with a specific adaptive function or action tendency. The function of fear is to motivate self-protective behavior in order to avoid a threat.

We also found an unanticipated direct relationship between television news exposure and intentions to engage in health actions (hypothesis 5). Our findings indicated that watching health content on television news was related to risk perceptions. Content analyses have suggested that news exposure might be related to low efficacy beliefs. Following the EPPM, we then predicted that high risk estimates combined with low efficacy beliefs would result in avoidance instead of intentions to take protective action.

There are a number of possible explanations for the positive association between news exposure and health promoting behavior. First, although content analyses have found that television news rarely mentions health prevention and treatment issues, this does not have to imply a strong correlation between watching health news and low efficacy beliefs. Our data suggest that correlations between television news exposure and efficacy beliefs are small and only marginally significant. Additional content analyses are needed to investigate the portrayal of health efficacy content on television news and future research should examine the relationship between exposure to these health messages and viewers' corresponding efficacy beliefs. Second, exposure to health content on television news and health promoting actions may be positively associated because they may both be considered to be health promoting behaviors. Recent studies have argued that information-seeking or scanning can be conceptualized as a form of self-protective behavior because it can lead to better knowledge and ultimately to changing health behaviors (29). It is possible that our measure of exposure to health content assessed conscious or unconscious information seeking or scanning instead of accidental exposure while watching. If information-seeking is a part of a cluster of health promoting behaviors, it seems plausible that individuals who seek information about their health and report exposure to health content messages in television news are also willing to engage in other health promoting actions.

This study had several limitations. First, although we hypothesised that TV viewing may lead to fear and fear may lead to higher estimates of risk, the cross-sectional nature of our data does not allow us to comment on the nature of the relationships between our variables. Whereas structural equation modeling is often used to make causal claims, it only tests whether a particular model is contradicted by reality in an empirical test or not. While a Cultivation model suggests that television exposure may result in the construction of health risk judgments (which is not contradicted by our data), it remains possible that health risk perceptions may lead to selective exposure to health content on television. Studies on risk perception and information-seeking have suggested that high risk perceptions will (under certain circumstances) predict exposure to health content to reduce anxiety about the health threat (29). Second, this study relied on self-reports. Despite advantages of face-to-face interviews, questions about anxiety or personal risk perceptions might be prone to socially desirable responding. Finally, based on previous studies (19) we hypothesised that fear precedes risk perception. It could, however, be argued that the causal pathway is the reverse and that risk perception is more likely to predict fear of health problems than vice versa. Nevertheless, research comparing both hypotheses offers support for the idea that affective judgments about hazards precede cognitive judgments (30).

In response to these concerns, future research on the relationship between television exposure and risk perception should include experiments to explore causal claims. In addition, these experiments can help to explore further the affective and cognitive processes underlying the construction of risk judgments and health behaviors.

Acknowledgments

This study was funded by the Fund for Scientific Research-Flanders (Grant No. G.0293.06).

References

[1] Brodie M, Foehr U, Rideout V, et al. Communicating health information through the entertainment media. Health Aff 2001; 20(1):192-9.

[2] Bahk CM. Drench effects of media portrayal of fatal virus disease on health locus of control beliefs. Health Comm 2001;13(2):187-204.

[3] Valente TW, Murphy S, Huang G, Gusek J, Greene J, Beck V. Evaluating a minor storyline on ER about teen obesity, hypertension, and 5 a day. J Health Comm 2007;12(6):551-66.

[4] Brodie M, Hamel EC, Altman DE, Blendon RJ, Benson JM. Health news and the American public, 1996-2002. J Health Polit Policy Law 2003; 28(5):927-50.

[5] Dutta-Bergman MJ. Primary sources of health information: Comparisons in the domain of health attitudes, health cognitions, and health behaviors. Health Comm 2004;16(3):273-88.

[6] Wang Z, Gantz W. Health content in local television news. Health Comm 2007;21(3):213-21.

[7] Pribble JM, Goldstein KM, Fowler EF, Greenberg MJ, Noel SK, Howell JD. Medical news for the public to use? What's on local TV news. Am J Manag Care 2006;12(3):170-6.
[8] Berry TR, Wharf-Higgins J, Naylor PJ. Sars wars: an examination of the quantity and construction of health information in the news media. Health Comm 2007;21(1):35-44.
[9] Green MC. Narratives and cancer communication. J Commun 2006; 56:S163-S183.
[10] Brewer NT, Weinstein ND, Cuite CL, Herrington JE. Risk perceptions and their relation to risk behavior. Ann Behav Med 2004; 27(2):125-30.
[11] Sjoberg L. The methodology of risk perception research. Qual Quant 2000;34(4):407-18.
[12] Kasperson RE, Kasperson JX. The social amplification and attenuation of risk. Ann Am Acad Pol Soc Sci 1996;545:95-105.
[13] Shanahan J, Morgan M. Television and its viewers. Cambridge: Cambridge University Press, 1999.
[14] Romer D, Jamieson KH, Aday S. Television news and the cultivation of fear of crime. J Commun 2003;53(1):88-104.
[15] Coleman CL. The influence of mass-media and interpersonal communication on societal and personal risk judgments. Communic Res 1993;20(4):611-28.
[16] Snyder LB, Rouse RA. The media can have more than an impersonal impact: the case of AIDS risk perceptions and behavior. Health Comm 1995;7(2):125-45.
[17] Morton TA, Duck JM. Communication and health beliefs: Mass and interpersonal influences on perceptions of risk to self and others. Communic Res 2001;28(5):602-26.
[18] Peters E, Mccaul KD, Stefanek M, Nelson W. A heuristics approach to understanding cancer risk perception: Contributions from judgment and decision-making research. Ann Behav Med 2006;31(1):45-52.
[19] Slovic P, Finucane ML, Peters E, Macgregor DG. Risk as analysis and risk as feelings: Some thoughts about affect, reason, risk, and rationality. Risk Anal 2004;24(2):311-22.
[20] Loewenstein GF, Weber EU, Hsee CK, Welch N. Risk as feelings. Psychol Bull 2001;127(2):267-86.
[21] Lerner JS, Keltner D. Fear, anger, and risk. J Pers Soc Psychol 2001; 81(1):146-59.
[22] Witte K, Allen M. A meta-analysis of fear appeals: Implications for effective public health campaigns. Health Educ Behav 2000; 27(5):591-615.
[23] Diefenbach MA, Weinstein ND, Oreilly J. Scales for assessing perceptions of health-hazard susceptibility. Health Educ Res 1993; 8:181-92.
[24] Smith MS, Wallston KA, Smith CA. The development and validation of the perceived health competence scale. Health Educ Res 1995; 10(1):51-64.
[25] Hu LT, Bentler P. Evaluating model fit. In: Hoyle RH. Structural equation modeling. Concepts, issues, and applications. London: Sage, 1995:76-99.
[26] Adoni H, Mane S. Media and the social construction of reality: Toward an integration of theory and research. Communic Res 1984; 11(3):323-40.
[27] Shrum LJ. Mainstreaming, resonance, and impersonal Impact: Testing moderators of the cultivation effect for estimates of crime risk. Hum Commun Res 2001;27(2):187-215.
[28] Lazarus RS. Emotion and adaptation. New York: Oxford Univ Press, 1991.
[29] Turner MM, Rimal RN, Morrison D, Kim H. The Role of anxiety in seeking and retaining risk information: Testing the risk perception attitude framework in two Studies. Hum Commun Res 2006; 32(2):130-56.
[30] Rundmo T. Associations between affect and risk perception. J Risk Res 2002;5:119-35.

Submitted: January 01, 2009.
Revised: February 15, 2009.
Accepted: February 18, 2009.

In: Public Health Yearbook 2009
Editor: Joav Merrick

ISBN: 978-1-61668-911-7

Chapter 17

Body esteem in British children: Differences due to weight status, ethnicity and gender

Michael J. Duncan, PhD*[*1], Yahya Al-Nakeeb, PhD[2], Lorayne Woodfield, PhD[2] and Alan M. Nevill, PhD[3]

[1]Department of Sport and Exercise Sciences, University of Derby, Derby, England
[2]Department of Physical Education and Sports Studies, Newman University College, Birmingham, England
[3]School of Sport, Performing Arts and Leisure, University of Wolverhampton, England

Abstract

Body esteem is an important variable that has been linked to a range of negative health outcomes including depression, negative affect, obesity and increased risk of suffering from eating disorders. However, little information is available regarding ethnic differences in body esteem in British children. Objective: To examine gender, ethnic and weight status differences in body esteem in a sample of British children. Methods: The study was cross sectional in design and assessed body esteem and weight status in 756 children (394 boys, 362 girls, mean age 11.4 ± 1.6 years). Body esteem was determined using the body esteem scale for children. Height and body mass were measured directly. Body mass index was determined as kg/m^2. Overweight/obesity status was determined using child-specific, International Obesity task force cut-off points. Results: A 2 (gender) X 3 (ethnicity) X 2 (weight status) ways analysis of variance (ANCOVA) controlling for age indicated that body esteem was higher for normal weight boys compared to girls whereas body esteem scores were similar for boys and girls in the overweight/obese category (P = 0.044). Body esteem scores were higher in boys compared to girls from white and black ethnic groups but this pattern was reversed for Asian boys and girls (P = 0.039). Conclusions: Findings of this study indicate that body esteem interacts with weight status and ethnicity across gender groups in British children after controlling for age. In the context of

* Correspondence: Michael J Duncan, Faculty of Education, Health and Science, University of Derby, Kedleston Road, Derby, England DE22 1GB. E-mail: m.duncan@derby.ac.uk

the current study overweight children and Asian boys may be particular populations where future research needs to focus.

Keywords: Obesity, body image, Asian, body mass index.

Introduction

Body image concerns in childhood are becoming increasingly prevalent in western society and have been linked to a number of social, psychological and physiological problems including increased incidence of eating disorders, use of illegal substances, cosmetic surgery, restricted eating, poor psychological well being, obesity and excessive exercise (1,2). Furthermore, weight status may be particularly important in the development of these concerns. The societal preference for leanness in the western world stigmatises overweight and obesity. This in turn places a social and psychological burden on children who are dissatisfied with their bodies that can lead to considerable negative health outcomes (3). Although levels of overweight and obesity are increasing worldwide (4,5) studies have also reported increasing body image problems in young people (6,7). Previous studies have indicated that girls express greater body dissatisfaction, lower body esteem and more negative body image than boys (1,8) and that black individuals have a more positive body image and greater body esteem than other ethnic groups (9,10). Franko and Streigel-Moore (9) go on to suggest that black individuals have different standards of attractiveness and place less emphasis on thinness for attractiveness compared to other ethnic groups. British Asian girls have also been identified as a group who may be at risk of developing eating disorders and body esteem problems (11). Hill and Bhatti (11) reported that Asian girls may be subjected to ethnic specific media (e.g. Hindu films) that result in low body esteem and that in all cases lower body esteem was related to higher eating restraint. They suggested that further research was needed examining body image in this group. However, the majority of studies examining ethnic differences in body image have been based on American samples and have tended to examine either adult populations or a restricted range of ethnic groups that may not be applicable to countries outside of North America.

For example, Jones, Fries and Danish (12) recently reported that Caucasian adolescent females were more dissatisfied with their bodies than African American females. While this work highlights a possible role of ethnicity on body image, further research on this topic is needed to provide information from other countries and on wider ranges or different ethnic groups. Additionally, those studies that have examined ethnic differences in children's body image do not appear to have directly assessed weight status and this has been highlighted as a future research need (12). Therefore, this study was designed to explore any ethnic and weight status differences in body image in British children.

Methods

Following institutional ethics approval and informed consent, 756 children (394 boys, 362 girls, mean age 11.4 ± 1.6 years SD) participated in the study. Participants were classified using methods currently employed by the Department for Education and Skills (13) when classifying ethnic group in schools as being from black (n = 62), white (n = 549) and Asian (n = 142) ethnic groups.

Procedures

Height and body mass were assessed using a Seca stadiometre and weighing scales (Seca Instruments, Germany) from which body mass index (BMI) was calculated and children were classified as 'normal weight' (n = 534) and 'overweight/obese' (n = 221) according to International criteria (14). Prior to collection of anthropometric data, body image was assessed individually using the Body Esteem Scale for Children (15).

Data analysis

Body esteem scores were analysed using a 2 (gender) X 3 (ethnicity) X 2 (weight status) ways analysis of variance (ANCOVA) controlling for age at a value of 11.4 years. The statistical Package for Social Sciences (SPSS version 15) was used for all analysis.

Results

Results from ANCOVA revealed a significant gender by weight status interaction (F1, 746 = 4.07, p = 0.044 Partial $\eta 2$ = 0.005) and a significant gender by ethnicity interaction (F2, 746 = 3.26, p = 0.039, Partial $\eta 2$ = 0.009). Body esteem was higher for boys compared to girls in the normal weight category whereas body esteem scores were similar for boys and girls in the overweight/obese category (see figure 1). Furthermore, body esteem scores were higher in boys compared to girls from white and black ethnic groups but this pattern was reversed for Asian boys and girls (see figure 2).

A significant main effect was also evident for weight status ($F_{1, 746}$ = 151.5, p = 0.0001, Partial η^2= 0.169) with normal weight children reporting significantly higher body esteem than their overweight/obese counterparts. Mean ± S.D. of body esteem scores were 16.33 ± 5.1 for normal weight children and 11.3 ± 5.2 for the overweight/obese children. The 'age' covariate also identified that as children got older physical activity declined (slope parameter ß = -.375; $F_{1, 746}$ = 10.52, p = 0.001, Partial η^2= 0.014).

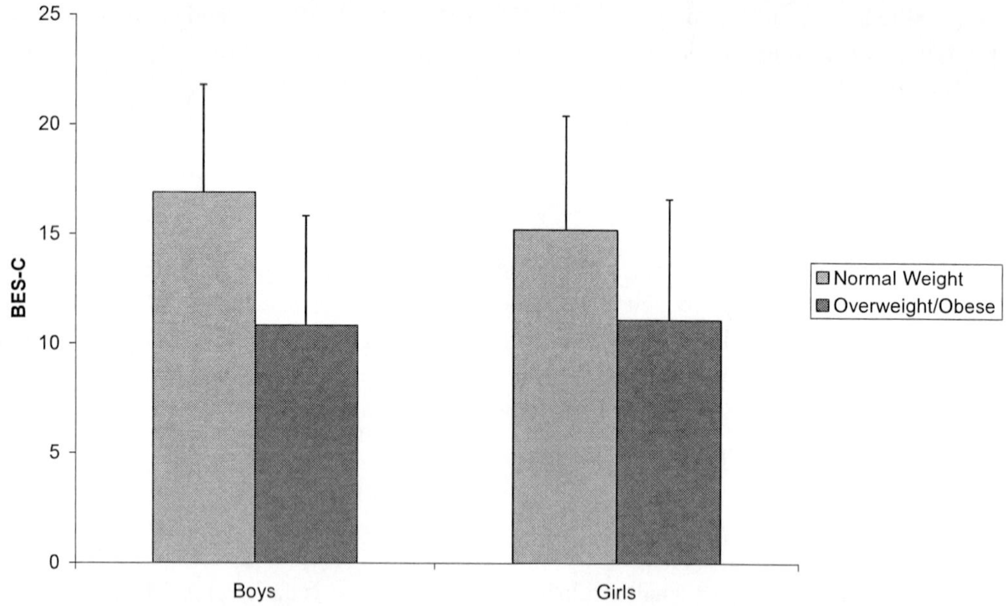

Figure 1. Mean ± S.D. of body esteem scores between boys and girls and across weight status groups.

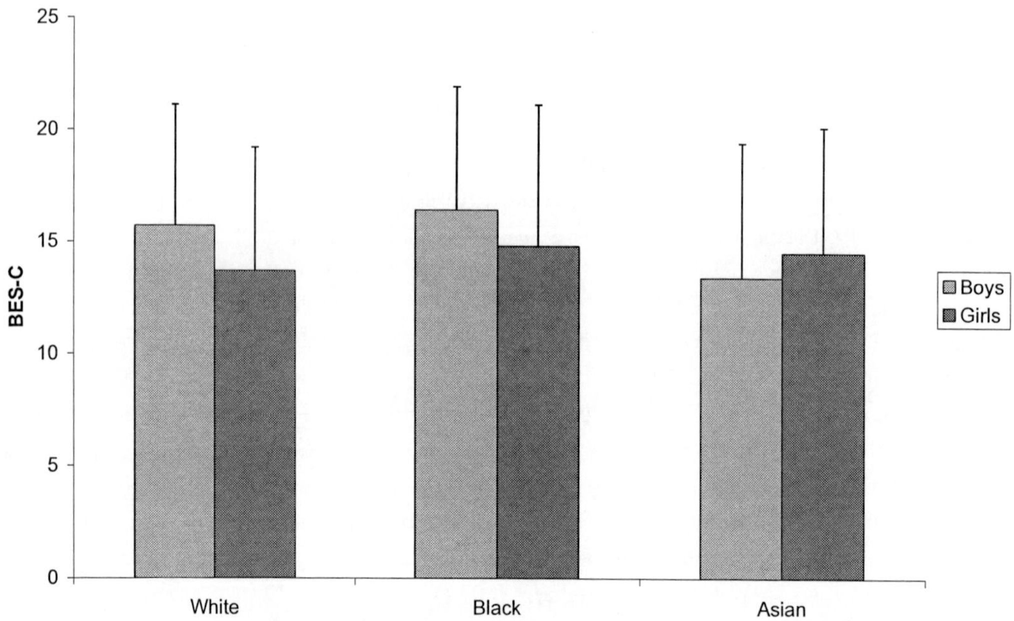

Figure 2. Mean ± S.D. of body esteem scores between boys and girls and across ethnic groups.

Discussion

Findings of this study indicate that body esteem interacts with weight status and ethnicity across gender groups in British children after controlling for age. Although the main effect for weight status found in this study is not surprising, this study present novel work in that at 'normal' weight status boys reported higher body esteem than girls, as has been reported widely in the literature (1,14). However, there was no difference in body esteem scores between boys and girls who were overweight/obese. This does not appear to have been specifically examined in prior studies although Presnell et al (16) have reported that boys report more body dissatisfaction than girls when they are above 'average' weight. This suggestion would seem to, at least partly, explain the findings of the current study although more research would be warranted to substantiate this claim. The second novel finding of this study was that body esteem was significantly lower in Asian boys compared to Asian girls, whereas the opposite was true of white and black children. This finding seems to support previous studies that have documented more positive body image in black individuals compared to those from other ethnic groups (9,10). These results also support research by Hill and Bhatti (11) that body image issues in Asian children may be a cause for concern. Hill and Bhatti (11) proposed that Asian children may be particularly influenced by ethnic specific media (e.g. Hindu films) that may shape body image in childhood. In the context of the current study Asian boys may be a particular population where future research needs to focus as they had the lowest values for body esteem than any other groups in the study irrespective of gender. The covariate of 'age' was also significant with older children reporting lower body esteem. This finding is not surprising and has been reported previously (1). However, the population in the current study were drawn from a relatively wide age range which possibly may have taken in preadolescent and adolescent children. The authors attempted to take account of this by controlling for age in their analysis. However, this could be viewed as a limitation of the study and as such, future research, that takes account for pubertal status, is needed to support the findings of the current study.

Conclusions

The results of this small, exploratory study suggest that weight status interacts with a number of other variables, notably gender and ethnicity when examining differences in body esteem. Further work is needed on this topic, possibly from a qualitative and quantitative standpoint, in order to really elucidate the nature of these interactions. This level of analysis was beyond the remit of the current study but is obviously an interesting and important avenue for future research and may be important in targeting interventions aimed at improving children's body image and/or weight status.

Acknowledgments

This research was partly supported by a small research grant from the British Academy.

References

[1] Grogan S. Body Image: Understanding body dissatisfaction in men, women and children. London, Routledge, 2007.

[2] Smolak L, Levine MP. Body Image in children. In: Thompson JK, Smolak L, eds. Body image, eating disorders and obesity in youth. Washington, DC: Am Psychol Assoc, 2001:41-66.
[3] Hills AP, Byrne NM. Exercise, daily physical activity, eating and weight disorders in children. In: Armstrong N, van Mechelen W, eds. Paediatric exercise science and medicine. Oxford, Oxford Univ Press, 2000:339-49.
[4] James WPT. Global trends of childhood obesity-long term consequences. Ann Nestle 2001;59: 49-58.
[5] Goodfellow S, Northstone K. Childhood overweight and obesity in the UK. A comparison of two environmentally distinct populations of 7-Year old children. Int J Ped Obesity 2008;3:117-9.
[6] Duncan M, Al-Nakeeb Y, Woodfield L. Relationships between body esteem, objectively measured physical activity and anthropometry in children. In: Simmons M, Foster L, eds. Sport and exercise psychology research advances. Hauppage, NY: Nova Science, 2008: 1-8.
[7] Duncan M, Al-Nakeeb Y, Jones M, Nevill A. Body dissatisfaction, body fat and physical activity in British children. Int J Ped Obesity 2006;1:89-95.
[8] McCabe MP, Ricciardelli LA, Finemore J. The role of puberty, media and popularity with peers to increase weight, decrease weight and increase muscle tone among adolescent boys and girls. J Psychosom Res 2002;52:145-53.
[9] Franko DL, Streigel Moore RH. The role of body dissatisfaction as a risk factor for depression in adolescent girls. Are the differences Black and White? J Psychosom Res 2002;53:1-9.
[10] Neumark-Sztainer D, Croll J, Story M, Hannan PJ, French SA, Perry C. Ethnic/racial differences in weight related concerns and behaviours among adolescent girls and boys. Findings from project EAT. J Psychosom Res 2002;53:963-74.
[11] Hill AJ, Bhatti R. Body shape perception and dieting in preadolescent British Asian girls: Links with eating disorders. Int J Eat Dis 1995; 17:175-83.
[12] Jones LR, Fries E, Danish SJ. Gender and ethnic differences in body image and opposite sex figure preference of rural adolescents. Body Image 2007;4:103-8.
[13] Department for Education and Skills. Guidance for local education authorities on schools' collection and recording data on pupils' ethnic background. London: DFES, Circular DfES/0002, 2002.
[14] Cole TJ, Bellizzi MC, Flegal KM, Dietz WH. Establishing a standard definition for child overweight and obesity worldwide: International Survey. BMJ 2000;320:1240-3.
[15] Mendelson BK, White DR. Relation between body-esteem and self-esteem of obese and normal children. Percep Mot Skills 1982;54: 899-905.
[16] Presnell K, Bearman SK, Stice E. Risk factors for body dissatisfaction in adolescent boys and girls: A prospective study. Int J Eat Dis 2004; 36:389-401.

Submitted: December 17, 2008.
Revised: February 15, 2009.
Accepted: February 22, 2009.

In: Public Health Yearbook 2009
Editor: Joav Merrick
ISBN: 978-1-61668-911-7

Chapter 18

CAUSES AND CONSEQUENCES OF CHILDHOOD BURN: EXPERIENCE FROM 100 CASES IN BANGLADESH

Selim Ahmed, MBBS, FCPS*[*1]*,
Aminur Rahman, MBBS, DCM, MMed[2],
Maleeha Hussain, MBBS, MPhil[3]
and Fazlur Rahman, MBBS, MPhil, PhD[2]

[1]Department of Pediatrics, Institute of Child and Mother Health, Dhaka, Bangladesh
[2]Centre for Injury Prevention and Research, Bangladesh (CIPRB), Dhaka, Bangladesh
[3]Dcpartment of Pathology, National Institute of Cancer Research and Hospital, Dhaka, Bangladesh

Abstract

Childhood burn in Bangladesh is a significant public health problem. Uncovered kerosene-lamp ("Kupi") for lighting and traditional earthen oven for cooking is commonly used in rural areas. The study was conducted to reveal the epidemiology of childhood burn and thereby help in planning future strategies for prevention of child burns in Bangladesh. Methods: A prospective study was conducted on a total of 100 consecutively enrolled patients admitted in the burn unit of Dhaka Medical College Hospital between January and June 2005. Data extracted included demographics; burn related causes as well as treatment related variables. Results: The results revealed preponderance of older girls burnt by flame, mainly from uncovered, kerosene-oil lamp used for house hold lighting in rural areas. There were two deaths in the series, both were victims of massive flame burn. The mean duration of hospital stay was 34 +/- 15 days, with higher treatment cost than the monthly income of the families. Almost all the cases had some sort of permanent disfigurement as the treatment outcome. Conclusion: Kerosene lamp, cooking in open oven, loose attires and lack of parental supervision and awareness were the most important risk factors identified in childhood burn.

---

* Correspondence: Selim Ahmed, MBBS, FCPS Assistant Professor of Pediatrics, Institute of Child and Mother Health, Matuail, Dhaka-1362 Bangladesh. Tel: +880-2-7542814 (office); Fax: +880-2-7542672; E-mail: drselim@gmail.com

Keywords: Children, burn, Bangladesh.

Introduction

Burn is a significant public health problem both in the developed and in the developing world. Globally in 2002, fire-related burns ranked among the 15 leading causes of death among children and young adults (1). In the United Kingdom, about 250,000 people are burnt each year; the incidence is higher in the United States (2). An estimated 128,000 persons died of burn injuries in the countries of the WHO's SEA Region in 2000. This burden accounts for more than half of the global burden of fire related burns (3,4). In Bangladesh, burn injuries have been identified as the fifth leading cause of child injury and second commonest cause of permanent disability from injury in children. About 474 children are burned everyday in Bangladesh. In 2004, About 340 children were burnt to death and over 3,400 burn victims became permanently disabled (5).

The risk factors of burn injury differ in different communities; so the analysis of the epidemiological factors in every community deserve attentions before formulating an effective prevention program. The study was conducted to reveal the epidemiology of pediatric burn and thereby helping in planning future strategies for prevention of child burns in Bangladesh.

Methods

The burn unit of Dhaka Medical College Hospital is the major referral centre for all burn cases in Bangladesh. The policy of the burn unit is to admit severe and complicated cases; the less severe cases are treated in the outpatient department. This prospective study was conducted on 100 consecutive cases of pediatric burn admitted to the burn unit from January to June 2005. Children in the age range of 1-15 years with burn injury were ascertained as the cases. These patients were either directly attended the hospital or were referred from other centers.

All cases were subjected to an interview on the day of admission by a pre-tested questionnaire. The respondents of the interview were either the patient himself/herself (older children and adolescent) or the attending person (parent, relative). All cases were followed up twice weekly until discharged. The principal investigator interviewed and collected the information. The following data were obtained:

- Hospital registration number, date and time of admission and address were collected from the hospital record.
- Demographic data: age, sex, residence, level of education of the patients and parents, occupation of the older children and of the parents, family members and family income.
- Circumstances of the injury: place and time, brief description of the event, agent of burn.
- First-aid measures and health seeking behavior after burn.

- Clinical assessment of the wound: depth of burns (superficial when only the outer layer and deep when the entire skin were involved in the burn process). The percentage of burn was determined according the hospital record.
- Chronological data: dates of admission and discharge.
- Treatment outcome was assessed according to the notes written in the hospital discharge certificate.
- Information about monthly family income, cost of treatment and the source of the money for treatment were recorded only according to the statement of either parent.

Statistical analysis

Descriptive statistics were applied to analyse the characteristics of burn patients. Mean, standard deviation (SD) and proportion were used where appropriate. All the descriptive analyses were carried out by using SPSS 11.0 software.

Results

In our study, almost half of the patients (49%) were in the age group of 1-6 years and 80% of them were in the age group of 1-10 years. The oldest patient was 15 years old and the youngest one was 13 months old. The mean age was 6.86 years (SD ± 3.76); the median was 7 years.

Females outnumbered (62%) the males (38%) in the studied patients. The female - male ratio was 1.63:1. Eighty percent of all types of burn injury happened in the rural areas. Among the cases burnt by flame, more than three quarters occurred in rural areas.

Sixty percent of the patients were from families whose monthly income was less than Taka 2,000 ($29.5) i.e. less than 1 US $ per day (1 US $=68 taka). The mean monthly income was Taka 3260 (SD 3761.3); and the median was Taka 2000(SD 3761.3).

Among the external causes of burn injury, flame was identified as the commonest (68%) cause of burn followed by electrocution injury (11%), burn by ash (9%) and by hot liquid (8%).

Table 1. Distribution of burn cases by age groups (n=100)

Age group in years	Percent
1-2 years	9
3-4 years	22
5-6 years	18
7-8 years	23
9-10 years	8
11-12 years	10
13-14 years	6
15 years	4
Total (1-15 years)	100

Flame was the major cause of burn in children of all age groups. It was highest (45%) in children 5-9 years. This was followed by the toddlers 1-4 years (31%).

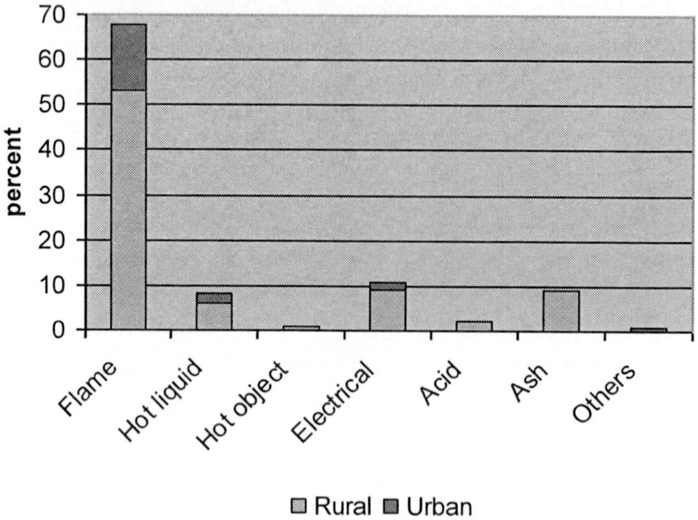

Figure 1. Type of burns by residence (n=100).

Flame burn and burn by hot liquid (scald) predominantly occurred in girls. Electric burn and burn by ash mainly happened in male children. Two cases of acid burn victims were found in the study. They were the members of the same family, and the acid was thrown by enemies at night when they were sleeping by the side of an open window.

About 39% of cases of flame burn, the children caught fire from uncovered, small, kerosene oil lamps ("Kupi") which are popular and cheaper means of lighting in low income families in villages and slums.

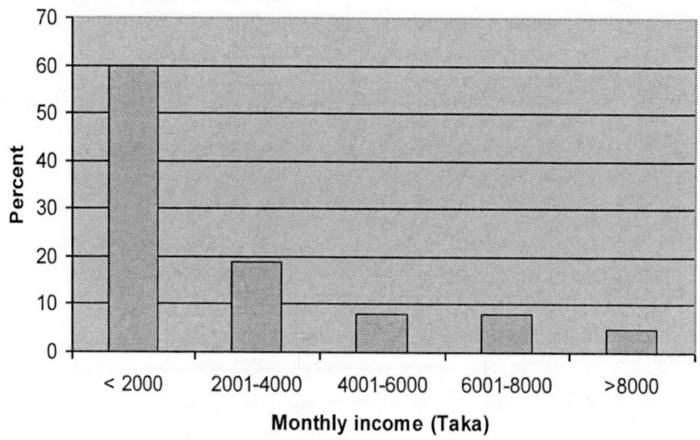

Figure 2. Distribution of the burn affected families by income

Other sources of flame were open earthen oven during cooking and open fire for body warming during winter. The proportions of these sources were 26 % each.

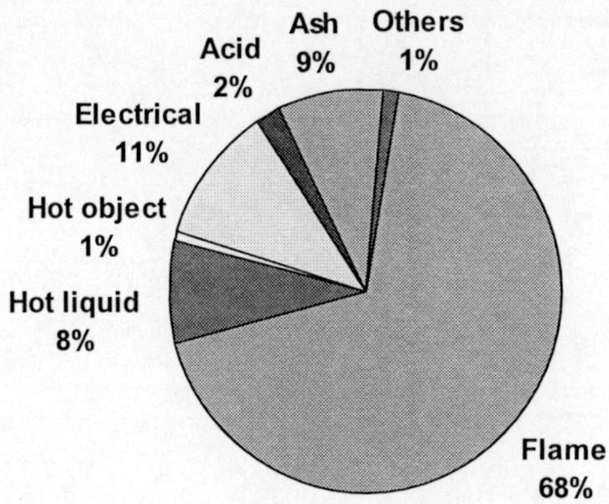

Figure 3. External causes of burn injury (n=100).

Out of the total patients 86% had superficial and 14% had deep burn. The mean percent of burn (in terms of body surface area affected) was about 26%.

The mean duration of hospital stay was 34 days (SD 14.81). Of the total patients 38% patients did not complete the treatment because of high treatment cost; prolong hospital stay, painful dressing, slow healing and or recurrent wound infection.

Among the enrolled patients, two patients died. Both of them were female and the victims of flame burn. Among the survivors, almost all patients had more than one treatment outcome like scar, post burn contracture, disfigurement of cosmetic area (collectively termed as permanent disfigurement in the hospital record). Out of 11 cases of electric burn, five cases (45.45%) needed amputation of the affected limb.

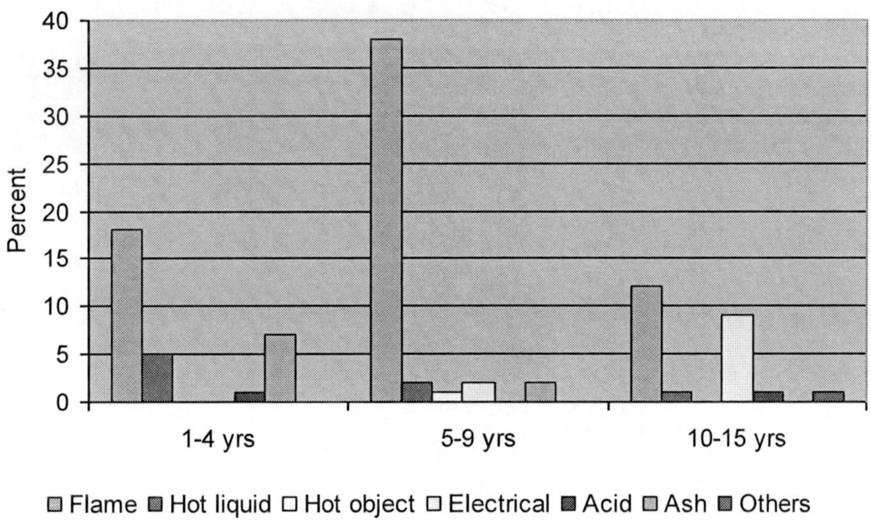

Figure 4. Distribution of different causes of burn in relation to age groups (n=100).

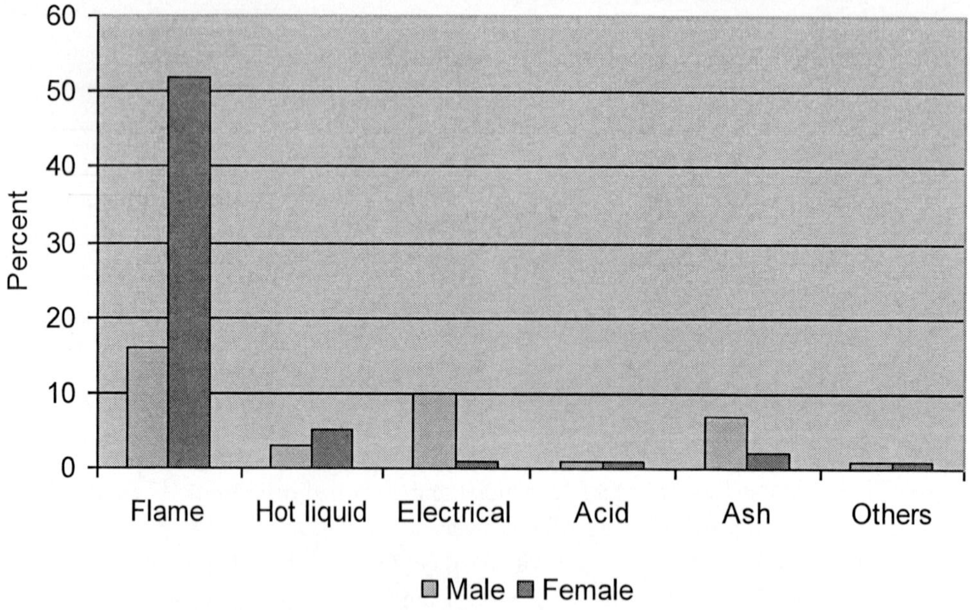

Figure 5. External cause of burn injury by sex (n=100).

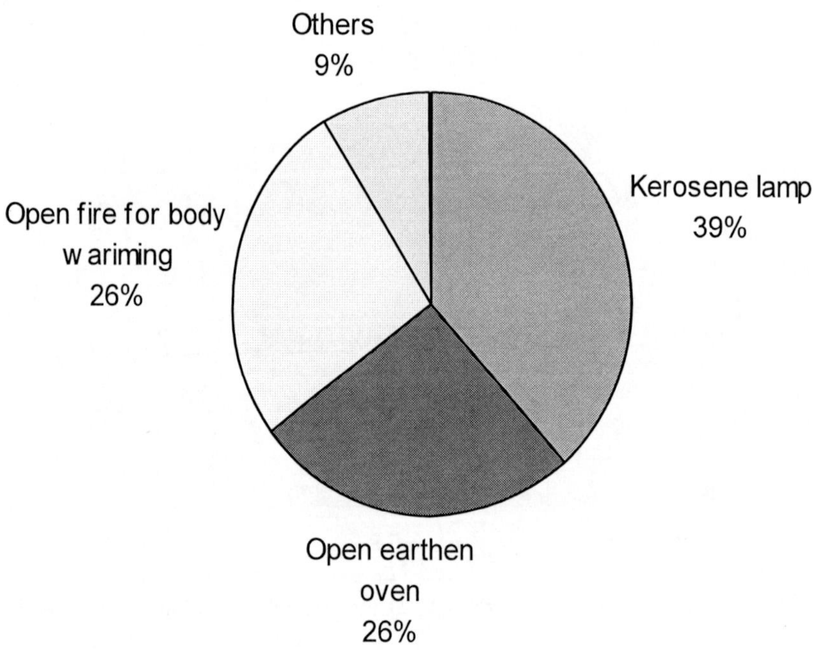

Figure 6. Distribution of sources of flame burn.

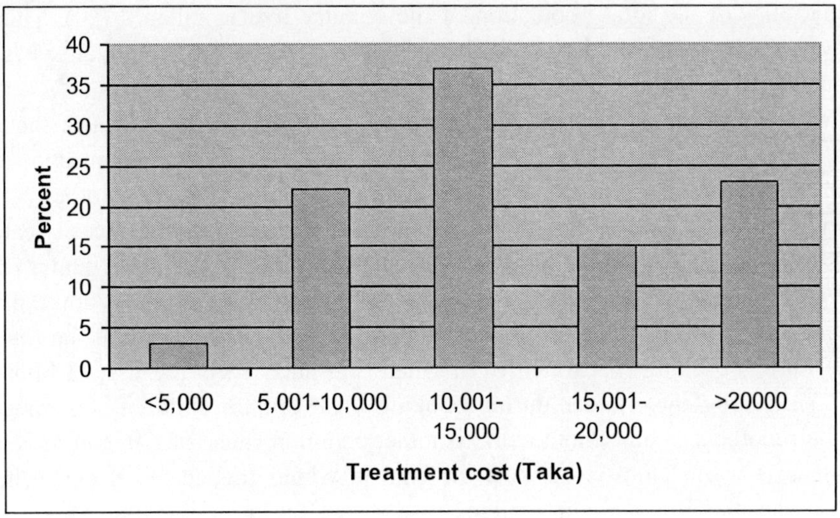

Figure 7. Treatment cost of burn victims.

The mean treatment cost was 15, 227 taka (SD 10,881). In about 60% of cases the treatment cost ranged between Taka 5,000 and 15,000. In 23% of cases, the figure was Taka 20,000 and above.

About the source of money to maintain the treatment expense, 84% of the parents had more than one sources of collection of money like selling personal goods/lands, burrowing from others, help from relatives, and support from the social welfare office in the hospital. All the house maids received full financial support from the families where they worked.

Discussion

Burn is an important, but preventable cause of child injury. A careful analysis of the epidemiological factors in every community is needed before the planning and implementation of a sound prevention program (6). This study identified a mixed picture of burn in relation to the cause with the age and sex. In our study, majority of the burn occurred in 1-10 years age group, this finding corroborates with other studies (7-12). The outstanding finding was identification of flame as the commonest cause of burn injury. Other studies also showed the similar picture (13-17). Comparable to this study the female preponderance of flame burn was also observed in the neighboring country, India, having similar socio-economic-cultural background (18). However, studies in the high income countries reveled scald as the major cause of burn (9,19). This can be explained by the facts that in developed countries scald burn is common due to use of water heaters.

From the study, it was also evident that small, kerosene oil lamp ("Kupi") is the single most important source of flame burn in children. In Bangladesh, only 25% of the rural households have electricity (20), so therefore the majority of the rural people use "Kupi" for lighting at night. These "Kupis" are popular, because they are cheap, easy to make, handy and fuel (Kerosene) consumption is low. The dangerous part of this lamp is its open flame. The majority (80%) of all types of burn happened in rural areas. This finding is in parallel with the fact that 80% of the total population of the country live in villages (20). This finding matched with the Bangladesh Health and Injury Survey - the largest community based study ever conducted in the country (7).

The female predominance in flame burn can be explained by the facts that in rural cultures of Bangladesh, the female children usually help their mothers in domestic works like cooking in ovens, carrying hot curries/water, lighting the lamp. For them, other risk factors are their loose attires (called "frock" and "orna" in local language) that can easily caught fire. Similar findings are also available in other studies on childhood burn in the country (21).

Some older female children got burnt while cooking in other's house as house maid. One of such patients died who was burnt during cooking in gas stoves. Many of the flame burns took place during cooking in earthen oven where bio-mass fuels are used. Children roam around or sit nearby the mother during cooking. The female children sometimes try to "mimic" their mothers in household work. Another common cause of flame burn is warming in winter. Loose warm cloths to protect the cold in winter (called "sweater", "chador" or "shall" etc), and men's loose attire called "loongi" are the most important risk factors for catching fire during warming.

Almost half of the patients were in the age group of 1-6 years and three-quarters in the age group of 1-10 years. Studies in other places (22-27) showed the same distribution of childhood burns in the similar age groups. The male predominance in ash burn can be explained by the fact that pre-school male children usually play in the outdoor, the reverse is usual for the same aged female children; they like to play inside the home with dolls and dummy kitchen utensils. Children unknowingly stepped into the ash that contained fire underneath.

It is interesting that despite scarcity of electric supply in rural areas, 82% of the electric burn happened in rural areas. Electric burn was also more common in the adolescent male.

This may be due to unsafe electric wiring in villages and lack of alertness or risk taking behavior among the adolescents. Electric burn is one of the important causes of permanent disability and almost half of the patients had to undergo amputation of the affected limb.

The mean cost of treatment of burn is much higher than the mean income of the affected families. This imposes enormous economic burden on the poor parents. To meet this huge treatment cost, the majority of the parents had to borrow, sale properties and to seek help from relatives.

Apart from the treatment cost, burn treatment needed prolonged hospital stay. During hospitalization, either parents (usually the mother) had to attend to the child. In two cases, the working mother lost her job due to the "long leave of absence" from her working place (garment factory). Lengthy hospital stay, painful dressing, high treatment cost, loss of working hours of the parents, all contributed for premature discharge or leave from the hospital against medical advice.

Limitations of the study

Small sample size and convenience sampling technique were the main limitations of the study. Mainly the lower and the lower middle class section of the population attended the burn unit of Dhaka Medical College hospital for treatment. The upper middle and higher class families usually attend private clinics or large national or multinational corporate hospitals. Therefore, this study does not represent the burn situation at the national level. However, the findings could be utilized to develop burn prevention strategies.

Conclusions

In terms of morbidity and mortality, burn in children is a significant public health problem in Bangladesh. We have derived data, which showed that flame burns from kerosene lamp and oven fire mainly victimize the poor rural girls and poses significant physical and financial constraints on the affected persons as well as their families.

From the comprehensive overview of this study, it can be recommended that many pediatric burn injuries can be avoided by simple awareness raising programs. This is particularly important for a country like Bangladesh, where cost of burn management is expensive and post burn rehabilitation is almost non-existent. The results highlight the following important aspects of prevention of burn in children:

- Awareness raising though mass media campaign, radio/TV message about the cautious use of oil lamps.
- Programs addressing the parents/caregivers about careful supervision of the children.
- The youngsters must not be allowed to carry kerosene lamp and also stay away form cooking oven.
- Pouring of water into ashes; avoiding dumping of ashes in the areas where the small kids play or move.
- Caution should be taken to keep the youngsters away from open fire warming in winter.
- Loose attires of the female children can better be modified to a tighter garment to avoid easy catch of fire in clothes. The social attitudes need modification in this regards.
- Safe electrification and wiring
- Technological conversion of uncovered, kerosene lamps into a low cost chimney lamp
- Further epidemiological study with larger sample size to grasp the problem more precisely is recommended

Acknowledgments

We acknowledge the cooperation from the studied burn patients and their parents, physicians, nurses and other staffs of the Burn Unit of Dhaka Medical College hospital, Bangladesh. We also declare that there was no formal funding agency for this study. The study was carried out by spending personal resources.

References

[1] World Health organization. World Health Report 2001 Database. Geneva: WHO, 2002

[2] Hettiaratchy S, Dziewulski P. ABC of burn. BMJ 2004;328: 1366-8.

[3] Mohan D, Varghese M. Injuries in the South-East Asia Region: Priorities for policy and action. New Delhi: WHO, SEA/Injuries/A1, 2002.

[4] World Bank. Investing in health: World development report 1993. New York: Oxford Univ Press, 1993.

[5] Rahman A, Shafinaz S, Linnan M, Rahman F. Bangladesh health and injury survey: Report on children. Dhaka: Dir Gen Health Serv, 2005.

[6] Bouter LM, Knipschild PG, van Rijn JL, Meertens RM. How to study the etiology of burn injury: The epidemiological approach. Burns 1989;15:162-6.

[7] Mashreky SR, Rahman A, Chowdhury SM, Giashuddin S, Svanström L, et al. Epidemiology of childhood burn: Yield of largest community based injury survey in Bangladesh. Burns 2008;34(6):856-62.

[8] http://www.keepkidshealthy.com/welcome/safety/burn_safety.html

[9] Verma SS, Srinivasan S, Vartak AM. An epidemiological study of 500 pediatric burn patients in Mumbai, India. Indian J Plast Surg 2007;40(2):153-7.

[10] Cheng JC, Leung KS, Lam ZC, Leung PC. An analysis of 1,704 burn injuries in Hong Kong children. Burns 1990;16:182-4.

[11] Ryan CA, Shankowsky HA, Tredget EE. Profile of the pediatric burn patients in a Canadian burn centre. Burns 1992;18:267-72.

[12] Mukerji G, Chamania S, Patidar GP, Gupta S. Epidemiology of paediatric burns in Indore, India. Burns 2001;27:33-8.

[13] Andrew ED, Eshobo EI, Lilian OO, Charles EO, Christopher EI, Jhon EOS. A five-year review of burn injuries in Irrua. BMC Health Serv Res 2007;7:171.

[14] Momoh MI, Okugbo SU, Ohanaka EC, Ugbeye ME. Causes and risk factors in burns; Experience from Benin city. Nigerian J Surg Sci 2000;10(2):103-11.

[15] Song C, Chua A. Epidemiology of burn injury in Singapore from 1997-2003. Burns 2005;31(suppl 1):18-26.

[16] Fasika OM. Changing pattern of burn epidemiology and the compliance factor in management at Ibadan. Nigerian Postgrad Med J 1997;4(2):7-10.

[17] Jaiswal AK, Aggarwal H, Solanki P, Lubana PS, Mathur RK, Odiya S. Epidemiological and socio-cultural study of burn patients in MY Hospital, Indore, India. Indian J Plast Surg 2007;40(2):158-63.

[18] Attia AF, Sherif AA, Massoud MN, Abou-Nazel MW, Arafa MA. Epidemiological and socio-cultural study of burn patients in Alexandria, Egypt. East Med Health J 1997;3(3):451-61.

[19] Zeitin R, Somppi E, Jarnberg J. Pediatric burn in central Finaland between the 1960s and the 1980s. Burns 1993;19:418-22.

[20] Statistical year book of Bangladesh Dahka: Bangladesh Bureau Stat, 2001.

[21] Daisy S, Mostaque AK, Bari TS, Khan AR, Karim S, Quamruzzaman Q. Socioeconomic and cultural influence in the causation of burns in the urban children of Bangladesh. J Burn Care Rehabil 2001;22(4): 269-73.

[22] Rossingnol M, Locke JA, Burke JF. Pediatric burn injures, New England, USA. Burns 1990;16:41-8.

[23] Gupta M, Gupata OK, Goil P. Pediatric burns in Jaipur, India: An epidemiological study. Burns 1992;18(1):63-7.

[24] Iregbulem LM, Nnabuko BE. Epidemiology of childhood thermal injuries in Enugu, Nigeria. Burns 1993;19(3):223-6.

[25] Dedovic Z, Boychta P, Koupilova I, Suchanek I. Epidemiology of childhood burns at the Burn Centre in Brno, Czech Republic. Burns 1996;22:125-9.

[26] Cronin KJ, Butles PEM, McHugh M, Edwards G. A 1 year prospective study of burns in an Irish pediatric burns unit. Burns 1996;22:221-4.

[27] Liao CC, Rossignol AM. Landmarks in burn prevention. Burns 2000;26:422-34.

Submitted: December 17, 2008.
Revised: February 15, 2009.
Accepted: February 22, 2009.

In: Public Health Yearbook 2009
Editor: Joav Merrick

ISBN: 978-1-61668-911-7

Chapter 19

Attitude of Secondary School Children towards People with HIV/AIDS. An Insight into the Stigma and Discrimination Problem in the English Speaking Caribbean

Alok Kumar, MBBS, MD*[*1], Geeta Kumari, MSW, MA (Couns Psychol)[2], Richard Carter, MSc[3] and Carmita Douglin, MSc[4]
[1]School of Clinical Medicine and Research, University of West Indies (Cave Hill), Barbados,
[2]Faculty of Social Sciences, University of West Indies (Cave Hill), Barbedos,
[3]Ministry of Education and Youth Affairs, Barbados and [4]National HIV/AIDS Commission, Government of Barbados, Barbedos, West Indies

Abstract

The objective was to explore the attitude of the secondary school children toward persons living with HIV/AIDS. Methods: This report is based on a cross section survey of the secondary school children in Barbados. Representative samples of these children were selected from the secondary schools across Barbados using a two stage randomization. The survey instrument consisted of a structured self administered questionnaire. Results: Respondents varied proportionately between 10 and 18 years coming from form (class) 1 to 5 of the secondary schools, 53% being males. Nearly a sixth of the respondents personally knew someone living with HIV/AIDS and nearly a third personally knew someone, who had died of AIDS. Around 50% of the respondents answered "ÿes", when asked whether HIV infected students and teachers should be allowed to attend school to learn and teach respectively.

* Correspondence: Alok Kumar, MBBS, MD, Lecturer, School of Clinical Medicine and Research, University of the West Indies (Cave Hill Campus) and Queen Elizabeth Hospital, Barbados, West Indies. E-mail: alokkumar.uwichill@gmail.com

However, only a tenth were willing to buy food from a vendor who was HIV infected. Majority of the children were willing to take care of relatives or get close to a class mate infected with the HIV. However, over a half of the respondent would prefer to maintain secrecy about one of their family member being HIV infected. Conclusions: It is clear that the issues of stigma and discrimination remain important in Barbados. However, compared to our previous survey of the same population, attitudes toward persons with HIV/AIDS have softened.

Keywords: HIV, AIDS, school, attitude, West Indies.

Introduction

HIV-related stigma refers to all unfavorable attitudes, beliefs and policies directed toward people perceived to have HIV/AIDS, as well as towards their significant others and loved ones, close associates, social groups, and communities. HIV infection fits the profile of a condition that carries a high level of stigmatization (1). The existence of HIV/AIDS-related stigma has been widely documented (2-4). HIV/AIDS-related stigma and discrimination rank among the biggest and most pervasive barriers to effective responses to the AIDS epidemic. Also, AIDS-related stigma and discrimination remains one of the most poorly understood aspects of the epidemic, because of its variations across cultures and limited theoretical frameworks for understanding how it is created, manifested, and maintained and how it affects upon health behaviors (5). Interventions to reduce stigma are therefore crucial for improving care, quality of life, and emotional health for people living with HIV and AIDS. HIV/AIDS-related stigma has been specifically identified as a domestic policy challenge that must be addressed to reduce the number of new HIV infections, and eliminating stigma is a crucial element of global efforts (6-9).

One of the ways to reduce stigma and discrimination toward people living with HIV/AIDS is by exploring beliefs and attitude and bringing about positive changes through education (10). Yong people are at the center of the global HIV/AIDS pandemics. They also are the world's greatest hope in the struggle against this fatal disease (11). During these years, youth learn, explore, and make decisions that will affect the rest of their lives. If they receive the information and services, they need to make informed choices, then they are more likely to change their attitudes and beliefs. In this paper we explore the attitude of secondary school children toward persons living with HIV/AIDS using a redesigned questionnaire during a behavioral surveillance survey.

Methods

This report is based on the findings from a nation wide behavioral surveillance survey of secondary school children in Barbados conducted in 2006. This survey was designed to study the HIV related knowledge, attitude and the risk taking behaviors among secondary school children. The survey instrument was a self-administered questionnaire comprised predominantly of closed-ended questions. The questionnaire was based on the WHO/KABP questionnaire for students (12), modified to suit local needs based on our own experience from a similar study conducted in 1991 (13). Of the 150 questions in the survey instrument, which was to be completed in 90 minutes, 25 questions were designed to investigate the attitudes of these children toward persons with HIV/AIDS. The original survey instrument designed by the author was further modified based on the suggestions by education experts at the Ministry of Education and Youth Affairs, Government of Barbados, primarily for appropriateness in respect of socio-cultural context and age of respondents. Further minor modifications were made after pre-testing of the questionnaire among a group of secondary school students.

Respondents were drawn from most of the secondary schools in Barbados based on random sample selection. The survey was based on a multi-stage systematic random sample of all secondary schools in Barbados – both public and private. The sample basically sought to select 1,500 respondents – 300 at each form (class) level from 1st to 5th. Based on a general average of 30 students per form, 10 schools were randomly selected for each form level hence 30 students x 10 schools x 5 form levels = 1,500 students.

In order to facilitate the survey at the school level the principals were circularized by the Chief Education Officer advising of the survey and seeking the support of the principals. Based on information derived from the schools concerning the designation of forms copies of a letter from the Chief Education Officer seeking the permission of the parents/guardians of children in the selected forms were forwarded to the principal to be taken home by the students and returned in advance of the survey. The conduct of the fieldwork at the schools (completion of the questionnaires) was coordinated by three research assistants recruited and trained by the Youth Affairs Department. It should be noted here that although the survey instrument was intended to be self-administered there were a number of cases, particularly in the lower forms of some schools, where children had to be assisted by the coordinator due to literacy challenges. In these cases the questions/items on the questionnaire were read by the coordinator and the respondents assisted in completion of the questionnaire.

The coding and data entry of completed questionnaires were completed by the coordinators themselves with data management and analysis being conducted by the Youth Affairs Department using the Statistical Package for the Social Sciences (SPSS 2006, Chicago, United States).

Results

Selected socio-demographics of the respondents are shown in table 1. Given that the survey targeted the first to fifth forms (class), the age of respondents varied proportionately between 10 and 18 years. Males constituted a slight majority of respondents 52.6 % as opposed to females 47.3%, which constituted some level of over-representation of males given the relatively even gender balance in the secondary school system in this country. Consistent with the racial distribution of Barbados' population the majority of respondents were black (80.7%). Mother was present in 86.1% of the households of respondents and the father was present in only 40.9%.

Many of the respondents personally knew someone who had died from AIDS and over one eighth of the respondents had personal exposure to persons living with HIV/AIDS (see figure 1). Respondents perception about tolerance toward persons living with the HIV/AIDS was assessed by questions on their acceptance of persons with HIV in various settings, where they were directly involved (see table 2). Nearly a third of the respondents were either not sure of the answer or did not answer the questions in this section. Caring attitude of these children were also elicited by questioning on their willingness to care for or their willingness to freely associate themselves with a relative or classmate infected with the AIDS virus (see table 3). Once again, one third of the respondents were either not sure or did not answer the questions in this section.

Table 1. Socio-demographics of the respondents

	Percentage
FORMS	
First and Second	39
Third and Fourth	30
Fifth and Sixth	31
AGE	
≤ 10 Years	4
11 – 13 Years	50
14 – 16 Years	38
> 16 Years	3
GENDER	
Male	53
Female	47
HOUSEHOLD COMPOSITION	
Mother	86
Father	41
Grandparents	18
Step father/mother	12

Table 2. Perception about persons living with HIV/AIDS

	Percent
Should students be allowed to attend school if he/she has HIV virus	
Yes	56
No	17
Not sure	21
No answer	6
If a teacher has the AIDS virus but is not sick, should he/she be allowed to continue teaching in school	
Yes	45
No	25
Not sure	23
No answer	7
If you knew that a shopkeeper or food seller had the AIDS virus, would you buy food from them?	
Yes	10
No	59
Not sure	23
No answer	8

Table 3. Caring attitude toward persons living with HIV/AIDS

	Percent
If a relative of yours became sick with AIDS, would you take care of him/her?	
Yes	64
No	9
Not sure	22
No answer	5
If you knew a classmate was infected with the AIDS virus, would you behave the same as usual with them?	
Yes	30
No, get closer and give him emotional support	27
No, be cautious and not get close because of fear of AIDS	10
Not sure	24
No answer	9
If the women in the next door neighbor who you used to visit frequently catches the AIDS virus, would you continue to visit her?	
Yes	23
No	19
Not sure	54
No answer	4

Figure 1. Social exposure to persons with HIV/AIDS

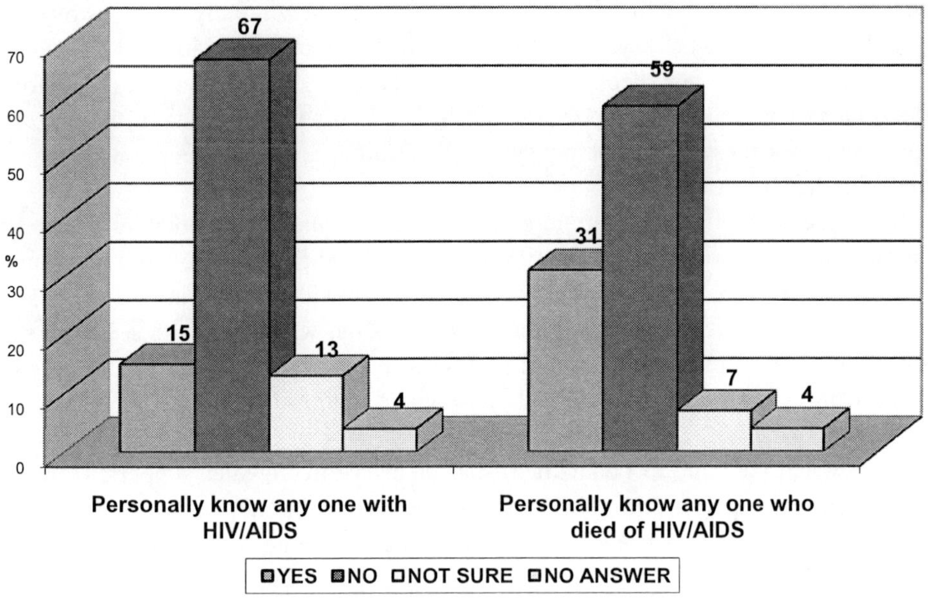

Figure 1. Social exposure to persons with HIV/AIDS.

In order to assess the perception of stigma and discrimination toward HIV/AIDS in this population, respondents were asked: "If a member of your family got infected with the AIDS virus, would you want it to remain a secret?" Fifty one percent of the respondents answered

"Yes", 19% answered "No", 22% were not sure of their answer and 8% did not answer this question. When asked: "If a person catches the AIDS virus he or she is to blame herself?", 67% answered "Yes", 22% answered "No", 8% were not sure and 3% did not answer this question.

Discussion

The Caribbean has the second highest prevalence of HIV/AIDS, after the Sub-Saharan Africa. Today's generation of schoolchildren have been born into a world, where AIDS is a harsh, unavoidable reality - a situation that their time at school can help them to prepare for. As well as providing an environment in which people can be educated about AIDS, schools often act as a centre-point for community discussion and activity; as such, they can be a vital tool in monitoring the epidemic and co-coordinating a response to it. With a capacity to reach large numbers of young people with information that can save their lives, basic school education can have such a powerful preventive effect that it has been described as a 'social vaccine'(14). While our children are seriously threatened by AIDS, they are also an invaluable tool in the fight to establish an environment where people living with HIV are well-supported and new infections are prevented.

Almost one third of respondents personally knew someone who had died from AIDS and 15% reported knowing someone who is HIV positive – figures that carries important implications for developing initiatives for the sensitization of this age group. Given that the over all prevalence of HIV in this country is quoted at 1.75% (15), over a seventh of students having known some one with AIDS may also reflect the how rapidly the news of HIV/AIDS in people spread in this society. This is often facilitated in closely-knit small societies such as in these Caribbean islands. People may be very curious to know who has AIDS for several reasons including the use these persons as subject of gossip, avoidance of these persons and blame game. All these would perpetuate stigmatization and discrimination of these people living with the HIV/AIDS.

It is somewhat refreshing that more than half the respondents felt that a student should be allowed to attend school if they had HIV (only 17% said an outright "no") and almost two-thirds would take care of a relative if they became sick with AIDS. Similarly almost half the respondents felt that if a teacher had the AIDS virus but was not sick then he/she should be allowed to continue teaching in school as against a quarter who disagreed. In similar vein, only 10% of respondents reported that they would be cautious and not get too close to an HIV infected classmate out of fear of infection whereas most of the other respondents indicated that they would continue to behave as usual or even offer greater support. However, it is worth noting that nearly a third of the respondents were either not sure of their answer or did not respond to many of these questions. It is likely that the discussion generated on this important social problem of HIV/AIDS is not enough to facilitate formation of favorable opinion and attitude among these students toward the persons living with the HIV/AIDS in this society.

It is clear that the issues of stigma and discrimination remain important in Barbados, because when respondents were asked whether they would want the infection of a family member with the AIDS virus to remain a secret 50.6% said "yes". In addition, less than a fourth of the respondents were willing to continue to visit their close neighbor with HIV. Similar findings have been reported from studies in other countries (16-18). Interestingly, however, an aggregated 56.2% of respondents said that if a classmate became infected they would either behave the same way towards them (29.6%) or get closer and provide emotional support (29.6%). Only 10.5% said that they would be cautious and not get too close for fear of infection and 24.3% were unsure as to their response. These findings indicated that despite their perception of the prevalent stigma and discrimination in the society they were willing to take a different and a more compassionate position toward their peer living with HIV/AIDS.

We compared the responses from this survey with those of a previous survey conducted in the same population group in the early 1990s (13). Although the instrument used in the previous survey was not exactly the same, comparisons of the findings from the two surveys suggest a softening of the level of stigma and discrimination among this segment of the population as personal experience of the disease increased. This may have been because of the school based HIV education introduced in this country following the recommendation from the previous survey. Similar findings have been reported in other studies (19-20). We did not find any other similar studies from the Caribbean for comparison.

There is a need for continuing HIV education in the schools. Sequential HIV education starting in the primary school will help to bring about desirable positive changes in the attitude and perception of these young people toward people living with the HIV/AIDS in this society.

References

[1] Herek GM. AIDS and stigma. Am Behav Scientist 1999; 42(7):1106-16.

[2] Centers for Disease Control and Prevention. HIV-related knowledge and stigma. United States, 2000. MMWR 2000;49(47):1062-4.

[3] Rankin WW, Brennan S, Schell E, Laviwa J, Rankin SH The stigma of being HIV-positive in Africa. PLoS Med 2005;2(8):247.

[4] Herek GM, Capitanio JP. AIDS stigma and sexual prejudice Am Behav Scientist 1999;42(7):1126-43.

[5] Parker R, Aggleton P. HIV/AIDS related stigma and discrimination: A conceptual framework and an agenda for action (New York: Population Council). 2002. Accessed 2008 Mar 01. URL: http://www.popcouncil. orgpdfs/horizons/sdcncptlfrmwrk.pdf

[6] Institute of Medicine. No time to lose: Getting more from HIV prevention. Washington, DC: Natl Acad Press, 2001.

[7] Joint United Nations Program on HIV/AIDS (UNAIDS). A conceptual framework and basis for action: HIV/AIDS stigma and discrimination. Geneva: UNAIDS, 2002.

[8] Henry J Kaiser Family Foundation. Policy brief: Critical policy challenges in the third decade of the HIV/AIDS epidemic. Menlo Park, CA: Henry J Kaiser Fam Foundation, 2002.

[9] Klein SJ, Karchner WD, O'Connell DA. Interventions to prevent HIV-related stigma and discrimination: findings and recommendations for public health practice. J Public Health Manage Pract 2002;8(6):44-53.

[10] Rutledge SE, Abell N. Awareness, acceptance, and action: an emerging framework for understanding AIDS stigmatizing attitudes among community leaders in Barbados. AIDS Patient Care STDS 2005;19(3):186-99.

[11] UN Special session on Children and HIV/AIDS. Accessed 2008 Feb 12. URL: http://www.unicef.org/specialsession/docs_new/documents/SSC-anniversary-report.pdf

[12] WHO/GPA. WHO/KAPB questionnaire for students. Geneva: WHO, 1986.

[13] Walrond E, Jones F, Hoyos M, Souder M, Ellis H, Roach T. An AIDS-related knowledge, attitudes, beliefs, and practices survey among schoolchildren in Barbados. Bull Pan Am Health Organ 1992;26(3):208-19.
[14] Boler T. and Jellema A. Deadly Inertia: A cross-country study of educational responses to HIV/AIDS, Global campaign for education, 2005. Accessed 2008 Jan 12. URL: http://aidsportal.org/store/1382.pdf
[15] Caribbean Epidemiology Centre/Pan American Health Organization/WHO. Status and trends: Analysis of the Caribbean HIV/AIDS epidemic 1982-2002. Caribbean Epidemiology Centre Publication 2004. Accessed 2007 Dec 05. URL: http://www.carec.org/pdf/status_trends.pdf
[16] Tavoosi A, Zaferani A, Enzevaei A, Tajik P, Ahmadinezhad Z. Knowledge and attitude towards HIV/AIDS among Iranian students.
[17] BMC Public Health 2004;4:17.
[18] Merakou K, Costopoulos C, Markopoulou J, Kourea-Kremastinou J. Knowledge, attitudes, and behavior after 15 years of HIV/AIDS prevention in schools. Eur J Public Health 2002;12:90-3.
[19] Chatterjee C. Baur B. Ram R. Dhar G. Sandhukhan S. Dan A. A study on awareness of AIDS among school students and teachers of higher secondary schools in north Calcutta. Indian J Public Health 2001;45(1):27-30.
[20] Ndeki SS. Klepp KI. Seha AM. Leshabari MT. Exposure to HIV/AIDS information, AIDS knowledge, perceived risk and attitudes toward people with AIDS among primary school-children in northern Tanzania. AIDS Care 1994;6(2):183-91.
[21] Caceres CF. Rosasco AM. Mandel JS. Hearst N. Evaluating a school-based intervention for STD/AIDS prevention in Peru. J Adolesc Health 1994;15(7):582-91.

Submitted: March 06, 2008.
Revised: June 01, 2008.
Accepted: June 08, 2008.

In: Public Health Yearbook 2009
Editor: Joav Merrick
ISBN: 978-1-61668-911-7

Chapter 20

DOES PROLONGED BOTTLE USE EFFECT OBESITY INDEXES AMONG PRESCHOOL CHILDREN?

Constantine I. Vardavas, RN, MPH*, Manolis Linardakis, MSc and Anthony G. Kafatos, MD, PhD
Department of Social Medicine, Faculty of Medicine, University of Crete, Greece

Abstract

To investigate a possible relationship between the way milk is consumed (defined as only bottle, only cup or combined both cup and bottle use) and obesity indexes among preschool children. Study Design: Cross-sectional. Methods: Body Mass Index (BMI), waist circumference (WC) and waist to length ratio (WtLR) where combined with parameters from a lifestyle questionnaire (n=1,755) and a 3-day dietary recall questionnaire (n=855) from preschool children (4-7 years old) in Crete, Greece. Results: Taking into account age, sex, nationality, mothers level of education, current energy intake and expenditure, children who consume milk only from a cup, were found to have lower mean BMI (16.44, 16.95 and 16.96 kg/m2, respectively, p=0.047), WC (55.5, 55.8 and 56.8 cm, respectively, p=0.024), and WtLR (0.480, 0.482 and 0.491, respectively, p=0.014) when compared to those who drank milk from either only a nursing bottle or from both a cup and nursing bottle. Prolonged bottle use was significantly related to obesity (OR of 2.14 [95%CI: 1.21 - 3.78]) and to having a waist circumference over the 90th percentile (OR of 1.88 [95%CI: 1.12 - 3.15]). Conclusions: Childhood obesity may be affected by prolonged bottle use during preschool years independently of current energy intake and expenditure. These current findings stress the imperative need for parental education on the effects of prolonged bottle use on child weight and health.

Keywords: Obesity, bottle-feeding, milk, nursing bottle, child.

* Correspondence: Constantine I Vardavas, Department of Social Medicine, Faculty of Medicine, University of Crete, PO Box 2208, Heraklion 71003, Crete, Greece. Tel: +30 2810 394599; Fax number: +30 2810 394604; E-mail: vardavas@edu.med.uoc.gr

Introduction

The prevalence of obesity both in adults and in children has increased dramatically worldwide (1). In Europe it is estimated that 18% of schoolchildren are overweight (which can be translated into almost 14 million children) with an increase of 0.55% to 1.65% every year (2).

Obesity results from an imbalance between energy intake and energy expenditure. In childhood it has a significant impact on both physical and psychological health. Type 2 diabetes, sleep apnea, hypertension, dyslipidemia, the metabolic syndrome as also depression, social isolation and peer problems are imminent consequences of childhood obesity that most often continue into adult life (3,4).

Prolonged bottle feeding has been associated previously with a number of conditions such as restricted diet, poor chewing techniques, food refusal, dental caries and iron deficiency anaemia (5-7). Although studies have evaluated the role of prolonged bottle-feeding on obesity (8-9) there is still insufficient data regarding the risk of overweight and obesity in regard to the milk drinking habits of older, preschool children.

The purpose of this study was to evaluate a possible relationship between the way milk is consumed (defined as only bottle, only cup or combined both cup and bottle use) and obesity indexes among preschool children.

Methods

The study was conducted during 2004-2005 in preschools in Crete, Greece (in the Chania area with a population of 150,000 or 25% of the population of Crete) as part of a health and nutrition educational intervention program planned to commence, when the preschool children entered primary education. The measurements were obtained during the children's baseline examinations to evaluate the nutritional, growth and health level of all preschoolers, including parental lifestyle and health habits.

From a total of 121 preschools, 118 participated in the study. Out of the other three, two did not operate that academic year and one was excluded due to its topographical inaccessibility and small number of children. A total of 2,630 children were enrolled in these 118 preschools, 77% of which accepted to participate (1,988 children) and due to technical reasons finally 1,755 were examined (67%). The examinations were performed by certified and specifically trained pediatricians from the General Hospital of Chania, Crete on site at the schools after parental informed written consent. The Greek Ministry of Education and the University of Crete's Ethics Research Council approved the study, while Chania's municipality and governing authorities granted funding.

Questionnaire

In addition to the clinical examinations, self-administered questionnaires were posted to the schoolteachers, headmasters and the board of Primary Education in Chania, who subsequently handed the questionnaires to the parents along with written instructions. Completed health habit questionnaires was returned and available for 934 children of the 1,755 examined (53% response rate). This self administered questionnaire was based on a previously designed questionnaire by our Preventive Medicine and Nutrition Clinic and collected information on the parents smoking habits, alcohol use, breastfeeding attempts and current way that they provide their child with milk (10).

Among the data collected we received 855 three-day dietary recall questionnaires (855/1,755=49% response rate) in order to gather information on daily calorie intake. Nutrient contents and calorie intake were analysed according to the food database developed at the Department of Social Medicine of the University of Crete in 1998 and updated in 2000 (11).

Basic characteristics like sex, age and BMI were compared between children that had completed the three-day dietary questionnaire and children that hadn't so as to investigate into the representativeness of the sample and the generalisabilty of the results. No significant difference in the distribution of sex (Chi square test, boys 50.2% and girls 47.3% versus boys 47.3% and girls 52.7%, respectively, $p=0.227$), age (t student test, mean age 5.36 versus 5.34 years, respectively, $p=0.387$) or BMI was found between those who had and those who had not completed three day dietary recall questionnaires (t-student test, mean BMI 16.67 versus 16.50 kg/m2, respectively, $p=0.147$).

Anthropometrical – physical activity assessment

Anthropometrical body measurements were taken from 1,755 of the children. Body weight was measured using a digital scale (± 100g), with the children without shoes and in light clothing. Body length was measured without shoes to the nearest 0.5cm using a measuring tape with the children lying down on a board, so that they could cooperate better and allow for a more accurate measurement. Waist circumference (WC) was measured at the level of umbilicus, and measurements were performed at minimal respiration to the nearest 0.1cm. Waist to length ratio (WtLR) was estimated dividing WC by length. The children were categorised as normal weight, overweight and obese according to the to the cut-offs for childhood overweight and obesity adopted by the International Obesity Task Force (IOTF) (12). Assessment of the children's moderate-to-vigorous physical activity out of school was performed using a standardised activity interview based on a questionnaire completed by the children's parents. Further details regarding the reliability and validity of the questionnaire are given elsewhere (13).

Statistical analysis

The SPSS, version 15.0, statistical program was used for all analyses and a p value of <0.05 was considered as statistically significant. Prevalence values were compared using the chi-square test. Continuous variables were tested for normality and were log-transformed if necessary. ANCOVA was used to check the differences between the three different ways of milk consumption ("cup", "nursing bottle" and "cup and nursing bottle") and the existence of a linear by linear association between them and obesity indices.

During the analysis, gender, age, nationality, maternal and paternal educational level, the child's weight at birth and current daily energy intake were accounted for. The child's birth weight and the father's level of education was not found to be statistical significant parameters in the analysis. Due to the smaller number of children in our study for which we had complete dietary information two models were used, one (Model 1) included the covariates: child's gender, age, nationality and maternal education and another (Model 2) also included the child's dietary intake. These two models were used to estimate the effect of current energy intake (derived from a three day dietary questionnaire) as a confounding factor in the analysis due to the smaller number of children (n=855 or 49% of the 1,755 examined) where we had information on their dietary calorie intake. Finally, logistic regression analysis was carried out to calculate the risk OR (Odds Ratio) and 95% CI (95% confidence interval) for overweight or obesity, for the categories of "nursing bottle" and "cup and nursing bottle" in relation to "cup" category as a reference.

Results

Table 1 depicts the descriptive characteristics of the preschool children of our study according to age, class, district of residence and current way of milk consumption and mean birth weight. Only the mean birth weight was found to differ according to the child's gender ($p<0.05$). Although approximately 52% of 1st grade preschool children (age of 4.8 ± 0.3 years old) and 68% of children in the 2nd grade of preschool (5.8 ± 0.4 years of age) drank milk only from a cup almost half of all 1st grade preschool children and a third of 2nd grade preschool children still drink milk sometime during the day from a nursing bottle, while up to almost 18% of 1st grade preschool children still drank milk only from a nursing bottle and never use a cup. No gender differences were noted in regards to the means of milk consumption.

Prolonged bottle-feeding and obesity indexes

As seen in table 2, 43.8% of children in the 2nd grade of preschool who consumed milk from both "cup and nursing bottle" were obese or overweight compared to only 28% of obese and overweight children that consumed milk from a "cup" and this difference was statistically significant ($p=0.008$).

Table 1. Descriptive characteristics and method of milk consumption of the study participants

	Boys	Girls
N	471	463
Mean birth weight in grams *	3341 ± 436 [1]	3230 ± 428
Age in years	5.4 ± 0.6	5.4 ± 0.6
Class in Preschool		
1st class	40.6 (191) [2]	41.3 (191)
2nd class	59.4 (280)	58.7 (272)
District of residence		
Urban	38.8 (183)	42.0 (198)
Sub-urban	6.1 (29)	7.8 (36)
Rural	55.1 (260)	49.5 (228)
Nationality		
Both Greek parents	88.1 (416)	91.3 (422)
One Greek parent	5.7 (27)	2.8 (13)
Both immigrants	6.1 (29)	5.8 (27)
Milk Consumption		
Preschool 1st class		
Cup	52.9 (101)	51.8 (99)
Nursing bottle	28.8 (55)	29.3 (56)
Cup and nursing bottle	18.3 (35)	18.8 (36)
Preschool 2nd class		
Cup	65.7 (184)	71.7 (195)
Nursing bottle	17.9 (50)	15.4 (42)
Cup and nursing bottle	16.4 (46)	12.9 (35)

1. Values are mean ± standard deviation. Student t-test.
2. Values are % (N). Chi-squared test.
* p-value <0.05.

Table 2. Milk Consumption of pre-school children in relation to categories of obesity indexes

	1st class Preschool			2nd class Preschool		
	Cup	Nursing bottle	Cup and nursing bottle	Cup	Nursing bottle	Cup and nursing bottle
		% (N)			% (N)	
Body Mass Index [a]						
Normal	76.0 (149)	69.7 (76)	70.4 (50)	72.0 (267)	74.4 (67)	56.3 (45)
Overweight	15.8 (31)	22.0 (24)	19.7 (14)	18.3 (68)	11.1 (10)	25.0 (20)
Obese	8.2 (16)	8.3 (9)	9.9 (7)	9.7 (36)	14.4 (13)	18.8 (15)
P-value [b]	0.344			0.008		
Waist Circumference [c]						
<90th percentile	88.7 (173)	91.7 (100)	84.5 (60)	88.1 (326)	86.7 (78)	80.0 (64)
≥90th percentile	11.3 (22)	8.3 (9)	15.5 (11)	11.9 (44)	13.3 (12)	20 (16)
P-value [b]	0.542			0.068		

a. According to IOTF criteria (BMJ 2000; 320:1240-3).
b. Chi-square test (χ^2) (liner by linear association).
c. Age-sex specific percentile.

This difference in obesity was also noticed among 1st grade preschool children but in a much smaller proportion (29.6% of obese and overweight drink milk both from "cup and nursing bottle" compared to 24% that drank milk only from a "cup", an this finding was not statistically significant).

As seen in table 3 according to the first model (taking into account age, gender, nationality and maternal education), children who consumed milk only from a "cup" were found to have lower mean BMI (16.45, 16.92 and 17.08 kg/m2, respectively, p=0.008), WC (55.5, 55.8 and 57.2 cm, respectively, p=0.004), and WtLR (0.480, 0.482 and 0.493, respectively, p=0.002) compared to those who drank milk from a "nursing bottle" and "cup and nursing bottle". The results do not differ using the second model (with energy intake added as a covariate to those of model 1), where children who consume milk only from a "cup", were still found to have a lower BMI, WC, and WtLR (p=0.047, p=0.024 and p=0.014 respectively).

Taking into account the fact that current energy intake did not significantly affect BMI, WC and WtLR in the analysis, the Odds Ratio (OR) of being overweight and obese according to the child's current way of drinking milk was estimated without taking current energy intake into concern (therefore increasing our sample size in this specific analysis to 1,755 children). As depicted in table 4 consuming milk only from a "nursing bottle" was found not to be statistically significantly related to overweight and obesity in children, with an OR of 1.04 [95%CI:0.65-1.66] and 1.37 [95%CI :0.78-2.42] respectively. On the other hand childhood obesity according to the IOTF cut-offs was found to be significantly related ($p<0.05$) to drinking milk both from a "cup and nursing bottle" with an OR of 2.14 [95%CI: 1.21 - 3.78] and 1.88 [95%CI: 1.12 - 3.15] respectively.

Table 3. BMI, waist circumference and waist-to-length ratio in relation to milk drinking

Milk Consumption	Model 1 [a]	Model 2 [b]
	Body Mass Index (kg/m^2)	
Cup	16.45±0.12 ‡ (522) [c]	16.44±0.11 †‡ (437)
Nursing bottle	16.92±0.19 (182)	16.95±0.21 † (158)
Cup and nursing bottle	17.08±0.21 ‡ (139)	16.96±0.23 ‡ (125)
P-value	0.010	0.036
Trend P-value	0.008	0.047
	Waist Circumference (cm)	
Cup	55.47±0.26 ‡	55.50±0.28 ‡
Nursing bottle	55.83±0.49	55.75±0.47
Cup and nursing bottle	57.20±0.50 ‡	56.82±0.52 ‡
P-value	0.009	0.079
Trend P-value	0.004	0.024
	Waist-to-length ratio	
Cup	0.480±0.002 ‡	0.480±0.002 ‡
Nursing bottle	0.482±0.003 †	0.482±0.004
Cup and nursing bottle	0.493±0.004 †‡	0.491±0.004 ‡
P-value	0.005	0.050
Trend P-value	0.002	0.014

a. Analysis of covariance: as covariates were used sex, age, nationality and mother's education.

b. Analysis of covariance: as covariates were used sex, age, nationality, mother's education and energy intake (kcal).

c. Values are mean ± standard error (N).

‡ Statistically significant difference ($p<0.05$) between *"Cup"* and *"Cup and nursing bottle"*.

† Statistically significant difference ($p<0.05$) between *"Nursing bottle"* and *"Cup and nursing bottle"*.

In BMI and Waist circumference the $\log_{10}$ transformations were used.

Table 4. Odds Ratio indexes of children with elevated BMI and waist circumference and in relation of milk drinking

	Body Mass Index (kg/m^2)[a]		Waist circumference [b]
	Overweight *Odds Ratio [95% CI]*	Obese *Odds Ratio [95% CI]*	≥90th perc *Odds Ratio [95% CI]*
Cup (reference)	1.00	1.00	1.00
Nursing bottle	1.04 [0.65-1.66]	1.37 [0.78-2.42]	1.01 [0.58-1.76]
Cup and nursing bottle	1.52 [0.94-2.45]	2.14 [1.21-3.78]*	1.88 [1.12-3.15]*

a. According to IOTF criteria (BMJ 2000; 320:1240-3).
b. Age-sex specific percentile.
Multiple Logistic regression analysis: as covariates were used sex, age, nationality and mother's education.
*p-value<0.05.

Table 5. Physical activity level and dietary intake and of certain variables in relation to current bottle weaning status

	Cup	Nursing bottle	Cup and nursing bottle	
	Mean ± SE (N)			*P* for trend *
Energy (kcal)	1749±18 (468)	1772±29 (173)	1814±33 (133)	0.082
Carbohydrates (% en)	45.1±0.2	43.7±0.4	43.4±0.5	<0.001
Total Fat (% en)	41.7±0.2	42.6±0.4	42.8±0.4	0.020
SFA (% en)	15.2±0.1	16.2±0.2	16.3±0.2	<0.001
MUFA (% en)	16.9±0.1	17.0±0.2	16.9±0.3	0.915
PUFA (% en)	4.7±0.1	4.7±0.1	4.6±0.1	0.770
Calcium (mg)	956.8±13.8	1124.8±22.8	1096.2±25.6	<0.001
Calcium per 1000 kcal (mg)	556.0±7.4	645.9±12.3	618.7±13.9	<0.001
Dairy products (g)	341±8	397±14	398±16	0.001
Milk (g)	267±8	327±13	326±15	0.001
Cheese (g)	26±1	23±2	26±2	0.925
Yogurt (g)	47±2	47±4	46±5	0.756
MVPA (mins/week)	54±4 (552)	58±7 (192)	55±8 (149)	0.957

* Analysis of covariance (sex, age & BMI were used as covariates) for linear trend.

Dietary intake

Although total daily calorie intake and level of physical exercise did not differ between the three groups as seen in table 5, the dietary intake of milk, calcium, total dairy products, total fat and saturated fat intake was found to differ. Children that drank milk either from just a "nursing bottle" or from both a "cup and nursing bottle" found to have a greater intake of the above in comparison to those who drank milk only from a "cup". Specifically, daily calcium and daily milk intake was greater in those who drank milk only from a bottle, while total fat, total dairy product and total saturated fat intake was greater in those that were in the phase of bottle weaning and drank milk from both. Additionally we investigated into the role of calcium intake on obesity as defined by IOTF. The daily calcium intake (mean ± SD) of those who were classified as normal-weight was 1,027 ± 321mg, those overweight 1,010 ± 273 mg and those obese 975 ± 290mg but these differences were not found to be statistically important.

Discussion

Our study implicates that both prolonged bottle-feeding and a prolonged transition phase between cup drinking and bottle-feeding may lead to a higher risk of obesity as shown in the obesity indexes, in comparison to drinking milk only from a cup. Additionally from an epidemiological point of view, the rates of bottle use among these 4-7 year old children were notably elevated, even though the actual quantity of milk consumed daily was below the recommendations. The American Academy of Pediatrics' Guidelines for Health Supervision II, recommended the introduction of the cup at six months of age and complete weaning by 15 to 18 months of age, therefore the one in two preschool children who still drink from a bottle is remarkably high (14).

Our study strengthen the fact that prolonged bottle use in young children in associated with increased body weight using an older Mediterranean population. Bonuck et al (9) analysed the NHANES III data and found that late bottle weaning was significantly associated with child overweight and obesity, and that each additional month of bottle use corresponded to an approximate 3% increase in the odds of being in a higher BMI category. Our findings regarding obesity are similar although we did not find any relation between being overweight and concurrent way of milk consumption.

Bonuck and Kahn (8) found that bottle use was significantly associated with obesity, which was also our experience. One additional point that we found was the negative effect of prolonged bottle-feeding dependant on the child's age and the relationship between obesity and bottle feeding found stronger among 2nd class preschool children in comparison to 1st class preschool children. A subsequent follow up study could determine such an age related difference.

The role of milk consumption on BMI in preschool children has been previously investigated (15, 16). Carruth and Skinner (17) followed a number of preschool children and found that the daily intake of dairy products were inversely associated with body fat accumulation and BMI, Barba et al (15,16) also found similar results when investigating the frequency of milk consumption even though they did not control for current energy intake. In our analysis, milk consumption, as well as calcium intake, differed according to the group the child was classified. Dietary calcium is known to play an important role in the regulation of blood pressure, insulin resistance and in the regulation of energy metabolism. High calcium diets have been found to reduce weight gain during periods of high-energy intake and increase lipolysis during periods of calorie restriction (18). In our case, dietary calcium intake was not found to differ according to the IOTF standards for overweight and obesity and thus could not explain the noted differences between the groups. As stated the contents and not the bottles themselves are of concern as they almost always contain milk or juice rather than water (19) and most likely prolonged bottle-feeding in preschool children may not induce obesity by itself, but probably acts in synergy with other psychological, behavioural or genetic factors and concurrent different eating and exercise habits. Television exposure, child food behaviours, parental role modelling and maternal knowledge of appropriate child nutrition have all been found to influence a preschool child's food intake and energy expenditure thus affecting the child's obesity indexes (20-23). These parental and environmental influences are stronger during early childhood as the parents act as both role models and providers of food and influence health habits (24).

It is possible that in our case the children who still, at the age of 5 or 7 years, drank milk from a bottle, did so before sleeping at night and thus, although differences in physical activity and calorie intake did not differ, the timing of the calorie intake did which could explain the difference noted, even though we have no such data to support this hypothesis. Research has shown that preschool children who skip breakfast, have a higher dinner time calorie consumption and have a higher risk of obesity, since the distribution of energy intake during the day is important to energy regulation and could possibly explain our findings (25).

Due to the study's cross sectional and ad-hoc design we could not examine a causal relationship between prolonged bottle-feeding and obesity indexes, although large population size increase the studies statistical strength. Further studies are needed to investigate the possible mechanisms both biological and behavioural, which relate prolonged bottle use to obesity.

This study implicates that prolonged bottle use into preschool years, can lead to a higher risk for obesity. Our study stress the necessity to improve maternal education regarding the negative effects of prolonged bottle-feeding, whether that is incorporated in the child's health booklet or transmitted by the health professionals during the child (well baby) check-up visits. Since childhood and adult obesity is on the rise globally, it is a must that we combat its predisposition from early in life, since obesity and its associated risk factors seems preventable through early intervention.

Acknowledgments

We would like to thank D Niaounaki from the Regional office of Primary Education in Crete, Dr E Balomenaki and Dr D Athanasopoulos from the paediatric clinic of the Chania General Hospital and the Prefecture's of Chania governing body for their support in funding the study. Funding: Obtained from the Prefecture's of Chania governing body. Competing interests: None declared.

References

[1] De Onis M, Blossner M. Prevalence and trends of overweight among preschool children in developing countries. Am J Clin Nutr 2000; 72:1032-9.

[2] Lobstein T, Baur L, Uauy R. Obesity in children and young people : a crisis in public health. Report to the World Health Organization by the International Obesity TaskForce. Obes Rev 2004;5(Suppl 1):5-104.

[3] Daniels SR, Arnett DK, Eckel RH, Gidding SS, Hayman LL, Kumanyika S, et al. Overweight in children and adolescents: pathophysiology, consequences, prevention, and treatment. Circulation 2005;111:1999-2012.

[4] Dietz WH. Health consequences of obesity in youth: childhood predictors of adult disease. Pediatrics 1998;101(suppl):518-25.

[5] Avery A, Baxter A. Change to cup: an audit to determine parental awereness and practices in changing from bottle to cup. J Hum Nutr Diet 2001;14:217-23.

[6] Marino RV, Bomze K, Scholl TO, Anhalt H. Nursing bottle caries: characteristics of children at risk. Clin Pediatr (Phila) 1989; 28:129-31.

[7] Brotanek JM, Halterman JS, Auinger P, Flores G, Weitzman M. Iron deficiency, Prolonged bottle feeding and racial/ethnic disparities in young children. Arch Pediatr Adolesc Med 2005;159:1038-42.

[8] Bonuck KA, Kahn, R. Prolonged bottle use and its association with iron deficiency anemia and overweight: A preliminary study. Clin Pediatr 2002;41:603-7.

[9] Bonuck K, Kahn R, Schechter C. Is late bottle-weaning associated with overweight in young children? Analysis of NHANES III data. Clin Pediatr 2004;43:535-40.

[10] Mammas I, Bertsias G, Linardakis M, Tzanakis NE, Labadarios D, Kafatos A. Cigarette smoking, alcohol consumption and serum lipid profile among medical students in Greece. Eur J Public Health 2003; 13:278-82.

[11] Kafatos AG, Verhagen H, Moschandreas J, Apostolaki I, Van Westerop J. Mediterranean diet of Crete: foods and nutrient content. J Am Diet Assoc 2000;100:1487-93.

[12] Cole TJ, Bellizzi MC, Flegal KM, Dietz WH. Establishing a standard definition for child overweight and obesity worldwide: international survey. BMJ 2000;320:1240-3.

[13] Manios Y, Kafatos A, Markakis G. Physical activity of 6 year old children: Validation of two proxy reports. Pediatr Exerc Sci 1998;10: 176-88.

[14] Korsch BM, Nelson KG, Reinhart JB, Willis D, Zuckerman BS. Feeding skills in infancy and early childhood. In: Guidelines for health supervision II. Elk Grove Village, Ill: Am Acad Pediatr, 1998: 127.

[15] Barba G, Russo P. Dietary foods, dietary calcium and obesity: A short review of the evidence. Nutr Metabol Cardiovasc Dis 2006;16: 445-51.

[16] Barba G, Troiano E, Russo P, Venezia A, Siani A. Inverse association between body mass and frequency of milk consumption in children. Br J Nutri 2005;93:15-9.

[17] Carruth BR, Skinner JD. The role of dietary calcium and other nutrients in moderating body fat in preschool children. Int J Obes 2001;25:559-66.

[18] Zemel M. Regulation of adiposity and obesity risk by dietary calcium: Mechanisms and implications. J Am Coll Nutr 2002;21:146s-51.

[19] Hammer LD, Bryson S, Agras S. Development of feeding practices in the first 5 years of life. Arch Pediatr Med 1999;153:189-94.

[20] Arenz S, Ruckerl R, Koletzko B, von Kries R. Breastfeeding and childhood obesity. A systematic review. Int J Obes Relat Metabol Disord 2004;28:1247-56.

[21] Coon KA, Goldberg J, Rogers BL, Tucker KL. Relationships between use of television during meals and Children's food consumption patterns. Pediatrics 2001;107: E7.

[22] Gibson EL, Wardle J, Watts CJ. Fruit and vegetable consumption, nutritional knowledge and beliefs in mothers and children. Appetite 1998;31:205-28.

[23] Hediger ML, Overpeck MD, Kuczmarski RJ, Ruan WJ. Association between infant breastfeeding and overweight in young children. J Am Med Assoc 2001;285:2453-60.

[24] Clark HR, Goyder E, Bissell P, Blank L, Peters J. How do parents' child feeding behaviours influence child weight? Implications for childhood obesity policy. J Public Health 2007;29:132-41.
[25] Dubois L, Girard M, Potvin Kent M, Farmer A, Tatone-Tokuda F. Breakfast skipping is associated with differences in meal patterns, macronutrient intakes and overweight among pre-school children. Public Health Nutr 2008;11(12):1267-79.

Submitted: January 03, 2009.
Revised: February 18, 2009.
Accepted: February 25, 2009.

In: Public Health Yearbook 2009
Editor: Joav Merrick

ISBN: 978-1-61668-911-7

Chapter 21

Psychological and Socio-Demographic Determinants of Obsessionality Ratings Among the General Population

***Bruce D. Kirkcaldy*[1]*, MA, PhD, FBPsS*[*]**
and Rainer Georg Siefen*[2]*, Priv. Doz, MD, Dipl Psychol
[1] International Centre for the Study of Occupational and Mental Health and
[2] Department of Pediatrics, St Josef-Hospital, Ruhr-University of Bochum, Bochum, Germany

Abstract

In a large scale European study of 1,250 adults, subjective reports of obsessive thinking was assessed using anonymous self-ratings. The incidence of frequent compulsive thinking was 3 percent, and a further 9.5% of the sample reported "often" experiencing compulsive thoughts. There were significant differences associated with age (obsessiveness decreased with age), gender (1:1.6 males to females) and educational status (obsessionals were likely to have higher educational status). There was no evidence that compulsivity rating was related to weekly hours worked nor with hours invested in physical exercise, or number of hours slept per night. An array of physical ailments emerged as major determinants of compulsivity including mental fatigue, sleeplessness, migraine and sickness or nausea. The mood predictors of compulsivity encompassed depression, apathy and fearfulness (as well as irritation, anger and anxiety). Persons rating themselves high on compulsive attitudes were more likely to display inferior mental well-being, dissatisfaction with physical health and with work relationships and job content. Despite inferior subjectively perceived physical health, persons displaying a high frequency of obsessive thoughts were not more likely to have been ill during the last year than those "free" of obsessive thinking. The implications of these findings for a better understanding of compulsive thinking/behaviour are discussed.

[*] Correspondence: Bruce D Kirkcaldy, MA, PhD, FBPsS, Director, International Centre for the Study of Occupational and Mental Health, Haydnstrasse 61, D-40593 Düsseldorf - Benrath, Germany.

Keywords: Compulsivity obsessive-compulsive disorder, incidence rates, self-report, gender differences, life satisfaction, anxiety, depression.

Introduction

Obsessions are the recurrent, "intrusive, unwelcome, distressing thoughts and mental images" that create fear and anxiety by "besieging" our minds, and they are frequently perceived as both intruding and repugnant (1). Obsessive thoughts are considered different from normal thoughts because they are repetitive, ruminative, irrelevant and distracting (2) and thus are likely to disrupt the attention and concentration ("narrowing of attention") (3).

More recently, Schuman (4) labeled it "drive(n) to distraction". Turner et al (5) argue that obsessional thoughts and worry represent different cognitive phenomena, and see worry and obsessive thinking as widespread cognitive activities amongst the general population as well as in types of psychopathology. They further suggest that worry is associated with generalised anxiety disorder and obsessions with obsessive-compulsive disorder. Some clinicians e.g. Clark (6) would further assert that mental intrusions (unwelcomed thoughts and images) are common among the general population, and are generally perceived as insignificant and non-threatening, and thus do not require a "response or action". Among obsessive-compulsive disordered persons, however, there is a "faulty appraisal" of these interfering thoughts, and they are more likely to be identified as highly significant and a threat. Consequently, the person feels mobilised to take some kind of action to "neutralise" or extinguish the potential menace. Compulsions refer to the behaviours that sufferers of obsessional disorders perform in the form of a ritual or rumination in response to the obsession so as to reverse or relieve the fear.

In an earlier publication of the World Health Organisation (7), obsessive-compulsive disorder (OCD) was ranked 20th among diseases in developed countries in terms of disability-adjusted life years lost. Hollander (8) asserted that the relatively high prevalence rates of OCD recently observed — has resulted in it being labelled a hidden epidemic. Its incidence is smaller than anxiety and mood disorders, but clinical researchers have suggested that in the past there was much shame and fear and a sense of secrecy with this ailment with patients avoid seeking treatment (9).

Many studies have attempted to come up with an accurate incidence or prevalence statistic (9-13). Estimates vary essentially from 1 to 4% of the population.

Socio-demographic factors

Epidemiological studies of obsessional compulsive disordered surveys tend to report a smaller preponderance of male to female (2.0% and 2.7% respectively) subjects (14,15). Furthermore, there is evidence that gender differences vary in the age of onset of the disorder OCD with males showing a higher prevalence pre-pubertally and females more likely to be affected post-pubertally (16). Bridgeman (17) showed OCD rates to be around 2-3% in the US population with the average age of onset being 14.5 years. Boys were shown to have earlier onset (peak onset 13-15 years of age) than girls (peak onset 20-24 yrs). Niehaus and Stein (18) suggest that although research indicates a somewhat higher incidence of OCD among women than men, the relationship is reversed among children, with boys displaying OCD rates outnumbering girls by 2 to 1. The majority of studies exploring gender differences in OCD are Anglo-American in origin. An Iranian study (19) reported a 1.8% prevalence rate of OCD, and a clear predominance of women to men (4:1) in the general population. Samuels and Nestadt (20) found OCD was less prevalent in older individuals. There are several claims that obsessionality is more common among people of higher education, IQ and socio-economic status. In a prospective, longitudinal study Petersen et al. (21) found that while attention-deficit/hyperactivity disorder was associated with lower IQ and lower social status among children, OCD was associated with higher IQ scores.

Personality correlates

Various theoretical models have been proposed which suggest an association between compulsivity and specific personality traits, behaviours and cognitions. For example, historically, Freud's psychoanalytical theory asserts that obsessional behaviour is frequently linked to revengefulness, defiance and conscientiousness. Obsessional thinking could be perceived as a defence against hostile and sexual impulses. Studies have shown that overt aggression may in fact be different among compulsive patients because of the obsessive fear of inflicting harm onto others (or self), a finding observed in childhood psychiatric disorders such as OCD (22,23). Yaryura-Tobias et al (24) examining self-injurious behaviour, anorexia and dysmenorrhoea in obsessive compulsive disordered individuals supposed the emergence of OCD, self-mutilation, dysorexia, and dysmenorrhea in a sequential manner might suggest the presence of an OCD subset. Others (e.g. 25) have found a relationship between specific forms of compulsive behaviour (e.g. body dysmorphic disorder) and social phobia.

Riggs and Foa (26) found obsessional compulsive disorders co-occur with anxiety, depression, phobic avoidance and excessive concern although "they typically do not show (other) symptoms of schizophrenia such as marked loosening of associations, prominent hallucinations, flat or grossly inappropriate affect, thought insertion or projection" (p. 194).

In a recent German study involving children and adolescents, Kirkcaldy et al. (27) used multiple regression analyses with trait compulsivity as a dimensional trait (outcome variable) and revealed the significant determinants were anxiety-depression, schizoid-compulsive and attention disordered. Furthermore, the somatic checklist scales most predictive of compulsivity were depression, anxiety, anger-hostility, phobic anxiety and psychoticism.

Quality of life

Bobes and colleagues (28) suggested that although the life prevalence of OCD is around 1.5% in the United States, there may be as many as 10 percent who are identified on the "obsessive-compulsive spectrum". They criticise lack of studies exploring the relationship between obsessionality and quality of life: Low quality of life was found most pronounced in social relationships. Eisen et al (29) addressed psychosocial functioning and quality of life among obsessives. They found significant correlations – between 0.4 to almost 0.8 – between severity of obsessionality (obsessive-compulsive scale) and quality of life enjoyment. Others e.g. Bystritsky et al (30) had also found too much focus on symptomatic at the expense of functional improvement ratings. They reported that comparison between admission and discharge of OCD patients showed changes in 3 of the 8 scales of quality of life – activities, social and health, and no changes on ratings of financial, employment, family support and disability. In a more recent study, Stengler-Wenzke et al (31), OCD patients displaying compulsions revealed reductions in the quality of life in the domains of physical health, psychological well-being and environment, whereas those with obsessions revealed no difference in quality of life.

Dissatisfaction with body image and an obsessed need for physical exercise have characteristics not unlike anorexia nervosa (32,33), with symptoms not unlike a psychological dependence (34). Kirkcaldy and Shephard (35) examined the literature on leisure, physical activity and personality. They discuss not only the benefits of exercise therapy on psychological and physical health, but also the risks associated with too frequent exercise. This negative addiction is witnessed when there is an inability to pursue high levels of physical activity to which the person has been habituated to and this can result in adverse emotional and psychological states, including hostility, frustration headache and tension (36), restlessness, irritability and guilt (37).

Machlowitz (38) was one of the earliest researchers to explore the nature of causes of excessive work attitudes, workaholism. On the positive side such persons are perceived as competitive, energetic and driven with a powerful work ethic. On the negative side they can be overly perfectionistic, poor at work-life balance, and plagued by self-doubt that only burning oneself in work appears to alleviate. Kirkcaldy et al (39) found that individuals working long hours were more likely to worry than those working fewer hours, "it may be that long hours lead to personal anxiety or that those who worry work longer hours. Ultimately, it is likely that these two dynamics are mutually reinforcing so that, for most individuals worrying and long hours feed off each other." Moreover, those working long hours were more likely to display Type A behaviour and have a high internal locus of control. They suggest "future research should distinguish between the involuntary and voluntary excessive worker. Whilst legal restrictions and legislation would seem essential in enhancing the long-term health and job satisfaction of the overall community, it may not prevent hard-driven managers from pursuing a self-destructive working pace. Certainly, compulsive attitudes to work ("workaholism") are a prevalent feature of management, driving individuals to maintain high levels of work" (39, p. 449) and such attitudes generally receive positive reinforcement in the workplace.

Nicolas (40) examined the frequent claim that OCD is associated with complaints of insomnia in part due perhaps to delays in sleeping through the endless compulsive rituals and mental regurgitations. This may result in impaired sleep continuity, intrusion of wake during sleep and reduction of sleep duration among obsessionals.

There are likely to be long term adverse effects of pursuing an addictive attitude towards work. Compulsive working styles may be counterproductive to healthy functioning both psychologically and physically. Looking at obsessive compulsive disorders – which may be related to excessive working attitudes - the economic and personal costs are wide ranging and long lasting (41) in terms of personal income, ability to work, impoverishment of quality of life and productive contribution to the national economy.

The aim of this study was an attempt to explore the incidence of self-reported obsessionality among a non-clinical adult working sample responding to an anonymous questionnaire over the internet. Our sample is mainly people from managerial positions in the public and private sector. This paper investigates the relationship between the subjective rating of the personality trait compulsiveness, and other socio-psychological variables (age, gender, educational status, psychological emotions, physical symptoms and outcome variables such as life satisfaction, illness during the last year, hours worked per week, sleeping behaviour, and hours spent exercising per week).

An attempt was made to create "quasi-groups" (OCD analogue patients) which are based not on psychiatric or other mental worker diagnosis but scores on subjective ratings of compulsive thinking. This has been done before (42,43). In this study we created groups based on a self-rating of psychological health including a measure of compulsiveness. High scores were thus treated as an analogue group of OCD patients and could be compared to average and low scores to investigate specific questions and hypotheses. This study examined personality, intelligence, and health outcomes (life and work satisfaction, sleeping, drinking and accident behaviour) in these various analogue groups. Based on findings on individual difference variables (e.g. 26), it was predicted that analogue OCD patients would be higher on negative affect, that is, anxiety and depression, interpersonally sensitive (phobic avoidance), and display deficits in attention (attention disordered). If cognitive functioning is impaired this may lead to deficits in intellectual functioning (IQ). Several hypotheses are addressed in this study:

- Prevalence of obsessionality may be around 2-3% for normal adult sample
- Obsessionality may be more frequent among women than men
- Obsessionality could be related to age and educational status, declining with age and being higher among the more educated persons
- Individuals rating themselves high on obsessionality are more likely to adhere to extreme of work (more working hours and/or excessive physical activity) and less hours (reduced) sleep
- Obsessives might be more likely to be ill off work during the last year
- Obsessionality may be associated with anxiety, depression and anger
- Obsessionality might be related to general levels of heightened sensitivity to physical symptoms
- Life satisfaction (Quality of life) will be less amongst the OCD analogue group, especially in relationships (family and working life)

Methods

A dual strategy was adopted of treating trait compulsivity either as a dimension of personality or as a analogue OCD clinical category. Since we had no clinically identifiable OCD patients, attempts were made to generate two groups (low and high scoring trait compulsives) derived to test our hypotheses. So, essentially we have two strategies using correlational analyses including all persons in the sample and an OCD-analogue group generated by those created by pseudo-groups requiring different analyses. The underlying rationale is that trait compulsiveness represents a dimension which may have pathologies at both extremes, a concept of a spectrum of disorders with perhaps dysfunctional disinhibition at one end and

OCD ("compulsive" control) at the other. A dimensional view of obsessionality has been explored by Thomsen and Jensen (44) and Harsányi et al (45). In addition, the association between obsessive-compulsive disorder and personality dimensions has been a focus of a study by Bogetto et al (46). As trait compulsive scores increase, individuals are likely to be functional but "handicapped procrastinators" (e.g. problems associated with obsessional worry about money, cleanliness and order) but when extremes are reached–deviating markedly from the population mean score–obsessive-compulsive disorder may be manifested.

In a three month period, an internet exploratory research study was performed collating data from the new psychometric instrument. Recent studies suggest that comparative analyses about internet questionnaires reveal findings generalisable across presentation formats and are not adversely affected by non-serious or repeat responders and produce results consistent with traditional methods of data collation (47). Internet certainly presents empirical researchers with tremendous opportunities for collecting large data bases on topics of contemporary interest (48). In addition to ratings of "obsessional thoughts" persons were required to respond on a 1-5 Likert scale the degree of endorsement of items associated with physical (somatic ailments) and psychological (emotions) health, satisfaction with specific areas of working and private life (family, partnership, work content, working relationships, physical health and mental health). The alpha-coefficients for the total scales were 0.854 for physical health, 0.934 for mental (ill)-health and 0.710 for life satisfaction. Moreover, a variety of questions were asked regarding number of hours worked, time invested in physical exercise, hours slept per day, etc, as well as details of socio-demographic data – age, gender, educational status, marital status, parenthood. Since it has frequently been asserted that obsessives are reluctant to admit to their less than rational behaviour, the advantages of using an anonymous internet administration of questionnaires may allow us to get better estimates of actual compulsive thinking among European adult workers.

One of the difficulties inherent in such data collection involves the issue of the quality of such data. In order to ensure good quality data sets in this study, the data was double-screened, checked through visually and through descriptive analyses filtering out multiple responders and removing those respondents with incomplete data or those who exhibited obvious outliers or response sets. Individuals were provided with a special coded number after completion of the questionnaire enabling them to obtain their detailed profile scores if requested. Description statistics of the sample are provided in table below. Over a period of approximately 6 months, there were 1275 persons who had completed the entire questionnaire in the complete sample. The average age was 35.54 years and average number of children – including those persons having "0" children - was 0.63 SD 0.99. Number of weekly hours worked was 45.1 SD 10.7. And the mean number of hours exercised per week was 3.98 SD 21.16 hrs.

Results

Persons who claim to be frequent (very often) obsessional thinkers accounted for 3% of our adult sample. The proportion of females to males yielding "frequent" obsessional thinking corresponded to 5.7:1.5. This implies that 3.8:1 or almost 4 times as many adult females as males expressed having more obsessional thoughts (chi-squared (4)=23.06 $p<0.001$). Looking at the frequency of males and females with high compulsive attitudes, we see that about 1 in 4 females displayed frequent compulsive thinking sets in contrast to 1 in 6 males. A ratio of approximately 1:1.6 adult males to females (chi-squared (1) = 8.68, p<0.003).

The next stage of analyses generated low and high scoring obsessional thinkers selecting those who never ("0") and those that often or frequently ("3" and "4") have compulsive thoughts. The middle scorers ("rarely" and "sometimes") were left out. Around 160 persons from 1275, 12.5 percent have often (9.5%) or very often (3.0%) problems associated with compulsive thinking. These groups were generated to compare their physical and emotional state. In effect we have selected those individuals at least one standard deviation either side of the mean. Again a distinction must be made between willingness to express frequent compulsive thoughts and manifestation of obsessive compulsive behaviour.

Table 1. Description of sample. Socio-demographic factors

	%	n
Gender		
Male	65.8%	843
Female	34.2%	433
Age		
	Mean 35.54 SD 9.01	
<20 years	1.3%	16
21-30	34.0%	434
31-40	37.3%	476
41-50	20.4%	260
51-60	6.4%	82
>60 years	0.6%	8
Educational status		
Secondary	23.5%	298
GCE A level	22.3%	283
First degree	23.7%	300
Higher degree	24.0%	304
Other	6.5%	82
Marital status		
Single	30.6%	388
Married /cohabiting	61.8%	782
Divorced	4.3%	55
Separated	2.8%	36
Widowed	0.5%	6
Parenthood		
No	65.7%	832
Yes	34.3%	435

Table 2. Distribution of responses - across the sample – for the item of degree of obsessional thinking

Response rating	Frequency	Percent	Cumulative Percent
never	608	47.6	47.7
rarely	309	24.2	71.9
sometimes	199	15.6	87.5
often	121	9.5	97.0
very often	38	3.0	100.0

Table 3. Distribution of low and high obsessionals (O) for men and women

	Gender			
	male		female	
	Count	%	Count	%
Low O	416	82.4%	192	73.3%
High O	89	17.6%	70	26.7%

A comparison of physical ailment profiles between low and high obsessionals was made incorporating stepwise linear discriminant analysis. This takes into account the degree of interrelationship between the scales and explores those predictors which yield the highest amount in explaining variance in compulsivity. The canonical variate was statistically significant (Rc=0.58, eigenvalue = 0.51, lambda = 0.66, chi-squared (10) = 311.61, $p<0.001$) showing that the somatic profiles were different between the two groups. The predictor variables with the highest loadings (standardised canonical discriminant function coefficient) were mental fatigue, sleeplessness, sickness or nausea, migraine, lack of appetite and breathlessness.

Table 4 shows the summary of the statistical analysis (largest predictors in bold print). The magnitude of the adjusted R-square was 0.58, thus almost sixty per cent of the variance in obsessionality could be explained by these variables.

Problems with blood pressure, breathlessness, backache and tension headaches were all significant determinants but less related to obsessionality. The following ratings had not be included in the stepwise regression analyses, that is, they were not significant predictors of group membership: chest pains, stomach upsets/bowel complaints, muscular aches and pains, allergies, physical exhaustion and sexual problems. A classification analysis followed in which the persons' scores were substituted in the specification equation (weighted by the standardised canonical discriminant function coefficients). This revealed that approximately 85 % of cases were accurately assigned to their groups (low and analogue OCD) based on the physical symptom profile.

The next stage of statistical analyses compared the low and high obsessional groups in terms of their psychological mood profiles (Table 5).

Table 4. Stepwise discriminant regression – profile analysis – of low and high obsessive persons

	F(10,756)=38.32	P<0.001	
Model	Standardized Coefficients	t	p
Tension headaches	-0.08	-2.10	0.04
Lack of appetite	0.12	3.34	0.001
Backache	-0.09	-2.73	0.01
Migraine	0.12	3.21	0.001
Sickness or nausea	0.14	3.65	0.001
Skin disorders	0.07	2.32	0.02
Mental fatigue	0.27	7.20	0.001
Sleeplessness	0.17	4.75	0.001
Breathlessness	0.09	2.55	0.02
High or low blood pressure	-0.09	-2.95	0.01

Over one half of the scales were not significant predictors of compulsivity. Previous research (e.g. 27) suggested that among children and adolescents the scale compulsivity may also reflect a general distress factor and thus only by regression analyses which takes into account the interrelatedness between scales can we arrive at a coherent picture of which specific facets of emotional and psychological distress are associated with compulsivity.

The psychological mood profile between low and high obsesionals was statistically significant (Rc = 0.69, eigenvalue =0.89, Wilk's lambda = 0.53, chi-squared (7) = 482.99, p<0.001). The magnitude of adjusted R2 (68.5%) was somewhat higher than for the physical ailment profiles (58%) suggesting that obsessional groups differed both in their somatic and psychological symptoms, but more so psychologically.

Table 5. Summary of stepwise linear multiple discriminant analyses using psychological mood descriptors

Low/High Obsessives		F(7,759)=96.93	P<0.001
	beta	t	p
(Constant)		-14.54	0.001
Depression	0.23	3.45	0.001
Fearfulness	0.34	5.65	0.001
Apathy	0.39	6.66	0.001
Irritation	0.17	2.58	0.01
Anger	0.15	2.42	0.05
Reduced interest in life	0.13	2.14	0.05
Anxiety	0.14	2.08	0.05

Standardised discriminant function coefficients revealed that fearfulness (0.34), apathy (0.39), depression (0.23), irritation (0.17), anxiety (0.14) anger (0.15) and a reduced interest in life (0.13) were those variables which best predicted obsessive thinking. The scales not entered into the regression were: frustration, lack of concentration, moodiness, indecisiveness, low self-esteem, dissatisfaction, emotional exhaustion, and agitation.

The percentage of accuracy in the classification analysis assignment increased to almost 90 percent.

Nonparametric Correlations - A series of Spearman rho's were computed between obsessional thinking scores and the various socio-demographic variables. Consistent with the previous analyses, obsessive thinking was associated with gender, women scoring higher ($r=0.082$, $n=1275$, $p<0.01$), age-older subjects ($r=-0.06$, $n=1275$, $p<0.04$) were somewhat less inclined to display obsessional thinking and education ($r=0.128$, $n=1275$), $p<0.001$) with higher levels of educational status being linked with more obsessional tendencies. Marital status and number of dependent children were unrelated to obsessional thinking ($r=-0.03$ and $r=0.01$, respectively, $p>0.05$).

Table 6. Comparison of time-related activity factors for both low and high obsessive groups

	Low obsessives	High obsessives	F(1,536)
Weekly hours worked	45.56 (11.19)	43.94 (9.13)	1.80 n.s.
Average numbers of hours slept per day	6.79 (1.18)	6.80 (1.25)	0.01 n.s.
Amount of exercise per week	3.80 (2.08)	3.44 (1.86)	2.70 n.s.
Days taken off ill during the last year	5.06 (13.48)	5.73 (11.57)	0.21 n.s.

Table 7. Comparison of specific quality of life (life satisfaction) scores between both groups

Satisfaction ratings	Non obsessive (n=608)	Quasi-obsessive (n=159)	
	Mean (sd)	Mean (sd)	F(1,765)
Health			
Physical health	3.48 (1.01)	3.09 (1.07)	17.88***
Mental well-being	3.57 (0.85)	2.99 (1.02)	52.01***
Family relationships			
Partnership	3.71 (1.22)	3.26 (1.17)	16.70***
Family	3.73 (0.93)	2.99 (1.15)	73.08***
Work			
Working climate	3.58 (1.06)	3.73 (1.20)	21.34***
Work content	3.68 (0.97)	3.18 (1.08)	32.56***

Educational status was confined to four categories secondary, GCE A- Level, first degree and higher degree (omitting 6.5% other). Differences were observed with a higher proportion of those individuals from progressively higher educational status displaying a greater proportion of compulsive thinking (chi-squared $(12)=35.40$, $p<0.001$). The number of often/frequent scores for obsessionality increased from 9.7%, 9.2%, to 13.0% and 13.8% for the first and higher degree graduates. Using the low and high compulsive scorers no difference was observed on number of hours worked weekly, duration of physical activity during the week (exercise), hours slept and absenteeism.

The correlation coefficient between physical ill-health and days ill off work was significant for non-compulsives ($r=0.09$, $n=602$, $p<0.05$), as it was for mental ill-health and for days off ($r=0.09$, $p<0.05$). For the high compulsive group correlations were not statistically significant.

The multivariate statistic comparison of satisfaction profiles showed that across all domains – physical and psychological health as well as family and work domain – the compulsive group revealed lower levels of satisfaction (Wilk's lambda (5, 761) =20.23, $p<0.001$). An examination of the magnitudes of F-test reveals that the differences were largest for satisfaction with family life and mental health.

Finally, a series of Pearson product-moment correlations were computed between the full-scales of life satisfaction, mental health and physical health, for both non-compulsives ($n=608$) and the analogue OCD ($n=159$) groups separately. Physical health was shown to be psychometrically independent of mental health (r's of 0.04 and 0.08 for the non-compulsives "NC" and analogue OCD group, $p>0.05$). Moreover, mental health was significantly correlated with life satisfaction for both groups (-0.33 and –0.54 for NC and OCD group, $p<0.001$). On the other hand, although physical health was significantly related to life satisfaction for the non-compulsive group ($r=0.27$, $p<0.001$), this was not so for the analogue OCD group ($r=0.08$, $p>0.05$). Indeed whereas the non-compulsive persons showed a significant correlation between physical health and absenteeism ($r=0.09$, $n=602$, $p<0.05$) this was not the case for the analogue OCD group ($r=0.09$, $n=159$, $p>0.05$).

Discussion

The prevalence of "severe" obsessive thinking – defined as endorsement of "very frequent" obsessional thoughts – among this adult working population suggests estimates consistent with other epidemiological studies. Persons who reported frequent compulsive thinking corresponded to 3 percent of the population, which would seem consistent with the epidemiological studies of 2-3% incidence rate of obsessive compulsive disorders, assuming these persons were severely impaired by their ailments. Another 9.5% admitted often experiencing obsessive thoughts and these may correspond to those individuals who are obsessive personality types but otherwise not especially "concerned" or disabled by their symptoms. Again this figure comes close to the estimates provided by Bobes et al (28). These may be the perfectionists who otherwise function well in their family and working lives. These results afford credence for the hypothesis that gathering data using internet would seem a reliable way of obtaining information about personality traits associated with psychological disorders (47), our incidence rates being fairly consistent with those from other non-clinical populations.

Gender age and intelligence differences - Correlational analyses revealed a decrease in compulsive thinking across age, with the older persons experiencing less compulsive attitudes. It may be that with increasing age, worry and rumination and indeed perfectionism, all facets of compulsive thinking become "diluted". Individuals become accustomed to concerns and have witnessed little impact of incessant worrying on daily life. Women were inclined to display higher levels of obsessional thinking compared to men. By selecting the more conservative criteria of "often and frequent" obsessional scores the proportion an was around 1.6 : 1, again a finding which would appear consistent with other research reports and demonstrates the cross-cultural stability of these findings. On the other hand if we select those 3% of the population who have described themselves as very frequently engaging in obsessional thinking – possibly most likely to be displaying clinical symptoms of OCD - then the proportion of females to males approaches 3.8:1. Only in Iran were the proportions larger (0.7% males and 2.8% females for the rate of OCD). Overall, it is plausible that women respond to the „dual" demands of running a household with family commitments, and occupational pressures by displaying more compulsive behavioural tendencies as a way of coping with stress. Finally, there was some indication that obsessional thinking was highly significantly correlated with educational status – defined as educational attainment (secondary school, college, university thru to postgraduate training) – and if we assume that educational attainment is itself related to intellectual capacity, it is indeed likely that obsessionality is associated with (superior) intellectual and cognitive functioning. Again findings are consistent with other studies e.g. Petersen et al (21).

Working hours, hours of sleep and time devoted to physical activity – Multivariate statistical analyses showed no evidence of compulsivity being associated with longer working hours or increased need for physical exercise. This appears to contradict other research which points to the strivings of obsessionals to perform persistently and perfectly investing much time and effort to perform work-related tasks. There was further, no evidence that those persons reporting high obsessional thinking were more likely to sleep less than those claiming "no" obsessive thinking. On the other hand, subjective reports of somatic ailments, more specifically difficulties/problems sleeping (sleeplessness) were associated with obsessionality. Finally, there was no support for the claim of obsessionals being more likely to have taken more days off illness during the last year – despite their showing inferior physical health. The non-significant correlation between physical health and life satisfaction among the analogue OCD group would tend to support the concept that obsessionals when physically ill are less inclined to display a "spill-over" in their daily lives. Indeed, analysis had shown that absenteeism (number of days taken ill during the last year) was unrelated to physical (ill) health among the analogue OCD group but was significantly related for the non-compulsive group.

The stepwise regression analyses had shown that diverse physical symptoms were significantly associated with obsessive thinking. Over one half of the variance in obsessionality could be explained by the physical symptom scales, including mental fatigue, sleeplessness, sickness or nausea, and lack of appetite. Apparently, heightened compulsivity would seem associated with those symptoms linked to chronic stress and exhaustion. Interestingly, tension headaches, backache and blood pressure problems were inversely related to compulsivity, suggesting that compulsive persons whilst inclined to report an array of physical ailments, were less likely to experience tension and headache pains.

Thus the aspects of mental fatigue, sleeplessness, sickness or nausea, and lack of appetite being central somatic complaints, suggest that clinicians focus some of their attention in differential diagnosis on those factors of chronic psychological and bodily stressors. It may be that sufferers of compulsive disorders somaticise their ailments and express reluctance about expressing their "obsessive" behaviour and cognitions in order to conceal the "personal embarrassment" or anxiety associated with their condition. It is the task of the diagnostician to identify such possible relationships.

Looking at the personality (emotional) correlates of obsessionality, negative affect appears more pronounced for those persons with higher scores on compulsivity. The major determinants of obsessive thinking were apathy, fearfulness, depression followed by irritation, anger, anxiety and reduced interest in life. These factors too, account for a significant proportion of the variance in self-reports of compulsivity. The comorbidity of negative affect and compulsivity has also been observed among clinical samples. One of the deficiencies of such a cross-sectional study is the difficulty in whether the compulsive thoughts and behaviour are an attempt to moderate the negative affect – functioning as a stress coping mechanism, or whether compulsivity is a further manifestation of a general threat or emotional disequilibrium.

A look at the profile differences across measures of life satisfaction (quality of life) suggests that in all three domains, general health (physical and mental), family relationships and work (climate and job content), the analogue OCD group appears to experience greater dissatisfaction. The magnitude of the differences seems largest for family relationships and psychological health. Again, this would suggest that clinicians be astutely aware of possible compulsive ailments for those individuals who more frequently report problems at work, and dissatisfaction in their marital and family relationships. The client who suffers from compulsive disorders may see his or her ailment as "ego-synton" and coping oriented, and/or negate such feelings and emotions preferring not to disclose them if not asked directly about them. Again, it is interesting that despite the observed reduction in quality of life (greater dissatisfaction) in various areas of life, the analogue OCD group didn't differ in terms of subjective reports of "quantity of time" devoted to work, sleep or other activities. Hence the differences in satisfaction could hardly be attributed to deficits in the work-life balance. The relationship may be different for "clinical" samples. For example, Nicolas (40) showed disruption in "quality and quantity" of sleep in OCD, but the insomnia may be associated with other factors not necessarily connected to obsessionality per se.

On concluding, ratings of compulsive thinking are not equivalent to the clinical diagnosis of obsessional compulsive disorder, nor indeed are they necessarily associated with obsessionality per se (49). On the other hand, because some clinical ailments such as OCD are comparatively rare, not just amongst non-clinical but also clinical populations, it would seem useful to look at predictors of a continuum of impulsivity vs. compulsivity considered as a scale (or single dimension). Certainly, it seems justifiable to view compulsiveness as a personality dimension in which the further we deviate from the norm (high scores) the higher the likelihood of low risk, cautious procrastinating behaviour (functional but not handicapped) and at the very extreme of the continuum, the emergence of the clinical disorder OCD. Clinical typologies could thus to some extent be derived from personality dimensions. That implies that the personality disorders are seen as extreme traits. In research trying to understand obsessive compulsive behaviour it may be useful to screen large general populations on subjective reports of compulsivity and then use extreme score to generate OCD analogue persons. By then going on to examine differences in working and leisure domains, physical and psychological health as well as diverse aspects of quality of life, we may gain an insight to the mechanisms underlying obsessionality and its impact on both subjective reports of physical and psychological health, and impairments in (social) functioning. In this way, we may be able to develop better ideas for constructing more efficient therapeutic programmes.

References

[1] Schwartz JM, Beyette B. Brain Lock - free yourself from obsessive-compulsive behaviour. New York: Harper Perennial, 1996.

[2] Rycroft C. A critical dictionary of psychoanalysis. Harmondsworth, Middlesex: Penguin, 1972.

[3] Schwartz JM, Begley S. The Mind and the Brain: Neuroplasticity and the Power of Mental Force. New York: HarperCollins /Regan Books, 2002.

[4] Schuman M. Driven to distraction: observations on obsessionality - adapted from a chapter in Cooper P (Ed.), Into the mountain stream: psychoanalysis and buddhist experience. Maryland: Rowman Littlefield, 2006.

[5] Turner SM, Beidel DC, Stanley M. Are obsessive thoughts and worry different cognitive phenomena. Clin Psychol Rev 1992;12(2):257-70.

[6] Clark DA. Intrusive thoughts in clinical psychology: theory, research and treatment. New York: Guilford, 2004.

[7] Murray CJL, Lopez AD. Global burden of disease: A comprehensive assessment of mortality and morbidity from diseases, injuries and risk factors from 1990 and projected to 2020, vol. 1. Harvard, MA: World Health Organisation, 1996.

[8] Hollander E. Obsessive-compulsive disorder - the hidden epidemic. J Clin Psychiatry 1997;58:S3-6.

[9] Heyman I, Fombonne E, Simmons H, Ford T, Meltzer H, Goodman R. Prevalence of obsessive-compulsive disorder in the British nationwide survey of child mental health. Int Rev Psychiatry 2003;15:178-84.

[10] Karno M, Golding JM, Sorenson, SB, Burnam MA. The epidemiology of obsessive-compulsive disorder in five US communities. Arch Gen Psychiatry 1988;45(12):1094-9.

[11] Valleni-Basile LA, Garrison CZ, Waller JL, Addy CL, McKeown RE, Jackson KL et al. Incidence of obsessive-compulsive disorder in a community sample of young adolescents. J Am Acad Child Adolesc Psychiatry 1996;35(7):898-906.

[12] Brynska A, Wolaczyk T. Epidemiology and phenomenology of obsessive-compulsive disorder in non-referred young adolescents - a Polish perspective. Eur Child Adolesc Psychiatry 2005;14(6):319-27.

[13] Thomsen PH, Mikkelsen HU. Children and adolescents with obsessive-compulsive disorder: the demographic and diagnostic characteristics of 61 Danish patients. Acta Psychiatr Scand 1991;83(4):262-6.

[14] Weissman MM. Cross-national epidemiology of obsessive-compulsive disorder. CNS Spectr 1998;3(5):S6-9.

[15] Weissman MM, Bland RC, Canino CJ, Greenwald S, Hwu HG, Lee CK, et al. The cross-national epidemiologist of obsessive-compulsive disorders. J Clin Psychiatry 1994;55:5-10.

[16] Penn JV, March J, Leonard HL. Obsessive-compulsive disorder in children and adolescents. In: Dickstein LJ, Riba MB, Oldham JM, eds. Review of psychiatry, vol. 16, section III. Washington, DC: Am Psychiatr Press, 1997:7-28.

[17] Bridgeman A. Pharmacologic treatment of obsessive compulsive disorders in children and adolescence. Pennsylvania State University, 2003. Available at: www.childadvocate.net/ocd_and_medication.htm

[18] Niehaus DJH, Stein DJ. Obsessive-compulsive disorder: diagnosis and assessment. In: Hollander E, Stein DJ (Eds.). Obsessive-compulsive disorders: diagnosis, etiology and treatment. New York: Marcel Dekker, 1997.

[19] Mohammadi MR, Ghanizadek A, Rahgazar M, Noorbala AA, Davidian H, Afzali HM et al. Prevalence of obsessional-compulsive disorder in Iran. BMC Psychiatry 2004;4:2.

[20] Samuels J, Nestadt G. Epidemiology and genetics of obsessive-compulsive disorder. Int Rev Psychiatry 1997;9(1):61-72.

[21] Petersen BS, Pine DS, Cohen P, Brook JS. Prospective, longitudinal study of tic, obsessive-compulsive and attention-deficit/hyperactivity disorders in an epidemiological sample. J Am Acad Child Adolesc Psychiatry 2001;40(6):685-95.
[22] Papolos D, Hennen J, Cockerham M. Obsessive fears about harm to self or others and overt aggressive behaviors in youth diagnosed with juvenile onset bipolar disorders. J Affect Disord 2005;89:99-105.
[23] Sekula SA. Self-injury of the nails and hands. Dermatol Online J 2000;6:1. http://dermatology.cdib.org/DOJvol6num1
[24] Yaryura-Tobias JA, Neziroglu FA, Kaplan S. Self-mutilation, anorexia and dysmenorrhea in obsessive-compulsive disorder. Int J Eat Disord 1995;17(1):33-8.
[25] Coles ME, Phillips KA, Menard W, Pagano ME, Fay C, Weisberg RB, et al. Body dysmorphic disorder and social phobias: Cross-sectional and prospective data. Depress Anxiety 2006;23(1):26-33.
[26] Riggs DS, Foa EB. Obsessive compulsive disorder. In: Barlow DH, ed. Clinical handbook of psychological disorders, 2nd ed. New York: Guilford, 1993.
[27] Kirkcaldy BD, Furnham AF, Siefen RG. Social, family and psychological predictors of obsessive-compulsive behaviour. School Psychol Internat, in press.
[28] Bobes J, Garcia-Portilla MP, Bascaran MT, Saiz PA, Bobes-Bascaran MT, Bousaño M. Quality of life in obsessive-compulsive disorders. In: Ritsner MS, Awad AG, eds. Quality of life impairment in schizophrenic, mood and anxiety disorders. Netherlands: Springer, 2007.
[29] Eisen J, Mancebo M, Pinto M, Coles M, Pagano R, Stout S et al. Impact of obsessive compulsive disorder quality of life. Compr Psychiatry 2003;47(4):270-5.
[30] Bystritsky A, Saxena S, Maidment K, Vapnik T, Tarlow G, Rosen R. Quality of life changes in patients with obsessive-compulsive disorders in a partial hospitalisation programme. Psychiatr Serv 1999;50:414.
[31] Stengler-Wenzke K, Kroll M, Riedel-Heller S, Matschinger H, Angermeyer MC. Quality of life in obsessive-compulsive disorders. The different impact of obsessions and compulsions. Psychopathology 2007;40:5.
[32] Yates E, Leehey K, Shisslak CM. Running – analogue of anorexia? N Engl J Med 1983;308:251-5.
[33] Weights LM, Noakes D. Is running an analog of anorexia? A survey of the incidence of eating disorders in female distance runners. Med Sci Sports Exerc 1987;19:213-7.
[34] Farrell PA, Gates WK, Maksund MG, Morgan WP. Increases in plasma beta-endorphin/beta-lipotropin immunoreactivity after the treadmill running in humans. J Appl Physiol 1982;52:1245-59.
[35] Kirkcaldy BD, Shephard RJ. Therapeutic aspects of leisure and sport - special edited issue. Int J Sport Psychol 1990;21(3):165-84.
[36] Glasser P. Positive addiction. New York: Harper Row, 1976.
[37] Robbins JM, Joseph P. Experiencing exercise withdrawal: possible consequences of therapeutic and mastery running. Int J Sport Psychol 1985;7:23-9.
[38] Machlowitz M. Workaholics. New York: Mentor, 1980.
[39] Kirkcaldy BD, Levine R, Shephard RJ. The impact of working hours on physical and psychological health of German managers. Eur Rev Appl Psychol 2000;50(4):443-9.
[40] Nicolas A. Sleep and quality of life in obsessive-compulsive disorder. In: Vester JC, Pandi-Perumal SR, Streiner DL, eds. Sleep and quality of life in clinical medicine. Totowa, NJ: Humana Press, 2008.
[41] Knapp M, Hendersen J, Patel A. Costs of obsessive-compulsive disorders - a review. In: Maj M, Sartorius N, Okasha A, Zahor J, eds. Obsessive-compulsive disorders. New York: Wiley, 2000.
[42] Kirkcaldy BD. Psychoticism and arousal organization: covariation between critical flicker frequency and frontalis electromyographic activity. *Revija za Psihologiju* 1990;20(1-2):35-8.
[43] Kirkcaldy BD, Siefen G. Depression, anxiety and self-image among children and adolescents. Sch Psychol Int 1998;19(2):135-49.
[44] Thomsen PH, Jensen J. Dimensional approach to obsessive-compulsive disorder in childhood and adolescence. Acta Psychiatr Scand 1991;83(3):183-7.
[45] Harsányi A, Csigo K, Demeter G, Németh A, Racsmany M. Dimensionality and neurocognitive symptoms of OCD. Psychiat Hung 2007;22(5):366-78.
[46] Bogetto F, Barzega G, Bellino S, Maina G, Ravizza L. Obsessive-compulsive disorder and personality dimension: a study report. Eur J Pers 1997;11(3):156-61.

[47] Gosling SD, Vazire S, Srivastava S, John OP. Should We Trust Web-based Studies? A Comparative Analysis of Six Preconceptions about Internet Questionnaires. Am Psychol 2004;59:93-104.
[48] Kraut RM, Olson J, Banaji M, Bruckman A, Cohen J, Couper M. Psychological Research Online: Report of Board of Scientific Affairs' Advisory Group on the Conduct of Research on the Internet. Am Psychol 2004;59(2):106-17.
[49] Woody SR, Steketee G, Chambless DL. The usefulness of the obsessive-compulsive scale of the symptom checklist-90-revised. Behav Res Ther 1995;33(5):607-11.

Submitted: January 01, 2009.
Revised: February 20, 2009.
Accepted: February 26, 2009.

In: Public Health Yearbook 2009
Editor: Joav Merrick
ISBN: 978-1-61668-911-7

Chapter 22

KNOWLEDGE AND ATTITUDES TOWARD ANOREXIA NERVOSA AND SELF BODY IMAGE AMONG YOUNG AND OLDER WOMEN IN ISRAEL

Liat Korn, PhD* and Racheli Magnezi, PhD, MBA
Department of Health Management, School of Health Science, Ariel University Center of Samaria, Ariel, Israel

Abstract

This study examines differences in knowledge of and the attitude toward anorexia nervosa among Israeli women. Methods: This study used data from a survey questionnaire answered by 360 Israeli women during the years 2007-2008. Data was split from two groups of 180 women, ages 45-65 and 15-25 years of age. Results: In contrast to the older age group the younger age group had a poorer understanding of the symptoms of AN; a more positive conception of being thin and a lower opinion of their body self-image. The younger women displayed higher percentages of socially beneficial elements considered outcomes of AN: finding jobs, having more friends, being popular and accepted and being the object of admiration. Discussion: Younger women viewed AN more positively than the older women. The distorted views of self and of the disease of AN among young Israeli women, warrants further investigation and implementation of intervention established.

Keywords: Anorexia nervosa, eating disorders, women, attitudes, Israel.

Introduction

Anorexia nervosa (AN) is considered to be a severe emotional disorder that expresses itself by an obsession to be thin and a distorted body image. Although many factors contribute

* Correspondence: Liat Korn, PhD, Researcher, Department of Health Management, School of Health Science, University Center of Ariel, Israel. Tel/Fax: 972 3 9066661; E-mail: kornli@zahav.net.il, Liatk@ariel.ac.il

to AN, definitive indicators are not currently known. However, multiple risk factors, which include biological, psychological, social and familial patterns, can suggest the possibility of developing AN (1). The mortality rate among people with anorexia has been estimated at 0.56 percent per year, or approximately 5.6 percent per decade, which is about 12 times higher than the annual death rate due to all causes of death among females ages 15-24 in the general population (2).

Some physical symptoms of anorexia include loss of menstrual periods, lack of energy and weakness, a continuous sensation of cold, dry yellowish skin, constipation, abdominal pain, restlessness, insomnia, dizziness, fainting, headaches, and growth of fine hair over the body and face. Symptoms like compulsive behavior, anxiety, and depression can be present as well. During weight loss, social closure and outbursts of anger may appear (3). Additional evidence of AN includes dental erosion, xerostomia, enlargement of the parotid gland, and other dental deterioration. Mottled teeth and heartburn were also observed (4). Anorexia nervosa is associated with bulimia nervosa, in which the use of laxatives and vomiting is resorted to in order to lose weight (3). Significant disagreement exists regarding the possible connection between the behavioral and cognitive dimensions of aggression, anorexia and bulimia disorder. In one study three groups of anorexic patients, bulimic patients and a control group were tested for aggression. The results confirm the higher propensity to anger in patients with bulimia nervosa; in patients with anorexia nervosa, difficulties in expressing anger and outward-directed aggressiveness (5).

Knowledge concerning anorexia nervosa symptoms in the general population was tested in a study of 106 college students. It was found that most students have general, but not specific information about anorexia nervosa symptoms, consequences, causes, duration, and cures. Subjects also indicated that they believe people with eating disorders tend to be young, white women (6).

Social and cultural factors have an important influence on this disorder. In one study, analysis indicated a high distortion of body image among elite female professional ballet dancers. Tests indicated that the mean rating for current body image was significantly higher than the rating for ideal, despite the fact that body-composition measures for all subjects were in an "ideal" range, according to normative standards (7). Another recent study investigated the influence of media exposure on body image in eating disorder patients. The results suggested that media exposure acted as a stimulus that triggers body-related issues. Both perceptual and attitudinal body image components changed markedly after media exposure for eating disorder patients, compared with normal control groups (8). Another recent study showed that the fashion models group and matching control female group did not differ significantly as regards self-report questionnaires testing attitudes toward thinness. However, in a detailed interview (the Eating Disorder Examination), models reported significantly more symptoms of eating disorders than controls, and a higher prevalence of partial syndromes of eating disorders was found in models than in controls. Also, a body mass index below 18 was found for 34 models (54.5%) as compared with 14 controls (12.7%) (9). These studies indicate that thinness, and anorexia nervosa behaviors are considered acceptable in order to pursue careers in dance, modeling, acting, and other arenas where beauty is a requirement.

Research revealed inaccurate body image by testing positive assessment of other people's bodies, specifically recognition of flaws in attractive features. Results indicated that normal control women subjects were significantly more accurate at detecting flaws than eating disorder women subjects (8). Clearly anorexic woman have a distorted body image not only of their own bodies, but also that of others. The question arises whether even healthy women have mistaken perceptions regarding the feminine ideal as regards thinness, and whether these perceptions lead to dissatisfaction with their own bodies.

The cultural influences impacting adolescent girls regarding healthy body image were revealed in a study of music videos, which featured scantily clad female models that have become the ultra-thin socio-cultural ideal for young women. After viewing the music videos, the study showed that 16-19 year old healthy, adolescent girls reported significantly elevated scores on an adaptation of the Body Image States Scale, indicating increased body dissatisfaction (10). In another study the ubiquitous Barbie doll was examined as a possible cause for young girls' body dissatisfaction. It was found that age 5 to age 8 girls exposed to the Barbie doll reported lower body esteem and greater desire for a thinner body shape than girls in the control group. The authors concluded that, even if dolls cease to function as inspirational role models for older girls, early exposure to dolls epitomizing an unrealistically thin body ideal may damage girls' body image, giving rise to an increased risk of disordered eating and weight cycling (11).

Data from the Rotterdam Youth Health Monitor, a publication for 9-13 year olds, was used to assess the association of psychosocial well-being with weight perception among young Dutch adolescents. The authors concluded that in 12-13 year old adolescents, feeling overweight, rather than being overweight, appears to be important (12).

In a study made in Japan, female college students aged 18 to 21 years-old were given questionnaires on ideal body shape. The questionnaire asked the subjects to report their current and ideal body shape, and to make a qualitative self-assessment of their weight. On average, the perceived ideal weight was 5.2 kg lower than the current weight. The results also revealed that young women have a tendency to misunderstand their body shape, and to regard themselves as heavier than they really were (13). These studies reveal that distorted body image exists predominantly in technologically advanced cultures which are influenced by media messaging.

Therapeutic intervention, for patients suffering from anorexia nervosa, focuses primarily on family therapy (14-17). The combination of nutritional supervision and family therapy targeting parental approval, specifically from the mother, enhances patient recovery. Internet based intervention for prevention of eating disorders to college-aged women, and specifically trained counselors at private universities were also found to be successful in the treatment of anorexia nervosa (18-20).

According to the Diagnostic and Statistical Manual of Mental Disorders (21), 0.5% to 1.0% of those in late adolescence and early adulthood meet the full criteria for anorexia nervosa (22). In Israel, the frequency values among adolescents are similar (23), but Israeli women have the highest frequency of dieting among 36 western countries according to a representative sample taken in the year 2002. 32% of high school girls reported bad eating patterns that could lead to eating disorders (24). Anorexia nervosa was found to be more common in urbanized women. Constant dieting, childhood abuse, and a history of being overweight are factors significantly associated with anorexia nervosa (25).

It is well known that approximately 90-95% of those suffering from anorexia are females (22). Recently however, anorexia nervosa has become evident in males, blacks, Latino, older people and even pregnant woman (26), which reveals the disturbing growth of this disorder. Anorexia is considered to be self-induced; so many questions arise regarding the "healthy" population's susceptibility to anorexia nervosa.

The following study concerns the knowledge and attitudes toward AN among different age groups of women in Israel. The questionnaire disclosed differences among younger and older Israeli women's knowledge and attitudes toward AN.

Methods

This study is based on quantative analysis of data from a survey conducted in the years 2007-2008 among Israeli women. The target population of this study was Israeli woman. The sample consisted of 360 women, divided into two groups: 180 older women in the age range of 45-65, and 180 younger women from the ages of 15-25.

The anonymous questionnaire included topics such as knowledge concerning anorexia nervosa, perceptions and attitudes toward the disorder, exposure to a person already suffering from anorexia, self esteem, self body image, nutrition, physical activity and demographic characteristics.

Variables

The dependent variable in this research is self body image. The answers were on a scale 1 to 5 ("agree very much" to "not agree at all"). Self body image results were obtained by counting the "agree" and "most agree" response to these two statements: "If I lose 2 kilos, I would be a happier person" and "It is important for me to be thin".

Independent variables were age recoded as (1=young, 0=old). BMI was recoded by height and weight variables, and calculated by the BMI (Body Mass Index) equation (Weight [kg]/ Height^2 [m^2]). Normal weight recoded as 18.6 to 24.9, overweight recoded as BMI 25 or more, and underweight recoded as BMI 18.5 or less. Knowledge included 10 symptoms of AN. Correct answers were tabulated, and a high score was given to any subject who answered true for 8 symptoms or more. Low scores were given to any subject who answered true for 7 or less symptoms. Exposure to a sick person recoded as 0=yes, 1=no.

Attitudes: The answers were on a scale 1 to 5 ("agree very much" to "not agree at all"). Attitudes recorded as counting the "agree" and "most agree" responses to the 7 positive statements: 1) "Thinness is pretty", 2)"Thinness opens doors", 3)" AN women can find jobs easily", 4) "Thin women are admirable", 5) " AN women have more friends", 6) " AN women are socially popular and accepted" and 7) " AN women are powerful and have self control".

Results

Table 1 presents the distribution of different variables in this study by age group. This table reveals an expected gap between the two age groups. More young women were underweight, had less knowledge of symptoms of AN, had exposure to a person afflicted with AN, agreed with positive perceptions toward AN and satisfied with their self body image in comparison to older woman. Figure 1 represents the knowledge of AN symptoms by age group. Both age groups of women were asked questions concerning their knowledge about anorexia nervosa, including ten of the most frequent symptoms. The table indicates insignificant differences between the two groups' knowledge for the first six symptoms. Loss of menstrual periods, anxiety, anger outburst, vomiting, hair loss, compulsive behavior are symptoms know to the two age groups in the same level. But the older women's group had a greater awareness of other AN symptoms than the younger group, such as the use of laxatives, mottled teeth, insomnia and compulsive exercising. Therefore, we conclude that the older group showed a higher knowledge of this disorder than the younger group.

Women were asked about their attitude toward thinness and AN. Figure 2 represents agreement with positive image statements of skinny and anorexic woman, and shows a significant differentiation between the two age groups in most of the statements. All of these seven statements were expressed positively and highly acceptable to the younger group. "Anorexic women are socially popular and accepted", "Thin women are admirable", "Thinness opens doors" and "Thinness is pretty" were statements most chosen by the younger group. Clearly, younger women tend to perceive AN as a positive trait.

Table 1. Distribution of variables by age groups

Measure	Young women	Old women	All
BMI			
1. % of normal BMI	68.7	57.1	62.9
2. % of overweight	5.1	41.8	23.5
3. % of underweight	26.1	1.1	13.6
Knowledge			
1. % of high knowledge (right in more than 7 symptoms)	48.9	71.7	60.3
2. % of low knowledge (right in 7 or less symptoms)	51.1	28.3	39.7
Exposure			
1. % of not exposed to sick person	47.2	61.1	54.2
2. % of exposed to sick person	52.2	38.9	45.6
Attitudes			
1. % of disagreement with positive perceptions toward AN	49.4	53.9	51.7
2. % of agreement with positive perceptions toward AN	50.6	46.1	48.3
Self body image			
1. % of satisfied with self body image	47.2	71.7	59.4
2. % of not satisfied with self body image	52.8	28.3	40.6
Total N	180	180	360

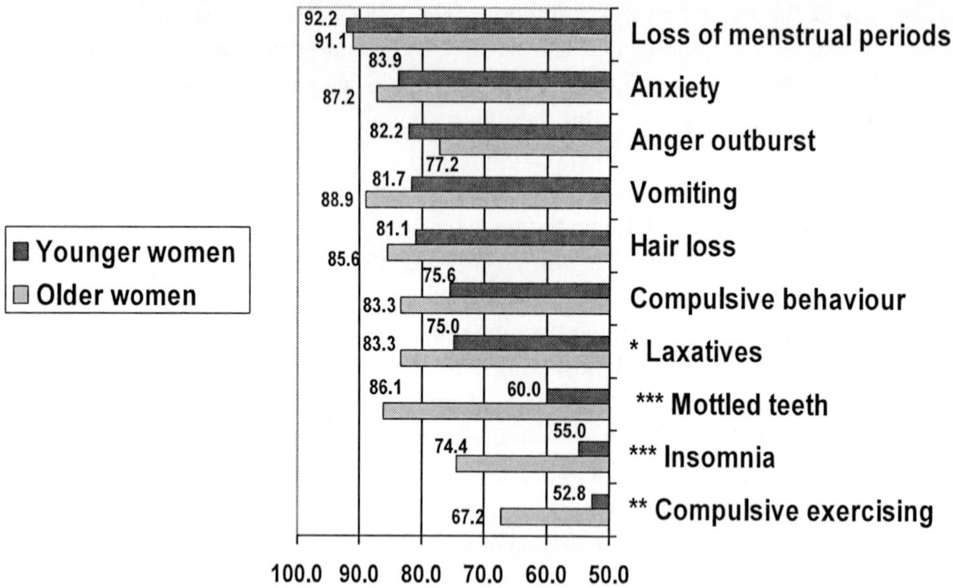

N=360, P<0.001***, P<0.01**, P<0.05*.

Figure 1. Knowledge of anorxia nervosa symptoms by age groups.

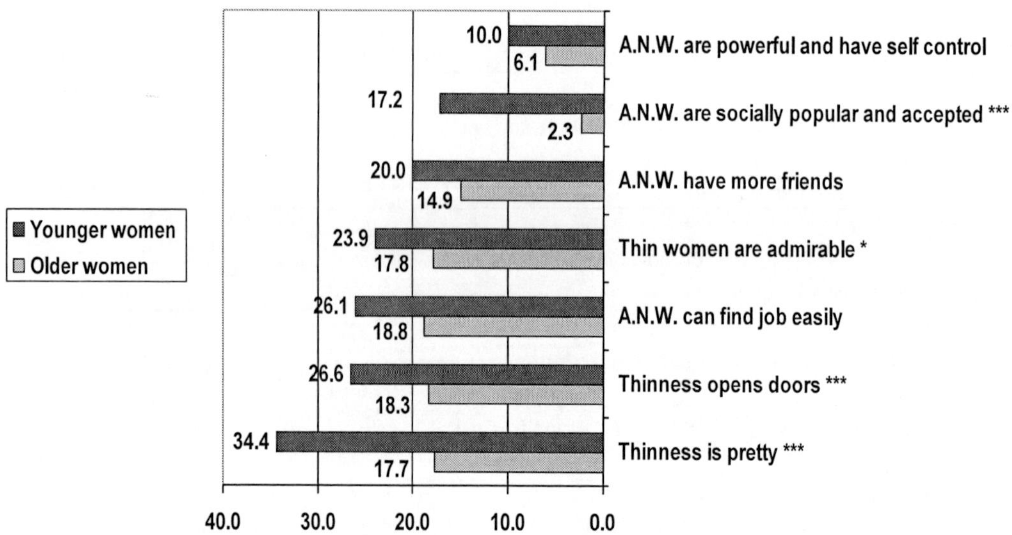

N=360, P<0.001***, P<0.01**, P<0.05*

Figure 2. Agreement with positive image statements on skinny and anorectic woman, by age group.

Women were asked about their attitude toward self body image. Younger women were expected to have lower self body image than older women. Figure 3 reveals the distribution of self body image by age group, and shows differences between the two age groups as expected. The statements "It is important for me to be thin" and "If I lose 2 kg.- I'll be a happier person" were reported most often by the younger group. Conversely, older women reported that it is preferable to be overweight than underweight, and that they feel satisfied with their weight as opposed to younger woman. Younger woman tend to perceive body thinness positively, consider being thin important and believe thinness contributes to their happiness, as opposed to the older group.

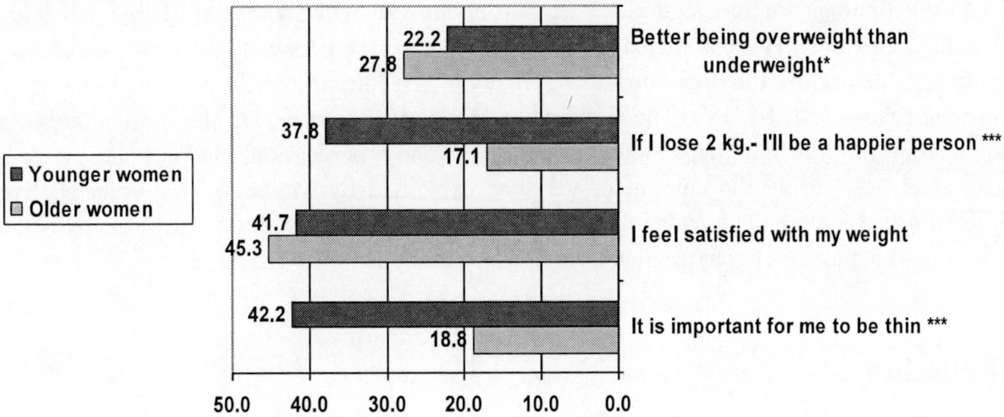

N=360, P<0.001***, P<0.01**, P<0.05*

Figure 3. Self body image by age group.

Table 2. Hierarchical Logistic regression models to predict low self body perception among women

Measures	I	II	III	IV	V
Demographic: Age: (0= Old, 1=Young)	**2.82*** **	**2.59*** **	**2.47*** **	**2.40*** **	2.59***
BMI (0= Weight OK, 1= Overweight or underweight)		1.07	1.08	1.09	1.31
Knowledge (0=high, 1=low)			1.22	1.22	1.12
Exposure (0= No, 1= Yes)				0.78	0.66
Attitudes: 0= Negative attitudes toward AN 1= Positive attitudes toward AN					5.32***
Adj R2	**%8.2**	**%7.3**	**%7.5**	**8.0%**	**24.8%**
N	**360**	**353**	**353**	**353**	**353**

The significant value: ***p<0.001, **p<0.01, *p<0.05.
* The value shown in the table is odd ratio.

Table 2 presents the outcomes of applying Hierarchical Logistic regression models to predict low self body perception among all women participating in this sample. The value shown in the table is odd ratio, and present the probability of the value "1" to be involve in this or to have that statement compare to the value "0". There are five distinct hierarchically ordered models presented:

I. Demographic model (age: 0= Old, 1=Young)
II. BMI (0=Weight OK, 1=Overweight or underweight)
III. Knowledge model (0=high, 1=low)
IV. Exposure to a sick person model (0= No, 1=Yes)

V. Full Model including attitudes toward thinness and AN model (0=Negative attitudes toward AN, 1= Positive attitudes toward AN

As the findings suggest, age alone explain about 8% of the variance of low self body perception. However, BMI, knowledge and exposure to a sick person do not have statistically significant odds ratios for predicting low self body perception, and do not add to variance explained (Models II, III, IV). The findings of Model V, however, are the most interesting and meaningful. For the dependent variable self body perception, the attitudes toward thinness and AN triple the amount of variance explained by Modal I: The Adjusted Rsq jumps from 8.2 to 24.8. The odds ratios from this table reveal that attitudes toward AN is the most powerful and significant predictor variable – with odds ratios of 5.3.

Discussion

This study examined the knowledge and attitudes toward anorexia nervosa among woman in Israel, and revealed the differences in attitude and knowledge between older and younger Israeli women. As expected, age is a significant factor in determining attitude, knowledge and healthy body image.

The young women group showed significantly ($p<0.001$) higher frequency of lower knowledge (51.1%) of anorexia nervosa symptoms as compared to the oldest women group (28.3%), and accordingly, showed significantly ($p<0.001$) lower frequency of superior knowledge (48.9%) as compared to the oldest women group (71.7%). Consistent with existing research, the results in this study support the conclusion that basic knowledge of AN symptoms exists in both groups. Both younger and older women were able to recognize symptoms such as loss of menstrual periods, anxiety, anger outburst, vomiting, hair loss and compulsive behavior as indicative of AN. The symptoms that made the difference in knowledge between the two groups were laxative use, mottled teeth, insomnia and compulsive exercising. The biggest gap (more than 25%) between the groups was in the symptom of mottled teeth. This finding is noteworthy because whereas mottled teeth are considered highly unattractive, young women regard anorexic women as beautiful. Anorexia is associated with models, dancers and celebrities and is, therefore, considered desirable. The general public's ability to recognize the symptoms of AN influences the likelihood of professional treatment. These findings show that Israeli women in the general population do have a basic knowledge of AN symptoms, most significantly amongst mature women. Knowledge of AN symptoms however was not found to be a significant variable to predict low self body image in this research.

Other outcomes of this research showed that social benefits, such as finding a job (26.1%), having more friends (20.0%), being popular and accepted (17.2%) and being admired (23.9%) were considered outcomes of anorexia in higher frequency among the youngest compare to the oldest group (18.8%, 14.9%, 2.3% and 17.8% accordingly). Anorexia nervosa is a phenomenon perceived positively among young women as compared to older women. Clearly the results from this study indicate that amongst young women AN is regarded as a positive trait. We learned from the studies presented in the introduction that women have a great concern about their looks. In cultures obsessed with image, women are affected most. Men do not have to be slim in order to get a job, be socially accepted, or to be considered attractive. In the workplace, women are frequently discriminated against if they are overweight, and the social stigma against fat women is often exploited for comic value in the media. Eating disorders are perceived to be the solution because thinness is considered feminine. Young women in particular have a greater concern about their appearance because of peer group pressure and their need to appear fashionable. These pressures appear to diminish with age.

Western culture's emphasis on appearance, money and power has impacted Israeli women with its view of the ideal body. The media has promulgated the message with ruthless thoroughness that "thin is in." The result is a relentless self-starvation that leads to an array of ailments, based on a distorted body image. It now appears that Israeli women are not immune to the allure of AN, and have joined legions of suffering women who believe that the self-destructive behavior of AN is not only acceptable, but desirable. Young women who suffer from low self body image and view AN as acceptable should be considered in the high risk category for developing AN (Odd ratio 5.3, $p<0.001$) of low self body image, as the findings suggest in this paper.

Exposure to a person afflicted with AN, significantly impacts young women (52.2%) as compared to older women (38.9%). This finding indicates that the problem is more acute during adolescence and young adulthood. However, exposure to someone suffering from AN did not substantially contribute to the prediction of low self body image. Also BMI was not found to be a significant variable contributing to low self body image. Logistic regression model outcomes reveal that age and attitudes were strong and significant variables to predict lower self body image. The results in this study strengthen the hypothesis that more young women suffer from low body image than older women, and that social pressure combined with unrealistic expectations can trigger AN behavior in young women.

Conclusions

Anorexia nervosa is a phenomenon perceived positively among younger woman compared to adult woman. Young girls have a greater concern of their social status among their peer group, and are more influenced by social and cultural factors than adult woman. Anorexia nervosa is perceived by young woman as an "easy way" to gain social benefits in order to become popular and successful in life. These young women perceive AN as a positive tool for success, and are therefore at risk. The results of this study should be greeted with alarm. More research needs to be devoted to AN, and preventive interventions must be developed. Efforts to educate young women to the physical, mental and emotional dangers of AN must be implemented to change distorted self image, and increase self-confidence based on factors other than appearance.

The frequency and severity of this disorder can not be attributed to an individual's particular genes or tendencies. Historically, only wealthy people could afford adequate food, so thin people were normally assessed as being poor. Yet in today's most abundant societies, an obsession with emaciation as fashion statement has triggered a disorder that threatens the health and happiness of vulnerable young women. Parents, educators, community leaders and counselors need to take an active role in encouraging young girls to aspire to goals in line with their natural talents and abilities. Allowing young women to fall victim to the message that only by being thin can they arouse admiration will condemn thousands more to an endless cycle of starvation, illness and self-hatred.

Acknowledgments

The authors would first like to thank to Ariel University Center of Samaria, School of Health Science, for funding and supporting this research. Second, to Mrs. Sharon Mendel for her contribution in the pilot phase of this research. Also to Ms. Maya Solomon, Mrs. Maya Arditi, Ms. Nataliya Lavonski, Mr. Abdelhai Ashraf and Ms. Sarsor Ehab for their hard work and contribution in data collecting and gathering. And finally, to Prof. Gabriell Abraham Amiti for his vast contribution in the writing phase of this paper.

References

[1] Kirkcaldy BD, Siefen GR, Kandel I, Merrick J. A review on eating disorders and adolescence. Minerva Pediatr 2007;59(3):239-48.
[2] Sullivan PF. Mortality in anorexia nervosa. Am J Psychiatry 1995;152(7):1073-4.
[3] Herpertz-Dahlmann B. Adolescent eating disorders: definitions, symptomatology, epidemiology and comorbidity. Child Adolesc Psychiatr Clin North Am 2009;18(1):31-47.
[4] Aranha AC, Eduardo CP, Cordas TA. Eating disorders. Part I: Psychiatric diagnosis and dental implications. J Contemp Dent Pract 2008;9(6):73-81.
[5] Miotto P, Pollini B, Restaneo A, Favaretto G, Preti A. Aggressiveness, anger, and hostility in eating disorders. Compr Psychiatry 2008;49(4):364-73.
[6] Hunt JS, Rothman AJ. College students' mental models for recognizing anorexia and bulimia nervosa. Appetite 2007;48(3):289-300.
[7] Pierce EF, Daleng ML. Distortion of body image among elite female dancers. Percept Mot Skills 1998;87(3Pt1):769-70.
[8] Legenbauer T, Kleinstäuber M, Müller T, Stangier U. Are individuals with an eating disorder less sensitive to aesthetic flaws than healthy controls? J Psychosom Res 2008;65(1):87-95.
[9] Preti A, Usai A, Miotto P, Petretto DR, Masala C. Eating disorders among professional fashion models. J Psychiatry Res 2008;59(1-2):86-94.
[10] Bell BT, Lawton R, Dittmar H.The impact of thin models in music videos on adolescent girls' body dissatisfaction. Body Image 2007;4(2):137-45.
[11] Dittmar H, Halliwell E, Ive S. Does Barbie make girls want to be thin? The effect of experimental exposure to images of dolls on the body image of 5-to 8-year-old girls. Dev Psychol 2006;42 (2):283-92.
[12] Jansen W, Van de Looij-Jansen PM, De Wilde EJ, Brug J. Feeling fat rather than being fat may be associated with psychological well-being in young dutch adolescents. J Adolesc Health 2008;42(2):128-36.
[13] Takasaki Y, Fukuda T, Watanabe Y, Kurosawa T, Shigekawa K. Ideal body shape in young Japanese women and assessment of excessive leanness based on allometry. J Physiol Anthropol Appl Human Sci 2003;22(2):105-10.
[14] Lock J, Agras WS, Bryson S, Kraemer HC. A comparison of short and long term family therapy for adolescent anorexia nervosa. J Am Acad Child Adolesc Psychiatry 2005;44(7):632-39.
[15] Lock J, Couturier J, Agras WS. Comparison of long-term outcomes in adolescents with anorexia nervosa treated with family therapy. J Am Acad Child Adolesc Psychiatry 2006;45(6):666-72.

[16] Eisler I, Dare C, Hodes M, Russell G, Dodge E, Le Grange D. Family therapy for adolescent anorexia nervosa: the results of a controlled comparison of two family interventions. J Child Psychol Psychiatry 2000;41(6):727-36.

[17] Eisler I, Simic M, Russel GF, Dare C. A randomised controlled treatment trial of two forms of family therapy in adolescent anorexia nervosa: a five-year follow up. J Child Psychol Psychiatry 2007;48(6):552-60.

[18] Manwaring JL, Bryson SW, Goldschmidt AB, Winzelberg AJ, Luce KH, Cunning D et al. Do adherence variables predict outcome in an online program for the prevention of eating disorders. J Consult Clin Psychol 2008;76(2):341-6.

[19] Celio AA, Winzelberg AJ, Wilfley DE, Eppstein-Herald D, Springer EA, Dev P, Taylor CB. Reducing risk factors for eating disorders: comparison of an internet- and a classroom-delivered psychoeducational program. J Consult Clin Psychol 2000;68(4):650-57.

[20] Low KG, Charanasomboon S, Lesser J, Reinhalter K, Martin R, Jones H, et al. Effectiveness of a computer-based interactive eating disorders prevention program at long-term follow-up. Eat Disord 2006;14(1):17-30.

[21] American Psychiatric Association. Diagnostic and Statistical Manual of Mental Disorders, 5th ed (DSM IV). Washington, DC: APA, 1997.

[22] Anorexia nervosa and related eating disorders, inc. Statistics: How many people have eating disorders? 2006. Accessed 2008 Dec 08. URL:http://www.anred.com/stats.html.

[23] Modan-Moses D, Yaroslavsky A, Novikov I, Segev S, Toledano A, Miterany E, Stein D. Stunting of growth as a major feature of anorexia nervosa in male adolescents J Pediatr 2003;111:270-6.

[24] Currie C, et al. Young people's health in context: international report from the HBSC 2001/02 survey. Copenhagen: WHO Regional Office Eur, 2004.

[25] Favaro A, Ferrara S, Santonastaso P. The spectrum of eating disorders in young women: a prevalence study in a general population sample. Psychosom Med 2003;65(4):701-8.

[26] Bennett J. It's not just white girls. Anorexics can be male, old, Latino, black or pregnant. A new book undercuts old stereotypes. Newsweek. 2008 Sep 15;152(11):96.

Submitted: January 12, 2009.
Revised: February 28, 2009.
Accepted: March 09, 2009.

In: Public Health Yearbook 2009
Editor: Joav Merrick

ISBN: 978-1-61668-911-7

Chapter 23

Detection of a Rare Hereditary Persistence of Fetal Hemoglobin in a Tribal Family in Orissa, India

Ranbir S. Balgir, M.Sc.Hons., Ph.D*

Department of Biochemistry, Regional Medical Research Centre for Tribals, Jabalpur, Madhya Pradesh, India

Abstract

In the normal newborn infants, human fetal hemoglobin (Hb F) is readily replaced by the adult hemoglobins A and A_2, and at the age of about six months only a small percentage of fetal hemoglobin is detectable. The failure of normal process of switching off the production of γ-chains during neonatal period leads to a high level of fetal hemoglobin in adult life without causing any anemia. This is called as a hereditary persistence of fetal hemoglobin (HPFH). The Hb F in general delivers less oxygen to tissues, shortens the life span of red cells, and makes red cells unsuitable to cope with physiological stress of life. The HPFH is an autosomal co-dominantly inherited condition of rare occurrence. The present study reports for the first time a Paraja-Bhuyan (tribal) family having HPFH in four members, i.e. a mother with her three children from Sundargarh district of Orissa. These four cases showed no apparent clinical or hematological abnormality except mild pallor observed in two younger children. The acid elution test revealed pancellular distribution of fetal hemoglobin in all cases of HPFH in the erythrocytes. The findings of the present study have been discussed in the light of a few case reports available in the literature.

Keywords: Hereditary persistence of fetal hemoglobin, hemoglobinopathies, pancellular distribution, Paraja-Bhuyan, tribal medicine, India.

---

* Correspondence: Ranbir S Balgir, M.Sc.Hons., Ph. D, Deputy Director (Senior Grade) and Head, Department of Biochemistry, Regional Medical Research Centre for Tribals, Indian Council of Medical Research, Nagpur Road, Jabalpur-482 003, Madhya Pradesh, Central India. E-mail: balgirrs@yahoo.co.in

Introduction

The fetal hemoglobin (Hb F) in human erythrocytes, which forms a bulk of hemoglobin during the later two trimesters of intrauterine life, is sometimes, found to be persistently high even in adult life. It is believed that the normal process of switching off the γ-chain production and turning on the β- and δ-chains fails to occur and a high level of fetal hemoglobin continues in adult life unassociated with anemia. The term hereditary persistence of fetal hemoglobin (HPFH) is used to describe a group of conditions in which there is a persistent fetal hemoglobin synthesis into adult life in the absence of any major hematological abnormality. These conditions are divided into pancellular HPFH, in which the Hb F is more or less uniformly distributed, and heterocellular HPFH in which the Hb F is heterogeneously distributed among the red cells (1). The fetal hemoglobin, in general, functionally delivers less oxygen to tissues because of high affinity for oxygen, shortens the life span of red cells, and unsuitable to bear the physiological stress of life (2).

It has been shown that the γ-chain of the fetal hemoglobin exists in two forms, i.e. with a glycine residue in the 136th position, and with an alanine residue in the same position of the polypeptide chain. Depending upon the nature of γ-chain of fetal hemoglobin, the carriers of HPFH may be classified as Hb $^{G}\gamma$, Hb $^{A}\gamma$ and Hb $^{G}\gamma$ Hb $^{A}\gamma$ by Schroeder and Coworkers (3). The commonest type of pancellular HPFH, the Black form, is due to deletion of a part or all of the δ and β regions of the β-globin gene complex, and in most cases resembles δβ–thalassemia. In the homozygous state, it shows a mild thalassemia like blood picture, and the hemoglobin consists entirely of hemoglobin F. Heterozygotes have a fetal hemoglobin level of 6-25%, and the only hematological abnormality is a slight reduction in mean cell hemoglobin (MCH). It is an autosomal co-dominantly inherited condition of rare occurrence.

The persistence of fetal hemoglobin in adult life was first described in West Africa and the term Hereditary Persistence of Fetal Hemoglobin (HPFH) was used when a case of persistent Hb F in adult life was seen along with sickle cell hemoglobin (Hb S) in a Jamaican family (4,5). Suspected case of HPFH was reported from Bombay area along with β-thalassemia in an East Indian Christian family (6). The first reported case showed Hb E and HPFH in three sibs of a Thai family (7). To the best of our knowledge, there is no study so far available which has reported the HPFH gene in the tribal population of Orissa (2). This is the first study reporting the occurrence of HPFH in a scheduled tribe, Paraja-Bhuyan family from Sundargarh district of Western Orissa.

Bhuyan Tribe

The Bhuyan tribe is an endogamous community, which is mostly confined to Sundargarh district of Orissa. This district is bordering district, surrounded by Jharkhand state in the North, Chhattisgarh state in the West, Keonjhar district in the East and Jharsuguda, Sambalpur, and Deogarh districts in the Southern part of the district (see figure 1). However, the sporadic families of Bhuyan tribe are also seen in Anugul, Deogarh, Jharsuguda and Keonjhar districts. Some of their families have also migrated to Assam to work in the tea plantation as labor force (8, 9). In the state of Orissa, the total population of Bhuyan tribe was

207,792 persons according to Census of 1981 which arose to 256,930 persons in the year 2001. The sex ratio of Bhuyan tribe was 1,016 females per 1,000 males. The literacy rate was 22.5% in the year 1981 which arose to 38.1% by the year 2001.

The Bhuyan tribe although originally belonged to one ethnic stock, but now divided into three social groups namely, the Hill Bhuyan (Pahari or Paudi Bhuyan), Paraja Bhuyan (Common People) and the Paik or Khandayat Bhuyan (Warrior Bhuyan), which are distinguished from each other on the basis of three grades of primitive culture in the state of Orissa. The Hill Bhuyan, the primitive and backward section, represents the hunting and food gathering stage of economic life along with the practice of rudimentary shifting cultivation and primitive culture. The Paraja Bhuyan section represents the more advanced culture with habit of plough-cultivation and food production. The Khandayat Bhuyans have the most advanced culture, which equates them with other nontribal population of the region. The inter-group marriages are not taking place at all. Reproductively and genetically, they are completely isolated from each other.

Methods

Out of a total 212 Paraja-Bhuyan screened from Gad Dwar village in Hemgiri block of Sundargarh district of Orissa, incidently one family of hereditary persistence of fetal hemoglobin was detected. About 2-3 ml. blood was intravenously collected after obtaining the informed/written consent in the presence of a doctor and community leaders. A medical doctor recorded signs and symptoms related to hemoglobinopathies after clinical examination on the pre-designed performa. Any other ailment present was treated/referred to local health facility. Blood samples so collected were transported to the laboratory at Bhubaneswar under ice-cold conditions within 24 hours of collection. Laboratory investigations were carried out following the standard procedures. Hematological parameters were studied by using an automated Blood Cell Counter (Model-MS4, Melet Schloesing Laboratories, Cergy-Pontoise Cedex, France).

The routine horizontal hemoglobin electrophoresis was carried out on cellulose acetate membrane (CAM) in Tris-EDTA-Borate buffer at pH 8.6 to identify abnormal hemoglobins by their differential mobility and quantitation of A_2 fraction of hemoglobin was performed by elution method at pH 8.6 (1, 10). Estimation of fetal hemoglobin (Hb F) was done as per the method of Betke and Coworkers (11) described in Weatherall (1). This method is the most reliable for the quantitation of low percentages of Hb F (below 10-15%). The subjects with HPFH have fetal Hb values ranging from 5% to as high as 35% without any other apparent hematological abnormalities. The acid elution-staining test of Kleihauer and Coworkers (12), which is based on the differential elution of fetal and adult hemoglobins, was used to demonstrate intra-cellular distribution of fetal hemoglobin containing erythrocytes.

The G-6-PD enzyme deficiency was detected by using Dichlorophenol Indophenol (DCIP) dye as described by Bernstein (13) and, subsequently, confirmed by WHO procedures (14) and Beutler and Coworkers (15). ABO and Rhesus blood groups typing were done by slide method, following the instructions of the manufacturer (Tulip Diagnostics Pvt. Ltd, Goa, India).

Table-1. Salient features of Paraja Bhuyan (Tribal) Family in Sundargarh District of Western Orissa

Code No.	6047	6048	6049	6050	6051	6052	6053
Name	SC	SK	HC	NC	NC	AC	DC
Age (Years)	59	55	36	30	09	08	06
Sex	M	F	M	F	F	M	M
Hb (g/dl)	10.9	11.3	13.5	12.5	12.1	11.9	10.6
RBC ($10^6/\mu l$)	5.3	5.3	5.7	4.9	5.1	5.1	4.6
MCV (fl)	78.2	78.1	73.9	83.7	76.0	76.0	79.6
HCT (%)	41.2	41.7	42.3	41.2	38.4	38.9	37.0
MCH (pg)	20.7	21.1	23.6	25.4	23.9	23.2	22.8
MCHC (g/dl)	26.4	27.0	31.9	30.3	31.5	30.6	28.6
WBC ($10^3/\mu l$)	8.9	4.6	6.7	8.1	10.7	8.4	8.7
Electrophoresis	$A+A_2$	$A+A_2$	$A+A_2$	$A+A_2$	$A+A_2$	$A+A_2$	$A+A_2$
Hb A (%)	97.6	97.1	97.2	89.4	84.4	90.6	87.9
Hb A_2 (%)	2.2	2.6	2.2	2.2	1.9	2.9	1.3
Hb F (%)	0.2	0.3	0.6	8.4	13.7	6.5	10.8
G-6-PD Enzyme	N	N	N	N	N	N	N
ABO Blood Group	B	B	O	O	O	O	O
Rhesus Blood Group	+ve	+ve	+ve	+ve	+ve	+ve	+ve

N= Normal

Results

Laboratory investigations of all family members are summarized in table 1. It is apparent from table 1 and figure 2 that the father (HC) and both grand parents (SC and SK) were found to have normal level of fetal hemoglobin (range 0.2-0.6%) and A_2 (range 2.2-2.6%). However, the mother (NC) showed raised fetal hemoglobin (8.4%), normal hemoglobin level (12.5%), normal A_2 (2.2%) and normal electrophoresis ($A+A_2$). Parents of this mother could not be tested. All of her three children had raised fetal hemoglobin (range 6.5-13.7%), transmitted from their mother as codominant fashion.

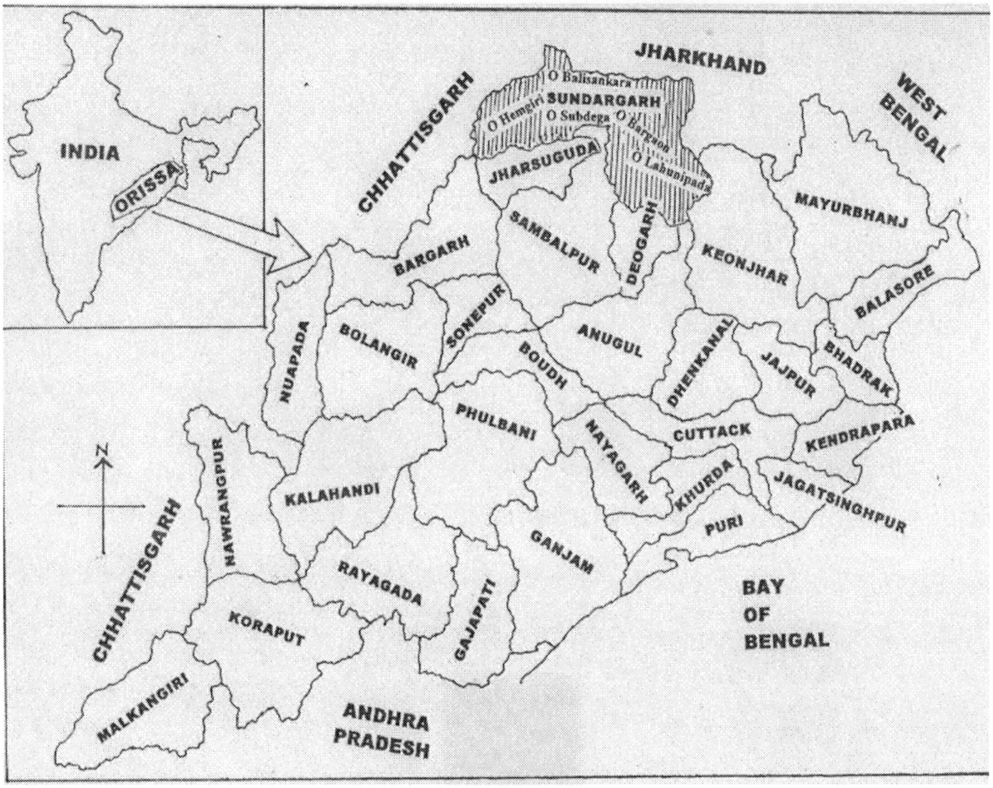

Figure 1. Map of Orissa showing the study area (shaded) and thirty districts.

It is an autosomal codominantly inherited condition. Neither other clinical nor hematological abnormality could be detected in all the four cases, except mild pallor was observed in two younger (AC and DC) children (see table 1). However, the low values of MCV and MCH noted in this family may suggest interaction with alpha-thalassemia. All had normal G-6-PD enzyme activity with O blood group and Rhesus (D) positivity.

Acid elution staining test revealed pancellular distribution of fetal hemoglobin in all the cases with HPFH in their red cells.

Discussion

The evidence for HPFH gene in this Paraja-Bhuyan tribe is established by the presence of high level of fetal hemoglobin in four family members without any apparent abnormal red cell morphology, except mild pallor in two of the three children and pancellular distribution of fetal hemoglobin in erythrocytes as demonstrated by acid elution staining test in all cases. These findings appear to exclude other known conditions causing elevation of Hb F such as beta-thalassemia and acquired hematological disorders. However, the present study is the first report of HPFH in a Paraja-Bhuyan (tribal) family from Sundargarh district of Orissa.

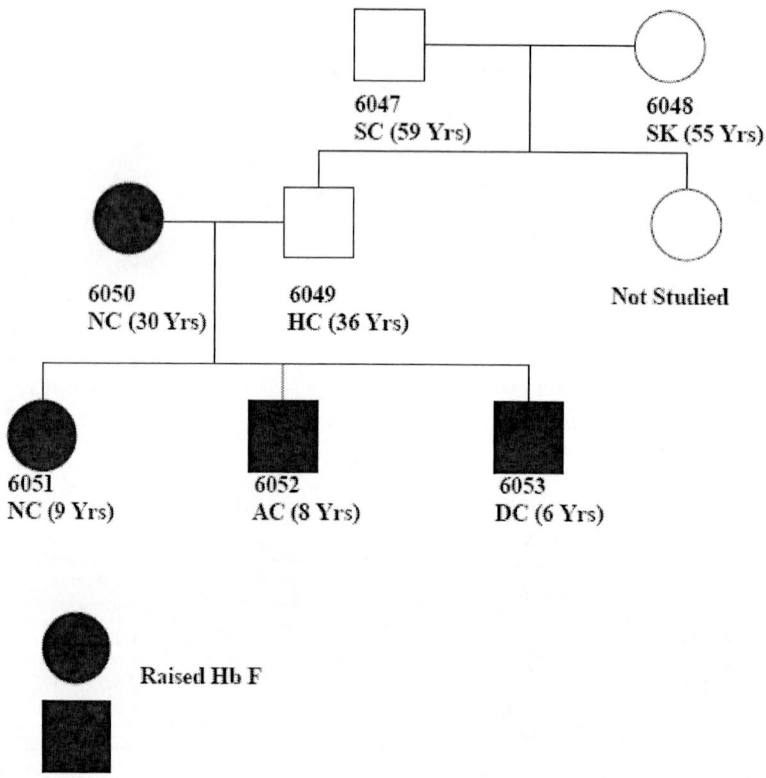

Figure 2. Family Pedigree of Hereditary Persistence of Fetal Hemoglobin of Paraja Bhuyan Tribe in Sundargarh District of Orissa, India.

The mother (NC) seems to have inherited a gene for HPFH from either of her parents, which she, subsequently, has passed on codominantly to her three children. It is now known from the structural analysis that normal γ-chain is duplicated. One is having glycine at 136th position and the other having alanine instead. Thus, broadly, there can be at least three different types of HPFH, i.e. $^{G}\gamma$, $^{A}\gamma$ or $^{G}\gamma^{A}\gamma$ types (16). Pancellular HPFH is an extremely heterogeneous condition, which is due to a deletion of the δ and β-globin genes, resulting in persistent $^{G}\gamma$ and $^{A}\gamma$ synthesis but not entirely well compensated form of δβ–thalassemia. Homozygotes have 100% fetal hemoglobin and red cell changes almost identical to those of heterozygous β-thalassemia (1). Heterozygotes have normal hematological findings and fetal hemoglobin homogeneously distributed among their red cells. The hemoglobin F is a mixture of $^{G}\gamma$ and $^{A}\gamma$ varieties in this condition. Further, molecular level investigations in the present family need to be done.

Both deletion and nondeletion forms of HPFH have been characterized (17). In the deletion variants, both $^{G}\gamma$ and $^{A}\gamma$-globin synthesis is increased, whereas only one or the other γ-globin gene is over-expressed in the nondeletion syndromes. Consequently, the nondeletion variants may be classified as $^{G}\gamma$ HPFH and $^{A}\gamma$ HPFH. The most prevalent deletion variants are those encountered in black Americans (HPFH-1) and black Ghanians (HPFH-2). Deletions in both variants are approximately 105 kb in length, with endpoints staggered by approximately 5 kb. The Indian and two Italian HPFH variants are characterized by smaller deletions. All of the 3' breakpoints of HPFH deletions fall adjacent to or within the 3' β-globin gene enhancer. Increased Hb F synthesis in the deletion forms of HPFH is thought to be a result of the transposition of enhancer sequences into proximity with the γ-globin genes (17).

Although less prevalent than deletion variants, nondeletion types of HPFH have been observed in many populations including the Italians, Greeks, Swiss, British, Chinese, Japanese and black Americans. Most of these types of HPFH result from base substitutions in the promoter regions 5' to the $^{G}\gamma$ and $^{A}\gamma$ genes. These substitutions are within DNA sequence motifs that bind regulatory proteins. Mutations at these sites are likely to alter the binding affinity for regulatory proteins, thereby influencing expression of the juxtaposed to γ-globin gene. Single base substitutions in the promoter region of the $^{A}\gamma$-globin gene include T→C at position -198 in the British $^{A}\gamma$ HPFH, C→T at -196 in Chinese, Greek, and Italian $^{A}\gamma$ HPFH, T→C at -175 in black American $^{A}\gamma$ HPFH, and G→A at -117 in Greek $^{A}\gamma$ HPFH. The $^{G}\gamma$ HPFH phenotype results from base substitutions at positions -202, -175, and -161 5' to the $^{G}\gamma$-globin gene. The genetic basis for Seattle HPFH remains to be elucidated. Although base substitutions in the enhancer region 3' to the $^{A}\gamma$-globin gene initially were implicated in increased Hb F synthesis, these mutations were later found to be prevalent polymorphisms not associated with the HPFH phenotype (17).

Relatively the studies pertaining to HPFH are very limited in India. Only a few cases have been reported from Western India and Kolkata (2). Cases of HPFH hemoglobin along with β-thalassemia have been reported from Bombay (18). One of them was first investigated with high fetal trait in 1953 in a Christian family and was reported as having interaction with thalassemia (6). Similar conditions were noticed in two Bengalee families (19), and a later study in Bombay revealed this type of double heterozygous condition in two cases (20). Barkhan and Adinolfi (21) in a family of mixed Indian and Portuguese ancestry in London and Bird and Coworkers (22) in an Indian boy at Pune have recorded similar cases of HPFH with beta-thalassemia. One Maratha family showing hemoglobin E with this gene (HPFH) has been described from Bombay (23, 24).

In view of the evidence of multiple structural genes for the γ-chain of human fetal hemoglobin, some of the HPFH already reported from Bombay were subjected to biochemical analysis. In one case in a 9-year-old boy, HPFH in homozygous state was found to have Hb F entirely of $^{G}\gamma$ type. In addition the case of Hb E with HPFH was also found to be $^{G}\gamma$ type (24, 25). A similar study of six individuals in four families showing HPFH were found to have two types of γ-chains (the $^{G}\gamma$–chain with glycine in 136th position and the $^{A}\gamma$ chain with alanine in the same position), which were present in the ratio of 70:30. It was suggested that these heterozygotes form a distinct sub-group of hemoglobin $^{G}\gamma^{A}\gamma$ class (16).

Some members of this family carried β-thalassemia gene along with the above abnormality (26, 27).

Conclusions

This paper is a small part of our major research project on "Intervention for hereditary common hemolytic disorders among the major tribals of Sundargarh district in Orissa". While screening a village of Bhuyan tribe for hemoglobinopathies and G-6-PD deficiency in order to intervene and provide genetic counseling to affected persons, this family with hereditary persistence of fetal hemoglobin (HPFH) was incidentally detected and studied in details. Unless molecular analysis is carried out, the interaction of α-thalassemia with HPFH cannot be ruled out by clinical studies only. However, the normal hemoglobin concentration, the slightly reduced MCV and MCH values, presence of target cells, low level of A_2 (1.3-2.9%), raised fetal hemoglobin (6.5-13.7%) and evenly distribution of Hb F in erythrocytes in the present family, all these aspects suggest not the cases of α-thalassemia, but the possibility of HPFH in Paraja-Bhuyan tribal family.

Acknowledgments

Author acknowledges the financial support from the Ministry of Health and Family Welfare through the Indian Council of Medical Research (ICMR), New Delhi. I am also grateful to Prof. N.K.Ganguly, Director General, ICMR, New Delhi for providing the necessary facilities. I am thankful to doctor of Primary Health Centre, Gopalpur and Community leaders of Paraja Bhuyan tribe for their kind cooperation during our fieldwork. Thanks are also due to Mr.R.K.Mishra, LT for his support in the field and laboratory work.

References

[1] Weatherall DJ. Methods in hematology: The thalassemias. Edinburgh: Churchill Livingstone, 1983:19.

[2] Balgir RS. The burden of hemoglobinopathies in India and the challenges ahead. Current Sci 2000; 79:1536-47.

[3] Schroeder WA, Huisman THJ, Shelton RJ, Shelton JB, Kleihaur EF, Dozy AM, Robberson B. Evidence for multiple structural genes for the γ-chain of human fetal hemoglobin. Proc Natl Acad Sci USA 1968; 60:537-44.

[4] Edington GM, Lehmann H. Expression of the sickle cell gene in Africa. BMJ 1955;1:1308.

[5] Went LN, McIver JE. An unusual hemoglobinopathy: sickle cell thalassemia disease. Blood 1958;13:559.

[6] Sukumaran PK, Bhatia HM, Sanghvi LD, Shah PN. Interaction of thalassemia and high fetal traits: a family study. Paper presented at Association of Teaching Pathologists, Bombay, June 1959.

[7] Wasi P, Pootrakul S, Na-Nakorn S. Hereditary persistence of fetal hemoglobin in a Thai family. Br J Hemat 1968;14:501.

[8] Balgir RS. Biomedical anthropological approaches in North Eastern India: A synthesis of the tea garden population of Assam. In: Sarthak Sengupta (Ed.). Peoples of North East India: Anthropological perspective. New Delhi: Gyan Publ House, 1996:91-104.

[9] Balgir RS. Emerging trends in genetic epidemiology of hemoglobinopathy in the seven sister States of North Eastern India. In: Kanti DR, Debashish B, eds. North East India in perspectives: Biology, social formation and contemporary problems. New Delhi: Akansha Publ House, 2005:17-37.

[10] Dacie JV, Lewis DJ. Practical hematology. 7th ed. Edinburgh: Churchill Livingstone, 1991.

[11] Betke K, Marti HR, Schlict L. Estimation of small percentages of fetal hemoglobin. Nature 1959;184:1877-8.

[12] Kleihauer E, Braun H and Betke K. Demonstration von fetalem haemoglobin in den erythrocyten eines Blutausstrichs. Klin Wochenschrift 1957;35:635-6. [German].

[13] Bernstein RE. A rapid screening dye test for detection of G-6-PD deficiency in red cells. Nature 1962; 194:192.

[14] WHO Report. Standardization of procedures for study of glucose-6-phosphate dehydrogenase. WHO Tech Rep Series 1967; 366:1-53.

[15] Beutler E, Blune EG, Kaplan JC, Lohr GW, Ramot B, Valentine WW. International committee for standardization in hematology recommended Screening test for glucose-6-phosphate dehydrogenase deficiency. Br J Hemat 1979; 43:465-7.

[16] Kutlar A, Gardiner MB, Headlee MG, Reese AL, Cleek MP, Nagle S, Sukumaran Huisman THJ. Heterogeneity in the molecular basis of three types of hereditary persistence of fetal hemoglobin and the relative synthesis of the $^{G}\gamma$ and $^{A}\gamma$ types of γ–chain. Biochem Genet 1984; 22:21-35.

[17] Lukens JN. The thalassemias and related disorders: Quantitative disorders of hemoglobin synthesis. In: Lee GR, Foerster J, Lukens J, Paraskevas F, Greer JP and Rodgers GM, eds. Wintrobe's clinical hematology, 10 ed. Philadelphia, PA: Lippincott Williams Wilkins, 1999:1413.

[18] Sukumaran PK, Randelia HP, Merchant SM. Thalassemia syndromes in Bombay. J Indian Med Assoc 1961; 9:477-88.

[19] Chatterjea JB. Hemoglobinopathies, glucose-6-phosphate dehydrogenase deficiency and allied problems in the Indian subcontinent. Bull World Health Org 1966; 35:837-56.

[20] Parekh JG, Sharma RS, Shah KM. Hereditary persistence of fetal hemoglobin in combination with thalassemia in two Indian families. Proc Annual Meeting Indian Soc Hemat 1963; 4:25-31.

[21] Barkhan P, Adinolfi M. Observations on the high fetal hemoglobin gene and its interaction with the thalassemia gene. J Clin Path 1962; 51:350-6.

[22] Bird GWG, Hasan MI, Malhotra OP, Lehmann H. Interaction of β-thalassemia and hereditary persistence of fetal hemoglobin. J Med Genet 1964; 1:24-6.

[23] Sukumaran PK, Vengsarkar AS. Hereditary persistence of fetal hemoglobin with hemoglobin E in a Maratha family from Bombay. Proc Ann Meet Indian Soc Hemat Blood Transf Madras, 1972:34-41.

[24] Desai SS, Master H, Chavan DS, Sukumaran PK. Hemoglobin D, E and Hereditary persistence of fetal hemoglobin in a Maratha family – Hemoglobin DE disease in two members. Indian J Hemat 1986; 4:71-4.

[25] Sukumaran PK, Merchant SM, Desai MP, Wiltshire BG, Lehmann H. Hemoglobin Q India (<64 (E13) Aspartic acid-Histidine) associated with beta-thalassemia observed in three Sindhi families. J Med Genet 1972; 9:436-42.

[26] Schroeder WA, Huisman THJ, Sukumaran PK. A second type of hereditary persistence of fetal hemoglobin in India. Br J Hemat 1973; 25:131-5.

[27] Sukumaran PK, Master HR. The distribution of abnormal hemoglobins in the Indian population. In: Sanghvi LD, Balakrishnan V, Bhatia HM, Sukumaran PK, Undevia JV, eds. Human population genetics in India. Bombay: Orient Longman, 1974: 91-111.

Submitted: January 13, 2009.
Revised: March 01, 2009.
Accepted: March 08, 2009.

SECTION THREE
POSITIVE YOUTH DEVELOPMENT

In: Public Health Yearbook 2009
Editor: Joav Merrick

ISBN: 978-1-61668-911-7

Chapter 24

Objective and Subjective Outcome Evaluation of Project P.A.T.H.S.: First Year Evaluation Findings

Daniel TL Shek, PhD, FHKPS, BBS, JP[*1,2,3]

[1]Department of Applied Social Sciences, The Hong Kong Polytechnic University, Hong Kong, PRC, [2]Department of Sociology, East China Normal University, Shanghai, PRC and [3]Kiang Wu Nursing College of Macau, Macau, PRC

Abstract

In the Tier 1 Program of the Project P.A.T.H.S., teaching units based on different positive youth development constructs are covered. A total of 24 experimental schools and 24 control schools were randomly selected to participate in a randomized group trial. Subjective outcome evaluation at posttest showed that the program participants generally had favorable perceptions of the program, workers and benefits of the program. Analyses of covariance and linear mixed models controlling for differences between the two groups in terms of pretest scores, personal variables and random effects of schools showed that participants in the experimental schools who perceived the program to be beneficial (N=1,888) had significantly higher positive youth development levels than did participants in the control schools (N=3,358) at posttest based on different indicators derived from the Chinese Positive Youth Development Scale. Both objective outcome and subjective outcome evaluation findings suggest that the Tier 1 Program of the Project P.A.T.H.S. was effective in promoting the holistic development of the program participants.

Keywords: Project P.A.T.H.S., objective outcome evaluation, subjective outcome evaluation, public health psychology.

[*] Correspondence: Professor Daniel TL Shek, PhD, FHKPS, BBS, JP, Chair Professor of Applied Social Sciences, Department of Applied Social Sciences, The Hong Kong Polytechnic University, Hunghom, Hong Kong. E-mail: danielshek@inet.polyu.edu.hk

Introduction

There are worrying trends and phenomena related to the development of adolescents in Hong Kong, such as mental health problems, abuse of psychotropic substances, suicide, school violence, and drop in family solidarity (1-3). For helping professionals, one relevant question is how such adolescent developmental problems can be prevented. A survey of literature shows that there are growing efforts to identify at-risk students at an early stage and to develop primary prevention programs that utilize the classroom-based curricular approach (4).

While it is important and meaningful to focus on prevention of adolescent developmental problems, there are several difficulties associated with this approach. First, one may criticize that over-emphasis of adolescent developmental problems represents a "pathological" approach in viewing adolescents. Second, in view of the existence of different developmental problems in adolescents, we need a huge number of separate preventive programs (e.g., prevention of bullying, substance abuse, gambling … etc.) and such programs will take up much time if they are implemented in the school context. Third, implementation of preventive programs in the school context would receive strong resistance from the school authority who might argue that their students do not have problems to be prevented. Similar resistance from the parents is also expected. Finally, consistent with the beliefs that "problem free is not fully prepared" (5) and that "young people are not problems to be solved but resources to be developed", one may counter-argue that it is more useful to consider how adolescents in Hong Kong can be cultivated using a more positive approach. As argued by Shek (6), instead of solely looking at adolescent developmental problems, it would be helpful to focus our attention on positive youth development programs (i.e., programs that attempt to cultivate the potentials and skills of adolescents).

To promote holistic development among adolescents in Hong Kong, The Hong Kong Jockey Club Charities Trust has invited academics of five local universities to form a Research Team with The Chinese University of Hong Kong being the lead institution and the author being the Principal Investigator to develop a multi-year universal positive youth development program in the territory (Project P.A.T.H.S.). There are two tiers of programs in this project. The Tier 1 Program is a universal positive youth development program designed for Secondary 1 to Secondary 3 students by the Research Team. There are 10 hours and 20 hours of training for the core program and full program, respectively, in each school year for each grade. The design of the program can be seen in the publications of the project (6, 7). For the Tier 2 Program, it is specifically designed for students who display greater psychosocial needs at each grade (i.e., selective prevention) by the social service agency serving the participating schools.

Catalano and his associates (8) reviewed the effectiveness of 77 positive youth development programs in North America. Results showed that only 25 programs were successful and different positive youth development constructs were incorporated in the successful programs. These constructs include: promotion of bonding, cultivation of resilience, promotion of social competence, promotion of emotional competence, promotion of cognitive competence, promotion of behavioral competence, promotion of moral competence, cultivation of self-determination, promotion of spirituality, development of self-efficacy, development of a clear and positive identity, promotion of beliefs in the future, provision of recognition for positive behaviour, provision of opportunities for prosocial involvement, and fostering prosocial norms. To help adolescents develop in a holistic manner, these 15 adolescent developmental constructs are covered in the Project P.A.T.H.S., particularly in the Tier 1 Program.

In terms of financial and manpower resources, the Project P.A.T.H.S. can be regarded as a huge project. The Hong Kong Jockey Club Charities Trust has earmarked HK$400 million for the project and more than 220 schools have participated in the project. Obviously, one basic question that one should ask is whether the program is helpful to the students. This question is important because not all positive youth development programs are effective. In the Western context, for instance, Catalano et al. (8) showed that only roughly one-third of the 77 programs under review were effective. In addition, Shek, Lam and Tsoi (9) pointed out that evidence-based social work practice was very weak in Hong Kong. As such, there is a need to accumulate research findings on the effectiveness of psychosocial intervention programs. Against this background, it is obvious that rigorous evaluation of the Project P.A.T.H.S. is indispensable.

To provide a comprehensive and complete picture regarding the effectiveness of the project, several evaluation strategies, including objective outcome evaluation, subjective outcome evaluation, qualitative evaluation based on focus groups, student diaries and in-depth interviews, process evaluation, and interim evaluation are employed. Based on the data collected in the Experimental Implementation Phase and Full Implementation Phase, there are results demonstrating the effectiveness of the program via objective outcome evaluation (10), subjective outcome evaluation (11, 12, 13, 14), process evaluation (15), interim evaluation (16), qualitative evaluation (17) and convergence of subjective outcome evaluation and objective outcome evaluation findings (18). Although the above mechanisms provided evidence supporting positive program effect and Shek (10) reported positive findings based on a one group pretest-posttest design, it is noteworthy that objective outcome evaluation based on experimental design can yield additional important information on the effectiveness of the program. Against this background, utilizing a randomized group trial approach, findings on the effectiveness of the Tier 1 Program of the Project P.A.T.H.S. based on the data collected from the first year of the Full Implementation Phase are reported in this paper. Besides, corresponding subjective outcome evaluation findings based on data collected at posttest were also reported.

Methods

Participants

Among the 227 schools joining the Project P.A.T.H.S., there were 131 schools adopting the full program (i.e., 20-hour program involving 40 units) and 96 schools adopting the core program (i.e., 10-hour program involving 20 units). With the help of the Education and Manpower Bureau (which was re-named as the Education Bureau in July 1, 2007), it was planned that 24 pairs of schools stratified by district with equivalent school characteristics, including district, banding (i.e., academic characteristics of the students), religion, and gender of the students, would be randomly selected from the participating schools adopting the 20-hour mode.

Reserve lists of schools were created for each pair of schools in the 24 pairs of schools drawn from the participating schools. For the potential experimental group schools, 31 participating schools were contacted with 24 schools accepted the invitation and 7 schools declined the invitation. For the potential control group schools, 36 participating schools were contacted with 20 schools accepting the invitation and 16 schools rejecting the invitation. The rejection rate was high because the schools were eager to join the project without delay for one year. As the reserve control school lists were exhausted for 4 pairs of schools, 4 equivalent schools not joining the Project P.A.T.H.S. were randomly selected and invited to join the control group by the Education and Manpower Bureau.

Eventually, 19 matched pairs of schools with identical background characteristics (with 3 schools not joining the Project P.A.T.H.S.), 4 matched pairs with similar background characteristics (with 1 school not joining the Project P.A.T.H.S.), and 1 pair of schools which could not be matched were included in the study. For the 20 control schools joining the research, the students admitted to Secondary 1 in 2006 did not join the Project P.A.T.H.S. in their secondary school years. However, the schools concerned could offer youth enhancement programs that were normally offered to these students. The design of the study is presented in Table 1. The number of students joining the pretest and posttest in the experimental group and control group can be seen in Table 2.

Procedures

At pretest and posttest, the purpose of the study was mentioned, and the confidentiality of the data collected was repeatedly emphasized to all of the students in attendance on the day of testing. Parental and student consent had been obtained prior to data collection. All participants responded to all scales in the questionnaire in a self-administration format. Adequate time was provided for the participants to complete the questionnaire. A trained research assistant was present throughout the administration process.

Instruments

The Chinese Positive Youth Development Scale (CPYDS)

At pretest and posttest, the participants were invited to respond to a questionnaire containing measures of positive youth development, including the Chinese Positive Youth Development Scale (CPYDS). Based on reliability analyses of both pretest and posttest data in the present study, there were some modifications in the composition of the items of the 15 subscales of the CPYDS as follows:

1. Bonding Subscale (6 items): α =.83 and .85 at pretest and posttest.
2. Resilience Subscale (6 items): α =.82 and .86 at pretest and posttest.
3. Social Competence Subscale (7 items): α =.83 and .86 at pretest and posttest.
4. Emotional Competence Subscale (6 items): α =.83 and .85 at pretest and posttest.

5. Cognitive Competence Subscale (6 items): α =.84 and .86 at pretest and posttest.
6. Behavioral Competence Subscale (modified 5 items): α =.76 and .80 at pretest and posttest.
7. Moral Competence Subscale (6 items): α =.78 and .78 at pretest and posttest.
8. Self-Determination Subscale (5 items): α =.76 and .80 at pretest and posttest.
9. Self-Efficacy Subscale (modified 2 items): α =.50 and .56 at pretest and posttest.
10. Beliefs in the Future Subscale (modified 3 items): α =.82 and .83 at pretest and posttest.
11. Clear and Positive Identity Subscale (7 items): α =.84 and .85 at pretest and posttest.
12. Spirituality Subscale (7 items): α =.88 and .90 at pretest and posttest.
13. Prosocial Involvement Subscale (5 items): α =.83 and .83 at pretest and posttest.
14. Prosocial Norms Subscale (5 items): α =.77 and .80 at pretest and posttest.
15 Recognition for Positive Behavior Subscale (4 items): α =.76 and .80 at pretest and posttest.

Table 1. Characteristics of the experimental schools (N=24) and control schools (N=24)

<table>
<tr><th>Pair</th><th>Experimental Group</th><th>Control Group</th><th>Characteristics</th></tr>
<tr><td>Pair 1</td><td>1A</td><td>1B</td><td rowspan="19">19 pairs of schools with identical banding. In each pair, one school was randomly assigned to the experimental group and one school was randomly assigned to the control group.</td></tr>
<tr><td>Pair 2</td><td>2A</td><td>2B</td></tr>
<tr><td>Pair 3</td><td>3A</td><td>3B</td></tr>
<tr><td>Pair 4</td><td>4A</td><td>4B</td></tr>
<tr><td>Pair 5</td><td>5A</td><td>5B</td></tr>
<tr><td>Pair 6</td><td>6A</td><td>6B</td></tr>
<tr><td>Pair 7</td><td>7A</td><td>7B</td></tr>
<tr><td>Pair 8</td><td>8A</td><td>8B</td></tr>
<tr><td>Pair 9</td><td>9A</td><td>9B</td></tr>
<tr><td>Pair 10</td><td>10A</td><td>10B</td></tr>
<tr><td>Pair 11</td><td>11A</td><td>11B</td></tr>
<tr><td>Pair 12</td><td>12A</td><td>12B</td></tr>
<tr><td>Pair 13</td><td>13A</td><td>13B</td></tr>
<tr><td>Pair 14</td><td>14A</td><td>14B</td></tr>
<tr><td>Pair 15</td><td>15A</td><td>15B</td></tr>
<tr><td>Pair 16</td><td>16A</td><td>16B</td></tr>
<tr><td>Pair 17</td><td>17A</td><td>17B</td></tr>
<tr><td>Pair 18</td><td>18A</td><td>18B</td></tr>
<tr><td>Pair 19</td><td>19A</td><td>19B</td></tr>
<tr><td>Pair 20</td><td>20A</td><td>20B</td><td rowspan="4">4 pairs of schools with similar banding and randomly assigned.</td></tr>
<tr><td>Pair 21</td><td>21A</td><td>21B</td></tr>
<tr><td>Pair 22</td><td>22A</td><td>22B</td></tr>
<tr><td>Pair 23</td><td>23A</td><td>23B</td></tr>
<tr><td>Pair 24</td><td>24A</td><td>N/A</td><td>1 pair of schools with similar banding but not randomly assigned.</td></tr>
</table>

Table 2. Number of questionnaires collected from pretest and posttest

Cases	Experimental Group	Control Group	Total
Pretest Questionnaire collected	4121	3854	7975
Pretest Questionnaire available for analysis	3792	4044	7863
Posttest Questionnaire collected	3915	3769	7684
Posttest Questionnaire available for analysis	3886	3722	7608
Successfully matched cases based on the unique identifier for each participant	3298 (49.5%)	3358 (50.5%)	6656 (100%)

Note: The number of participants in the Experimental Group who perceived the program to be beneficial = 1,888.

Table 3. Items in the Trimmed Scale involving 15 items

Domain	Item
Bonding	When I need help, I trust my friend will help me.
Resilience	When I face adversity, I remain optimistic.
Social Competence	I understand the rules and expectations in interacting with others.
Emotional Competence	When I am angry, I can rationally describe my feelings.
Cognitive Competence	I know how to find the causes of and solutions to a problem.
Behavioral Competence	I can face criticisms with an open mind.
Moral Competence	I have the habit of self-evaluation.
Self-Determination	I am able to make wise choices.
Self-Efficacy	I can finish almost everything that I am determined to do.
Spirituality	Regarding my life goals, there is no progress *versus* total achievement.
Beliefs in the Future	I have confidence that I will be a useful person when I grow up.
Clear and Positive Identity	I am a person with self-confidence.
Prosocial Involvement	In this school, classmates are encouraged to have mutual help.
Prosocial Norms	If I do something wrong, I will feel shameful.
Recognition for Positive Behavior	When I help others, my classmates will recognize my behavior.

Two composite indices based on the above measures were utilized in this study. According to Shek et al. (19), the mean of the total mean score based on all 15 subscales could be used as an overall measure of positive development (Indicator 1: α =.94 and .93 at pretest and posttest). Second, based on conceptual analyses of the items, 1 item was derived from each domain which resulted in a 15-item key measure (Indicator 2: α =.88 and .89 at pretest and posttest). The 15 items in this indicator can be seen in Table 3.

Subjective outcome evaluation scale

Twenty items were used to assess the participants' satisfaction with the program and instructor as well as their perceived benefits of the program at posttest. Reliability analysis showed that this measure is reliable ($\alpha = .97$; mean inter-item correlation = .62).

Data analytic strategies

In their discussion of the statistical analyses for change data, Allison, Gorman and Primavera (20) pointed out that there were four basic strategies. The first strategy was to examine difference between the experimental group and control group at posttest only. As this strategy did not take into account of all information, it was not a recommended approach. The second strategy was to conduct a two-way ANOVA (with group and time as the main effect) and examine the interaction effect between group and time. As this approach was often misinterpreted, it was also not recommended. The third strategy was to look at gain scores. However, as the correlation between pretest and posttest scores seldom equals to 1.0, there would be biases in this analysis. The final recommended strategy is to use analyses of covariance to compare posttest scores of the experimental group and control group after controlling pretest scores. In this study, the final strategy based on analysis of covariance was used. Furthermore, as students in this study were recruited from schools, it could be argued that variations in the outcome measures across groups may also be due to variations in the school characteristics across groups. As such, there is a need to adjust for the random effect of schools when examining the effect of treatment on the outcome variables (21-23).

In an earlier objective outcome evaluation paper, findings showed that the experimental group had better developmental outcomes than did the control group (24). Although school banding was not different across schools in the experimental group and control group using schools as the units of analysis, school banding at the individual level was included as a covariate in this paper. Furthermore, as participants' motivation and perception may confound the program effect, only participants who perceived the Tier 1 Program to be effective were included in the analyses to highlight the effects of the experimental group (if any).

Results

Regarding the participants' perceptions of the program, instructor and perceived benefits of the Tier 1 Program, the percentage findings in Table 4 revealed several observations. First, most of the participants perceived that the program could help them to do reflection. Second, the respondents were appreciative of the encouragement given by the instructor. Third, a high proportion of the participants regarded the program as helpful to them. These findings generally showed that the subjective outcomes regarding the program were very favorable.

Using schools as the units of analysis, results showed that the 24 experimental schools and 24 control schools did not differ in the banding of the schools, district, religion, gender of the students and source of funding. For the personal characteristics of the participants, results showed that there were no statistically significant differences between the two groups in their socio-demographic background, except age (see Table 5). In short, except that the mean age of the control group was higher than that of the experimental group, the background characteristics of the experimental schools and control schools were highly comparable at pretest. However, to remove the effect of school banding at the individual level, school banding at the individual level was included as a covariate in this study.

As motivation and perception of the students are crucial to the success of positive youth development programs such as the Project P.A.T.H.S., only students who perceived the program to be beneficial were included in the analysis. Operationally speaking, participants who responded in the agreement direction on item 20 of the subjective outcome evaluation scale (i.e., ratings of 4, 5 or 6) were included in the analysis. For the findings based on analyses of covariance, results in Table 6 showed that there were significant differences between the experimental group and control group participants in terms of two global indicators. For the linear mixed models, the hypothesized models were significantly better than the intercept models ($p < .01$ in all cases). In addition, the findings based on the hypothesized models were generally positive. For the estimates of the fixed effects, the experimental group (reference category with a value of 0) performed better than the control group on CPYDS-15 (estimate = -.11, $p < .0001$) and KEY15 (estimate = -.14, $p < .0001$). These findings generally showed that the experimental group performed better than the control group in terms of the global positive youth development indicators after controlling for pretest scores and age as well as adjusting for the random effect of schools.

Discussion

The findings based on the subjective outcome evaluation strategy or client satisfaction survey showed that a very high proportion of the respondents had positive perceptions of the program and worker. Most importantly, roughly 82.4% of the respondents regarded the program as helpful to them (see Table 4). The use of subjective outcome indicators or the client satisfaction approach in evaluation has a long history in human services in different cultures. Although there are arguments against the use of subjective outcome assessment, there is evidence showing that subjective outcome measures were correlated with objective outcome measures (18). The subjective outcome evaluation findings in this study provide support for the positive program effects of the Tier 1 Program of the Project P.A.T.H.S..

Table 4. Findings based on the subjective outcome evaluation strategy

		Percentage of Responses (%)								
		1	2	3	A	4	5	6	B	Total
1.	The atmosphere of the class was good. (N=3854)	6.2	6.0	13.1	25.3	32.0	29.1	13.5	74.6	99.9
2.	There were many opportunities for students to exchange ideas during class. (N=3847)	4.4	4.9	11.5	20.8	34.3	32.2	12.7	79.2	100
3.	I often had encouragement from the responses of classmates. (N=3841)	4.5	4.4	13.5	22.4	35.3	30.7	11.6	77.6	100
4.	I think students actively participated in the class activities. (N=3842)	4.2	4.9	12.7	21.8	32.1	33.1	13.0	78.2	100

		Percentage of Responses (%)								
		1	2	3	A	4	5	6	B	Total
5.	I think I actively participated in the class activities. (N=3845)	4.1	5.2	12.5	21.8	31.9	33.1	13.2	78.2	100
6.	I think the discipline in class was good. (N=3832)	6.0	8.1	17.2	31.3	31.6	27.0	10.2	68.8	100.1
7.	I think this course is very interesting. (N=3843)	5.7	5.9	12.6	24.2	33.0	29.6	13.2	75.8	100
8.	I think this course encouraged me to reflect. (N=3840)	4.8	4.7	11.7	21.2	35.4	30.7	12.7	78.8	100
9.	I like this course very much. (N=3840)	5.5	5.7	13.0	24.2	32.6	28.3	14.9	75.8	100
10.	The instructor could arouse my interest in the course. (N=3832)	4.9	5.0	12.1	22.0	32.8	30.9	14.4	78.1	100.1
11.	The instructor could arouse my learning motivation. (N=3845)	5.0	5.1	13.0	23.1	33.2	30.6	13.0	76.8	99.9
12.	The instructor knew how to promote discussion and participation among the students. (N=3841)	4.5	3.8	9.8	18.1	33.7	33.6	14.6	81.9	100
13.	I could get encouragement from the responses of the instructor. (N=3832)	4.7	3.9	12.6	21.2	33.6	31.9	13.5	79.0	100.2
14.	I often share the things I have learned from the course with my friends. (N=3841)	7.8	7.5	15.8	31.1	31.0	26.2	11.7	68.9	100
15.	I often share the things I have learned from the course with my family members. (N=3835)	10.0	9.2	17.5	36.7	27.9	23.9	11.6	63.4	100.1
16.	I think this course can strengthen my ability to face the challenge of life. (N=3837)	4.8	4.6	13.0	22.4	32.9	31.5	13.2	77.6	100
17.	I think this course can strengthen my ability to face adversity. (N=3835)	4.9	4.0	11.8	20.7	34.0	31.6	13.7	79.3	100
18.	I think this course can increase my understanding about myself. (N=3843)	4.6	3.9	9.2	17.7	34.3	32.9	15.0	82.2	99.9
19.	I think this course can promote my overall development. (N=3844)	4.7	3.9	10.6	19.2	33.3	32.6	14.8	80.7	99.9
20.	Overall speaking, I think this course is helpful to me. (N=3821)	5.1	3.5	8.8	17.4	31.5	32.3	18.6	82.4	99.8

Note: 1=Strongly Disagree. 2=Disagree. 3=Slightly Disagree. 4=Slightly Agree. 5=Agree. 6=Strongly Agree. A=Sum of the disagree responses (i.e., negative responses). B=Sum of the agree responses (i.e., positive responses).

For the analyses of covariance and linear mixed model analyses, the findings generally showed that compared with participants in the control group, participants in the experimental schools who perceived the program to be beneficial (using item 20 on the subjective outcome evaluation scale) performed better on different indicators of positive youth development.

Adopting a more liberal perspective, findings based on CPYDS-15 suggest that the experimental subjects performed better than the control subjects on the global indicator comprising the 15 domains of positive youth development assessed by the scale, including bonding, resilience, social competence, emotional competence, cognitive competence, behavioral competence, moral competence, self-determination, self-efficacy, beliefs in the future, spirituality, clear and positive identity, prosocial norms, prosocial involvement and recognition for positive behavior. Analyses based on the 15 key items also showed similar findings. The differences between the two groups were more pronounced as compared to those reported previously (24).

Table 5. Differences between the experimental group and control group in terms of personal characteristics

Socio- demographic Variables	Control Group	Experimental Group	Differences
Age group	Mean = 3.31	Mean = 3.17	Z = 5.63, $p <$ .05
Gender ratio	Male = 54.77%	Male =53.32%	$X^2 = 1.06$, $p >$ .05
Number of persons in the family	Mean = 4.19	Mean = 4.23	Z = -0.93, $p >$ .05
Marital status of parents	Intact families = 82.16%	Intact families = 83.33%	$X^2 = 2.74$, $p >$ .05
Family on welfare	Yes = 14.79%	Yes = 14.89%	$X^2 = 0.01$, $p >$ .05

Note: Age group (age 10 or less=1, age 11=2, age 12=3, age 13=4, age 14=5, age 15=6, age 16=7, age 17=8, age 18=9, age 19=10, age 20 or above=11).

Table 6. Differences between the experimental group and control group based on the different indicators derived from the Chinese Positive Youth Development Scale (CPYDS)

Findings Based on Analyses of Covariance			
Global Indicator	Estimated Marginal Mean (Control Group)	Estimated Marginal Mean (Experimental Group)	*F* value
CPYDS-15	4.45	4.61	63.73, $p < .0001$ $(\eta_P^2) = .012$
KEY15	4.34	4.53	79.70, $p < .0001$ $(\eta_P^2) = .015$
Linear Mixed Model Findings Adjusting for the Random Effect of Schools			
Global Indicator	Estimated Marginal Mean (Control Group)	Estimated Marginal Mean (Experimental Group)	*F* value
CPYDS-15	4.47	4.58	24.99, $p < .0001$
KEY15	4.36	4.50	28.20, $p < .0001$

Note: CPYDS-15 (Mean of the mean scores in 15 subscales). KEY15 (Mean total score based on 15 key items).

In conjunction with the previous findings based on objective outcome evaluation, subjective outcome evaluation, qualitative evaluation via focus groups, qualitative evaluation via diaries, process evaluation, and interim evaluation, the existing evaluation findings surrounding the Project P.A.T.H.S. basically suggest that the program is an effective one (25). This is an encouraging finding, particularly in view of the fact that the implementation period of the program was not long. Nevertheless, as only one year was involved in the program, only the short-term effect of the program was revealed. Obviously, it would be exciting to examine the program effect over a longer period of time. Although the schools did not differ in their background characteristics (when schools were used as units of analyses) and student characteristics, it would be helpful to examine the differences between the two groups in terms of the other school-related variables. With the collection of such information via the School Background Questionnaire, further analyses of the findings along this line will be carried out in the future.

Acknowledgments

The preparation for this paper and the Project P.A.T.H.S. were financially supported by The Hong Kong Jockey Club Charities Trust.

References

[1] Shek DTL. Adolescent developmental issues in Hong Kong: relevance to positive youth development programs in Hong Kong. Int J Adolesc Med Health 2006;18(3):341-54.

[2] Shek DTL, Lam CM. Adolescent cough medicine abuse in Hong Kong: implications for the design of positive youth development programs in Hong Kong. Int J Adolesc Med Health 2006;18(3):493-503.

[3] Shek DTL, Lee TY. Perceived parental control processes in Chinese adolescents: implications for positive youth development programs in Hong Kong. Int J Adolesc Med Health 2006;18(3):505-19.

[4] Weissberg RP, Kumpfer KL, Seligman MEP. Prevention that works for children and youth: an introduction. Am Psychol 2003;58:425-32.

[5] Pittman KJ. Promoting youth development: strengthening the role of youth-serving and community organizations. Report prepared for the U.S. Department of Agriculture Extension Services. Washington, DC: Center Youth Dev Policy Res, 1991.

[6] Shek DTL. Conceptual framework underlying the development of a positive youth development program in Hong Kong. Int J Adolesc Med Health 2006;18(3):303-14.

[7] Shek DTL, Ma HK. Design of a positive youth development program in Hong Kong. Int J Adolesc Med Health 2006;18(3):315-27.

[8] Catalano RF, Berglund ML, Ryan JAM, Lonczak HS, Hawkins JD. Positive youth development in the United States: research findings on evaluations of positive youth development programs. Prev Treatment 2002. Accessed 2008 Nov 01. URL: http://aspe.hhs.gov/hsp/PositiveYouthDev99/

[9] Shek DTL, Lam MC, Tsoi KW. Evidence-based practice in Hong Kong. In: Thyer B, Kazi MAF, editors. International perspectives on evidence-based practice in social work. London: Venture Press, 2004:167-81.

[10] Shek DTL. Effectiveness of the Tier 1 Program of the Project P.A.T.H.S.: preliminary objective and subjective outcome evaluation findings. ScientificWorldJournal 2006;6:1466-74.

[11] Shek DTL, Ma HK. Subjective outcome evaluation of the Project P.A.T.H.S.: findings based on the perspective of the program participants. ScientificWorldJournal 2007;7:47-55.

[12] Shek DTL, Siu A, Lee TY. Subjective outcome evaluation of the Project P.A.T.H.S.: findings based on the perspective of the program implementers. ScientificWorldJournal 2007;7:195-203.
[13] Shek DTL, Sun RCF. Subjective outcome evaluation of the Project P.A.T.H.S.: qualitative findings based on the experiences of program participants. ScientificWorldJournal 2007;7:686-97.
[14] Shek DTL, Sun RCF. Subjective outcome evaluation of the Project P.A.T.H.S.: qualitative findings based on the experiences of program implementers. ScientificWorldJournal 2007;7:1024-35.
[15] Shek DTL, Ma HK, Lui JHY, Lung DWM. Process evaluation of the Tier 1 Program of the Project P.A.T.H.S. ScientificWorldJournal 2006;1:300-9.
[16] Shek DTL, Sun RCF. Implementation of the Tier 1 Program of the Project P.A.T.H.S.: interim evaluation findings. ScientificWorldJournal 2006;6:2274-84.
[17] Shek DTL, Lee TY, Siu A, Lam CM. Qualitative evaluation of the Project P.A.T.H.S. based on the perceptions of the program participants. ScientificWorldJournal 2006;1:290-9.
[18] Shek DTL, Lee TY, Siu AMH, Ma HK. Convergence of subjective outcome and objective outcome evaluation findings: insights based on the Project P.A.T.H.S. ScientificWorldJournal 2007;7:258-67.
[19] Shek DTL, Siu AMH, Lee TY. The Chinese Positive Youth Development Scale: a validation study. Res Soc Work Prac 2007;17(3):380-91.
[20] Allison DB, Gorman BS, Primavera LH. Some of the most common questions asked of statistical consultants: our favourite responses and recommended readings. Genet Soc Gen Psychol Monogr 1993;119:153-85.
[21] Peugh JL, Enders CK. Using the SPSS mixed procedure and fit cross-sectional and longitudinal multilevel models. Educ Psychol Meas 2005;65:717-41.
[22] Tabachnick BG, Fidell LS. Using multivariate statistics. Boston: Pearson Education, 2007.
[23] West BT, Welch KB, Galecki AT. Linear mixed models: a practical guide using statistical software. Boca Raton: Chapman and Hall/CRC, 2007.
[24] Shek DTL, Siu AMH, Lee TY, Cheung CK, Chung R. Effectiveness of the Tier 1 Program of the Project P.A.T.H.S.: objective outcome evaluation based on a randomized group trial. ScientificWorldJournal 2008;8:4-12.
[25] Shek DTL, ed. Special Issue: evaluation of the Project P.A.T.H.S. in Hong Kong. ScientificWorldJournal 2008;8:1-94.

Submitted: December 15, 2008.
Revised: December 30, 2008.
Accepted: January 21, 2009.

In: Public Health Yearbook 2009
Editor: Joav Merrick
ISBN: 978-1-61668-911-7

Chapter 25

QUALITATIVE EVALUATION OF THE PROJECT P.A.T.H.S. (SECONDARY 1 PROGRAM) BASED ON THE PERCEPTIONS OF THE PROGRAM IMPLEMENTERS

Daniel TL Shek, PhD, FHKPS, BBS, JP [*1,2,3]
and Rachel CF Sun, BSocSc, PhD [4]

[1]Department of Applied Social Sciences, The Hong Kong Polytechnic University, Hong Kong, PRC, [2]Department of Sociology, East China Normal University, Shanghai, PRC [3]Kiang Wu Nursing College of Macau, Macau, PRC and [4]Department of Social Work, The Chinese University of Hong Kong, Hong Kong, PRC

Abstract

Nine focus groups involving 61 instructors recruited from nine schools were conducted to understand the perceptions of the program implementers of the Tier 1 Program of the Project P.A.T.H.S. via a qualitative approach. The informants generally described the program in a positive manner, although suggestions for improvement were proposed. When the informants were invited to name some metaphors that could stand for the program, the related metaphors and related explanation were generally positive in nature. Finally, the program implementers perceived many beneficial effects of the program in different domains. Intra-rater and inter-rater reliability analyses revealed that the coding of the positive or negative nature of the responses and the categorization was reliable. The present study provides qualitative support for the effectiveness of the Tier 1 Program of the Project P.A.T.H.S. in promoting holistic development among Chinese adolescents in Hong Kong.
Keywords: Project P.A.T.H.S., qualitative evaluation, positive youth development program, program implementers, effectiveness.

* Correspondence: Professor Daniel TL Shek, PhD, FHKPS, BBS, JP, Chair Professor of Applied Social Sciences, Department of Applied Social Sciences, The Hong Kong Polytechnic University, Hunghom, Hong Kong. E-mail: danielshek@inet.polyu.edu.hk

Introduction

There are two main approaches in the field of evaluation – quantitative paradigm and qualitative paradigm (1). For the quantitative or experimental paradigm, there are several characteristics including quantitative data (use of numbers and statistics), experimental designs, treatment and control groups, deductive hypothesis testing, objective perspective, evaluator aloof from the program, independent and dependent variables, linear and sequential modeling, pre-post focus on change, probabilistic and random sampling, standardized and uniform procedures, fixed and controlled designs, statistical analysis, as well as generalizations. On the other hand, there are several attributes of the qualitative or naturalistic paradigm, including qualitative data (e.g., narratives), naturalistic inquiry, case studies, inductive analysis, subjective perspective, evaluator close to the program, holistic contextual portrayal, systems perspective focused on interdependencies, dynamic and ongoing view of change, purposeful sampling of relevant cases, focus on uniqueness and diversity, emergent and flexible designs, thematic content analysis, and extrapolations.

An examination of the evaluation literature shows that although there is a strong preference for the use of quantitative or experimental approach to evaluate the effectiveness of prevention programs for adolescents, the number of qualitative evaluation studies in this area is increasing (2). Moreover, regardless of the general impression that quantitative evaluation is the "mainstream" evaluation approach, there is a growing emphasis on the use of qualitative methods in evaluation. For instance, Chatterji (3) criticized the sole reliance on experimental methods and argued for the use of more diverse types of evaluation strategies, particularly in the context of education. Slayton and Llosa (4) also remarked that "qualitative methods should be an essential part of large-scale program evaluations if program effectiveness is to be determined and understood" (p. 2543).

The Project P.A.T.H.S. (**P**ositive **A**dolescent **T**raining through **H**olistic **S**ocial Programmes) is a youth enhancement program that attempts to promote holistic youth development in Hong Kong (5). There are two tiers of programs (Tier 1 and Tier 2) in this project. The Tier 1 Program is a universal positive youth development program based on 15 positive youth development constructs (6) in which students in Secondary 1 to 3 will take part. Obviously, to enable researchers to claim that the Tier 1 Program of the project is effective, research evidence is needed.

Based on the principle of triangulation, evaluation data based on different strategies and sources have been collected to understand the program effectiveness and effect. These include objective outcome evaluation utilizing a randomized group trial (7), subjective outcome evaluation based on quantitative and qualitative data collected from the program participants and instructors (8-11), process evaluation involving systematic observations of the delivery of program (12,13), interim evaluation (14), and qualitative evaluation, including focus groups based on students and program implementers (15,16), case study (17,18), in-depth interviews with program implementers, student logs and student products (19). While the above evaluation findings were encouraging, it should be noted that they were primarily based on the responses and perceptions of the program participants. Obviously, evaluation data based on qualitative methodology should also be conducted to examine the program implementers' perceptions of the program and program effects.

In their review of the common problems intrinsic to qualitative evaluation studies in the social work literature, Shek, Tang and Han (20) suggested that 12 principles should be maintained in a qualitative evaluation study. These include: explicit statement of the philosophical base of the study (Principle 1), justifications for the number and nature of the participants of the study (Principle 2), detailed description of the data collection procedures (Principle 3), discussion of the biases and preoccupations of the researchers (Principle 4), description of the steps taken to guard against biases or arguments that biases should and/or could not be eliminated (Principle 5), inclusion of measures of reliability, such as inter-rater reliability and intra-rater reliability (Principle 6), inclusion of measures of triangulation in terms of researchers and data types (Principle 7), inclusion of peer checking and member checking procedures (Principle 8), consciousness of the importance and development of audit trails (Principle 9), consideration of alternative explanations for the observed findings (Principle 10), inclusion of explanations for negative evidence (Principle 11), and clear statement of the limitations of the study (Principle 12). In this qualitative evaluation study, the above principles were upheld as far as possible.

The purpose of this paper is to describe some of the qualitative findings based on focus group interviews with implementers of the Tier 1 Program. Although there are many strands of qualitative research (21), the most commonly-used approach in qualitative research is the general qualitative approach in which the general strategies of qualitative research are employed (e.g., collection of qualitative data, respecting the views of the informants, data analysis without preset coding scheme) but a specific qualitative approach is not adhered to (22). The exposition of the nature of this qualitative study is consistent with the view of Shek, Tang and Han (20) that there should be an explicit statement of the philosophical base of the study (Principle 1).

Methods

Participants

Among the 207 schools joining the Full Implementation Phase, there were 112 schools adopting the full program (i.e., 20-hour program involving 40 units) and 95 schools adopting the 10-hour core program. Nine randomly selected schools joining the full program and two randomly selected schools joining the core program were invited to participate in the focus group interviews. As the time for conducting the interviews was near the end of the school term, two schools joining the full program declined our invitation. As a result, a total of nine schools joined the focus group interviews. However, the research team discovered at the time of the interview that untrained teachers had implemented the program in one of these schools since the trained staff had resigned in the period of program implementation. As this practice seriously violated the program requirement and it possibly negatively influenced the implementation quality of the program, additional analyses that disregarded the interview data based on that school were carried out. The results of analyses including and excluding the interview data based on that school were both reported in Table 2 to Table 4.

A total of 61 instructors participated in nine focus group interviews. The number of informants in each focus group ranged between 2 to 14 instructors. Although only 4% of the participating schools were selected for this study, the strategy of random sampling helped to enhance the generalizability of the findings. Also, with the limitation of resources, the number of instructors joining the focus group discussion could be regarded as on the high side in qualitative research. These arguments can satisfy Principle 2 (i.e., justifications for the number and nature of the participants of the study) proposed by Shek, Tang and Han (20).

Procedures

The focus group interviews were conducted by the second author and trained research assistants of the project. As they either had training in group work and/or substantial group work experience, they were conscious of the importance of encouraging the informants to verbalize their views and perceptions of the program and to express views of different nature, including both positive and negative ones. They were also conscious of the importance of adopting an open attitude to accommodate both positive and negative experiences expressed by the program implementers in the interviews. With respect to Principle 3 (i.e., detailed description of the data collection procedures) suggested by Shek, Tang and Han (20), the broad interview guide of the focus group interviews conducted is presented in Table 1. The interview questions were designed with reference to the CIPP model (23) and previous research (24). After obtaining the consent of the respondents, the focus group interviews were audio-taped.

Data analysis

The interviews were tape-recorded, and the content of the interviews was fully transcribed by student helpers and checked for accuracy by a research assistant and four trained helpers. To enhance reliability in the coding process, two research assistants and the first author were involved in the data analyses of the narratives. The unit of analysis was a meaningful unit instead of a statement. For example, the statement that a program was "meaningful and amusing" would be broken down into two meaningful units or attributes, namely, "meaningful" and "amusing". Furthermore, descriptions with the same meaning (e.g., "good quality" and "high quality") were grouped into the same attribute category.

Table 1. Interview guide for the focus group involving program implementers
A. Context Evaluation

- How much do you know about "Positive Youth Development Programs" (e.g., "Life Skills Education")? What is your overall impression of these programs?
- Have you taught programs that are similar to the Project P.A.T.H.S. before?
- If yes, how effective do you feel they are?
- From your perspective, what are the differences between the Project P.A.T.H.S. and other similar programs?
- Do you agree with the vision of the Project P.A.T.H.S.? Why?

B. Input Evaluation

- What kind of effects do you feel that the implementation of the Project P.A.T.H.S. have on the school's normal operation?
- If the school incorporates the Project P.A.T.H.S. curriculum into the normal curriculum (e.g., Life Education, Integrated Humanities, etc.), from your perspective, what are the advantages and disadvantages of this arrangement?
- If the school *does not* incorporate the Project P.A.T.H.S. curriculum into the normal curriculum (e.g., homeroom, extra-curricular activities, etc.), do you feel that this arrangement is successful?
- To accommodate the implementation of the Project P.A.T.H.S., did the school make special arrangements?
- Do you feel that the principal and administrative staff support the implementation of the Project P.A.T.H.S. at your school? Why or Why not?
- Do you feel that the training you received is adequate for you to carry out the program requirements?

C. Process Evaluation

1. General Impression of the Program

- What is your overall impression of the program? What are your feelings?
- All in all, did you enjoy leading the program?
- Regarding the program, what has given you a lasting impression?
- While implementing the program, did you have any unforgettable experiences?

2. Comments on the Program Content

- Regarding the program, what are the things you like? And what are the things you dislike?
- What are your views on the different units and content of the program?
- Which units do you like the most? Why?
- From your recollection, are there any activities that aroused students' interest to participate in the program?

3. Comments on the Program Implementation

- While implementing the program, did you encounter any difficulties?
- Do you feel that the program implementation was successful?
- To what degree/extent did you follow the program curriculum manuals? Why?
- What are your thoughts on the students' responses to the program?

D. Product Evaluation

1. Evaluation of the General Effectiveness of the Program

- Do you feel that the program is beneficial to the development of adolescents?
- Have you noticed any changes in students after their participation in the program? If yes, what are the changes? (free elicitation)
- If you noticed changes in students, what do you think are the factors that have caused such changes?
- If you *have not* noticed changes in students, what do you think are the factors that have caused students *not* to change?

2. Evaluation of the Specific Effectiveness of the Program

- Do you think that the program can promote students' self-confidence/ability to face the future?
- Do you think that the program can enhance students' abilities in different areas?

Optional Questions

- Do you think that the program can enhance students' spirituality aspect?
- Do you think that the program can promote the students' bonding with family, teachers and friends?
- Do you think that the program can establish students' compassion and care for others?
- Do you think that the program can promote students' participation and care for the society?
- Do you think that the program can promote students' sense of responsibility to the society, family, teachers and peers?

3. The Program's Impact on the Instructor

- Do you feel you have gained something by leading this program? And have you lost something?
- If you have the opportunity in future, do you wish to lead similar programs again?

4. Other Comments

- If you are invited to use three descriptive words to describe the program, what are the three words that you would use?
- If you are invited to use one incident, object/thing or feeling (e.g., indigestion, enjoyment, child at heart, etc.) to describe the program, how would you describe the program?

Table 2. Categorization of the descriptors used by the instructors to describe the program

Descriptions	Nature of the Response				Total
	Positive	Neutral	Negative	Undecided	
Positive	4				4
Interactive	4				4
Fun and Relaxed	9				9
Happy	3				3
Diverse	6				6
Systematic	3				3
Enlightening	1				1
Meaningful	4				4
Novel	4				4
Chaotic			5		5
To be improved			1		1
Difficult			6		6
Descriptions	Nature of the Response				Total
Innovative	3				3
Useless			2		2
Practical	2				2
Confused			1		1
Worried			1		1
Clear	1				1
Focused	1				1

Superficial			8		8
In-depth	1				1
Helpless			2		2
Inadequate			1		1
Rush			1		1
Overlapping			2		2
Lack of connection			1		1
All-rounded	6				6
Over-generalized			1		1
Zealous	4				4
Prospective	2				2
Not practical			3		3
Senseless			1		1
Too rich content within insufficient time			1		1
Intensive	1				1
Too aggressive			3		3
Demanding and inept			1		1
Could not meet students' needs			4		4
Having a heart but no strength		1			1
Headache			1		1
Lack of reflection			1		1
Total Count (N):	59	1	47	0	107
Total Count (%):	55.14%	0.93%	43.93%	0%	100
(Disregarded the school without trained instructor) Total Count (N):	57	1	45	0	103
(Disregarded the school without trained instructor) Total Count (%):	55.34%	0.97%	43.69%	0%	100

Table 3. Categorization of the metaphors used by the instructors to describe the program

Metaphors	Number of Metaphor and Its Nature				Total	Number of Codes Derived from the Metaphor and Its Nature				Total
	Positive	Neutral	Negative	Undecided		Positive	Neutral	Negative	Undecided	
Teachers give hands to students	1				1	1				1
Street light	1				1	2		1		3
Crystal	1				1	2				2
The Sun		1			1		1			1
Compass	1				1	1				1
Water and stone		1			1		1			1
Tasteless water			1		1					0

Metaphors	Number of Metaphor and Its Nature				Total	Number of Codes Derived from the Metaphor and Its Nature				Total
Hand in class work		1			1					0
Wine		1			1		1			1
Rowing upstream			1		1					0
Pulling a cow up to a tree			1		1					0
Better than nothing		1			1		1			1
Piggy cashbox	1				1	1	1			2
Big bowl feast		1			1	1	1	1		3
Box		2			2		2			2
TV		1			1	1	1	1		3
Swimming	1				1	2	1			3
Praising life	1				1	1				1
Sunrise	1				1	2		1		3
Sashimi	1				1	2		1		3
Walking in the mist	1				1	1				1
Planting vegetables		1			1		1			1
Buying		1			1		1			1
Doraemon		1			1		1			1
Collective memory of experiences	1				1	1				1
Magician		1			1		1			1
Fighting a battle		1			1		2			2
Apple	1				1	5				5
Skipping rock		1			1		1			1
Principles of Bible *	1				1	2				2
Product builder *	1				1	1	1			2
Total Count (N):	14	15	3	0	32	26	18	5	0	49
Total Count (%):	43.75%	46.88%	9.38%	0%	100%	53.06%	36.73%	10.20%	0%	100%
(Disregarded the school without trained instructor) Total Count (N):	12	15	3	0	30	23	17	5	0	45
(Disregarded the school without trained instructor) Total Count (%):	40.00%	50.00%	10.00%	0%	100%	51.11%	37.78%	11.11%	0%	100%

* The responses from the school without trained instructor.

Table 4. Categorization of instructors' responses on perceived benefits for the students

Level of Competence	Subcategory	Benefits	Nature of the Response				Total	N in Subcategory
			Positive	Neutral	Negative	Undecided		
Familial level	Family relationships	Improved communication and relationship with family members	2				2	2
Interpersonal level	Communication and relationship among peers	Improved communication with peers	5				5	
		Improved relationship with peers	8				8	13
	Social skills	Learned how to handle conflicts	2				2	
		Learned how to treat people and deal with issues	3				3	
		Learned to share and express oneself	10				10	
		Learned to respect others	2				2	17
	Teacher-student relationship	Enhanced teacher-student relationship	9				9	9
Personal level	Reflection	Enhanced self-reflection	2				2	
		Enhanced understanding of purpose of life	3				3	5
	Cognitive competence	Enhanced critical thinking	5				5	
		Benefit to study	1				1	6
	Ways to face adversity	Be more persistent when facing difficulties	1				1	1
	Positive self-image	Enhanced self-understanding	5				5	
		Promoting self enrichment	3				3	
		Promoting personal growth	3				3	
		Enhanced self-confidence	10				10	
		Be more initiative	2				2	
		Became more active	2				2	25
	Emotional competence	Enhanced ability in handling emotions	2				2	2

Table 4. (Continued)

Level of Competence	Subcategory	Benefits	Nature of the Response				Total	N in Subcategory
			Positive	Neutral	Negative	Undecided		
	Behavioral competence	Promoted presentation skills	3				3	3
	Moral competence	Enhanced sense of equality	3				3	3
Others	General impression on effectiveness	Could not learn anything			4		4	
		Unhelpful / not very helpful			9		9	
		Not many changes in students		2	5		7	
		Students' changes were doubtful		16	8		24	
		Could not assess the effectiveness in a short time		15			15	
		Neutral impression towards program effectiveness		5			5	
		Positive impression towards program effectiveness	33				33	
		Broadened students' horizon	1				1	98
	Benefits to instructors	Enhanced instructors' understanding towards students	7				7	
		Instructors learned a lot from the program content / teaching experiences	7				7	14
	Others	Gained recognitions and encouragement from instructors	3				3	3
Total Count (N):			139	38	26	0	203	
Total Count (%):			68.47%	18.72%	12.81%	0%	100 %	
(Disregarded the school without trained instructor) Total Count (N):			128	35	21	0	184	
(Disregarded the school without trained instructor) Total Count (%):			69.57%	19.02%	11.41%	0%	100 %	

The present coding system was developed after much consideration of the raw data and several preliminary analyses. After initial coding, the positive or negative nature of the codes was determined, with four possibilities (positive code, negative code, neutral code and undecided code). To enhance the reliability of the coding of the positive or negative nature of the raw codes, both intra-rater and inter-rater reliability were carried out. Because of space limitation, qualitative findings on three areas are presented in this paper: a) descriptors that were used by the informants to describe the program; b) metaphors (i.e., incidents, objects or feelings) that were used by the informants to stand for the program; and c) implementers' perceptions of the benefits of the program to students.

Ideological biases and preoccupations as well as strategies to deal with them

Shek, Tang and Han (20) argued for the importance of discussing the ideological biases and preoccupations of the researchers in a qualitative evaluation report (Principle 4). As program developers, the authors might have the preoccupation that the implemented program was good and it was beneficial to the students. In addition, the researchers might have the tendency to look at positive evidence rather than negative evidence. Thus, it is important to discuss how such biases were addressed in this study (20). Several safeguards against the subtle influence of such ideological biases and preoccupations were included in the process of the study (Principle 5). First, the researchers were conscious of the existence of ideological preoccupation (e.g., positive youth development programs are beneficial to adolescents) and carried out data collection and analyses procedures in a disciplined manner. Second, although the analyses and interpretations were mainly carried out by the first author with the assistance of the two research assistants, apart from conducting intra-rater reliability, inter-rater reliability checks on the coding were also carried out, i.e., 20 responses were randomly selected from raw responses by the first author and were recoded by two other research assistants who did not know the original codes given at the end of the scoring process (Principle 6). Third, multiple researchers and research assistants were involved in the data collection and analyses processes (Principle 7). Fourth, the tapes, transcriptions, and steps involved in the development of coding system and interpretations were properly documented and systematically organized for audit trails (Principle 9).

Results

For the descriptors used by the informants to describe the program, there were 107 raw descriptors and they could be further categorized into 40 categories (see Table 2). Among these descriptors, 59 (55.14%) of them were coded as positive descriptors. After discarding the data from the school implementing the program without trained instructor, there were 57 (55.34%) raw descriptors coded as positive among 103 raw descriptors. Analyses showed that intra-rater agreement percentage was 90% and inter-rater agreement percentage was 85%, which suggested that the reliability of coding of the positivity of the responses was high in this part of analyses.

For the metaphors that were used by the informants to stand for the program, there were 32 raw "objects" involving 49 related attributes (see Table 3). The findings showed that 14 metaphors (43.75%) could be regarded as positive metaphors and 26 attributes (53.06%) could be regarded as positive attributes. If the data from the school implementing the program without trained instructor were discarded, there were 30 raw "objects" involving 45 related attributes. And the findings showed that 12 metaphors (40%) could be regarded as positive metaphors and 23 attributes (51.11%) could be regarded as positive attributes. The reliability of coding of the positivity of the responses was high because analyses showed that intra-rater agreement percentage and inter-rater agreement percentage were 80% and 85%, respectively.

Regarding the perceived benefits of the program for the program participants, 203 responses were recorded involving 35 attribute categories (see Table 4). The findings showed that 139 responses (68.47%) were coded as positive responses. If discarding the data from the school implementing the program without trained instructor, there were 128 responses (69.57%) were coded as positive among 184 raw responses. Analyses showed that intra-rater agreement percentage and inter-rater agreement percentage were 85% and 90%, respectively, which suggested that the reliability of coding of the positivity of responses was very high in this part of the analyses.

Discussion

This paper attempts to examine the perceptions of the program instructors regarding the qualities and effectiveness of the Tier 1 Program of the P.A.T.H.S. Project. Two major conclusions can be drawn from the qualitative evaluation findings obtained in this study. First, both positive and negative perceptions of the program were observed (see Table 2). While some informants regarded the program to be fun and relaxed, some perceived the program to be superficial. However, it is noteworthy that positive responses basically outnumbered negative ones. Similarly, although both positive and negative responses were found for the question on metaphor (see Table 3), positive responses outnumbered the negative ones.

Second, although the findings related to respondents' perception of program were not altogether positive, it is noteworthy that the findings in Table 4 suggest that most of the program implementers perceived the program to be beneficial to students, with 68% (the result of this part was 70% when disregarding the interview data based on the school without trained instructor) of the responses coded as positive responses. Based on the analyses, the benefits on the personal level were most significant among the three levels of competence. For instances, positive self-image (e.g., enhanced self-confidence, enhanced self-understanding), cognitive competence (e.g., enhanced critical thinking), reflection (e.g., enhanced understanding of purpose of life), moral competence (e.g., enhanced sense of equality) and behavioral competence (e.g., promoted presentation skills) were observed. In addition, the benefits on the interpersonal level, especially social skills (e.g., learned to share and express oneself) were also reported by many informants. Furthermore, benefits in family relationships (e.g., improved communication and relationship with family members) on familial level were also observed. These observations are consistent with the objective outcome evaluation findings of Shek (25) that the students changed in the positive direction in various outcome indicators. With reference to the principle of triangulation, the present study and the previous findings suggest that based on quantitative and qualitative evaluation findings, evidence on the positive effect of the Tier 1 Program on holistic youth development among the program participants is present.

However, it should be noted that some negative responses were recorded in the present study. For example, some program instructors perceived the program as superficial, difficult and chaotic (see Table 2), some used negative metaphors to stand for the program (e.g., tasteless water, see Table 3), and some rated the program as not helpful to the students (see Table 4). In response to Principle 11 proposed by Shek, Tang and Han (20), there are explanations for these negative evidences. First, since only two of the interviewed schools had familiarized themselves with the implementation of Project P.A.T.H.S. through participating in the Experimental Implementation Phase, it was the first year for the program implementers of the other seven schools to launch the program in the Full Implementation Phase. Therefore, negative comments were inevitable due to the fact that instructors might need time to adopt a new program in their schools. Second, as the program implementers were teachers and social workers who were specialized in classroom teaching and field/group work, respectively, both of them might feel challenging to adjust their professional skills in order to carry out a manual-based positive youth program in the classroom context. Third, as the respondents were encouraged to voice out both positive and negative viewpoints in the focus group interviews, it is normal to receive negative comments.

Shek, Tang and Han (20) suggested that it is important to consider alternative explanations in the interpretations of qualitative evaluation findings (Principle 10). There are several possible alternative explanations for the present findings. First, the findings can be explained in terms of demand characteristics. However, this explanation is not likely because the informants were encouraged to voice out their views without restriction and negative voices were in fact heard. The second alternative explanation is that the findings are due to selection bias. However, this argument is not strong as the schools and program implementers were randomly selected. The third alternative explanation is that the positive findings are due to ideological biases of the researchers. As several safeguards were used to reduce biases in the data collection and analysis processes, this possibility is not high. Finally, it may be argued that the perceived benefits are due to other youth enhancement programs. However, this argument can be partially dismissed as none of the schools in this study participated in the major youth enhancement programs in Hong Kong, including the Adolescent Health Project. In addition, respondents in the focus group interviews were specifically asked about the program effects of the Project P.A.T.H.S. only.

With reference to the argument of Shek, Tang and Han (20) that the authors should discuss the limitations of the qualitative evaluation studies conducted (Principle 12), the limitations of the study are outlined below. First, although the number of schools and program implementers participating in the study can be regarded as acceptable using standards in the mainstream qualitative evaluation studies, it would be helpful if more schools and instructors could be recruited. Second, in addition to the one-shot focus group interviews, it would be illuminating if regular and on-going qualitative evaluation data could be collected. Third, although observation data has been collected (12), the inclusion of other qualitative evaluation strategies such as in-depth individual interviews would be helpful to further understand the subjective experiences of the program implementers. Finally, although eleven principles proposed by Shek, Tang and Han (20) were upheld in this study, peer checking and member checking (Principle 8) were not carried out in this study because of time and manpower constraints. Despite these limitations, this study provides pioneering qualitative evaluation findings supporting the positive nature of the Project P.A.T.H.S. and its effectiveness in promoting holistic youth development among Chinese adolescents in Hong Kong.

Acknowledgments

The preparation for this paper and the Project P.A.T.H.S. were financially supported by The Hong Kong Jockey Club Charities Trust.

References

[1] Patton MQ. Utilization-focused evaluation: the new century text. Thousand Oaks, CA: Sage, 1997.

[2] Shek DTL, editor. Special Issue: evaluation of Project P.A.T.H.S. in Hong Kong. ScientificWorldJournal 2008;8:1-94.

[3] Chatterji M. Applying the Joint Committee's 1994 standards in international contexts: a case study of education evaluations in Bangladesh. Teach Coll Rec 2005;107(10):2372-400.

[4] Slayton J, Llosa L. The use of qualitative methods in large-scale evaluation: improving the quality of the evaluation and the meaningfulness of the findings. Teach Coll Rec 2005;107(12):2543-65.

[5] Shek DTL. Adolescent developmental issues in Hong Kong: relevance to positive youth development programs in Hong Kong. Int J Adolesc Med Health 2006;8:341-54.

[6] Catalano RF, Berglund ML, Ryan JAM, Lonczak HS, Hawkins JD. Positive youth development in the United States: research findings on evaluations of positive youth development programs. Prev Treatment 2002. Accessed 2008 Nov 01. URL: http://aspe.hhs.gov/hsp/PositiveYouthDev99/

[7] Shek DTL, Siu AMH, Lee TY, Cheung CK, Chung R. Effectiveness of the Tier 1 Program of Project P.A.T.H.S.: objective outcome evaluation based on a randomized group trial. ScientificWorldJournal 2008;8:4-12.

[8] Shek DTL, Ma HK. Subjective outcome evaluation of the Project P.A.T.H.S.: findings based on the perspective of the program participants. ScientificWorldJournal 2007;7:47-55.

[9] Shek DTL, Siu AMH, Lee TY. Subjective outcome evaluation of the Project P.A.T.H.S.: findings based on the perspective of the program implementers. ScientificWorldJournal 2007;7:195-203.

[10] Shek DTL, Sun RCF. Subjective outcome evaluation of the Project P.A.T.H.S.: qualitative findings based on the experiences of program implementers. ScientificWorldJournal 2007;7:1024-35.

[11] Shek DTL, Sun RCF. Subjective outcome evaluation of the Project P.A.T.H.S.: qualitative findings based on the experiences of the program participants. ScientificWorldJournal 2007;7:686-97.

[12] Shek DTL, Ma HK, Sun RCF, Lung DWM. Process evaluation of the Tier 1 Program (Secondary 1 Curriculum) of the Project P.A.T.H.S.: findings based on the Full Implementation Phase. ScientificWorldJournal 2008;8:35-46.

[13] Shek DTL, Lee TY, Sun RCF. Process evaluation of the implementation of the Secondary 2 program of Project P.A.T.H.S. in the Experimental Implementation Phase. ScientificWorldJournal. 2008;8:83-94.

[14] Shek DTL, Sun RCF. Implementation of the Tier 1 Program of the Project P.A.T.H.S.: interim evaluation findings. ScientificWorldJournal 2006;6:2274-84.

[15] Shek DTL, Shik AWY. Qualitative evaluation of the Project P.A.T.H.S. in Hong Kong: findings based on program implementers. Int J Adol Med Health, in press.

[16] Shek DTL, Lee TY, Siu A, Lam CM. Qualitative evaluation of the Project P.A.T.H.S. based on the perceptions of the program participants. ScientificWorldJournal 2006;6:2254-63.
[17] Shek DTL, Sun RCF. Implementation of a positive youth development program in a Chinese context: the role of policy, program, people, process, and place. ScientificWorldJournal 2008;8:960-96.
[18] Shek DTL, Chak YLY, Chan CWY. School-related factors in the implementation of a positive youth development project in Hong Kong. ScientificWorldJournal 2008;8:997-1009.
[19] Shek DTL, Sun RCF, Lam CM, Lung DWM, Lo SC. Evaluation of Project P.A.T.H.S. in Hong Kong: utilization of student weekly dairy. ScientificWorldJournal 2008;8:13-21.
[20] Shek DTL, Tang V, Han XY. Quality of qualitative evaluation studies in the social work literature: evidence that constitutes a wakeup call. Res Soc Work Prac 2005;15:180-94.
[21] Denzin K, Lincoln YS. The Sage handbook of qualitative research. Thousand Oaks, CA: Sage, 2005.
[22] Shek DTL, Lam MC, Lam CM, Tang V. Perceptions of present, ideal, and future lives among Chinese adolescents experiencing economic disadvantage. Adolesc 2004;39:779-92.
[23] Stufflebeam DL. The CIPP model for evaluation. In: Stufflebeam DL, Medaus GF, Kellaghan T, editors. Evaluation models: viewpoints on educational and human services evaluation. Boston: Kluwer, 2000:279-318.
[24] Shek DTL, Ng HY, Lam CW, Lam OB, Yeung KC. A longitudinal evaluation study of a pioneering drug prevention program (Project Astro MIND) in Hong Kong. Hong Kong: Univ Hong Kong, 2003.
[25] Shek DTL. Evaluation of Project P.A.T.H.S. in Hong Kong: triangulation of findings based on different evaluation strategies. ScientificWorldJournal 2008;8:1-3.

***Submitted*:** December 11, 2008.
Revised: December 30, 2008.
Accepted: January 28, 2009

In: Public Health Yearbook 2009
Editor: Joav Merrick

ISBN: 978-1-61668-911-7

Chapter 26

Evaluation of Project P.A.T.H.S. using Students' Weekly Diaries: Replication based on Secondary 2 Students

Daniel TL Shek, PhD, FHKPS, BBS, JP*[*1,2,3]
and Ching Man Lam, BSSc, MSW, PhD[4]

[1]Department of Applied Social Sciences, The Hong Kong Polytechnic University, Hong Kong, PRC, [2]Department of Sociology, East China Normal University, Shanghai, PRC [3]Kiang Wu Nursing College of Macau, Macau, PRC and [4]Department of Social Work, The Chinese University of Hong Kong, Hong Kong, PRC

Abstract

Four schools participating in the Experimental Implementation Phase of the Project P.A.T.H.S. (Secondary 2 Level) were randomly selected to join this qualitative evaluation study. After completion of the Tier 1 Program, 260 secondary 2 (Grade 8) students in these four participating schools were invited to write a reflective journal in the form of weekly diary to reveal their perceptions and feelings regarding the Tier 1 Program and the related benefits. Results of the qualitative data analyses showed that most of the respondents (a) had positive views on the program, (b) had positive views on the instructors, and (c) stated that they had acquired competencies at societal, familial, interpersonal and personal levels after joining the program. The present qualitative findings based on students' weekly diaries are generally consistent with the previous evaluation findings using students' diaries and other evaluation strategies.

Keywords: Project P.A.T.H.S., weekly diaries, qualitative evaluation; positive youth development program.

* Correspondence: Professor Daniel TL Shek, PhD, FHKPS, BBS, JP, Chair Professor of Applied Social Sciences, Department of Applied Social Sciences, The Hong Kong Polytechnic University, Hunghom, Hong Kong. E-mail: danielshek@inet.polyu.edu.hk

Introduction

The use of diaries or "documents of life" is common within the historical and anthropological tradition. For example, "Anne Frank: The Diary of a Young Girl" is a famous book that records the events, thoughts, feelings and dreams of a Jewish teenage girl who had fled and hid in Amsterdam with her family when Nazi Germany conquered the Netherlands. This diary is popular because it is a documentation reflecting an adolescent's development, and at the same time revealing the historical events of the Holocaust living during World War II. Other famous autobiographies are "The diary of Virginia Woolf" and "The Stone diaries".

According to Allport (1), diary is a "self-revealing record that intentionally or intentionally yields information regarding the structure, dynamics and functioning of the author's mental life" (p.xii). In the context of social sciences research, diaries for analyzing human behavior, discovering history or evaluating a program represent an attractive research approach. In diary studies, people provide reports on the events and experiences of their lives and these reports capture the particulars of experiences in a way that is not possible using traditional research design. The use of diary in non-experimental research becomes popular and this method is used to collect data on human behavior. For example, Leigh (2) asked the participants to record the time, quantity and type of drinking and sexual activity over 10 weeks in order to examine the temporal relationships of alcohol consumption to sexual behavior. Behavioral diary has also been used in behavioral modification programs (3). Social interaction diaries have also been used to examine the relationship between attachment styles and social activity (4). However, there are researches showing the strengths and weaknesses of using daily diaries as a research strategy (5-6) and the debate has continued in the literature (7-8).

In the field of education and social work training, teachers and social workers are generally trained to be reflective practitioners. Teachers are expected to keep diary or reflective journal which records their lesson planning and reflection on the teaching processes, and student social workers are encouraged to write recordings or logs to reflect on their practice. According to Hobson (9), a reflective journal "suggests questions, identifies new areas to explore, reveals meaningful absences, and uncovers recurring patterns" (p.16). Some researchers utilized teachers' reflective diaries as a kind of data collection methods to investigate the essential components of effective teaching practice (10) or pedagogy (11), and to examine ways contributing to professional development (12). Similarly, students are seen as active learners under the reflective practice movement where reflection is seen as an indispensable process in translating concrete experiences to concepts and action (13-14). As such, keeping diary is considered as an opportunity for personal reflection that in turn enhances students' autonomy and develops an ownership of their learning process (15). This process invariably leads to increased self-awareness, increased sensitivity to the environment and a change in conceptual perspective.

There are different ways of using diaries or reflective journals as a form of student learning. The most common form is to encourage students to be critical and reflective learners by recording their thoughts and opinions (16). The second form is the reflective practice type in which dairy is used for the purpose of strengthening students' ability in integrating theory with field practice (17). The third one is future-oriented where the current practices are analyzed and synthesized and new directions are explored (18). Chaloner (19) affirmed that "using a personal journal implies that the learner will construct a memory of the learning experience and how it can be applied to the workplace by using a personal narrative. Through such an individualized and personal approach, it is hoped that the learner will be motivated enough to assume the autonomy that he/she is being offered" (p. 22).

The use of diaries as the method of choice for qualitative research in the field of social science is relatively rare (20), either internationally or locally. In Hong Kong, there are very few researches using diary as a form of data collection, particularly in the education field (21). Although primary and secondary schools commonly require students to write weekly diaries, teachers only read and write down comments after reading and the wealth of data and resources has not been utilized. With the ease of collecting students' weekly diaries in the secondary schools in Hong Kong, the present study utilized students' weekly diaries as a research strategy to evaluate the effectiveness of the Project P.A.T.H.S. The aim of the study was to make explicit students' experiences, feelings and thoughts after participating in the program and to solicit students' view of the project. Schools joining the Project P.A.T.H.S. were invited to ask their students to write down their perceptions and feelings in their weekly dairies. As the project had already collected students' views on the program in terms of quantitative data generated from structured questionnaires, as well as qualitative data generated from the open-ended questions from questionnaires and focus group interviews, it is hoped that the information collected from weekly diaries can act as another kind of qualitative data for understanding the students' perceptions of the program in a comprehensive manner.

Methods

There were 49 schools joining the Tier 1 Program (Secondary 2 level) of the Experimental Implementation Phase of the Project P.A.T.H.S. (Positive Adolescent Training through Holistic Social Programmes) in 2006/2007. In the Tier 1 Program, 21 schools adopted the full program (i.e., 20-hour program involving 40 units) and 28 schools adopted the core program (i.e. 10-hour program involving 20 units).

After completion of the Tier 1 Program, four schools were randomly selected to join this research study. The school teachers were asked to randomly invite some Secondary 2 students to write a journal in the form of weekly diary to reveal their perceptions and feelings after joining the Tier 1 Program. Although the students' identity was revealed when they handed in the weekly diaries to their teachers, their identity remained anonymous when a copy of their work was sent to the Research Team.

The students were informed of the purpose of this study, and that the information they had given would be kept confidential for research use only. The students' willingness to join the study was respected and their consent of participation was sought.

All of the four schools were co-educational schools which had adopted the full program. The mean number of Secondary 2 students in these schools was 180.25 (ranged from 160 to 201), and each school had 4 to 5 classes.

The mean number of teachers and social workers who taught the Tier 1 Program per school were 4.55 (ranged from 0 to 12) and 2.27 (ranged from 0 to 6), respectively. The total number of students' weekly diaries received was 260, which was about 36% of the total

Secondary 2 students in these four schools. As the number of cases in qualitative study is commonly not high, the number of weekly diaries collected in this study can be regarded as respectable.

Instruments

The students were randomly selected by the school concerned. In order to ensure consistency of the data collecting procedure, a clear guideline of data collection was given to the teachers concerned. The students were asked to write a reflective journal with the title of *"Participating in the Tier 1 Program of Project P.A.T.H.S: Experiences and feelings"*. The length of the reflection journal was not less than 200 words (in Chinese) and it should be related to the students' experiences, feelings and comments after joining the Tier 1 Program. There was no specific requirement on how to write it. The students could either complete it at their home or during class time.

Data analyses

The data were analyzed using general qualitative analyses techniques (22) by two trained research assistants, one with a Bachelor degree in Social Work and another with a Bachelor degree in Psychology. The primary analyses were counter-checked by another trained research assistant who had a Master degree in Social Work. There were three steps in the data analysis process. First, relevant raw codes were developed for words, phrases and/or sentences that formed meaningful units at the raw responses level. Second, the codes were further combined to reflect higher-order attributes at the category of codes level. Third, the categories of codes were further analyzed to reveal the broader themes at the thematic level. For example, the response of "the program content is practical" at the raw response level could be subsumed under the category of "program content" which could further be subsumed under the broad theme of "views about program" (see Table 1).

In the present qualitative analyses, as the researchers designed the program in the Project P.A.T.H.S., they were conscious of their own biases and expectations of the program to be effective. As such, they were not directly involved in the first few steps of the data analyses. In addition, to minimize the possible biases involved, both intra-rater and inter-rater reliability on the coding was calculated.

Table 1. Views about program and instructors

Area	Subcategory	Item	N	N in Subcategory	Total
Views about program	Overall impression	Appreciate the program/activities/format	105	295	684
		The project is meaningful	37		
		Rewarding	34		
		Change in perception	21		
		Like the program	16		
		Perfect/excellent/very good	16		
		Matches adolescents' need	15		
		Better than other programs	11		
		The program is good	7		
		Glad to participate in the program	6		
		Satisfied with the program	4		
		The program is special	2		
		Fair	3		
		The program is meaningless (Negative)	6		
		Not interested in the program (Negative)	6		
		Dislike the program (Negative)	4		
		The program is bad (Negative)	2		
	Program content	Program content is practical	46	76	
		Diverse topics/rich content	13		
		Program content is interesting	5		
		Program content can be easily understood	4		
		Dissatisfied (Negative)	8		
	Learning process	Happy	47	203	
		Students' active participation	21		
		Interesting	20		
		Relaxed/Free	15		
		Funny	2		
		Not dull	2		
		Boring (Negative)	51		
		Uninvolved in the program (Negative)	12		
		Discontent with length and number of sessions (Negative)	12		
		Nonsense (Negative)	11		
		Discontent with implementation (Negative)	4		
		Too many worksheets (Negative)	3		
		Little interaction (Negative)	3		
	Other comments and suggestions	Suggestions	54	110	
		Wish to join P.A.T.H.S. again	32		
		Hope others can participate in P.A.T.H.S.	1		
		Unwilling to join (Negative)	3		
		Positive comments	10		
		Neutral comments	7		
		Negative comments (Negative)	3		

Table 1. (Continued)

Area	Subcategory	Item	N	N in Subcategory	Total N
Views about instructors	Overall impression	Appreciate instructor	24	44	159
		Instructor was pleasing	14		
		Wish to be taught by the instructor again	3		
		Instructor often blamed (Negative)	3		
	Teaching performance	Instructor was well prepared for the program	16	37	
		Professional teaching	12		
		Instructor's performance was excellent	6		
		Teaching was boring (Negative)	3		
	Teaching attitude	Enthusiastic	21	40	
		Will/able to help students	8		
		Instructor was caring and encouraging	7		
		Involved	4		
	Teaching process	Teaching was interesting and vivid	17	18	
		Teaching pace was too fast (Negative)	1		
	Other comments and suggestions	Suggestions	12	20	
		Positive	3		
		Neutral	2		
		Negative (Negative)	3		
TOTAL					843

Note. Twenty coded raw descriptors were randomly selected from examining intra- and inter-rater reliability. The raters were required to code the randomly selected descriptors into two categories (i.e., views about program and views about instructors) without knowing the original codes given.

For intra-rater reliability, the research assistants individually coded 20 randomly selected responses for each question. For inter-rater reliability, another two research assistants (one with a Master degree and another with a Bachelor degree) coded 20 randomly selected responses for each question without knowing the original codes given at the end of the scoring process with reference to the codes finalized by the first author.

Following the principles of qualitative analyses (23), the following attributes of the study regarding data collection and analyses are highlighted: 1) a general qualitative orientation was adopted; 2) recruitment process for the participants and justifications for the number of participants are clearly described; 3) details of the data collection are given; 4) issues of biases and ideological preoccupation are addressed; 5) inter-rater and intra-rater reliability information is presented; 6) the categorized data were kept in by a systematic filing system in order to ensure that the findings are auditable.

Results

As shown in Table 1, 843 meaningful units regarding the students' perceptions of the Tier 1 Program and the instructors could be categorized into two categories (i.e., views about program and views about instructors). In the aspect of "views about program", there were 684 responses which could be categorized into "overall impression", "program content", "learning process", and "other comments and suggestions". Most of the respondents had positive views on the "overall impression" (N=277), such as "appreciate the program/activities/format" (N=105) and "the project is meaningful" (N=37), while some had negative impression, such as "the program is meaningless" (N=6). Many respondents showed their views about the "learning process" (N=203), with both positive comments such as "happy" (N=47) and negative views such as "boring" (N=51).

Table 2. Perceived benefits to students

Level of Competence	Subcategory	Item	N	N in Subcategory	Total N
Societal level	Social norms	Following social norms	3	3	11
	Social responsibility and affairs	Prosocial involvement	4	8	
		Citizen's responsibilities	3		
		Knowledge about China and Hong Kong	1		
Familial level	Family relationships	To get along with family members	12	12	12
Interpersonal level	General interpersonal competence	To get along with others	41	147	175
		Connection between people	22		
		Social competence	21		
		Team spirit	18		
		Communication skills	18		
		Presentation ability	15		
		Making friends	6		
		Handling love affairs	4		
		To differentiate between healthy and unhealthy friends	2		
	Specific interpersonal competence	Respect	10	28	
		Caring for and helping others	9		
		Empathy	6		
		Politeness	3		
Personal level	Cherishing life	To enrich/cherish life	41	53	429
		To treasure people and things	12		
	Reflection	Wisdom of life	28	37	
		Self-reflection	9		
	Cognitive competence	Rational thinking and analytical thinking	26	54	
		Problem solving	22		
		Cognitive competence	6		
	Ways to face adversity	Optimism	9	33	
		Resilience	24		
	Positive self-image	Personal growth	34	88	
		Self-understanding	28		
		Self determination	15		
		Self-confidence	9		
		Self-efficacy	2		
	Emotional competence	Emotional management	28	28	
	Goal setting	Goal setting	29	29	
	Responsibility	Responsibility	7	7	
	Healthy life	Healthy life	12	12	

Table 2. (Continued)

Level of Competence	Subcategory	Item	N	N in Subcategory	Total N
	Moral competence and virtues	Personal ethics	25	47	
		To distinguish between right and wrong	19		
		To correct bad habits / defects	3		
	Learning and knowledge	Learnt a lot of knowledge	31	41	
		Interest in learning	10		
Others			8	8	8
TOTAL					635

Note. Twenty coded raw descriptors were randomly selected from examining intra- and inter-rater reliability. The raters were required to code the randomly selected descriptors into four categories (i.e., societal, familial, interpersonal and personal) without knowing the original codes given.

On the other hand, there were 159 responses of "views about instructors", which were categorized into "overall impression" (N=44, e.g., "the instructor was pleasing"), "teaching performance" (N=37, e.g., "instructor's performance was excellent"), "teaching attitude" (N=40, e.g., "involved"), "teaching process" (N=18, e.g., "teaching was interesting and vivid") and "others" (N=20). In total, there were 83.63% positive responses regarding the students' perceptions of the program and instructors. The intra-rater agreement percentage was 100% and inter-rater agreement percentage was 85% as far as the positivity of the responses are concerned.

The perceived benefits of the program to the students are shown in Table 2. There were a total of 635 meaningful units which could be categorized in five categories (i.e., societal, familial, interpersonal, personal levels of competence and others). Most of the respondents reported that they had learnt personal competence (N=429), particularly in the subcategory of "positive self-image" (N=88, e.g., "personal growth"), following by "cognitive competence" (N=54, e.g., "rational thinking and analytical thinking"), "cherishing life" (N=53, e.g., "to enrich /cherish life"), and "moral competence and virtues" (N=47, e.g., "personal ethics"). In addition, many respondents reported that they had acquired interpersonal competence (N=175), which could be categorized into "general interpersonal competence" (N=147, e.g., "get along with others") and "specific interpersonal competence" (N=28, e.g., "respect"). The intra-rater agreement percentage was 95% and inter-rater agreement percentage was 95% regarding the coding on the areas of competence.

Furthermore, the perceived changes in the students can be seen in the following three cases:

- *Student A in School 1*: "I understand there is a purpose in one's life and one should not give up his/her life easily. In this program, I have not only re-discovered myself and my strengths through the activities, but also learnt how to appreciate others, get along with others and listen to others. The most important thing is that I have had more friends and understood things and people around myself. After participating in this program, I have become happier and more open to accept my strengths and weaknesses. I thought of ending my life before. But when I think of my significant others, I know this would make them very sad. Therefore, I accept many things with an optimistic view now."

- *Student B in School 2:* "After the lessons, I always reflect on the program contents and think about whether I have practiced the principles involved. I also reflect on my life and I wish I could try my best to take up my responsibility. I will not give up easily. These useful teachings can be the energy in my daily life."
- *Student C in School 3*: "I think Life Education (P.A.T.H.S. lessons) let us learn many things. The learning is closely related to us, but we did not learn it specifically before. As such, this program can meet our needs (e.g., how to get along with others, how to distinguish "good" and "bad", and how to handle emotional problems). These are the things we face commonly and we can apply what we have learnt. It is really "putting what I learnt into practice". I think the things I learnt in Life Education (P.A.T.H.S. lessons) are useful not only at this moment, but also in the future (such as working attitudes, how to get along with new colleagues). These things are beneficial for me."

Discussion

Shek, Lam and Tsoi (24) pointed out that evidence-based social work practice is poorly developed in Hong Kong where systematic evaluation of social work services is lacking. As such, systematic and comprehensive evaluation can be seen as a unique feature of Project P.A.T.H.S. The research team conducted multi-year evaluation based on different strategies, including the use of weekly diaries (25). Generally speaking, both quantitative and qualitative evaluation findings suggest that different stakeholders perceive the program to be positive and effective.

Based on the weekly dairies collected from students in four randomly selected schools participating in the Experimental Implementation Phase of the Project P.A.T.H.S. (Secondary One Level), Shek, Sun, Lam, Lung and Lo (26) showed that most of the respondents had positive views on the program and the instructors and they stated that they had acquired competencies at societal, familial, interpersonal and personal levels after joining the program. An examination of the findings based on the weekly diaries written by the Secondary 2 students was identical to that of the Secondary 1 students. Both groups of students had positive perceptions of the program and the instructors, and they overwhelmingly regarded the program as beneficial to their own development. Furthermore, the present findings basically concur with both the quantitative and qualitative findings related to subjective outcome evaluation (25).

The present findings reveal that "program" and "people" factors are most significant to program success. Students' appreciation of the program, including its meaningfulness and practical nature can be regarded as program characteristics that promote student involvement. This observation is consistent with other qualitative evaluation findings that program characteristics including fun, meaningfulness and utility are valued by the program participants (27-28). Besides, the present findings highlight the importance of teacher/instructor quality. Consistent with other studies (29-31), the finding affirm that quality of the program implementer is the key to program success. Students express their appreciation of the instructors and their enthusiasm. The findings inform us that well-designed programs which can promote the involvement of students and instructors' willingness to implement the program in turn contribute to effective program implementation (32). Besides, training provided to teachers can familiarize teachers with the program philosophy and content, necessary teaching strategies, the need for fidelity, as well as cultivation of their enthusiasm and support for the program which in turn contribute to the program implementation quality (33).

According to Shek, Sun, Lam, Lung and Lo (26), there are several strengths of the diary method. The first strength is that reflective journal can consolidate learning experiences of the learners and allow students to experience behavior change. Unfortunately, due to resource constraint, this aspect had not been examined in the present study. The second strength is that in contrast to other artificial evaluation methods such as the use of self-report measurers in experimental designs, weekly diary is a naturalistic research method that has high ecological validity. The third strength is that reflective journals such as weekly diaries can act as a good tool for educational evaluation. In addition to the information collected from students' responses for course evaluation, teachers can also be invited to be researchers to record students' changes in several phases of the course in the format of weekly diaries in order to collect multiple data from different data sources. The final strength is that reflective journals capture the particulars of experiences and switch from measures based on between-person differences to those within-person changes (34). It helps to explain why people differ in variability rather than mean level. Besides, keeping the diary for a longer period of time allows studying change processes during major events and transitions, and is able to study interpersonal process using dyadic and group diary methods which yield richer and deeper understandings. Obviously, the second, third and fourth strengths of the diary method are clearly revealed in this study.

The present findings have significant implications to the development of youth research. The present study underscores the utility of using diaries to reveal experiences of the participants and the diary research method captures the particulars of experiences in a way that is not possible using traditional designs. The study supports the meaning of using diaries as an evaluation method and confirms that diary studies as a research method is particularly suitable for youth research. In fact, youths are eager to provide reports on experiences of their dairy life through various means (i.e. diary, log, personal blog, face book) and these documents are constructed within the diarist's own frame of reference. In future, researchers can consider using researcher-driven diaries, semi-private documents (personal blog) and other electronic forms of dairy for data collection and data triangulation when conducting youth research.

It is noteworthy that there are several weaknesses of weekly diaries as a qualitative evaluation method. First, students may have difficulties in writing down and disclosing their inner world to others. In particular, this method may not be a sensitive measure if the students are not good at using verbal techniques to express their experiences, such as students with poor academic performance and/or behavioral problems. Second, writing weekly diaries requires students' competencies on reflection and critical thinking but the students may lack experience and know-how for doing reflection. Third, Chinese people may lack the language to describe their feelings, the use of weekly diary technique may not be a sensitive tool that can gauge the feelings of the students. Fourthly, as a qualitative technique, weekly diaries inherit the basic problems of qualitative methods (23). In particular, biases generated by the workers and program participants should be addressed.

As an evaluation study utilizing student weekly diaries, the findings can be interpreted as evidence supporting the effectiveness of the Tier 1 Program of the Project P.A.T.H.S. Nevertheless, there are several possible explanations that should be considered. First, the findings are not representative. However, as the schools and participants were randomly selected, this alternative explanation can be dismissed. Second, the participants tried to play the role of good participants to please the teachers. Third, the positive findings may be a result of the threats from the teachers and social workers. Regarding the latter two explanations, as we have not checked with the participants, these two explanations are plausible. However, as students are encouraged to report their experience and there are no particular reasons for pleasing the workers, this possibility is not high. In future study, it is proposed that instead of asking the participants to write the reflective journal after the completion of the program, it would be more illuminating if the participants could be invited to engage in writing weekly diaries after each unit in a longitudinal manner.

Acknowledgments

The preparation for this paper and the Project P.A.T.H.S. were financially supported by The Hong Kong Jockey Club Charities Trust.

References

[1] Allport G. The use of personal documents in psychological science. New York: Soc Sci Res Council, 1943.

[2] Leigh BC. Alcohol consumption and sexual activity as reported with a diary technique. J Abnorm Psychol 1993;102(3):490-3.

[3] Peterson L, Tremblay G, Ewigman B, Popkey C. The parental daily diary: a sensitive measure of the process of change in a child maltreatment prevention program. Behav Modif 2002;26(5):627-47.

[4] Tidwell MC, Reis HT, Shaver PR. Attachment, attractiveness and social interaction: a diary study. Pers Soc Psy 1996;71(4):729-45.

[5] Leigh BC. Using daily reports to measure drinking and drinking patterns. J Subst Abuse 2000;12:51-65.

[6] Morrison DM, Leigh BC, Gillmore MR. Daily data collection: a comparison of three methods. J Sex Res 1999;36(1):76-81.

[7] Gillmore MR, Gaylord J, Hartway J, Hoppe MJ, Morrison DM, Leigh BC, Rainey DT. Daily data collection of sexual and other health-related behaviors. J Sex Res 2001;38(1):35-42.

[8] Stone AA, Kessler RC, Haythornthwaite JA. Measuring daily events and experiences: decisions for the researcher. J Pers 1991;59: 575-607.

[9] Hobson D. Beginning with the self: using autobiography and journal writing in research. In: Burnaford G, Fischer J, Hobson D. Teacher doing research: practical possibilities. Mahwah NJ: Erlbaum, 1996:1-17.

[10] Bartholomew H, Osborne J, Ratcliff M. Teaching students "ideas-about-science": five dimensions of effective practice. Sci Edu 2004;88(5):655-82.

[11] Reali AMMR, Mizukami MGN. Teachers construct a knowledge base for a Brazilian elementary school: analyzing a teaching-learning experience developed through university–public school partnership. Proceed Ann Meet Am Educ Res Assoc. New Orleans, LA, 2000.

[12] Mizukami MGN, Reali AMMR, Reysa CR, de Lima EF, Tancredi RMSP. Promoting and investigating professional development of elementary school teachers: contributions of a six-year public school-university collaborative partnership. Proceed Am Educ Res Assoc. Chicago, IL, 2003.
[13] Kolb DA. Experiential learning. Englewood Cliffs, NY: Prentice Hall, 1984.
[14] Lam CM, Wong H, Leung TTF. An unfinished reflexive journey: social work students' reflection on their placement experiences. Br J Soc Work 2007;37:91-105.
[15] Deci EL, Flaste R. Why we do what we do: understanding self-motivation. New York: Penguin, 1996.
[16] Rothwell A, Ghelipter S. The developing manager: reflective learning in undergraduate management education. Reflect Pract 2003;4(2):241-54.
[17] Ame N, Diepstra SA. Using intergenerational oral history service-learning projects to teach human behavior concepts: a qualitative analysis. Educ Gerontol 2006;32:721-35.
[18] McAllister L, McEwen E, Williams V, Frost N. Rural attachments for students in the health professions: are they worthwhile? Aust J Rural Health 1998;6:194-201.
[19] Chaloner B. An evaluative study on building the bridge between the training room and the workplace. Eva Res Educ 2006;19(1):21-37.
[20] Elliott H. The use of diaries in sociological research on health experience. Sociol Res Online 1997;2:2.
[21] Kember D. Interpreting student workload and the factors which shape students' perceptions of their workload. Stud High Educ 2004;29(2):165-184.
[22] Miles MB, Huberman AM. Qualitative data analysis. Thousand Oaks, CA: Sage, 1994.
[23] Shek DTL, Tang V, Han XY. Quality of qualitative evaluation studies in the social work literature: evidence that constitutes a wakeup call. Res Soc Work Pract 2005;15:180-94.
[24] Shek DTL, Lam MC, Tsoi KW. Evidence-based practice in Hong Kong. In: Thyer B, Kazi MAF. International perspectives on evidence-based practice in social work. London: Venture Press, 2004:167-81.
[25] Shek DTL, editor. Special Issue: evaluation of Project P.A.T.H.S. in Hong Kong. ScientificWorldJournal 2008;8:1-94.
[26] Shek DTL, Sun RCF, Lam CM, Lung DWM, Lo SC. Evaluation of Project P.A.T.H.S. in Hong Kong: utilization of student weekly dairy. ScientificWorldJournal 2008;8:13-21.
[27] Shek DTL, Ma HK. Subjective outcome evaluation of the Project P.A.T.H.S.: findings based on the perspective of the program participants. ScientificWorld Journal 2007;7:47-55.
[28] Shek DTL, Sun RCF. Subjective outcome evaluation of the Project P.A.T.H.S.: qualitative findings based on the experiences of the program participants. ScientificWorldJournal 2007;7:686-697.
[29] Kozol J. Savage inequalities. New York: HarperPerennial, 1991.
[30] Stringfield S. Attempting to enhance students' learning through innovative programs: the case for schools evolving into high reliability organizations. Sch Eff Sch Improv 1995;6:67-96.
[31] Teven JJ, Hanson TL. The impact of teacher immediacy and perceived caring on teacher competence and trustworthiness. Commun Q 2004;52:39-53.
[32] Ringwalt CL, Ennett S, Johnson R, Rohrback LA, Simons-Rudolpy A, Vincus A, Thorne J. Factors associated with fidelity to substance use prevention curriculum guides in the nation's middle school. Health Educ Behav 2003;30:375-91.
[33] Shek DTL, Wai CLY. Training workers implementing adolescent prevention and positive youth development programs: what have we learned from the literature? Adolesc 2008;43(172):823-46.
[34] Bolger N, Davis A, Rafaeli E. Dairy methods: capturing life as it is lived. Annu Rev Psychol 2003;54:579-616.

***Submitted*:** December 17, 2008.
Revised: December 30, 2008.
Accepted: January 31, 2009.

In: Public Health Yearbook 2009
Editor: Joav Merrick

ISBN: 978-1-61668-911-7

Chapter 27

INTERIM EVALUATION OF THE SECONDARY 3 PROGRAM OF PROJECT P.A.T.H.S.: INSIGHTS BASED ON THE EXPERIMENTAL IMPLEMENTATION PHASE

Daniel TL Shek, PhD, FHKPS, BBS, JP*[*1,2,3]*,
Rachel CF Sun, BSocSc, PhD[4] and Suet Yan Tam, BSSc, MPhil[4]
[1]Department of Applied Social Sciences, The Hong Kong Polytechnic University, Hong Kong, PRC, [2]Department of Sociology, East China Normal University, Shanghai, PRC, [3]Kiang Wu Nursing College of Macau, Macau, PRC and
[4]Department of Social Work, the Chinese University of Hong Kong, Hong Kong, PRC

Abstract

To evaluate the implementation quality of the Tier 1 Program (Secondary 2 Curriculum) of the Project P.A.T.H.S. in the Full Implementation Phase, 100 schools were randomly selected and participated in personal and/or telephone interviews regarding the implementation details of the Tier 1 Program. In the interviews, participants expressed their views on the students' responses and benefits of the program, appraisal of the positive and negative features of the program, and difficulties encountered during program implementation. Participants generally perceived that students had positive responses to the program and the program was perceived to be beneficial to the students, though negative comments and difficulties of program implementation were observed. They also perceived the Co-Walker Scheme to be beneficial. Consistent with previous findings, the present findings showed that the Tier 1 Program is generally perceived as helpful to the students and has positive global evaluation.

* Correspondence: Professor Daniel TL Shek, PhD, FHKPS, BBS, JP, Chair Professor of Applied Social Sciences, Department of Applied Social Sciences, The Hong Kong Polytechnic University, Hunghom, Hong Kong. E-mail: danielshek@inet.polyu.edu.hk

Keywords: Project P.A.T.H.S., interim evaluation, adolescents, positive youth development program.

Introduction

Positive **A**dolescent **T**raining through **H**olistic **S**ocial Programmes Project (P.A.T.H.S.) is a positive youth development program financially supported by The Hong Kong Jockey Club Charities Trust (1,2). The programs provide training to Secondary 1 to 3 students in Hong Kong. There are two implementation phases in the programs – Experimental Implementation Phase (2005/06 to 2007/08 school years) and Full Implementation Phase (2006/07 to 2008/2009 school years). A set of curriculum manuals are developed for the Tier 1 Program (1-3) which includes materials based on 15 positive youth development constructs identified from the existing successful positive youth development programs (4) Relevant research findings and experiences from existing programs in both local and foreign contexts were also taken as references in the development of the program manuals. Apart from program manuals and training workshops provided to program implementers, a "Co-Walker Scheme" has been launched since December 2006 to provide support to the implementers of the Tier 1 Program. The ultimate objective of this scheme is to provide ongoing support and guidance to the participating schools and their implementers and to promote communication between the Research Team and the program implementers.

One of the elements of a successful program is whether it achieves its objectives. Apparently, evaluation of programs is important which helps to assess whether the program achieves its goals. A series of evaluation programs were conducted to report the effects of the Tier 1 Program of Secondary 1 Curriculum (5-20) and Secondary 2 Curriculum (21-24) of the Project P.A.T.H.S. However, the evaluation reports of Secondary 2 Program mainly concentrated on programs conducted in the Experimental Implementation Phase. Only a few evaluation reports of Secondary 2 Program in the Full Implementation Phase have been published. Similar to the evaluation of the Secondary 1 Curriculum in the first year of the Experimental Implementation Phase (15) and Full Implementation Phase (16), an interim evaluation of the Secondary 2 Curriculum was conducted to examine the views of workers regarding the implementation of the Tier 1 Program during the Full Implementation Phase based on a random sample of schools joining the second year of the Full Implementation Phase in 2007/08 school year.

While it is important to examine outcomes of human service programs, there is increasing attention paid to the importance of looking at how intervention programs are implemented. As such, an interim evaluation during program implementation helps to enhance our understanding on the effectiveness and reactions of both workers and the targeted participants. In this study, information of the following areas was collected through interviews with implementers of the Tier 1 Program, 1) perceived students' responses, 2) perceived helpfulness of the program to students, 3) perceived positive aspects of the program, 4) suggestions for improvement of the program, 5) perceptions of difficulties encountered, 6) perceptions of the Co-Walker Scheme and 7) overall evaluation of the program.

Methods

Participants

There were 196 schools joining the Secondary 2 Program of the Project P.A.T.H.S. in the Full Implementation Phase in 2007/08 school year. Among these schools, 80 adopted the 20-hour full program that involving 40 teaching units and 116 adopted the 10-hour core program that involving 20 teaching units. Among the 100 participating schools, 61 schools joining the full program and 39 schools joining the core program were randomly selected to participate in this study. The instructors of the program (either school teachers or social workers) were invited to voluntarily participate in a face-to-face interview during a school visit. If the respondents were not available for interviews during the school visit, they were invited to participate in telephone interviews. Otherwise, they were invited to complete self-administered questionnaires and return via email or fax. Among these 100 schools, 55 of them participated in the face-to-face interviews, 30 participated in telephone interviews and 15 completed self-administered questionnaires. The respondents included 64 teachers and 50 social workers. Following Principle 2 regarding implementation of qualitative research suggested by Shek, Tang and Han (25), the number of schools participated in this research can be regarded as respectable as over half of the participating schools of the project in the Full Implementation Phase were randomly selected to join the interviews. Moreover, the generalizability of the findings could be guaranteed based on a set of randomly selected sample.

Procedures

The procedures for data collection are clearly presented below, and this satisfied Principle 3 in the procedures of conducting a qualitative research (25). The data collection was conducted between December 2007 and June 2008. This period can be regarded as midway of the implementation process, as the Full Implementation Phase took place from September 2007 to July 2008. In the face-to-face interviews, the responses of the respondents might be affected due to the social desirability effect. However, it is unlikely to happen because the interviewers were the co-walkers of the participating schools in which friendly rapport and mutual trust had been built. Also, the respondents were encouraged to freely express their positive and negative views.

A self-constructed semi-structured interview guide with five closed-ended questions and seven open-ended questions was used to collect information on the program implementation process. The open-ended questions were:

- Question 1: What are the responses of the students to this program?
- Question 2: Do you think this program is beneficial to the students? If yes, what are the benefits?
- Question 3: What are the good aspects of the program?
- Question 4: Which areas of the program require improvement?
- Question 5: Have you encountered any difficulties during the program implementation process? If yes, what problems have you encountered?

- Question 6: What are your perceptions of the "Co-Walker Scheme"?
- Question 7: Do you have other opinions?

Informed consent was obtained from the respondents and they participated in the study in a voluntary basis. The interviews were conducted by six co-walkers who were registered social workers with substantial working experience. After each interview, the interviewers were required to fill in the questionnaires. The completed questionnaires were then transcribed and analyzed.

Data analyses

For the quantitative data (closed-ended questions), frequencies and percentages of responses were calculated. The qualitative data (open-ended questions) were analyzed using general qualitative analyses techniques (26). There were three steps in the process. First, relevant raw codes were developed for words, phrases and/or sentences that formed meaningful units at the raw responses level. Second, the codes were further combined to reflect higher-order attributes at the category of codes level. Third, the categories of codes were further analyzed to reveal the broader themes at the thematic level. For instance, the response to "involved in discussion" at the raw response level could be subsumed under the category of "high student involvement" which could be further subsumed under the broad theme of "positive responses" of the students to the program (see table 2). Following the principles of qualitative analyses (25), the raw data and categorized data were kept in a systematic filing system in order to ensure that the findings are auditable.

The qualitative data were coded and categorized by a trained staff with a Master degree of Social Work and they were further checked by the second author. In the present analyses, as the researchers designed the program in the Project P.A.T.H.S., they were conscious of their own biases and expectations of the program to be effective. In addition, in order to minimize the possible biases involved, both intra-rater and inter-rater reliability on the coding was calculated. For intra-rater reliability, the trained staff and the second author individually coded 20 randomly selected responses for each question. For inter-rater reliability, one research assistant with a Master degree and one research assistant with a Bachelor degree who had not been involved in the data collection and analyses process coded 20 randomly selected responses for each question without knowing the original codes given at the end of the scoring process with reference to the codes finalized by the first author. This met the Principles 4, 5, 6, 7, 8, and 9 of conducting a qualitative study advocated by Shek, Tang and Han (25).

Results

Results showed that over 96% of the respondents reported that the students were involved and liked the program (Table 1) and about 73% of them perceived students' responses were positive (Table 2). The intra-rater agreement percentage on the positivity of coding was 97.5% and the inter-rater agreement percentage on the positivity of coding was 90% for the categorization of the responses reported in Table 2.

Table 1. Instructors' ratings of the Secondary 2 curriculum (N and Percentage)

1. Perceived degree of student involvement

	Totally not involved	Not involved	Involved	Totally involved	No response	Total
N	0	4	89	7	0	100
%	4%		96%		0%	100%

2. Perceived degree of students' liking of the Secondary 2 curriculum

	Strongly dislike	Dislike	Like	Strongly like	No response	Total
N	0	2	95	3	0	100
%	2%		98%		0%	100%

3. Perceived degree of helpfulness of the Secondary 2 curriculum

	Unhelpful	Not very helpful	Slightly helpful	Helpful	Very helpful	No response	Total
N	0	5	51	38	4	2	100
%	5%		93%			2%	100%

4. Perceived degree of workers' liking of Co-walker scheme

	Strongly dislike	Dislike	Like	Strongly like	No response	Total
N	0	1	83	10	6	100
%	1%		93%		6%	100%

5. Perceived degree of workers' overall satisfaction of the Secondary 2 curriculum

	Very dissatisfied	Dissatisfied	Slightly dissatisfied	Slightly satisfied	Satisfied	Very satisfied	No response	Total
N	0	0	4	28	66	2	0	100
%	4%			96%			0%	100%

Regarding the perceived benefits of the program to the students, nearly all respondents (95%) regarded the Tier 1 program of the Secondary 2 Curriculum was helpful (Table 1) and most of responses presented in Table 3 were positive in nature. The intra-rater agreement percentage on the positivity of coding was 90%, and the inter-rater agreement percentage on the positivity of coding was 82.5% for the categorization of the responses.

Table 2. Workers' perceptions of the responses of the students to the Secondary 2 curriculum

	Total Count
Positive Responses • High student involvement (e.g., "involved in discussion", "eager to participate", "willing to express their opinion", "actively responded to instructors' questions") (n=69) • Welcomed by students (e.g., "liked the program", "liked the class activities", "looking forward to attend the lessons") (n=27) • Attractive to students (e.g., "interested in the topics", "interested in the class activities", "the content could attract students", "felt happy/ relaxed in class") (n=18) • Other responses (e.g., "good responses", "satisfactory performance", "practical", "elicited self-reflection") (n=29)	143 (72.96%)

Table 2. (Continued)

Neutral Responses • "It depends on the content/ topics" (n=7) • "Some of the students were involved, some of them felt bored" (n=6) • "It depends on students' ability/ age/ gender" (n=6) • "Unable to have group activities" (n=1) • "Students refuse to self-disclose although they are involved in the program" (n=1)	21 (10.71%)
Negative Responses • Diminishing motivation (e.g. "Refused to/ seldom participate in class", "Negligent in class activities") (n=10) • Feeling bored (e.g., "students were not interested in some topics", "the content was not interesting") (n=8) • Other responses (e.g., "the content did not match student's need", "too rush", "too superficial") (n=14)	32 (16.33%)
Total (%)	196 (100%)

Table 3. Workers' perceptions of the benefits of the Secondary 2 curriculum

	Total Count (%)
Facilitating Students' Holistic Development/ Self-development • "It allows student to discuss/share growth issues" (n=2) • "The content caters students' growth need" (n=4) • "It helps students to understand themselves" (n=6) • "Improved self-efficacy" (n=1)	13 (9.22%)
Strengthening Students' Social Competence • "Building up interpersonal relationship" (n=26) • "Improving communication skills" (n=3) • "Strengthening social identity" (n=4)	33 (23.40%)
Strengthening Students' Behavioral, Cognitive, Emotional and Moral Competence • "It promotes students' thinking / reflection skills" (n=21) • "It promotes students' emotional management" (n=9) • "It promotes students' moral development" (n=15) • "It promotes students' positive behavior" (n=4)	49 (34.75%)
Facilitating Students' Learning	7 (4.96%)
• *"Active responses in class" (n=4)* • *"Strengthen knowledge in different area" (n=3)*	
Other Responses	39 (27.66%)
• *"Generally beneficial to students" (n=19)* • *"The benefits could not be determined" (n=8)* • *"No to minimal benefits" (n=12)*	
Total (%)	141 (100%)

Based on findings in Table 4, there were 137 meaningful units regarding the positive aspects of the program. The intra-rater agreement percentage of the categorization of the responses was 80%, and the inter-rater agreement percentage of the categorization of the responses was 82.5%. Furthermore, there were 150 meaningful units concerning the aspects of the program requiring improvement (Table 5). Nearly half of the responses indicated the "curriculum content and activity design" needed to be modified (48.67%), over one-fifth proposed improving the "teaching manuals and resources" (22.67%), over one-tenth of them suggested improving the "implementation time" (12%). The intra-rater agreement percentage of the categorization of the responses was 92.5%, and the inter-rater agreement percentage of the categorization of the responses was 87.5%. There were 155 meaningful units reported on workers' perception of difficulties encountered in program implementation (Table 6). Major responses were related to difficulties in "administration and co-ordination" (26.45%), which was followed by the perceived difficulties in handling "students' responses" (22.58%), "teachers' responses" (16.77%), as well as "time management" (14.84%). The intra-rater agreement percentage of the categorization of the responses was 87.5% and the inter-rater agreement percentage of the categorization of the responses was 82.5%.

Table 4. Workers' perceptions of the positive aspects of the Secondary 2 curriculum

	Total Count (%)
None /No Comment	4 (2.92%)
Teaching Manuals and Resources • Diverse and good teaching aids (e.g., "various multi-media resources", "attractive and diversified teaching aids", "creative and interesting activities") (n=24) • Good teaching manuals (e.g., "clear", "systematic", "user-friendly") (n=17) • Sufficient resources (n=1)	42 (30.66%)
Curriculum Content and Activity Design • Good curriculum content (e.g., "the content caters students' needs", "the topics are practical", "rich content", "comprehensive coverage", "clear instruction") (n=35) • Good activity design (e.g., "interesting", "attractive", "various activities") (n=29)	64 (46.72%)
Philosophy • "It meets student's needs" (n=4) • "Good theoretical basis" (n=4)	8 (5.84%)
Beneficial to Teachers and Students • "It improves relationship between teacher and students" (n=4) • Beneficial to students (e.g., "creativity", "reflection", "moral value') (n=9)	13 (9.49%)
Other Responses • "Training workshops/ co-walker scheme are good" (n=4) • "Provide informal civil education" (n=1) • "It is good to give presents to students as reinforcement" (n=1)	6 (4.38%)
Total (%)	137 (100%)

Regarding the workers' perception of the "Co-Walker Scheme" (Table 7), over 50% of the responses were positive, about 30% were "no comment", and only about 2% were negative comments. The intra-rater agreement percentage of the categorization of the responses was 90% and the inter-rater agreement percentage of the categorization of the responses was 82.5%. Generally, there were about 93% and 96% of the respondents expressed that they liked the program and felt satisfied, respectively (Table 1). The responses to the open-ended question of other opinions of the project were shown in Table 8. The responses were generally about suggestions on improvement on the curriculum content and activity design as well as comments on human and financial resources. The intra-rater agreement percentage of the categorization of the responses was 87.5%, and the inter-rater agreement percentage of the categorization of the responses was 80%.

Table 5. Workers' perceptions of the aspects of the Secondary 2 curriculum that require improvement

	Total Count (%)
None	11 (7.33%)
Curriculum Content and Activity Design • "The content/ activities does not suit students' need" (n=9) • "The content is too broad / too superficial/ too difficult/ outdated" (n=38) • "Too many activities/ add more activities/ increase variety/ revise activity format" (n=17) • Other responses (e.g., "growth puzzle is helpless", "discussion topic is not suitable for students", "difficult to carry out some activities") (n=9)	73 (48.67%)
Teaching Manuals and Resources • "Add more multi-media teaching aids/ insufficient teaching aids" (n=15) • "The video/ powerpoint/ teaching materials are boring / simple / naive" (n=5) • "Teaching manuals are not clear/ user-friendly/ suitable for all schools" (n=10) • Other responses (e.g., "upload updated video/ content onto the web", "teaching manual contains wrong information", "to have WORD document version") (n=4)	34 (22.67%)
Implementation Time • "There is insufficient time for running the activities" (n=9) • "Time is pressing" (n=4) • Other responses (e.g., "difficult to arrange time-table", "the teaching schedule should be more flexible") (n=5)	18 (12.00%)
Other Responses	14 (9.33%)
• *Need improvement in school administration (e.g., "classroom is too small for class activities", "not enough manpower", "incorporate into formal curriculum") (n=4)* • *"Give more flexibility to school" (n=3)* • *"Need more training workshops/ training workshops hold on September" (n=3)* • *"Too many Tier 2 participants needed for school chosen core program" (n=1)* • *"Need better collaboration with NGO" (n=1)* • *"Need guidelines for the usage of funding" (n=1)* • *"Revise the content of Tier 1 with reference to opinion collected" (n=1)*	
Total (%)	150 (100%)

Table 6. Workers' perceptions of the difficulties encountered in Secondary 2 curriculum implementation

	Total Count
None / No Comment	20 (12.90%)
Administration and Co-ordination • "It was difficult to arrange the teaching time-table" (n=12) • "There were difficulties in arranging manpower" (n=13) • "The physical classroom setting/ facilities were limited for running activities" (n=7) • Other responses (e.g., "little support from NGOs", "had to tailor make the teaching materials", "difficult to arrange teachers for training") (n=9)	41 (26.45%)

Time Management • "There was insufficient time to run the program" (n=11) • "Time was pressing" (n=8) • Other responses (e.g., "too much time for one unit", "insufficient time for competing the entire program") (n=4)	23 (14.84%)
Teachers' Responses • "Teachers had to spent much time for preparation" (n=5) • "Teachers did not identify with the rationale of the program" (n=7) • "Lacked of trained staff" (n=4) • "Too heavy workload" (n=4) • Other responses (e.g., "it was difficult to arrange cooperation", "teachers had role confusion", "some topics were difficult to teach in class") (n=6)	26 (16.77%)
Students' Responses • "Classroom discipline was a problem" (n=9) • "Students were not attentive / not involved" (n=15) • "Students did not understand/ were not interested in the content" (n=7) • Other responses (e.g., "some students dominated in discussion", "students completed the growth puzzle/ worksheets carelessly") (n=4)	35 (22.58%)
Other Responses • "The content was boring/ not interesting/ not helpful/ not suitable for students" (n=6) • "The program could not facilitate reflection" (n=1) • "It was difficult to find related prayers for each unit" (n=1) • "Not enough quota for training" (n=1) • "The number of students required for Tier 2 should be reduced for schools chose core program" (n=1)	10 (6.45%)
Total (%)	155 (100%)

Table 7. Workers' perceptions of the "Co-Walker Scheme" (Secondary 2 curriculum)

	Total Count
None / No Comment	33 (29.46%)
Positive Responses • "It is generally good" (n=3) • "It can strengthen communication" (n=22) • "It enables understanding to the needs of schools" (n=13) • "It gives supports to the schools" (n=8) • "The co-walkers give good suggestions to the schools" (n=5) • "The co-walkers/ workers can know more about the program implementation in different schools" (n=4) • "The workers can get more information about the program" (n=3) • "The co-walker is helpful/ warm-hearted" (n=2)	60 (53.57%)
Neutral Responses • "Do not know the effectiveness of co-walker scheme, though it provides channel for communication" (n=4) • "Not thoroughly understand the scheme and the co-walker" (n=2) • "No arrangement for the school visit yet" (n=1) • "The suggestions given by co-walker may not be successfully applied in school though they are very good" (n=1)	8 (7.14%)

Table 7. (Continued)

Negative Responses • "It is unable to arrange school visit" (n=2)	2 (1.97%)
Other Responses • "It is hoped that the co-walker can provide demonstration or school-based training" (n=3) • "It is hoped that the co-walker can provide more support/ carry out the suggestions given by schools" (n=3) • Others (e.g., "co-walker could participate in students' activities", "community-based visits or meetings could be arranged", "contact the school in the middle of the school year") (n=3)	9 (8.04%)
Total (%)	112 (100%)

Table 8. Other opinions of the project (Secondary 2 curriculum)

	Total Count (%)
None	72 (66.06%)
Curriculum Content and Activity Design • "The content is boring/ not suitable for students" (n=5) • "The content should be revised/ updated/ shortened" (n=6) • "Flexibility in teaching should be allowed" (n=2) • Other responses (e.g., "the design is good", "growth puzzle is not helpful", "invite students to involve in the content design") (n=3)	16 (14.68%)
Human and Financial Resources • "Increase/ do not reduce the funding allocation" (n=2) • "Better to have guidelines for the usage of funding and manpower distribution" (n=2) • "More flexibility in the usage of funding" (n=1) • "It is hoped that the funding can be continued" (n=1)	6 (5.5%)
Other Comments and Suggestions • "It is hoped that the Project P.A.T.H.S. can be continued" (n=5) • "Reduce the required number of participants for Tier 2 program" (n=2) • "It is suggested that the training workshops be arranged flexibly" (n=2) • "Evaluation/ revision of proposals are suggested at the end of academic year" (n=2) • Other responses (e.g., "encourage the students to participate", "give guidelines on schools' and teachers' role", "Tier 1 and Tier 2 program be carried out at the same time") (n=4)	15 (13.76%)
Total (%)	109 (100%)

Discussion

Several phenomena could be observed from the present study. First, the respondents expressed that most of the students and themselves had positive responses to the program, as based on the findings of Table 1-4. These observations are consistent with other previous findings in the Tier 1 Program (Secondary 1 Curriculum) in the Experimental Implementation Phase (2005/06 school year) and Full Implementation Phase (2006/07 school year) and the Tier 1 Program (Secondary 3 Curriculum) in the Experimental Implementation Phase (2006/07 school year) that both students and workers had positive perceptions of the program, and the program was beneficial to the students (15,16,24,27). The effectiveness of the Tier 1 Program of the Project P.A.T.H.S. is supported by the evaluation findings from different methods, different data, and different sources of information.

Although the perception to the Tier 1 Program (Secondary 2 Curriculum) was generally positive, several aspects of the program were suggested to be improved and difficulties were also reported. Consistent with previous findings from Experimental Implementation Phase (21), most of the responses proposed that the curriculum content and activity design required modifications. It is suggested that program content and activities should be tailor made to fit the special needs of certain students among different schools. However, the Tier 1 Program adopted a general approach and with program manuals designed for all secondary schools. Therefore, the schools were allowed to make minor adjustment according to their students' unique needs (and seek prior consent from the Research Team if substantial adjustment is needed). Nevertheless, it is worth noting that the overall adherence in other process evaluation studies showed that the adherence of the program was around 85% which was a very favorable observation (13,22).

Regarding the difficulties encountered by the implementers, most of them reported that administration and coordination as well as students' responses were the major difficulties. These two aspects are in fact the hardware and software of a successful program implementation. The hardware is about the manpower, resources (time and money) and support, while the software is about the program implementers and targeted program receivers. Based on respondents' expressions, time, manpower, school settings as well as support from schools and organizations were the major difficulties for program implementation. For program implementers, they found the program added extra workload to them and some of them did not identify themselves with the program rationale. Furthermore, classroom discipline was a problem and students were not involved and showed no interest to the program. These findings indicated that further coordination should be conducted, such as more resources should be added in order to ease the difficulties of program implementation.

Regarding the suggestions on program improvement, programs may need further modification in order to fit students' need as well as arouse students' interest. The Research Team will seriously consider these comments and suggestions. It is worthwhile in conducting the interim evaluation as it enhances our understanding about the process of program implementation. It also reflected how the hardware (coordination among teachers and schools) and software (program implementers and targeted participants) of the program implementation could be improved to enhance program effects.

Concerning the "Co-Walker Scheme", over half of the respondents (53.57%) had positive comments about this scheme and reported the benefits received from the scheme. Among the comments, respondents generally perceived that this supporting scheme provides channel for communication between implementing schools and the Research Team. Through this communicating channel, implementing schools could get support, constructive suggestions and information about program implementation; while the Research Team could have more understanding on the needs of the implementing schools. This further indicated that the co-walkers play the role of supporters and resource persons for the implementers in the process of program implementation, and this kind of tangible or mental support were welcomed by the workers. As there are few studies examining the effect of support provided to workers implementing positive youth development programs, this study can be regarded as pioneering in nature.

Shek and Sun (28) carried out cross-case analyses of factors that influence the process and implementation quality of the Tier 1 Program of the Project P.A.T.H.S. based on seven cases. They found that several factors related to policy, people, program, process, and place (5 "P"s) were conducive to the successful implementation of the Tier 1 Program in the schools. Besides, there were obstacles and difficulties with reference to the 5 "P"s that impeded the quality of implementation. Furthermore, policy support and people (especially commitment and passion of the principals, senior school administrators, and program implementers) are two main groups of factors that influence the quality of program implementation. Although there were different arrangements for program implementation, incorporation of the Tier 1 Program into the formal curriculum was a sound and viable strategy. Finally, the program implementers perceived the program to be beneficial to the program participants. Obviously, some of the findings based on these seven cases are consistent with the present interim evaluation findings and they provide a useful framework to interpret the interim evaluation findings. For example, support from the senior administrators in the school is an important factor affecting the quality of program implementation.

Following the Principle 10 of conducting a qualitative study (25), three possible alternative explanations were put forward from the present findings, including demand characteristics, selection bias, and ideological biases of the researchers. These possible alternative explanations were similar to those in the previous study (21), and again, these explanations are not likely because (i) the respondents were encouraged to voice out their views without restriction and negative voices were in fact heard, (ii) the schools were randomly selected, and (iii) several safeguards were used to reduce biases in the data collection and analysis process, such as multiple colleagues were involved which provided checking for individual biases, as well as both intra-rater and inter-rater reliability checks were carried out to safeguard consistency in coding.

Similar to the interim evaluation of the Secondary 2 Program (21), there were several limitations of the present study. Description of these limitations meets the Principle 12 proposed by Shek, Tang and Han (25). First, as each interview was brief and some data were collected through self-administrated questionnaires, the researchers were not able to collect in-depth information and construct "thick descriptions". Therefore, in-depth individual or focus group interviews had been conducted to further understand the subjective experiences of the program implementers and participants. Second, this interim evaluation was a kind of process evaluation of a program with the program implementers only. As such, another qualitative study which utilized students' weekly diaries to collect students' perceptions of the Secondary 2 Program had also been conducted at the end of the program to further explore the program implementation quality. Despite these limitations, this study conducted in the second year of the Full Implementation Phase provides interim findings that support the positive attributes of the Project P.A.T.H.S. and its effectiveness in promoting holistic youth development among Chinese adolescents in Hong Kong.

Acknowledgments

The preparation for this paper and the Project P.A.T.H.S. were financially supported by The Hong Kong Jockey Club Charities Trust.

References

[1] Shek DTL. Construction of a positive youth development program in Hong Kong. Int J Adolesc Med Health 2006;18:299-302.
[2] Shek DTL, Ma HK. Design of a positive youth development program in Hong Kong. Int J Adolesc Med Health 2006;18:315-27.
[3] Shek DTL, Ma HK, Merrick J., editors. Positive youth development: development of a pioneering program in a Chinese context. London: Freund, 2007.
[4] Catalano RF, Berglund ML, Ryan JAM, Lonczak HS, Hawkins JD. Positive youth development in the United States: research findings on evaluations of positive youth development programs. Prev Treatment 2002. Accessed 2008 Nov 01. URL: http://aspe.hhs.gov/hsp/PositiveYouthDev99/
[5] Shek DTL. Effectiveness of the Tier 1 Program of the Project P.A.T.H.S.: preliminary objective and subjective outcome evaluation findings. ScientificWorldJournal 2006;6:1466-74.
[6] Shek DTL, Siu AMH, Lee TY, Cheung CK, Chung R. Effectiveness of the Tier 1 Program of Project P.A.T.H.S.: objective outcome evaluation based on a randomized group trial. ScientificWorldJournal 2008;8:4-12.
[7] Shek DTL, Ma HK. Subjective outcome evaluation of the Project P.A.T.H.S.: findings based on the perspective of the program participants. ScientificWorldJournal 2007;7:47-55.
[8] Shek DTL, Siu AMH, Lee TY. Subjective outcome evaluation of the Project P.A.T.H.S.: findings based on the perspective of the program implementers. ScientificWorldJournal 2007;7:195-203.
[9] Shek DTL, Sun RCF. Subjective outcome evaluation of the Project P.A.T.H.S.: qualitative findings based on the experiences of program implementers. ScientificWorldJournal 2007;7:1024-35.
[10] Shek DTL, Sun RCF. Subjective outcome evaluation of the Project P.A.T.H.S.: qualitative findings based on the experiences of the program participants. ScientificWorldJournal 2007;7:686-97.
[11] Shek DTL, Sun RCF. Evaluation of Project P.A.T.H.S. (Secondary 1 Program) by the program participants: findings based on the Full Implementation Phase. Adolesc 2008;43:807-22.
[12] Shek DTL, Ma HK. Evaluation of Project P.A.T.H.S. (Secondary 1 Program) by the program implementers: findings based on the Full Implementation Phase. ScientificWorldJournal 2008;8:492-501.
[13] Shek DTL, Ma HK, Lui JHY, Lung DWM. Process evaluation of the Tier 1 Program of the Project P.A.T.H.S. ScientificWorldJournal 2006;6:2264-73.
[14] Shek DTL, Ma HK, Sun RCF, Lung DWM. Process evaluation of the Tier 1 Program (Secondary 1 Curriculum) of the Project P.A.T.H.S.: findings based on the Full Implementation Phase. ScientificWorldJournal 2008;8:35-46.
[15] Shek DTL, Sun RCF. Implementation of the Tier 1 Program of the Project P.A.T.H.S.: interim evaluation findings. ScientificWorldJournal 2006;6:2274-84.
[16] Shek DTL, Ma HK, Sun RCF. Interim evaluation of the Tier 1 Program (Secondary 1 Curriculum) of the Project P.A.T.H.S.: first year of the full implementation phase. ScientificWorldJournal 2008;8:47-60.
[17] Shek DTL, Lee TY, Siu A, Lam CM. Qualitative evaluation of the Project P.A.T.H.S. based on the perceptions of the program participants. ScientificWorldJournal 2006;6:2254-63.
[18] Shek DTL, Lee TY. Qualitative evaluation of the Project P.A.T.H.S.: findings based on focus groups with student participants. Int J Adolesc Med Health 2008;20(4):449-62.
[19] Shek DTL, Sun RCF, Lam CM, Lung DWM, Lo SC. Evaluation of Project P.A.T.H.S. in Hong Kong: utilization of student weekly dairy. ScientificWorldJournal 2008;8:13-21.

[20] Shek DTL, Sun RCF. Implementation of a positive youth development program in a Chinese context: the role of policy, program, people, process, and place. ScientificWorldJournal 2008;8:960-96.
[21] Shek DTL, Sun RCF, Siu AMH. Interim evaluation of the Secondary 2 program of Project P.A.T.H.S.: insights based on the Experimental Implementation Phase. ScientificWorldJournal 2008;8:61-72.
[22] Shek DTL, Lee TY, Sun RCF. Process evaluation of the implementation of the Secondary 2 program of Project P.A.T.H.S. in the Experimental Implementation Phase. ScientificWorldJournal 2008;8:83-94.
[23] Shek DTL, Sun RCF, Chan CWY. Evaluation of Project P.A.T.H.S. (Secondary 2 Program) by the program participants: findings based on the Experimental Implementation Phase. ScientificWorldJournal 2008;8:526-35.
[24] Shek DTL, Sun RCF, Lung DWM. Evaluation of Project P.A.T.H.S. (Secondary 2 Program) by the program implementers: findings based on the Experimental Implementation Phase. ScientificWorldJournal 2008;8:536-46.
[25] Shek DTL, Tang V, Han XY. Quality of qualitative evaluation studies in the social work literature: evidence that constitutes a wakeup call. Res Soc Work Pract 2005; 15:180-94.
[26] Miles MB, Huberman AM. Qualitative data analysis. Thousand Oaks, CA: Sage, 1994.
[27] Shek DTL, Sun RCF. Interim evaluation of the Secondary 3 program of Project P.A.T.H.S.: insights based on the Experimental Implementation Phase. Int Public Health J, in press.
[28] Shek DTL, Sun RCF. Implementation quality of a positive youth development program: cross-case analyses based on seven cases in Hong Kong. ScientificWorldJournal 2008;8:1075-87.

Submitted: December 22, 2008
Revised: January 4, 2009
Accepted: February 21, 2008.

In: Public Health Yearbook 2009
Editor: Joav Merrick

ISBN: 978-1-61668-911-7

Chapter 28

Interim Evaluation of the Secondary 3 Program of Project P.A.T.H.S.: Insights Based on the Experimental Implementation Phase

Daniel TL Shek, PhD, FHKPS, BBS, JP[*1,2,3]
and Rachel CF Sun, BSocSc, PhD[4]

[1]Department of Applied Social Sciences, The Hong Kong Polytechnic University, Hong Kong, PRC, [2]Department of Sociology, East China Normal University, Shanghai, PRC, [3]Kiang Wu Nursing College of Macau, Macau, PRC and [4]Department of Social Work, The Chinese University of Hong Kong, Hong Kong, PRC

Abstract

An interim evaluation was conducted to understand the implementation quality of the Tier 1 Program (Secondary 3 Curriculum) of the Project P.A.T.H.S. in the Experimental Implementation Phase. Twenty-five schools were randomly selected to provide information on the implementation details of the program via interviews and/or self-completed questionnaires. Results showed that a majority of the workers perceived that the students had positive responses to the program and the program was helpful to the students, although negative comments on the program design and difficulties in the implementation process were also recorded. In conjunction with previous findings, the present findings suggest that the three-year Tier 1 Program of the Project P.A.T.H.S. is well-received by different stakeholders and the program implementers perceive that the program can promote the holistic development of secondary school students in Hong Kong.

---

* Correspondence: Professor Daniel TL Shek, PhD, FHKPS, BBS, JP, Chair Professor of Applied Social Sciences, Department of Applied Social Sciences, The Hong Kong Polytechnic University, Hunghom, Hong Kong. E-mail: danielshek@inet.polyu.edu.hk

Keywords: Project P.A.T.H.S., weekly diaries, qualitative evaluation; positive youth development program.

Introduction

As indicated by the project name, "P.A.T.H.S. to Adulthood: A Jockey Club Youth Enhancement Scheme" (**P**ositive **A**dolescent **T**raining through **H**olistic **S**ocial Programmes), Project P.A.T.H.S. is a positive youth development program, which provides training to Secondary 1 to Secondary 3 students in Hong Kong with the ultimate goal to promote holistic adolescent development (1,2). In 2007/08 school year, there were 48 schools participated in the Secondary 3 Program in the third year of the Experimental Implementation Phase. In addition, there were 196 schools and 216 schools participated in the Secondary 2 Program and Secondary 1 Program, respectively, in the Full Implementation Phase. All junior students in these schools were required to attend the Tier 1 Program, which was a manual-based curriculum designed by the Research Team (3) based on 15 positive youth development constructs identified from the existing successful positive youth development programs (4), and had taken reference to relevant research findings and existing programs in both local and foreign contexts. All the instructors (mainly teachers and social workers) were required to attend a three-day 20-hour training workshop before implementing the program in schools. To provide support to colleagues who implement the Tier 1 Program, the Research Team has launched a "Co-Walker Scheme" since December 2006, which aimed to provide ongoing support and professional consultation to the participating schools.

Although there are papers documenting the positive program effects of the Tier 1 Program of Secondary 1 Program (5-20) and Secondary 2 Program (21-24), no evaluation findings pertinent to the Secondary 3 Program have been reported. As mentioned by Shek et al (25), although junior secondary school students are encountering several developmental challenges, such as adjustment to puberty, cognitive maturation, rapid expansion of social circle, increased stress, higher levels of social expectations, and gradual detachment from the family, there are comparatively more developmental challenges for Secondary 3 students as compared with their Secondary 1 and 2 counterparts in Hong Kong. Furthermore, they also pointed out that when students reach Secondary 3, they have poorer psychological well-being and adaptation skills, and they perceive family functioning to be poorer and parental control to be looser. As such, it is important to ask whether Secondary 3 students would have unique reactions to positive youth development programs and whether the program implementers would have certain feelings and comments about teaching Secondary 3 students.

Similar to the evaluation of the Secondary 1 and 2 Programs (15,16,21), an interim evaluation of the Secondary 3 Program was carried out to examine the views of the workers regarding the implementation of the Tier 1 Program, based on a random sample of schools joining the third year of the Experimental Implementation Phase in 2007/08 school year. Since there were several advantages of conducting process evaluation for program evaluation (26-29), understanding the reactions of the students and the program implementers in the process of program implementation is important. Moreover, the findings obtained from the present study can be regarded as invaluable in understanding the implementation process and program effect of the Tier 1 Program of the Project P.A.T.H.S.

Methods

Participants

There were 48 schools joined the Secondary 3 Program of the Project P.A.T.H.S. in the Experimental Implementation Phase in 2007/08 school year. Among these schools, 17 adopted the 20-hour full program that involving 40 teaching units and 31 adopted the 10-hour core program that involving 20 teaching units. Among these participating schools, 12 schools joining the full program and 13 schools joining the core program were randomly selected to participate in this study. In these selected schools, the instructors of the program (either school teachers or social workers) were invited to participate in face-to-face interviews on a voluntary basis during a school visit. If the respondents were not available for interviews during the school visit, they were invited to participate in telephone interviews. Otherwise, they were invited to fill in self-administered questionnaires and return via email or fax. Among these 25 schools, 14 of them took part in face-to-face interviews, 7 participated in telephone interviews and 4 completed self-administered questionnaires. The respondents included 11 teachers and 18 social workers. With reference to Principle 2 in the implementation of qualitative evaluation research proposed by Shek, Tang and Han (30), the number of schools participated in this research can be regarded as respectable as about half of the participating schools of the project in the third year of the Experimental Implementation Phase were randomly selected to join the interviews. Moreover, because the schools were randomly selected, the generalizability of the findings could be enhanced.

Procedures

The procedures for data collection are systematically described below, and this satisfied Principle 3 in the procedures of conducting a qualitative research (30). The data collection was conducted between December 2007 and May 2008. This period can be regarded as midway of the implementation process, as the Experimental Implementation Phase took place from September 2007 to July 2008. While the presence of interviewers may affect the responses of the respondents (e.g., social desirability effect) in face-to-face interviews, it is unlikely to happen because the interviewers were the co-walkers of the interviewed schools with which a friendly rapport and mutual trust had been built. Also, the major advantage of face-to-face interviews is having the opportunity to clarify any doubts instantly. On the other hand, while telephone interviews and self-administered questionnaires have the problems of psychological distance and inability to observe the non-verbal cues of the respondents, their major advantage is efficiency in collecting the data within time limit. In addition, follow-up calls could be arranged if there was a need to clarify the responses of the respondents. Therefore, these data collection methods basically complemented each other.

A self-constructed semi-structured interview guide with five closed-ended questions and seven open-ended questions was used to collect information on the program implementation process.

The open-ended questions were:

- Question 1: What are the responses of the students to this program?
- Question 2: Do you think this program is beneficial to the students? If yes, what are the benefits?
- Question 3: What are the good aspects of the program?
- Question 4: Which areas of the program require improvement?
- Question 5: Have you encountered any difficulties during the program implementation process? If yes, what problems have you encountered?
- Question 6: What are your perceptions of the "Co-Walker Scheme"?
- Question 7: Do you have other opinions?

Informed consent was obtained from the respondents and they participated in the study in a voluntary manner. The interviews were conducted by six co-walkers who were registered social workers with substantial working experience. After each interview, the interviewers were required to fill in the questionnaires. The completed questionnaires were then transcribed and analyzed.

Data analyses

For the quantitative data (closed-ended questions), frequencies and percentages of responses were calculated. The qualitative data (open-ended questions) were analyzed using general qualitative analyses techniques (31). There were three steps in the process. First, relevant raw codes were developed for words, phrases and/or sentences that formed meaningful units at the raw responses level. Second, the codes were further combined to reflect higher-order attributes at the category of codes level. Third, the categories of codes were further analyzed to reveal the broader themes at the thematic level. For example, the response to "involved in discussion" at the raw response level could be subsumed under the category of "high student involvement" which could be further subsumed under the broad theme of "positive responses" of the students to the program (see Table 2). Following the principles of qualitative analyses (30), the raw data and categorized data were kept in by a systematic filing system in order to ensure that the findings are auditable.

The qualitative data were coded and categorized by a trained staff with a Master degree of Social Work and they were further checked by the second author. In the present analyses, as the researchers designed the program in the Project P.A.T.H.S., they were conscious of their own biases and expectations of the program to be effective. In addition, in order to minimize the possible biases involved, both intra-rater and inter-rater reliability on the coding was calculated. For intra-rater reliability, the trained staff and the second author individually coded 20 randomly selected responses for each question (except nine randomly selected responses for question 7 because there were only nine different types of responses for that question). For inter-rater reliability, two research assistants with a Master degree and one research assistant with a Bachelor degree who had not been involved in the data collection and analyses process coded 20 randomly selected responses for each question (except 9 randomly selected responses for question 7) without knowing the original codes given at the end of the scoring process with reference to the codes finalized by the first author. This met the Principles 4, 5, 6, 7, 8 and 9 of conducting a qualitative study advocated by Shek, Tang and Han (30).

Results

Results showed that over four-fifths of the respondents reported that the students were involved and liked the program (Table 1) and 66.07% of the perceived students' responses were positive (see table 2). The intra-rater agreement percentage was 95%, and the inter-rater agreement percentage was 85% for the categorization of the responses reported in Table 2. Concerning the perceived benefits of the program to the students, all respondents regarded the Tier 1 Program of the Secondary 3 Curriculum was helpful to the students (see Table 1) and most of responses presented in Table 3 were positive in nature. The intra-rater agreement percentage was 82.5%, and the inter-rater agreement percentage was 85% for the categorization of the responses.

As shown in Table 4, there were 32 meaningful units regarding the positive aspects of the program. The intra-rater agreement percentage was 80%, and the inter-rater agreement percentage was 82.5% for the categorization of the responses. On the other hand, there were 31 meaningful units concerning the aspects of the program requiring improvement (see Table 5). About two-fifths of the responses indicated the "curriculum content and activity design" needed to be modified (41.94%), with about one-fifth suggested improving the "teaching manuals and resources" (22.58%), or adjusting the "implementation time" (22.58%). The intra-rater agreement percentage was 85%, and the inter-rater agreement percentage was 92.5% for the categorization of the responses. As shown in Table 6, there were 28 meaningful units indicating the workers' perception of the difficulties encountered during program implementation. Among them, most of the responses were related to difficulties in "administration and co-ordination" (28.57%), which was followed by the perceived difficulties in "time management" (14.29%), and then in handling "quantity and quality of instructors" (10.71%) and "students' responses" (10.71%). The intra-rater agreement percentage was 87.5%, and the inter-rater agreement percentage was 85% for the categorization of the responses.

For the workers' perceptions of the "Co-Walker Scheme" (Table 7), about 63% responses were positive and about 19% were "none / no comment". The intra-rater agreement percentage was 92.5%, and the inter-rater agreement percentage was 97.5% for the categorization of the responses. Finally, there were about 96% and 92% of the respondents stating that they liked the program and felt satisfied, respectively (Table 1). The responses to the open-ended question of other opinions of the project were shown in Table 8. The intra-rater agreement percentage was 88.34%, and the inter-rater agreement percentage was 77.78% for the categorization of the responses.

Discussion

Several phenomena could be highlighted from the present study. First, the respondents felt that most of the students and themselves had positive responses to the program, as shown in the findings reported in Table 1-4. These findings are similar to the interim evaluation findings of the Secondary 1 and 2 Programs (15,16,21). These observations are consistent with other findings reported previously in the Tier 1 Program (Secondary 1 Curriculum) in the Experimental Implementation Phase (2005/06 school year) and Full Implementation Phase (2006/07 school year) and the Tier 1 Program (Secondary 2 Curriculum) in the Experimental Implementation Phase (2006/07 school year) that both the students and workers had positive perceptions of the program, and the program was beneficial to the students (5-24).

Table 1. Instructors' ratings of the Secondary 3 curriculum (N and Percentage)

1. Perceived degree of student involvement

	Totally not involved	Not involved	Involved	Totally involved	No response	Total
N	0	3	20	1	1	25
%	12%		84%		4%	100%

2. Perceived degree of students' liking of the Secondary 3 curriculum

	Strongly dislike	Dislike	Like	Strongly like	No response	Total
N	0	2	22	0	1	25
%	8%		88%		4%	100%

3. Perceived degree of helpfulness of the Secondary 3 curriculum

	Unhelpful	Not very helpful	Slightly helpful	Helpful	Very helpful	No response	Total
N	0	0	15	9	1	0	25
%	0%		100%			0%	100%

4. Perceived degree of workers' liking of the Secondary 3 curriculum

	Strongly dislike	Dislike	Like	Strongly like	No response	Total
N	0	0	21	3	1	25
%	0%		96%		4%	100%

5. Perceived degree of workers' overall satisfaction of the Secondary 3 curriculum

	Very dissatisfied	Dissatisfied	Slightly dissatisfied	Slightly satisfied	Satisfied	Very satisfied	No response	Total
N	0	0	2	9	13	1	0	25
%	8%			92%			0%	100%

Table 2. Workers' perceptions of the responses of the students to the Secondary 3 curriculum

	Total Count
Positive Responses	37 (66.07%)
• High student involvement (e.g., "involved in discussion", "enthusiastic", "eager to participate", "willing to share", "active to voice out opinions") (n=16) • Welcomed by students (e.g., "liked the program", "looking forward to attending the lessons") (n=4) • Attractive to students (e.g., "interested in the topics", "interested in discussion topics", "attracted by teaching materials") (n=5) • Other responses (e.g., "good responses", "perceived the program as fruitful", "enhanced self-reflection") (n=12)	
Neutral Responses • "It depends on the content/topics"	3 (5.36%)
Negative Responses	16 (28.57%)
• Feeling bored (e.g., "students were not interested in some topics", "students found the content did not match their need") (n=6)	
• Incapability (e.g., "students could not understand some topics", "difficult to have group discussion, sharing and self-reflection", "students did not change") (n=4)	
• Other responses (e.g., "diminishing student motivation", "too rush", "too superficial", " too many worksheets") (n=6)	
Total (%)	56 (100%)

Table 3. Workers' perceptions of the benefits of the Secondary 3 curriculum

	Total Count
Strengthening Students' Social Competence • "Building up interpersonal relationship" (n=1) • "Improving communication skills" (n=1) • "Students learn how to choose friends" (n=3)	5 (15.63%)
Strengthening Students' Behavioral, Cognitive, Emotional and Moral Competence • "It promotes students' thinking / reflection skills" (n=8) • "It promotes students' emotional management" (n=1) • "It promotes students' moral development" (n=8) • "It promotes students' positive behavior" (n=1)	18 (56.26%)
Enhancing Students' Personal Growth • "It helps students to understand their career interest/self-development" • "It allows student to discuss/share growth issues"	2 (6.25%)
Facilitating Students' Learning • "It arouses students' active responses" (n=1) • "It facilitates application of knowledge" (n=3)	4 (12.5%)
Other Responses • Generally beneficial to students (n=1) • No to minimal benefits (n=2)	3 (9.38%)
Total (%)	32 (100%)

Table 4. Workers' perceptions of the positive aspects of the Secondary 3 curriculum

	Total Count
None / No Comment	1 (3.13%)
Teaching Manuals and Resources • Diverse and good teaching aids (e.g., "various multi-media resources", "teaching aids are attractive and diversified") (n=5) • Sufficient resources (e.g., "rich resources") (n=7)	12 (37.5%)
Curriculum Content and Activity Design • Good curriculum content (e.g., "the topics are practical and lively", "rich content", "comprehensive coverage") (n=10) • Good activity design (e.g., "the activity design is interesting", "sufficient activities") (n=3)	13 (40.63%)
Philosophy • "It meets students' needs" (n=2) • "Good theoretical basis" (n=1)	3 (9.38%)
Other Responses • "It enhances understanding between teacher and students"(n=2) • "Good opportunities for students to share with and to learn from teachers" (n=1)	3 (9.38%)
Total (%)	32 (100%)

Table 5. Workers' perceptions of the aspects of the Secondary 3 curriculum requiring improvement

	Total Count
None	2 (6.45%)
Curriculum Content and Activity Design • "The content does not suit students'/ schools' need" (n=3) • "The content is too board / too superficial/ outdated" (n=4) • Other responses (e.g., "growth puzzle is helpless", "increase flexibility") (n=6)	13 (41.94%)
Teaching Manuals and Resources • "Add more multi-media teaching aids" (n=3) • "The quality of video has to be improved" (n=4)	7 (22.58%)
Implementation Time • "There is insufficient time for running the activities" (n=4) • "Time is pressing" (n=3)	7 (22.58%)
Other Responses • "Workers need to tailor-make the program to attract students" • "It depends on workers' personal qualities/familiarity of students"	2 (6.45%)
Total (%)	31 (100%)

Table 6. Workers' perceptions of the difficulties encountered in Secondary 3 curriculum implementation

	Total Count (%)
None / No Comment	9 (32.14%)
Administration and Co-ordination • "It is difficult to arrange the teaching time-table" (n=3) • "The program was not incorporated into formal curriculum" (n=3) • Other responses (e.g., "little support from school", "complicated school administration") (n=2)	8 (28.57%)
Time Management • "There is insufficient time to run the program" (n=2) • "There is insufficient time for group discussion" (n=2) • "It is difficult to allocate time for different activities" (n=1)	4 (14.29%)
Quantity and Quality of Instructors • "There is not enough teacher to teach the program" (n=1) • "It is hard to prepare lessons" (n=1) • "Not every teacher is capable/ willing to teach the program" (n=1)	3 (10.71%)
Students' Responses • "Students are not attentive / not involved" (n=2) • "Students learned some of the content previously" (n=1)	3 (10.71%)
Other Responses • "It is difficult to evaluate students' performance"	1 (3.57%)
Total (%)	28 (100%)

Table 7. Workers' perceptions of the "Co-Walker Scheme" (Secondary 3 curriculum)

	Total Count (%)
None / No Comment	5 (18.52%)
Positive Responses • "It is generally good" (n=3) • "It can strengthen communication" (n=9) • "It enables understanding to the needs of schools" (n=1) • "The co-walkers/ workers can know more about the program implementation in different schools" (n=2) • "Workers' skills can be improved" (n=2)	17 (62.96%)
Neutral Responses • "It is difficult to arrange school visits though the scheme is generally good" • "The scheme is good, but there is insufficient time for school to cooperate with co-walker"	2 (7.41%)
Negative Responses	0 (0%)
Other Responses • "It is hoped that the co-walkers can arrange community-based meetings with schools in the same district" • "The effectiveness of co-walker scheme depends on whether the co-walkers can convey the schools' message to pertinent parties" • "It is hoped that the co-walkers can have a better understanding of information related to funding allocation, proposal and evaluation"	3 (11.11%)
Total (%)	27 (100%)

Table 8. Other opinions of the project (Secondary 3 curriculum)

	Total Count
None	17 (68%)
Curriculum Content and Activity Design • "The content is all-rounded" • "The curriculum should be more flexible in the number of sessions" • "The content should be revised"	3 (12%)
Human and Financial Resources • "Limited manpower was provided" • "It is suggested that the funding allocation would match with the actual expenses"	2 (8%)
Other Comments and Suggestions • "Due to the engagement of other extra-curricular activities, the attendance rate of Tier 2 Program was low" • "It would be better for school to be the main body of the program" • "It is hoped that the schools could be more involved in the entire program"	3 (12%)
Total (%)	25 (100%)

Based on the principle of triangulation (31), evaluation findings based on different methods, different data and different sources of information generally provide evidence for the effectiveness of the Tier 1 Program of the Project P.A.T.H.S.

Besides, the respondents also pointed out several aspects of the program that require improvement and difficulties encountered in the implementation process (see Tables 5, 6 and Table 8). Similar to previous findings (16, 21), most of the responses referred to the curriculum content and activity design requiring modifications.

Although the curriculum and activities were designed with reference to foreign and local literature and programs, and had been trial-taught in actual school contexts in order to suit the needs of the general secondary school students, it is understandable that some activities might need further tailor-making to meet the special needs of students in some schools. Hence, the schools were allowed to make minor adjustment in accordance to the unique needs of their students (and seek prior consent from the Research Team if substantial adjustment is needed). However, it is noteworthy that the overall adherence in several process evaluation studies showed that the adherence of the program was around 85% which was a very favorable observation (13, 14, 22).

It was observed that a substantial percentage of the respondents reported having difficulties in administration, co-ordination and time management. As it was the third year of program delivery in the Experimental Implementation Phase, it is possible that some schools had difficulties in deploying suitable or sufficient manpower and arranging appropriate time-slots for running the program across three grades. Moreover, although the project had offered training for the instructors, some instructors might encounter difficulties in managing time for running different activities in a lesson and handling unexpected students' responses in the actual classroom context, particularly for those who were the first time to implement the program. Since the above findings were quite similar across three years of program implementation (15,16,21), these comments made by the respondents provide invaluable feedback on further improvement of the program, and the Research Team would seriously consider the comments collected and recorded. Also, it is noteworthy that the present findings provide an opportunity for the school or agency administrators and workers to reflect on how their administration and co-ordination, time management, teaching skills and attitudes could be further improved.

Regarding the "Co-Walker Scheme", as it had been launched for more than a year, many respondents (62.9%) had positive comments about this scheme and reported the benefits received from the scheme. It indicated that the co-walkers could play the role of supporters and resource persons for the instructors in the process of program implementation, and this kind of tangible or mental support were welcomed by the workers.

Following the Principle 10 of conducting a qualitative study (30), three possible alternative explanations were put forward for the present findings – demand characteristics, selection bias and ideological biases of the researchers. These possible alternative explanations were similar to those in the previous study (21), and again, these explanations are not likely because (i) the respondents were encouraged to voice out their views without restriction and negative voices were in fact heard, (ii) the schools were randomly selected, and (iii) several safeguards were used to reduce biases in the data collection and analysis process, such as multiple colleagues were involved which provided checking for individual biases, as well as both intra-rater and inter-rater reliability checks were carried out to safeguard consistency in coding.

Similar to the interim evaluation of the Secondary 2 Program (21), there were several limitations of the present study. Description of these limitations meets the Principle 12 proposed by Shek, Tang and Han (30).

First, as each interview was brief and some data were collected through self-administrated questionnaires, the researchers were not able to collect in-depth information and construct "thick descriptions". Therefore, in-depth individual or focus group interviews had been conducted to further understand the subjective experiences of the program implementers and participants.

Second, this interim evaluation was a kind of process evaluation of a program with the program implementers only.

As such, another qualitative study which utilized students' weekly diaries to collect students' perceptions of the Secondary 3 Program had also been conducted at the end of the program to further explore the program implementation quality.

Despite these limitations, this study in the third year of the Experimental Implementation Phase provides interim evaluation findings that support the positive attributes of the Project P.A.T.H.S. and its effectiveness in promoting holistic youth development among Chinese adolescents in Hong Kong.

Acknowledgments

The preparation for this paper and the Project P.A.T.H.S. were financially supported by The Hong Kong Jockey Club Charities Trust.

References

[1] Shek DTL. Construction of a positive youth development program in Hong Kong. Int J Adolesc Med Health 2006;18:299-302.

[2] Shek DTL, Ma HK. Design of a positive youth development program in Hong Kong. Int J Adolesc Med Health 2006;18:315-27.

[3] Shek DTL, Ma HK, Merrick J, eds. Positive youth development: development of a pioneering program in a Chinese context. London: Freund, 2007.

[4] Catalano RF, Berglund ML, Ryan JAM, Lonczak HS, Hawkins JD. Positive youth development in the United States: research findings on evaluations of positive youth development programs. Prev Treatment 2002. Accessed 2008 Nov 17 URL: http://aspe.hhs.gov/hsp/
PositiveYouthDev99/

[5] Shek DTL. Effectiveness of the Tier 1 Program of the Project P.A.T.H.S.: preliminary objective and subjective outcome evaluation findings. ScientificWorldJournal 2006;6:1466-74.

[6] Shek DTL, Siu AMH, Lee TY, Cheung CK, Chung R. Effectiveness of the Tier 1 Program of Project P.A.T.H.S.: objective outcome evaluation based on a randomized group trial. ScientificWorldJournal 2008;8:4-12.

[7] Shek DTL, Ma HK. Subjective outcome evaluation of the Project P.A.T.H.S.: findings based on the perspective of the program participants. ScientificWorldJournal 2007;7:47-55.

[8] Shek DTL, Siu AMH, Lee TY. Subjective outcome evaluation of the Project P.A.T.H.S.: findings based on the perspective of the program implementers. ScientificWorldJournal 2007;7:195-203.

[9] Shek DTL, Sun RCF. Subjective outcome evaluation of the Project P.A.T.H.S.: qualitative findings based on the experiences of program implementers. ScientificWorldJournal 2007;7:1024-35.

[10] Shek DTL, Sun RCF. Subjective outcome evaluation of the Project P.A.T.H.S.: qualitative findings based on the experiences of the program participants. ScientificWorldJournal 2007;7: 686-97.

[11] Shek DTL, Sun RCF. Evaluation of Project P.A.T.H.S. (Secondary 1 Program) by the program participants: findings based on the Full Implementation Phase. Adolesc 2008;43:807-22.

[12] Shek DTL, Ma HK. Evaluation of Project P.A.T.H.S. (Secondary 1 Program) by the program implementers: findings based on the Full Implementation Phase. ScientificWorldJournal 2008;8:492-501.

[13] Shek DTL, Ma HK, Lui JHY, Lung DWM. Process evaluation of the Tier 1 Program of the Project P.A.T.H.S. ScientificWorldJournal 2006;6:2264-73.

[14] Shek DTL, Ma HK, Sun RCF, Lung DWM. Process evaluation of the Tier 1 Program (Secondary 1 Curriculum) of the Project P.A.T.H.S.: findings based on the Full Implementation Phase. ScientificWorldJournal 2008;8:35-46.

[15] Shek DTL, Sun RCF. Implementation of the Tier 1 Program of the Project P.A.T.H.S.: interim evaluation findings. ScientificWorldJournal 2006;6:2274-84.

[16] Shek DTL, Ma HK, Sun RCF. Interim evaluation of the Tier 1 Program (Secondary 1 Curriculum) of the Project P.A.T.H.S.: first year of the Full Implementation Phase. ScientificWorldJournal 2008;8:47-60.

[17] Shek DTL, Lee TY, Siu A, Lam CM. Qualitative evaluation of the Project P.A.T.H.S. based on the perceptions of the program participants. ScientificWorldJournal 2006;6: 2254-63.

[18] Shek DTL, Lee TY. Qualitative evaluation of the Project P.A.T.H.S.: findings based on focus groups with student participants. Int J Adolesc Med Health 2008;20(4);449-62.

[19] Shek DTL, Sun RCF, Lam CM, Lung DWM, Lo SC. Evaluation of Project P.A.T.H.S. in Hong Kong: utilization of student weekly dairy. ScientificWorldJournal 2008;8:13-21.

[20] Shek DTL, Sun RCF. Implementation of a positive youth development program in a Chinese context: the role of policy, program, people, process, and place. ScientificWorldJournal 2008;8:960-96.

[21] Shek DTL, Sun RCF, Siu AMH. Interim evaluation of the Secondary 2 program of Project P.A.T.H.S.: insights based on the Experimental Implementation Phase. ScientificWorldJournal 2008;8:61-72.

[22] Shek DTL, Lee TY, Sun RCF. Process evaluation of the implementation of the Secondary 2 program of Project P.A.T.H.S. in the Experimental Implementation Phase. ScientificWorldJournal 2008;8:83-94.

[23] Shek DTL, Sun RCF, Chan CWY. Evaluation of Project P.A.T.H.S. (Secondary 2 Program) by the program participants: findings based on the Experimental Implementation Phase. ScientificWorldJournal 2008;8:526-35.

[24] Shek DTL, Sun RCF, Lung DWM. Evaluation of Project P.A.T.H.S. (Secondary 2 Program) by the program implementers: findings based on the Experimental Implementation Phase. ScientificWorldJournal 2008;8:536-46.

[25] Shek DTL, Ma HK, Sun RCF, Yu FSY. Users' manual. In: Shek DTL, Ma HK, Lee TY, Lau PSY, Tsang SKM, Sun RCF, editors. P.A.T.H.S. to Adulthood: A Jockey Club Youth Enhancement Scheme. Secondary Three Curriculum. Users' Manual and Activity Handbook 1. Hong Kong: Soc Welfare Pract Res Centre, Dept SocWork, Chinese Univ Hong Kong, 2007:5-104.

[26] Scheirer MA. Designing and using process evaluation. In: Wholey JS, Hatry HP, Newcomer KE, eds. Handbook of practical program evaluation. San Francisco: Jossey-Bass,1994:40-68.

[27] Linnan L, Steckler A. Process evaluation for public health interventions and research: an overview. In: Steckler A, Linnan L, eds. Process evaluation for public health interventions and research. San Francisco: Jossey-Bass, 2002:1-23.

[28] Weinbach RW. Evaluating social work services and programs. Boston: Allyn Bacon, 2005.

[29] Meyer A, Miller S, Herman M. Balancing the priorities of evaluation with the priorities of the setting: a focus on positive youth development programs in school settings. J Primary Prev. 1993;14:95-113.

[30] Shek DTL, Tang V, Han XY. Quality of qualitative evaluation studies in the social work literature: evidence that constitutes a wakeup call. Res Soc Work Pract 2005;15: 180-94.

[31] Miles MB, Huberman AM. Qualitative data analysis. Thousand Oaks, CA: Sage, 1994.
[32] Singleton RA, Straits BC. Approaches to social research. New York: Oxford Univ Press, 2005.

Submitted: December 30, 2008.
Revised: January 20, 2009.
Accepted: February 25, 2009

In: Public Health Yearbook 2009
Editor: Joav Merrick
ISBN: 978-1-61668-911-7

Chapter 29

PROCESS EVALUATION OF THE SECONDARY 2 CURRICULUM OF THE PROJECT P.A.T.H.S.: FINDINGS BASED ON THE FULL IMPLEMENTATION PHASE

***Daniel TL Shek, PhD, FHKPS, BBS, JP*[*1,2,3]**
***and Rachel CF Sun, BSocSc, PhD*[4]**

[1]Department of Applied Social Sciences, The Hong Kong Polytechnic University, Hong Kong, PRC, [2]Department of Sociology, East China Normal University, Shanghai, PRC, [3]Kiang Wu Nursing College of Macau, Macau, PRC and
[4]Department of Social Work, The Chinese University of Hong Kong, Hong Kong, PRC

Abstract

To understand the implementation quality of the Tier 1 Program (Secondary 2 Curriculum) of the Project P.A.T.H.S. in the Full Implementation Phase, observers carried out process evaluation in the form of systematic observations of 21 units in 14 randomly selected schools. Results showed that the overall level of program adherence was generally high, ranging from 70% to 100%, with an average of 89.3%. The implementation quality of the program regarding student interest, student participation and involvement, classroom control, use of interactive delivery method, instructors' familiarity with the students, degree of achievement of the objectives, time management, lesson preparation, overall implementation quality, and success of implementation was also found. The present findings are consistent with those based on the Experimental Implementation Phase, suggesting that the implementation quality of the Tier 1 Program (Secondary 2 Curriculum) was generally high.

* Correspondence: Professor Daniel TL Shek, PhD, FHKPS, BBS, JP, Chair Professor of Applied Social Sciences, Department of Applied Social Sciences, The Hong Kong Polytechnic University, Hunghom, Hong Kong. E-mail: danielshek@inet.polyu.edu.hk

Keywords: Project P.A.T.H.S., weekly diaries, qualitative evaluation, positive youth development program.

Introduction

In the review of the public health literature, Linnan and Steckler (1) commented that there is "a plethora of reports about interventions that have successful outcomes. A limited number of studies, however, disentangle the factors that ensure successful outcomes, characterize the failure to achieve success, or attempt to document the steps involved in achieving successful implementation of an intervention" (p. 1). This phenomenon is also commonly found in the context of evaluation of positive youth development programs, since findings on program implementation quality are rarely reported by researchers (2-4). The problems of this negligence are twofold. First, it is theoretically and practically important to understand the process of program implementation because research findings suggest that program implementers do not implement the program as planned (i.e., low program fidelity). Second, understanding the process of program implementation can help to improve the quality of the program by identifying program weaknesses and gaps.

In view of this gap in the literature, an increasing number of studies have started to investigate process variables that determine the success of adolescent prevention programs (5-8), and they consistently found that the use of a wide range of teaching methods, the use of interactive methods, high peer interaction, support from school principal, and adherence to the program would facilitate the positive effects of the programs. As such, in assessing program success, examination of the quality of program implementation through conducting process evaluation is as important as investigating the program effects via outcome evaluation.

Process evaluation, according to Scheirer (9), is "the use of empirical data to assess the delivery of programs Process evaluation verifies what the program is, and whether or not it is delivered as intended to the targeted recipients and in the intended dosage" (p. 40).

There are several arguments for conducting process evaluation (9). First, process evaluation can tell the program developers whether Type III error (i.e., existence or non-existence of program effect because of occurrence of activities different from those intended by the program developers) has occurred. Second, fidelity in program implementation can be promoted by feedback collected in the implementation process. Third, process evaluation can help program developers to understand whether the intended targets receive the program. Fourth, process evaluation can help identifying factors that contribute to program success or failure. Finally, program developers can use process evaluation findings to understand how the developed program can be successfully implemented in human organizations and communities which are always complex in nature.

In regard of this, both process evaluation and outcome evaluation utilizing different evaluation methods and data sources were carried out in assessing the program effects of the Project P.A.T.H.S. (**P**ositive **A**dolescent **T**raining through **H**olistic **S**ocial Programmes). The Project P.A.T.H.S. is a positive youth development program in Hong Kong financially supported by The Hong Kong Jockey Club Charities Trust (10). To promote holistic development among adolescents, a total of 15 adolescent developmental constructs are covered in the project (11,12).

These include: promotion of bonding, cultivation of resilience, promotion of social competence, promotion of emotional competence, promotion of cognitive competence, promotion of behavioural competence, promotion of moral competence, cultivation of self-determination, promotion of spirituality, development of self-efficacy, development of a clear and positive identity, promotion of beliefs in the future, provision of recognition for positive behaviour, provision of opportunities for prosocial involvement, and fostering prosocial norms.

There are several lines of evidence that supports the effectiveness of the Tier 1 Program of the Project P.A.T.H.S., such as findings of the evaluation based on randomized group trial (13), subjective outcome evaluation (14-21), qualitative findings based on focus group interviews with program implementers and participants (22, 23), interim evaluation (24-26), analyses of the students' weekly dairies (27), case studies (28) and process evaluation based on systematic classroom observations (29-31).

In the aspect of the process evaluation of the Secondary 2 Program, although the findings obtained in the Experimental Implementation Phase gave a favorable picture about the implementation quality of the Tier 1 Program (31), there was no guarantee that the implementation quality in the Full Implementation Phase was acceptable. As such, process evaluation was carried out to examine the implementation quality of the Tier 1 Program based on a random sample of schools for the second year of the Full Implementation Phase.

METHODS

Participants

Among the 196 schools joining the Secondary 2 Program in the Full Implementation Phase in 2007/08, there were 116 schools adopting the full program (i.e., 20-hour program involving 40 units) and 80 schools adopting the core program (i.e., 10-hour program involving 20 units). Among these schools, nine schools adopting the full program and 5 schools adopting the core program were randomly selected to conduct the observations. The characteristics of the schools joining the process evaluation study can be seen in Table 1.

Table 1. Overall ratings on each unit observed in the different schools

School	A	B	C	D	E	F	G
Background Characteristics of the Schools:							
Location (District)	Sha Tin	Kwai Tsing	Yuen Long	Kwai Tsing	Yuen Long	Sha Tin	Tuen Mun
Finance Mode	Aided	Aided	Aided	DSS	Aided	Aided	Aided
Sex Composition	Co-ed	Co-ed	Co-ed	Co-ed	Co-ed	Co-ed	Co-ed
Religious Background	Buddhism	Catholicism	Catholicis m	Protestantism/ Christianity	Protestantism / Christianity	Nil	Taoism

Table 1. (Continued)

School	A	B	C	D	E	F	G
Context of Observation:							
Choice of Program	10 hours	20 hours	20 hours	20 hours	20 hours	10 hours	20 hours
Mode	10 sessions (1 hour per session)	40 sessions (30 minutes per session)	20 sessions (1 hour per session)	40 sessions (30 minutes per session)	20 sessions (1 hour per session)	20 sessions (30 minutes per session)	20 sessions (1 hour per session)
Integration with School Curriculum	Teacher's Period	Teacher's Period	Personal Growth Lesson	Teacher's Period	Teacher's Period	Personal Growth Lesson	Liberal Studies
No. of Students in the Class	27	38	27	27	46	36	43
Instructor(s)	Teacher	Teacher	Teacher	Teacher	Teacher	Teacher	Social Worker
Duration of Observation	60 minutes	50 minutes	30 minutes	30 minutes	60 minutes	30 minutes	65 minutes
Unit(s) Observed	CC2.1 and CC2.2	PN2.1	SE2.1	SE2.1	RE2.4	CC2.1	EC2.1 and EC2.2

H	I	J	K	L	M	N
Background Characteristics of the Schools:						
Kowloon City	Kwun Tong	Chai Wan	Sha Tin	Sai Kung	Tsuen Wan	Wan Chai
Government	Government	Aided	Aided	Aided	Government	Aided
Co-ed	Boys	Co-ed	Co-ed	Co-ed	Co-ed	Co-ed
Nil	Nil	Protestantism/ Christianity	Protestantism/ Christianity	Catholicism	Nil	Nil
Context of Observation:						
20 hours	10 hours	10 hours	10 hours	20 hours	20 hours	20 hours
20 sessions (1 hour per session)	2 sessions (2.5 hours per session) & 5 sessions (1 hour per session)	10 sessions (1 hour per session)	10 sessions (1 hour per session)	20 sessions (1 hour per session)	20 sessions (1 hour per session)	40 sessions (30 minutes per session)
PATHS Lesson	Teacher's Period	Teacher's Period	Civic Education	Teacher's Period	PATHS Lesson	Liberal Studies
37	40	22	40	33	36	31
Social Worker	Social Worker	Social Worker	Teacher and Social Worker	Social Worker	Teacher	Teacher and Social Worker
60 minutes	81 minutes	75 minutes	75 minutes	35 minutes	65 minutes	55 minutes
EC 2.1 and EC 2.4	SE2.1 and SE2.2	EC2.1 and EC2.4	EC2.1 and EC2.2	SD2.1	SP2.1 and SP2.2	SP2.1

Procedures

For each school joining the process evaluation study, systematic observations of one teaching unit or two teaching units were conducted. There were 21 units under observation, which covered seven positive youth development constructs, including self-efficacy, prosocial norms, cognitive competence, emotional competence, resilience, self-determination, and spirituality (see Table 1). The learning targets of these units can be seen in Table 2. The observers were one pair of the project colleagues who were registered social workers having a Master Degree.

Table 2. Summary of the objectives of the observed units

Schools	Units	Constructs	Objectives
A	CC2.1	Cognitive Competence	To identify the characteristics of different types of thinking styles To identify different thinking styles pertaining to various occupations
	CC2.2	Cognitive Competence	To apply different thinking styles in creative problem solving
B	PN2.1	Prosocial Norms	To understand that social norms may or may not apply to people with different identities when faced with the same social issue or situation To understand that people of different age groups and/or backgrounds have different social responsibilities
C	SE2.1	Self-efficacy	To explore different learning tactics To discover suitable learning tactics
D	SE2.1	Self-efficacy	To explore different learning tactics To discover suitable learning tactics
E	RE2.4	Resilience	To identify the difficulties and challenges that may help students become mature To judge the value behind significant life events as a learning opportunity
F	CC2.1	Cognitive Competence	To identify the characteristics of different types of thinking styles To identify different thinking styles pertaining to various occupations
G	EC2.1	Emotional Competence	To be empathetic toward others' feelings To understand the importance of respecting others' emotions
	EC2.2	Emotional Competence	To understand how improper negative emotional expressions affect interpersonal relationships To recognize the importance of properly expressing negative emotions
H	EC2.1	Emotional Competence	To be empathetic toward others' feelings To understand the importance of respecting others' emotions
	EC2.4	Emotional Competence	To identify characteristics of friends for secure sharing and factors to consider in sharing To develop basic active-listening and response skills

Table 2. (Continued)

Schools	Units	Constructs	Objectives
I	SE2.1	Self-efficacy	To explore different learning tactics To discover suitable learning tactics
	SE2.2	Self-efficacy	To identify distorted thoughts To learn to penetrate and deal with distorted thoughts
J	EC2.1	Emotional Competence	To be empathetic toward others' feelings To understand the importance of respecting others' emotions
	EC2.4	Emotional Competence	To identify characteristics of friends for secure sharing and factors to consider in sharing To develop basic active-listening and response skills
K	EC2.1	Emotional Competence	To be empathetic toward others' feelings To understand the importance of respecting others' emotions
	EC2.2	Emotional Competence	To understand how improper negative emotional expressions affect interpersonal relationships To recognize the importance of properly expressing negative emotions
L	SD2.1	Self-determination	To sharpen decision-making skills To handle peers' opinions and peer pressure by making use of decision-making skills To understand that one should be responsible for one's decisions and accept the consequences
M	SP2.1	Spirituality	To understand the plight of the deprived To treasure what we have and live a meaningful life
	SP2.2	Spirituality	To reflect on the meaning of money To understand that material possessions may not necessarily lead to happiness
N	SP2.1	Spirituality	To understand the plight of the deprived To treasure what we have and live a meaningful life

During the observations, each colleague observed how the units were implemented and was required to complete a rating form covering four major areas, including basic information, integration with the school formal curriculum, program fidelity and adherence, and quality of program delivery in an independent manner. For program fidelity and adherence, the observers rated the degree of adherence and recorded the time used to implement the unit. For the quality of program delivery, student interest, student participation and involvement, classroom control, use of interactive delivery method, use of strategies to enhance student motivation, use of positive and supportive feedback, instructors' familiarity with the students, opportunity for reflection, degree of achievement of the objectives, time management, quality of preparation, overall implementation quality, and success of implementation were rated. The colleagues did not have any discussion and they were "blind" to the ratings of their partner when they completed the rating forms.

RESULTS

For every unit, the ratings of each item by the two independent observers were averaged. To obtain an overall picture, the ratings for each item across all units were again averaged. As the ratings of the observers were averaged, it is necessary to know whether the ratings were reliable. Based on the overall adherence ratings across the 21 units, Pearson correlation analyses showed that the ratings across the observers in the observed units (N =21) were highly reliable (r = .85, p < .01). The average overall adherence to the Curriculum Manuals was 89.3% (ranging from 70% to 100%), which was quite remarkable (see Table 3). For those units where modifications had been made, the observers generally regarded the changes to be reasonable.

The findings on the program implementation quality can be seen in Table 3. As the ratings were averaged across observers, it is necessary to know whether the scale and the ratings were reliable. Based on the mean overall ratings across the 21 units, Pearson correlation analyses showed that the ratings across the two observers in the observed units (N =21) were highly reliable (r =.85, p < .01), and reliability analysis showed that the 13 items of the program implementation quality scale were internally consistent (alpha =.91, mean inter-item correlation =.47).

Regarding the ratings for the quality of delivery, results in Table 3 revealed that the quality of implementation as assessed by the two observers was high (over 5 on a 7-point rating scale). An examination of the different areas showed that the mean ratings were generally high, except the ratings of the use of motivation strategies, use of positive and supportive feedback and provision of opportunities for reflection were lower as compared to other dimensions of the program implementation quality.

Table 3. Overall ratings on each unit observed in the different schools

School	A		B	C	D	E	F	G	
Unit observed	CC2.1	CC2.2	PN2.1	SE2.1	SE2.1	RE2.4	CC2.1	EC2.1	EC2.2
Overall Adherence (%)	100	80	90	90	90	70	95	90	100
Ratings on a 7-point Scale. The percentages of responses with ratings of 5 and above are in brackets.									
1.Student Interest	5 (100)	4 (0)	6.5 (100)	5 (100)	3 (0)	6 (100)	5 (100)	5.5 (100)	5.5 (100)
2. Student Participation and Involvement	4 (0)	4 (0)	7 (100)	6 (100)	4 (0)	5.5 (100)	6 (100)	5.5 (100)	5.5 (100)
3. Classroom Control	6 (100)	6 (100)	6 (100)	5 (100)	4 (0)	6 (100)	6 (100)	5.5 (100)	6 (100)
4. Interactive Delivery Method	4 (0)	4 (0)	6 (100)	6 (100)	4 (0)	5 (100)	4.5 (50)	5 (100)	4 (0)
5. Strategies to Enhance Student Motivation	4 (0)	4 (0)	5.5 (100)	5 (100)	4 (0)	5 (100)	5 (100)	4.5 (50)	4 (0)
6. Use of Positive and Supportive Feedbacks	5 (100)	6 (100)	4.5 (50)	5 (100)	5 (100)	5 (100)	4.5 (50)	3.5 (0)	3 (0)
7. Familiarity with the Students	6.5 (100)	6.5 (100)	6 (100)	4 (0)	6 (100)	6.5 (100)	6.5 (100)	5.5 (100)	6 (100)
8. Opportunity for Reflection	5 (100)	4.5 (50)	6 (100)	5 (100)	4 (0)	6 (100)	5 (100)	4 (0)	4 (0)
9. Degree of Achievement of the Objectives	5 (100)	4 (0)	6 (100)	5 (100)	4 (0)	6 (100)	5 (100)	5 (100)	5 (100)
10. Time Management	6 (100)	6.5 (100)	6 (100)	6 (100)	5 (100)	5.5 (100)	5 (100)	6 (100)	6 (100)

Table 3. (Continued)

School	A		B	C	D	E	F	G	
11. Lesson Preparation	5 (100)	5 (100)	6 (100)	5 (100)	5 (100)	6 (100)	6 (100)	5 (100)	5 (100)
12. Overall Implementation Quality	5 (100)	5 (100)	6.5 (100)	6 (100)	4 (0)	6 (100)	5 (100)	4.5 (50)	4 (0)
13. Success of Implementation	5 (100)	5 (100)	6.5 (100)	5 (100)	3.5 (0)	6 (100)	5 (100)	5 (100)	5 (100)

H		I		J		K		L	M		N	Average / Mean
EC2.1	EC2.4	SE2.1	SE2.2	EC2.1	EC2.4	EC2.1	EC2.2	SD2.1	SP2.1	SP2.2	SP2.1	
90	90	90	90	77.5	77.5	90	95	80	100	100	90	89.29
6 (100)	5 (100)	4 (0)	4 (0)	5 (100)	5 (100)	5 (100)	5 (100)	5 (100)	5.5 (100)	6 (100)	6 (100)	5.10
6 (100)	6 (100)	4 (0)	5 (100)	5.5 (100)	6 (100)	4.5 (50)	5 (100)	5 (100)	6 (100)	6 (100)	5 (100)	5.31
6 (100)	6 (100)	3 (0)	4 (0)	6 (100)	5.5 (100)	6 (100)	5.5 (100)	5 (100)	6 (100)	5.5 (100)	6 (100)	5.48
6 (100)	6 (100)	4 (0)	5 (100)	5 (100)	5 (100)	5 (100)	5.5 (100)	5 (100)	6 (100)	6 (100)	6 (100)	5.10
5 (100)	5 (100)	5 (100)	5 (100)	5 (100)	5 (100)	5 (100)	4.5 (50)	5 (100)	5.5 (100)	5.5 (100)	5 (100)	4.83
5 (100)	5 (100)	5 (100)	4 (0)	5 (100)	5 (100)	4.5 (50)	4.5 (50)	5 (100)	5 (100)	5.5 (100)	5 (100)	4.76
5 (100)	5 (100)	3 (0)	3 (0)	4.5 (50)	4.5 (50)	4 (0)	4.5 (50)	4 (0)	6.5 (100)	6.5 (100)	6 (100)	5.24
6 (100)	5 (100)	4 (0)	4 (0)	5 (100)	5 (100)	4.5 (50)	5 (100)	5 (100)	5.5 (100)	6 (100)	6 (100)	4.98
6 (100)	6 (100)	4 (0)	4 (0)	6 (100)	6 (100)	5 (100)	4.5 (50)	5 (100)	6 (100)	6 (100)	6 (100)	5.21
6 (100)	6 (100)	4 (0)	4 (0)	4 (0)	4.5 (50)	6 (100)	5 (100)	4.5 (50)	6.5 (100)	6 (100)	4 (0)	5.36
6 (100)	6 (100)	5 (100)	5 (100)	5.5 (100)	5.5 (100)	5.5 (100)	5 (100)	5 (100)	6 (100)	5.5 (100)	6 (100)	5.43
6 (100)	6 (100)	4 (0)	4 (0)	5 (100)	5 (100)	5 (100)	5.5 (100)	5.5 (100)	6 (100)	6 (100)	6 (100)	5.24
6 (100)	5 (100)	4 (0)	4 (0)	5.5 (100)	5.5 (100)	5 (100)	5.5 (100)	5.5 (100)	6 (100)	6 (100)	6 (100)	5.24

DISCUSSION

This paper attempts to examine the adherence and quality of implementation of the Tier 1 Program (Secondary 2 Curriculum) of the Project P.A.T.H.S. in the second year of the Full Implementation Phase. With reference to the adherence of the program, results showed that the overall degree of adherence to the teaching units assessed by the two observers was on the high side. This observation is generally consistent with the previous findings generated from process evaluation conducted by observers (29-31) and subjective outcome evaluation reported by the program implementers (19, 21). All these findings suggested that the need for modifying the units in the implementation process was not high. These findings would dispute the common myth that curricula-based positive youth development programs cannot be easily used and major modifications must be made for different adolescent populations. This demystification provides an evidence-based justification for following the teaching manuals in an authentic manner.

The second major conclusion of the study is that the different aspects of the program delivery were perceived to be very positive. These aspects include: a) student interest and involvement (item 1 and item 2); b) classroom management and interactive teaching strategies used by the instructors (items 3, 4 and 10); and c) instructors' relationship with the students and effort (item 7 and item 11). In addition, the two observers perceived that the objectives of the units implemented could be achieved (item 9) and the overall quality of implementation was high (item 12). Most important of all, the implementation was regarded as successful by the observers (item 13).

Nevertheless, there were relatively low average ratings on three teaching strategies, including utilization of strategies to enhance student motivation (item 5), offering positive and supportive feedback (item 6), and provision of opportunities for reflection (item 8). These findings were similar to those based on the Experimental Implementation Phase (31). There are two possible explanations for these observations. First, it may be due to the didactic teaching in Hong Kong, where instructors are less used to giving positive feedback, appreciation and encouragement to students. Second, it may be due to the over-packing of the curriculum where instructors might not be able to arrange sufficient time for students to carry out reflection on their learning. Obviously, receiving supportive feedback and practicing reflection can strengthen students' positive behavior, guide them to make improvement and raise their self-esteem and intrinsic motivation in learning. Therefore, these teaching strategies have been highly addressed in the training workshops provided to the instructors before they implement the program. To further promote these teaching strategies, it is suggested that the co-walkers could remind or encourage the instructors during school visits or regular contacts.

The present findings are generally consistent with those findings based on the Experimental Implementation Phase and Full Implementation Phase. Based on systematic observations of 12 units in the Secondary 1 Curriculum (N = 6 schools) in the Experimental Implementation Phase, results showed that the overall level of program adherence was generally high, ranging from 50% to 95%, with an average of 84.5%. High implementation quality of the program was also observed (29). Based on systematic observations of 22 units in the Secondary 1 Curriculum (N = 14 schools) in the Full Implementation Phase, results showed that the overall level of program adherence was generally high, ranging from 45% to 100%, with an average of 86.3%. High implementation quality of the program was also observed (30). Based on systematic observations of 7 units in the Secondary 2 Curriculum (N = 4 schools) in the Full Implementation Phase, results showed that the overall level of program adherence was generally high, ranging from 70% to 95%, with an average of 83.6%. High implementation quality of the program was also observed (31). It is obvious that these findings generally converge and they suggest that the quality of program implementation was high in the project.

There are several limitations of the study. First, because of manpower constraints, only 14 schools were randomly selected to participate in this study. Although the number of schools participating in the study can be regarded as respectable, it would be desirable to include more schools with different characteristics to participate in the study.

Second, besides adherence and the quality of implementation, process evaluation with reference to other dimensions such as context of the implementation and the involvement of other stakeholders (32) would help the program developers to further understand the quality of the program implementation process.

Finally, consistent with the intrinsic problem of all observation studies where time sampling is involved, one needs to be conscious of the degree of generalizability of the present findings to other temporal and spatial contexts. One possible confounding effect is that the students may become more cooperative when there are visitors and outside observers. Of course, the use of ethnographic strategies with prolonged engagement and observations would be helpful.

Despite these limitations, process evaluation findings suggest that the quality of implementation of the Tier 1 Program was high, which would facilitate the achievement of the ultimate project goal in promoting the holistic development of the youths in Hong Kong.

Acknowledgments

The preparation for this paper and the Project P.A.T.H.S. were financially supported by The Hong Kong Jockey Club Charities Trust.

References

[1] Linnan L, Steckler A. Process evaluation for public health interventions and research: an overview. In: Steckler A, Linnan L, eds. Process evaluation for public health interventions and research. San Francisco: Jossey-Bass, 2002:1-23.

[2] Durlak JA. Successful prevention programs for children and adolescents. New York: Plenum, 1997.

[3] Dane AV, Schneider BH. Program integrity in primary and early secondary prevention: are implementation effects out of control? Clin Psychol Rev 1998;18:23-45.

[4] Domitrovich CE, Greenberg MT. The study of implementation: current findings from effective programs that prevent mental disorders in school-aged children. J Educ Psychol Cons 2000;11:193-221.

[5] Ringwalt CL, Ennett S, Johnson R, Rohrbach LA, Simons-Rudolph A, Vincus A et al. Factors associated with fidelity to substance use prevention curriculum guides in the nation's middle schools. Health Educ Behav 2003;30:375-91.

[6] Nation M, Crusto C, Wandersman A, Kumpfer KL, Seybolt D, Morrissey-Kane E et al. What works in prevention: principles of effective prevention programs. Am Psychol 2003;58:449-56.

[7] Harachi TW, Abbott RD, Catalano RF, Haggerty KP, Fleming CB. Opening the black box: using process evaluation measures to assess implementation and theory building. Am J Community Psychol 1999;27:711-31.

[8] Tobler NS, Lessard T, Marshall D, Ochshorn P, Roona M. Effectiveness of school-based drug prevention programs for marijuana use. Sch Psychol Int 1999;20:105-37.

[9] Scheirer MA. Designing and using process evaluation. In: Wholey JS, Hatry HP, Newcomer KE, eds. Handbook of practical program evaluation. San Francisco: Jossey-Bass, 1994:40-68.

[10] Shek DTL, Ma HK, Merrick J, eds. Positive youth development: development of a pioneering program in a Chinese context. London: Freund, 2007.
[11] Shek DTL. Construction of a positive youth development program in Hong Kong. Int J Adolesc Med Health 2006;18:299-302.
[12] Shek DTL, Ma HK. Design of a positive youth development program in Hong Kong. Int J Adolesc Med Health 2006;18:315-27.
[13] Shek DTL, Siu AMH, Lee TY, Cheung CK, Chung R. Effectiveness of the Tier 1 Program of Project P.A.T.H.S.: objective outcome evaluation based on a randomized group trial. ScientificWorldJournal 2008;8:4-12.
[14] Shek DTL, Ma HK. Subjective outcome evaluation of the Project P.A.T.H.S.: findings based on the perspective of the program participants. ScientificWorldJournal 2007;7:47-55.
[15] Shek DTL, Siu AMH, Lee TY. Subjective outcome evaluation of the Project P.A.T.H.S.: findings based on the perspective of the program implementers. ScientificWorldJournal 2007;7:195-203.
[16] Shek DTL, Sun RCF. Subjective outcome evaluation of the Project P.A.T.H.S.: qualitative findings based on the experiences of program implementers. ScientificWorldJournal 2007;7:1024-35.
[17] Shek DTL, Sun RCF. Subjective outcome evaluation of the Project P.A.T.H.S.: qualitative findings based on the experiences of program participants. ScientificWorldJournal 2007;7:686-97.
[18] Shek DTL, Sun RCF. Evaluation of Project P.A.T.H.S. (Secondary 1 Program) by the program participants: findings based on the Full Implementation Phase. Adolesc 2008;43:807-22.
[19] Shek DTL, Ma HK. Evaluation of Project P.A.T.H.S. (Secondary 1 Program) by the program implementers: findings based on the Full Implementation Phase. ScientificWorldJournal 2008;8:492-501.
[20] Shek DTL, Sun RCF, Chan CWY. Evaluation of Project P.A.T.H.S. (Secondary 2 Program) by the program participants: findings based on the Experimental Implementation Phase. ScientificWorldJournal 2008;8:526-35.
[21] Shek DTL, Sun RCF, Lung DWM. Evaluation of Project P.A.T.H.S. (Secondary 2 Program) by the program implementers: findings based on the Experimental Implementation Phase. ScientificWorldJournal 2008;8:536-46.
[22] Shek DTL, Lee TY, Siu A, Lam CM. Qualitative evaluation of the Project P.A.T.H.S. based on the perceptions of the program participants. ScientificWorldJournal 2006;1:290-99.
[23] Shek DTL, Shik AWY. Qualitative evaluation of the Project P.A.T.H.S. in Hong Kong: findings based on program implementers. Int J Adol Med Health, in press.
[24] Shek DTL, Sun RCF. Implementation of the Tier 1 Program of the Project P.A.T.H.S.: interim evaluation findings. ScientificWorldJournal 2006;1:310-20.
[25] Shek DTL, Ma HK, Sun RCF. Interim evaluation of the Tier 1 Program (Secondary 1 Curriculum) of the Project P.A.T.H.S.: first year of the Full Implementation Phase. ScientificWorldJournal 2008;8:47-60.
[26] Shek DTL, Sun RCF, Siu AMH. Interim evaluation of the Secondary 2 Program of Project P.A.T.H.S.: insights based on the Experimental Implementation Phase. ScientificWorldJournal 2008;8:61-72.
[27] Shek DTL, Sun RCF, Lam CM, Lung DWM, Lo SC. Evaluation of Project P.A.T.H.S. in Hong Kong: utilization of student weekly dairy. ScientificWorldJournal 2008;8:13-21.
[28] Shek DTL, Sun RCF. Implementation of a positive youth development program in a Chinese context: the role of policy, program, people, process, and place. ScientificWorldJournal 2008;8:960-96.
[29] Shek DTL, Ma HK, Lui JHY, Lung DWM. Process evaluation of the Tier 1 Program of the Project P.A.T.H.S. ScientificWorldJournal 2006;1:300-9.
[30] Shek DTL, Ma HK, Sun RCF, Lung DWM. Process evaluation of the Tier 1 Program (Secondary 1 Curriculum) of the Project P.A.T.H.S.: findings based on the Full Implementation Phase. ScientificWorldJournal 2008;8:35-46.
[31] Shek DTL, Lee TY, Sun RCF. Process evaluation of the implementation of the Secondary 2 Program of Project P.A.T.H.S. in the Experimental Implementation Phase. ScientificWorldJournal 2008;8:83-94.

[32] Saunders RP, Evans MH, Joshi P. Developing a process-evaluation plan for assessing health promotion program implementation: a how-to guide. Health Promot Pract 2005;6:134-47.

***Submitted*:** December 28, 2008.
Revised: January 22, 2009.
Accepted: February 28, 2009.

In: Public Health Yearbook 2009
Editor: Joav Merrick

ISBN: 978-1-61668-911-7

Chapter 30

PROCESS EVALUATION OF THE IMPLEMENTATION OF THE SECONDARY 3 PROGRAM OF THE PROJECT P.A.T.H.S. IN THE EXPERIMENTAL IMPLEMENTATION PHASE

Daniel TL Shek, PhD, FHKPS, BBS, JP*[*1,2,3], Rachel CF Sun, BSocSc, PhD[4] and Catalina SM Ng, BA, MEd, MA, PhD[4]

[1]Department of Applied Social Sciences, The Hong Kong Polytechnic University, Hong Kong, PRC, [2]Department of Sociology, East China Normal University, Shanghai, PRC, [3]Kiang Wu Nursing College of Macau, Macau, PRC and [4]Department of Social Work, The Chinese University of Hong Kong, Hong Kong, PRC

Abstract

This study examined the implementation quality of the Tier 1 Program (Secondary 3 Curriculum) delivered in the Experimental Implementation Phase of the Project P.A.T.H.S. (**P**ositive **A**dolescent **T**raining through **H**olistic **S**ocial Programmes). Process evaluation was conducted in the form of systematic observations of curriculum units in four randomly selected schools. Results indicated that the overall level of program adherence was high, ranging from 80% to 100%, with an average of 90%. The mean ratings of the program implementation quality were high, and the inter-rater reliability on these ratings across the observers was highly reliable. Despite limitations, the findings of this study suggest that the implementation of the Secondary 3 Program (Tier 1 Program) of the Experimental Implementation Phase was of very high quality. This provides strong evidence to account for the successful and encouraging outcomes of a major positive youth development program in Hong Kong.

Keywords: process evaluation, observational study, adolescents, positive youth development program.

---

* Correspondence: Professor Daniel TL Shek, PhD, FHKPS, BBS, JP, Chair Professor of Applied Social Sciences, Department of Applied Social Sciences, The Hong Kong Polytechnic University, Hunghom, Hong Kong. E-mail: danielshek@inet.polyu.edu.hk

Introduction

In the context of evaluation of positive youth development programs, reviews of the existing literature indicate that findings on program implementation quality are under-reported (1-3). Durlak (1), in a review of over 1,200 published prevention studies, found that less than 5% of these studies provided data on program implementation. In a meta-analysis of evaluation studies of primary and early secondary prevention programs published between 1980 and 1994, Dane and Schneider (2) reported that only 39 out of 162 evaluation studies documented procedures of fidelity. Similarly, Domitrovich and Greenberg (3) ascertained that among the 34 effective prevention programs under review, only 21% examined whether the effective intervention was related to outcomes.

Evidently, the sparse number of reported studies on the evaluation of positive youth development programs hinders our understanding of what constitutes the effectiveness or failure of the program implementation. Shek et al (4) highlighted several serious consequences of under-estimating the importance of the quality of the implementation of a program. In the first place, our knowledge of the process of the program success or failure could be hampered by the 'black box' approach. Second, given the newness of a program, the lack of process evaluation would prevent the program implementers from recognizing the strengths and weaknesses of the programs, and both anticipated and unanticipated consequences (3). Another grave consequence is both the program developers and implementers could not conclude how the program would be more effective if replicated again. Finally, without process evaluation, if program developers wish to fine-tune the program, they will have to wait until the outcome data are collected as implementation data provide a source of ongoing feedback that is useful for continuous quality improvement.

To advance our knowledge, substantial efforts should be channelled into disentangling the factors that result in successful or unsuccessful outcomes of a program. Process evaluation which can throw light on the mechanisms and processes responsible for the result (success or failure) can assist in making these discoveries (5). In substantiation of the use of process evaluation for further program development and improvement, Scheirer (6) states that first, process evaluation can inform the program developers whether a Type III error (i.e., existence or non-existence of program effect because of occurrence of activities different from those intended by the program developers) has occurred. Next, fidelity in program implementation can be promoted by feedback collected in the implementation process. Third, process evaluation can help immensely program developers to comprehend whether the program clientele receives the program. The fourth reason is, clearly, process evaluation can help to identify factors that contribute to program success or failure. Ultimately, information from a process evaluation is valuable because the results document how the program is being implemented; such information can be utilized by program developers to understand how the program can be implemented successfully in human organizations and communities, which are always complex in nature. Added to this, Weinbach (7) gave two more reasons to underscore the importance of process evaluation: initially, it provided some invaluable insights about a program that might be overlooked by the program developers and another reason is it unfolds how a program generally works.

Given the avowed importance of process evaluation research in fully understanding how and under what conditions programs may be effective, one of the aims of the present study is to complement and extend the published literature which the process evaluation is rarely reported.

While it is agreed that positive youth development programs are gaining prominence as a way to help adolescents become competent, engaged, and responsible adults, much remains to be done in Hong Kong as there are very few systematic and multi-year positive youth development programs. Even if such programs exist, they are limited in scope as they primarily focus on isolated problems and issues in youth development (i.e., deficits-oriented programs). Furthermore, most notably, they are relatively short-term in nature (4) and systematic and long-term evaluation of the available programs is lacking. In view of this, primary prevention programs targeting specific adolescent developmental problems and positive youth development programs are immensely needed in Hong Kong (8) as consistent findings from both published and unpublished studies demonstrated that Hong Kong adolescents face a number of developmental problems, such as mental health problems like depression (9), abuse of psychotropic substances (10), adolescent suicide (11), deliberate self-harm (12), school violence (13) and erosion of family solidarity (9).

Against this background, there is a pressing need to call for programs that promote holistic development among adolescents in Hong Kong. The Hong Kong Jockey Club Charities Trust funded a project entitled P.A.T.H.S. to Adulthood: A Jockey Club Youth Enhancement Scheme (P.A.T.H.S. denotes **P**ositive **A**dolescent **T**raining through **H**olistic **S**ocial Programmes). The Trust invited academics of five universities in Hong Kong to form a research team, with The Chinese University of Hong Kong as the lead institution, to develop a multi-year universal positive youth development program (Tier 1 Program) to promote holistic adolescent development in Hong Kong.

There are two implementation phases in this project, namely Experimental Implementation Phase (EIP) and Full Implementation Phase (FIP). For the EIP (January 2006 to August 2008), 52 secondary schools were invited to participate in the project with the aims of accumulating experience in program implementation, and helping front-line workers to familiarize themselves with the program design and philosophy. In the 2006/07 academic year, the programs were implemented on a full scale at the Secondary 1 level (FIP-S1: 2006-07). In the 2007/08 school year, the programs were being implemented at the Secondary 1 and 2 levels. In the 2008/09 academic year, the programs are implemented at the Secondary 1, 2, and 3 levels.

The Tier 1 Program is a universal positive youth development program where students of Secondary 1 to 3 will participate in the program, normally with 20 hours of training in the school year at each grade. The program was designed based on the 15 positive youth development constructs described in Catalano et al (14). A summary of the constructs, aims, and learning targets of the curriculum units for Secondary 3 is presented in Table 1. Apart from the positive youth development constructs, the ecological perspective was also adopted in the Project P.A.T.H.S. in designing the curriculum units that are intended to cultivate students' development in five different domains: individual, family, peer, school, and society.

The effectiveness of the Tier 1 Program of the Project P.A.T.H.S. both in the EIP (Experimental Implementation Phase) (EIP-S1: 2005-06; EIP-S2: 2006-07; EIP-S3: 2007-08) and FIP (Full Implementation Phase) (FIP-S1: 2006-07; FIP-S2: 2007-08) was supported by several lines of evidence. First, evaluation findings based on the one group pre-/post-test design indicated that there were positive changes in the program participants after participating in the program (15,16). Second, subjective outcome evaluation findings based on different studies, sources, and data types consistently demonstrated that the program participants and implementers had positive perceptions of the program and they generally felt that the program had a positive influence on the participants as a whole (17-21). The third evidence is research findings showed a close linkage between subjective and objective outcome evaluation findings, with those perceiving higher benefits of the program indicating greater positive changes on the different indicators of positive youth development (22,23). Fourth, qualitative findings based on focus group interviews indicated that the program participants enjoyed the program and they experienced positive changes in themselves (24). Fifth, interim evaluation findings showed that the respondents had positive perceptions of the program and it had a beneficial influence on the program participants (25,26). In addition, analyses of the students' weekly diaries showed that the students perceived that the program had helped them in many areas and the participants generally enjoyed the program (27). Finally, process evaluation studies based on systematic observations demonstrated that the quality of implementation and program adherence were high (4, 28).

Though good implementation quality of the Tier 1 Program was indicated by the process evaluations based on both the EIP, there was no guarantee that the implementation quality of the Secondary 3 curriculum in the EIP (EIP-S3: 2007-08) was acceptable. Concerns about the quality of program implementation, coupled with the fact that there is a dearth of information pertaining to the process evaluation of positive youth development programs in the published literature, make research in this area particularly important. Since the process evaluation is an invaluable tool that can meticulously answer the focal question of the quality of program implementation, part of the dilemma then involves the type of evaluation methodology used to conduct it.

In evaluating the data collection techniques, Bouffard, Taxman, and Silverman (29) stated that the more completely a process evaluation technique adheres to the fundamental scientific principles of observation and replication, the more likely the information about the program implementation gathered with that technique will be reliable and valid. Furthermore, techniques that allow evaluators to observe the operation of the program first-hand, rather than relying on stakeholders' report or understanding of the operations, provide a more valuable process evaluation. Given that observation techniques are more amenable to replication, clearly, independent confirmation of the results of an evaluation is possible by other observers. Observation techniques which meet both criteria for scientific study can help to shed light on the effectiveness of the program's implementation. Similarly, Mastrofski and colleagues' (30) stance on the use of observational technique is researchers using observation method can make and record their observations using systematized, replicable procedures. More importantly, data is gathered independent of any influence of the individuals and their behaviour in the natural setting. Added to this, observational studies serve a wide range of purposes, on a continuum from the discovery of new findings to the confirmation or refutation of previous findings (31).

The study reported here provides a more in-depth understanding of the implementation quality of the Tier 1 Program (Secondary 3 Curriculum) based on a random sample of schools for the third year of the EIP (EIP-S3: 2007-08). To explore this, process evaluation with systematic observations was used.

Table 1. An Overview of the 20-h full program of Secondary 3 curriculum

Construct	Unit	Unit Aims	Learning Targets
1. Bonding	Modern Love Stories (BO3.1) (30 min)	To understand qualities of a healthy love relationship	To examine one's attitude toward love relationships; to identify the essential elements of love
	What is Freedom of Love? (BO3.2) (30 min)	To construct the proper attitudes toward love relationships	To differentiate the proper and improper attitudes that appear during the initial stage of love relationships; to generalize the do's and don'ts of dating
2. Social Competence	"She" Comes from China (SC3.1) (30 min)	To establish a sense of connectedeness with China	To develop a sense of connectedeness with China by understanding the relationship between China and Hong Kong; to identify concrete examples on how Chinese culture and custom affect the day-to-day life of Hong Kong people
	Siblings of Hong Kong (SC3.2) (30 min)	To establish the vision of contributing to one's country	To identify the educational situation and needs of China; to reflect on how we can contribute to China
	Who's Right? Who's Wrong? (SC3.3) (30 min)	To analyze the reasons for conflict among siblings and suggest solutions	To understand the reasons for conflict among siblings; to learn the proper attitude to get along with siblings
	A Blog Post A Day (SC3.4) (30 min)	To understand the reasons for conflict among friends and how to handle such conflict, and learn to distinguish good company from bad company	To understand the reasons for conflict among friends; to learn how to face and handle conflict with friends
3. Emotional Competence	What Are My Feelings? (EC3.1) (30 min)	To understand the causes and consequences of our emotional problems	To examine the dynamic interactions between emotions and physiological responses; to experience the impact of relaxation strategies in relieving pressure and negative emotions
	Changing Emotions through Positive Thinking (EC3.2) (30 min)	To learn to handle negative emotions with positive thinking	To manage negative emotions by applying rational and positive thinking
4. Cognitive Competence	Truth or Myth? (CC3.1) (30 min)	To cultivate critical thinking to enable students to analyze information to which they are exposed in daily life	To learn to distinguish between fact and opinion; to analyze information in its context by differentiating between fact and opinion
	The Truth Behind Advertisements (CC3.2) (30 min)	To apply critical thinking in tackling information promoting materialism and consumerism	To apply critical thinking in analyzing advertising messages; to reflect on what has to be considered before consumption

Table 1. (Continued)

Construct	Unit	Unit Aims	Learning Targets
5. Behavioral Competence	The Key to Happiness (BC3.1) (30 min)	To learn how to express and accept appreciation	To understand that appreciation brings joy to oneself and others; to learn how to observe and appreciate people and things around us, and to express sincere appreciation; to learn how to respond to appreciation in a proper manner
	Revenge or Forgiveness? (BC3.2) (30 min)	To teach students to forgive those who have offended them	To understand the importance of sincere forgiveness; to understand the negative influence of taking revenge on those who have offended us
6. Moral Competence	Ideals and Reality (MC3.1) (30 min)	To discover the different aspects of fairness in our ideals and in reality	To discuss the differences between fairness in our ideals and in reality; to understand that a system or situation of "absolute fairness" does not exist in reality
	Am I a Superhero? (MC3.2) (30 min)	To reflect on how to help others, and understand the importance and ways of giving help	To learn how to exercise self-reflection and how to help others; to discuss ways of helping others in society
	Lovers' Codes (MC3.3) (30 min)	To help students to build up proper attitudes and positive values about love relationships	To learn to cherish love relationships and to love with commitment instead of quitting easily; to discuss the proper attitudes to end a love relationship
	The Stolen PIN (MC3.4) (30 min)	To understand the importance and impact of honesty	To understand the relationship between honesty and personal credibility; to understand how interpersonal relationships affect the practice of honest behavior; to learn to take responsibility for one's behavior and its consequences
7. Self-efficacy	Who is the Richest? (SE3.1) (30 min)	To cultivate students' self-efficacy in wealth management	To understand that successful wealth management relies on the ability to exercise self-control and delayed gratification; to understand the importance of controlling desires for unnecessary material things
	My Dream! My Way! (SE3.2) (30 min)	To motivate oneself to live according to one's dreams through an appropriate vision of the future	To understand the meaning of dreams and their importance in life; to identify the personal qualities that help one overcome environmental constraints and realize dreams

Construct	Unit	Unit Aims	Learning Targets
8. Prosocial Norms	Who Makes the Call? (PN3.1) (30 min)	To teach students to incorporate moral considerations into decisions	To understand that prosocial and moral consideration and analysis are essential when making decisions
	Stand Up, Speak Up (PN 3.2) (30 min)	To develop students' critical thinking when facing socially accepted behaviors that conflict with one another	To understand that society has different expectations of different roles; to investigate the potential conflicts between being prosocial and socially accepted behaviors
9. Resilience	A Contented Heart Is a Joyful Heart (RE3.1) (30 min)	To promote optimism through positive thinking	To describe experience and how people can be our treasures; to develop an optimistic view of life among students
	From Crisis to Opportunity (RE3.2) (30 min)	To cultivate the ability to face and handle crisis	To demonstrate how to face crisis; to identify crisis as an opportunity of growth
	Life Springs from Sorrow and Calamity (RE3.3) (30 min)	To introduce traditional values of the Chinese in relation to adversity so as to enhance students' resilience	To state how Mencius looked at adversity; to reflect upon oneself and how Mencius' teachings can be applied in daily life
	From Dream to Reality (RE3.4) (30 min)	To promote a sense of hope towards the future	To construct a vision of one's future family; to recognize that one needs to work hard and use resources properly so as to achieve their aspirations
10. Self-determination	Look Further and Wider (SD3.1) (30 min)	To learn how to make important decisions through simulating a choice of further studies or a career	To learn the importance of collecting comprehensive information before making choices; to identify the most important factors in decision-making
	Let Me Say It! (SD3.2) (30 min)	To enhance students' ability to gain parental support for personal decisions	To discuss the proper way to seek parental support for personal decisions; to understand the ways in which different actions and tones of voice affect the outcome of a discussion
11. Spirituality	Fortune's Favorite (SP3.1) (30 min)	To enable students' discovery, from different perspectives, of "the master" in their lives	To explore the meaning of "master" through "fortunate" and "unfortunate" stories
	Where Does Value Lie? (SP3.2) (30 min)	To help students understand life values from different perspectives	To reflect life values from the stories of people who have suffered; to understand the importance of belief in life
	Why? (SP3.3) (30 min)	To deepen students' understanding of the meaning of life	To introduce the work and life values of people who are committed volunteers and to explore how their beliefs influence their commitments; to deepen students' understanding on how beliefs influence behavior
	The Life Novel (SP3.4) (30 min)	To help students search for their own meanings of life	To integrate and consolidate the content learned in previous units; to apply the knowledge and experiences gained from daily life

Table 1. (Continued)

Construct	Unit	Unit Aims	Learning Targets
12. Clear and Positive Identity	Unshakable Me! (ID3.1) (30 min)	To identify the core competences for success and ways of cultivating them	To identify the core competences which help establish a foothold in different careers; to explore ways to develop core competences in one's own life
	Men and Women, Past and Present (ID3.2) (30 min)	To examine gender stereotypes and their impact on Hong Kong society	To discuss the gender-role expectations in contemporary Hong Kong; to reflect on the effect of these concepts on individuals' perceptions of gender roles
13. Beliefs in the Future	What Will Your Future Be? (BF3.1) (30 min)	To assist students to choose a realistic but optimistic way of life	To adopt a realistic and positive attitude in exploring future careers
	Job Market (BF3.2) (30 min)	To put students in touch with the job market and let them understand different jobs	To understand that different jobs have different requirements; to be aware of the issue of gender stereotypes and their impact(s) on career choices
	Gifts from Heaven (BF3.3) (30 min)	To enhance students' aspirations for higher education and future careers	To identify one's interest, ability and attainable career options; to identify pathways for higher education and vocational training
	Looking Forward (BF3.4) (30 min)	To cultivate students' abilities to plan for future education and careers, and to monitor and motivate their goal-pursuing behavior	To make both short- and long-term career plans; to set up evaluating and rewarding thinking patterns to strengthen one's perseverance in the process of goal-attainment
14. Prosocial Involvement	Across Generations (PI3.1) (30 min)	To develop students' abilities to design and plan prosocial activities	To learn to plan the activity with the W5H1 method
	All Hands on Deck (PI3.2) (30 min)	To develop students' ability to analyze people's motives in participating in prosocial activities	To understand the common barriers to participation; to devise feasible strategies to promote an activity and attract participants
	Secret Recipe PI3.3 (30 min)	To improve students' discussion techniques required for planning and organizing prosocial activities	To learn and practice how to lead a discussion by asking questions in appropriate ways
	Gathering Opinion PI3.4 (30 min)	To enhance the students' abilities to plan and evaluate prosocial activities	To utilize critical thinking and evaluate the success of an activity from the participants' point of view; to consider the needs of the participants in the planning process for community or prosocial activities

Note: The fifteenth construct of recognition for Positive Behaviour is spread over the other 14 constructs. This construct is used as teaching strategies and no teaching activity is assigned for this construct. The 10-hour Core Program consists of the units from Constructs 1-8. The units MC 3.1 and MC 3.2 were observed in School A, the units BF 3.1 and BF 3.2 were observed in School B, the units PI 3.3 and PI 3.4 were observed in School C, and the unit MC 3.4 was observed in School D. (Schools are identified in Table 2).

Methods

Participants

A total of 48 schools participated in the Secondary Three Curriculum of the Project P.A.T.H.S. in the Experimental Implementation Phase (EIP) in 2007-2008 academic year (EIP-S3: 2007-2008). Among these schools, 17 adopted the 20-hour full program which consists of 40 teaching units and 31 adopted the 10-hour core program which is composed of 20 teaching units. Among these participating schools, four schools which joined the full program were randomly selected to join the present study. The characteristics of the schools participating in this process evaluation study (Secondary Three Curriculum) can be seen in Table 2.

Procedures

For each school joining the process evaluation study, systematic observations of one or two teaching units were conducted. There were seven units under observation, which encompasses three positive youth development constructs, including moral competence, beliefs in the future and prosocial involvement (see Table 2). The learning objectives of these units can be seen in Table 1. The observation team is composed of two research assistants of the Project P.A.T.H.S. who are registered social workers. During the observations, each colleague observed how the units were implemented and was required to complete a rating form covering four major areas, including basic information, integration with the school formal curriculum, program fidelity and adherence, and quality of program delivery in an independent manner. For program fidelity and adherence, the observers rated the degree of adherence and recorded the time used to implement the unit. For the quality of program delivery, students' interest, participation and involvement, classroom control, use of interactive delivery method, use of strategies to enhance student motivation, use of positive and supportive feedback were the areas for assessment. Instructors' familiarity with the students, opportunity for reflection, degree of achievement of the objectives, time management, quality of preparation, overall implementation quality, and success of implementation were also rated. The research assistants did not have any discussion and they were blind to the ratings of their partner when they completed the rating forms. The standardized form for process evaluation can be seen in previous studies (4,5).

Results

For each unit, the ratings of every item by the two independent observers were averaged. To obtain a more comprehensive picture, the ratings for each item across all units were again averaged. In order to test the reliability of the averaged ratings, Pearson correlation was conducted based on the overall adherence ratings across the seven units and the analyses demonstrated that the ratings across the observers in the observed units (N =7) were highly reliable (r =0.96, p <0.01). The average overall adherence to the curriculum manuals was

90% (range from 80% to 100%, see Table 3), which was quite remarkable. Reliability analysis showed that the 13 items of the program implementation quality scale were internally consistent (alpha =0.97, mean inter-item correlation =0.72). For those units where modifications had been made, the observers generally regarded the changes to be reasonable.

Table 2. Summary of the characteristics of schools joining the process evaluation study (S3 curriculum)

School	A	B	C	D
Background Characteristics of the Schools:				
Location (district)	Tuen Mun	Tseung Kwan O	North Point	Sham Shui Po
Finance mode	Aided	Aided	Aided	Aided
Sex composition	Co-ed	Co-ed	Co-ed	Co-ed
Religious background	Buddhism	Buddhism	Nil	Nil
Context of Observation:				
Choice of program	20 hours	20 hours	20 hours	20 hours
Mode	20 sessions (1 hour per session)	20 sessions (1 hour per session)	20 sessions (1 hour per session)	20 sessions (1 hour per session)
Integration with school curriculum	Teacher's Period	Counseling Lesson	Liberal Studies and Life Education	Personal Growth Lesson
No. of students in the class	42	39	35	27
Instructor(s)	1 Social Worker	1 Social Worker	1 Social Worker	1 Teacher and 1 Social Worker
Teaching medium of the unit observed	Chinese	Chinese	Chinese	Chinese
Duration of observation	75 minutes	40 minutes	72 minutes	45 minutes
Unit observed	MC3.1 and MC3.2	BF3.1 and BF3.2	PI3.3 and PI3.4	MC3.4

The findings on the program implementation quality can be seen in Table 3. Pearson correlation was conducted based on the mean overall ratings across the seven units and the analyses indicated that the ratings across the two observers in the observed units (N =7) were also reliable (r =0.88, p <0.01). An examination of the different areas of the delivery quality showed that the mean ratings were generally high (over 5 on a 7-point rating scale). In particular, the two observers rated highly positive in the following areas: lesson preparation, classroom control, overall implementation quality and success of implementation. The findings demonstrated that the quality of delivery as assessed by the two independent observers was very good.

Table 3. Overall ratings on each unit observed in the different schools

School	A		B		C		D	Average / Mean
Unit observed	MC3.1	MC3.2	BF3.1	BF3.2	PI3.3	PI3.4	MC3.4	
Overall Adherence (%)	97.5	100	82.5	80	80	95	95	90
Ratings on a 7-point scale. The percentages of responses with ratings of 5 and above are in brackets.								
1. Student Interest	6 (100)	6 (100)	5.5 (100)	5.5 (100)	4.5 (50)	4 (0)	6 (100)	5.36
2. Student Participation and Involvement	6 (100)	6 (100)	6 (100)	5.5 (100)	4.5 (50)	5 (100)	5.5 (100)	5.50
3. Classroom Control	6 (100)	5.5 (100)	6 (100)	6 (100)	5 (100)	5 (100)	6 (100)	5.64
4.Interactive Delivery Method	6 (100)	5.5 (100)	6 (100)	5.5 (100)	4 (0)	5 (100)	6 (100)	5.43
5. Strategies to Enhance Student Motivation	6 (100)	5.5 (100)	5.5 (100)	5.5 (100)	4 (0)	5 (100)	6 (100)	5.36
6. Use of Positive and Supportive Feedback	5.5 (100)	5 (100)	5 (100)	5.5 (100)	5 (100)	5 (100)	5.5 (100)	5.21
7. Familiarity with the Students	6 (100)	5.5 (100)	5 (100)	5 (100)	5 (100)	5 (100)	7 (100)	5.50
8. Opportunity for Reflection	5.5 (100)	5.5 (100)	6 (100)	5.5 (100)	4.5 (50)	4.5 (50)	6 (100)	5.36
9. Degree of Achievement of the Objectives	6 (100)	6 (100)	6 (100)	5 (100)	5 (100)	5 (100)	6 (100)	5.57
10. Time Management	5.5 (100)	5 (100)	6 (100)	6 (100)	5 (100)	4 (0)	5.5 (100)	5.29
11. Lesson Preparation	6 (100)	6 (100)	6 (100)	6 (100)	5 (100)	5 (100)	6.5 (100)	5.79
12. Overall Implementation Quality	6 (100)	6 (100)	6 (100)	5.5 (100)	5 (100)	5 (100)	6 (100)	5.64
13. Success of Implementation	6 (100)	6 (100)	6 (100)	5.5 (100)	5 (100)	5 (100)	6 (100)	5.64

Discussion

This current study focuses on one specific aspect of process evaluation, i.e., program monitoring (7,32,33) with a central aim to assess the program fidelity and quality of program implementation. Results, using an observational design with four schools, largely support the findings of previous research (34). First, the findings did indicate that the overall degree of adherence to the teaching units assessed by the observers was higher than the previous two years (84.5% (EIP-S1: 2005-06) and 83.6% (EIP-S2: 2006-07)) when examining the adherence and quality of implementation of the Tier 1 Program (Secondary 3 Curriculum) of the Project P.A.T.H.S. in the third year of the EIP (EIP-S3: 2007-08). This finding is very encouraging as it suggests that the need for modifying the units in the implementation phase was not high. This further supports that curricula-based positive youth development programs can be easily utilized without making major modifications for different adolescent populations. This finding is imperative as there is a common myth among the program implementers that the program must be substantially modified before it can be meaningfully implemented.

The second major conclusion of the study is that different aspects of the program delivery were perceived to be very positive. These aspects include: effort in lesson preparation (item 11; rating: 5.79), the overall quality of implementation (item 12; rating: 5.64), and the success of implementation (item 13; rating 5.64).

Nevertheless, the use of positive and supportive feedback (item 6; rating: 5.21) was the lowest among all items, even though the rating reached 5 in a 7-point scale. There are several plausible explanations for this. First, although it is generally agreed that positive feedback or verbal praise has important influence on students' intrinsic motivation, praise is relatively infrequent in Hong Kong classrooms as Hong Kong teachers often adopt a more authoritarian role in teaching. An alternative explanation is that teachers might not possess good time management skills and so, they might not have sufficient time to give feedback to students. The poor time management skills could be reflected by the rating of time management (item 10; rating: 5.29) which was the second lowest among all. Since positive feedback is an invaluable part in the learning process that increases students' motivation, which in turn enables their growth and development, it should be further emphasized in subsequent instructors' and teachers' training.

Among the four schools observed, the scores on curriculum delivery of one school were far from satisfactory (School C: 4 out of 7). Based on the observations of the observers, several factors contributed to this situation: less interactive delivery method and limited strategies to enhance students' motivation. A plausible justification for this phenomenon is the didactic teaching style in Hong Kong.

This study had several limitations. First, because of manpower and resource constraints, only four schools were randomly selected to participate in this research and the data collection was carried out by the research team of the Project. It would be desirable to include more schools with different characteristics to join this study, and to involve as many staff at every level and stakeholder groups as possible in the day-to-day tasks of program monitoring because it will give everyone a sense of shared ownership in the monitoring process (7). Nonetheless, it is noteworthy that data collection must not hinder the functioning of the program and its implementers. Second, only seven curriculum units were observed. Due to limitation of resources, the evaluation design did not provide an ongoing activity to monitor the program to keep it on track, and the evaluators neither collected data over an extended period of time during the course of the program nor conducted ongoing process over the life cycle of the program. Third, besides adherence and the quality of implementation, process evaluation with reference to other dimensions, such as the context of the implementation (35) would help the program developers to further understand the quality of the program implementation process. With reference to the recommendation made by Linnan and Steckler (5) on gaps in current knowledge about process evaluation, future studies should refine on the concept of process, and the related assessment and interpretation methods.

Finally, one should be cautious when generalizing the present findings as the picture of a specific school cannot be shared with other schools because schools are under different management and evaluation results may place a specific school in jeopardy. Also, consistent with the intrinsic problem of all observational studies where time sampling is involved, we need to be conscious of the degree of generalizability of the present findings to other temporal and spatial contexts needs. Of course, this issue was partially addressed by the procedure that the schools were randomly selected from the participating schools. Nevertheless, it is noteworthy that one possible confounding effect is that the students might become more cooperative when there were visitors and outside observers. In addition, it is also possible that the instructors might be more motivated to teach well when being observed. Most obviously, the use of ethnographic strategies with prolonged engagement and observations would be desirable (36).

To conclude, despite these limitations, our study strongly suggests that the quality of implementation of the Secondary 3 Curriculum of the Tier 1 Program in the EIP was high and the program participants found the program offered to be of great value. Further, the present study provides unique information of program evaluation which is presently lacking in the field and it also attempts to illuminate certain blind spots that program implementers (i.e., school teachers and social workers), who have more personal investment in the program activities, are likely to have. The present findings will be made known to all implementers through publications and future staff training sessions. Similar to all formative evaluations, they are conducted when the program is underway with a goal to improve the overall project in its FIP as well.

Acknowledgments

The preparation for this paper and the Project P.A.T.H.S. were financially supported by The Hong Kong Jockey Club Charities Trust.

References

[1] Durlak JA. Successful prevention programs for children and adolescents. New York: Plenum, 1997.

[2] Dane AV, Schneider BH. Program integrity in primary and early secondary prevention: are implementation effects out of control? Clin Psychol Rev 1998; 18:23-45.

[3] Domitrovich CE, Greenberg MT. The study of implementation: current findings from effective programs that prevent mental disorders in school-aged children. J Educ Psychol Cons 2000;11:193-221.

[4] Shek DTL, Ma HK, Lui JHY, Lung DWM. Process evaluation of the Tier 1 Program of the Project P.A.T.H.S. ScientificWorldJournal 2006;1:300-9.

[5] Linnan L, Steckler A. Process evaluation for public health interventions and research: an overview. In: Steckler A, Linnan L, eds. Process evaluation for public health interventions and research. San Francisco: Jossey-Bass, 2002:1-23.

[6] Scheirer MA. Designing and using process evaluation. In: Wholey JS, Hatry HP, Newcomer KE, eds. Handbook of practical program evaluation. San Francisco: Jossey-Bass, 1994:40-66.

[7] Weinbach RW. Evaluating social work services and programs. Boston: Allyn Bacon, 2005.

[8] Shek DTL. Adolescent developmental issues in Hong Kong: relevance to positive youth development programs in Hong Kong. Int J Adolesc Med Health 2006;18:341-54.

[9] Lee MTY, Wong BP, Chow BWY, McBride-Chang C. Predictors of suicide ideation and depression in Hong Kong adolescents: perceptions of academic and family climates. Suicide Life Threat Behav 2006;36:82-96.

[10] Shek DTL. Tackling adolescent substance abuse in Hong Kong: where we should go and should not go. ScientificWorldJournal 2007;7:2021-30.

[11] Yip P, Yu A. Teenage suicide in Hong Kong 1981-1992: age trend, time and geographical distribution. Educ Res J 1993;8:32-9.

[12] Ng SMC. The role of psychological and environmental risk factors in self-harm amongst adolescents in Hong Kong. Dissertation. London: London Univ, 2007.

[13] Wong DSW. School bullying and tackling strategies in Hong Kong. Int J Offender Ther Comp Criminol 2004;48:537-53.

[14] Catalano RF, Berglund ML, Ryan JAM, Lonczak HS, Hawkins JD. Positive youth development in the United States: research findings on evaluations of positive youth development programs. Accessed 2008 Nov 15. URL: http://aspe.hhs.gov/hsp/PositiveYouthDev99/

[15] Shek DTL. Effectiveness of the Tier 1 Program of the Project P.A.T.H.S.: preliminary objective and subjective outcome evaluation findings. ScientificWorldJournal 2006;6:1466-74.

[16] Shek DTL, Siu AMH, Lee TY, Cheung CK, Chung R. Effectiveness of the Tier 1 Program of Project P.A.T.H.S.: objective outcome evaluation based on a randomized group trial. ScientificWorldJournal 2008;8:4-12.

[17] Shek DTL, Ma HK. Subjective outcome evaluation of the Project P.A.T.H.S.: findings based on the perspective of the program participants. ScientificWorldJournal 2007;7:47-55.

[18] Shek DTL, Siu AMH, Lee TY. Subjective outcome evaluation of the Project P.A.T.H.S.: findings based on the perspective of the program implementers. ScientificWorldJournal 2007;7:195-203.

[19] Shek DTL, Sun RCF. Subjective outcome evaluation of the Project P.A.T.H.S.: qualitative findings based on the experiences of program implementers. ScientificWorldJournal 2007;7:1024-35.

[20] Shek DTL, Sun RCF. Subjective outcome evaluation of the Project P.A.T.H.S.: qualitative findings based on the experiences of program participants. ScientificWorldJournal 2007;7:686-97.

[21] Shek DTL. Evaluation of the Tier 1 Program of Project P.A.T.H.S.: secondary data analyses of conclusions drawn by the program implementers. ScientificWorldJournal 2008;8:22-34.

[22] Shek DTL, Lee TY, Siu AMH, Ma HK. Convergence of subjective outcome and objective outcome evaluation findings: insights based on the Project P.A.T.H.S. ScientificWorldJournal 2007;7:258-67.

[23] Shek DTL, Sun RCF. Linkage between subjective outcome evaluation findings and objective outcome evaluation findings: a pioneer study in the Chinese culture. In: Columbus F, editor. Educational evaluation: 21st century issues and challenges. New York: Ed. Nova Science Publishers, in press.

[24] Shek DTL, Lee TY, Siu AMH, Lam CM. Qualitative evaluation of the Project P.A.T.H.S. based on the perceptions of the program participants. ScientificWorldJournal 2006;1:290-99.

[25] Shek DTL, Sun RCF. Implementation of the Tier 1 Program of the Project P.A.T.H.S.: interim evaluation findings. ScientificWorldJournal 2006;1:310-20.

[26] Shek DTL, Ma HK, Sun RCF. Interim evaluation of the Tier 1 Program (Secondary 1 Curriculum) of the Project P.A.T.H.S.: first year of the full implementation phase. ScientificWorldJournal 2008;8:47-60.

[27] Shek DTL, Sun RCF, Lam CM, Lung DWM, Lo SC. Evaluation of Project P.A.T.H.S. in Hong Kong: utilization of student weekly diary. ScientificWorldJournal 2008;8:13-21.

[28] Shek DTL, Ma HK, Lui JHY, Lung DWM. Process evaluation of the Tier 1 Program (Secondary 1 Curriculum) of the Project P.A.T.H.S.: findings based on the full implementation phase. ScientificWorldJournal 2008;8:35-46.

[29] Bouffard JA, Taxman FS, Silverman R. Improving process evaluation of correctional programs by using a comprehensive evaluation methodology. Eval Program Plann 2003;26:149-61.

[30] Mastrofski SD, Parks RB, Reiss AJ, Worden RE, DeLong C, Snipes JB, Terrill W. Systematic observation of public police: applying field research methods to policy analysis. Washington, DC: Natl Inst Justice, 1998.

[31] Elm EV, Altman DG, Egger M, Pocock SJ, Gotzsche PC, Vandenbroucke JP for the STROBE Initiative. The strengthening the reporting of observational studies in epidemiology (STROBE) statement: guidelines for reporting observational studies. PLoS Med 2007;4:1623-27.
[32] Unrau Y, Gabor P, Grinnell R. Evaluation in the human services. Itasca, IL: FE Peacock, 2001.
[33] Nugent W, Sieppert J, Hudson W. Practice evaluation for the 21st century. Belmont, CA: Brooks/Cole, 2001.
[34] Shek DTL, Lee TY, Sun RCF. Process evaluation of the implementation of the Secondary 2 Program of Project P.A.T.H.S. in the experimental implementation phase. ScientificWorldJournal 2008;8:83-94.
[35] Saunders RP, Evans MH, Joshi P. Developing a process-evaluation plan for assessing health promotion program implementation: a how-to guide. Health Promot Pract 2005;6:134-47.
[36] Patton MQ. Qualitative evaluation and research methods. Newbury Park, CA: Sage, 1990.

Submitted: December 30, 2008.
Revised: January 23, 2009.
Accepted: March 4, 2009

In: Public Health Yearbook 2009
Editor: Joav Merrick
ISBN: 978-1-61668-911-7

Chapter 31

PROCESS EVALUATION OF PROGRAM IMPLEMENTATION BASED ON THE CO-WALKER SCHEME

Daniel TL Shek, PhD, FHKPS, BBS, JP*[*1,2,3], Rachel CF Sun, BSocSc, PhD[4], Cathy NK Hang, BSocSc[4] and Christina YP Tang, BSocSc[4]

[1]Department of Applied Social Sciences, The Hong Kong Polytechnic University, Hong Kong, PRC, [2]Department of Sociology, East China Normal University, Shanghai, PRC, [3]Kiang Wu Nursing College of Macau, Macau, PRC and [4]Department of Social Work, The Chinese University of Hong Kong, Hong Kong, PRC

Abstract

This study examined the implementation quality of the Secondary 2 Program of the Project P.A.T.H.S. in the Experimental Implementation Phase. Classroom observations of 15 units implemented in ten schools were conducted under the Co-Walker Scheme, an initiative which attempts to provide support for the program implementers. Results showed that the overall level of program adherence was generally high (mean = 81.9%) and implementation quality of the program in terms of students' interest and involvement, instructors' use of time, classroom management and interactive teaching strategies as well as their relationship with the students was good. Results also revealed that different aspects of program implementation were significantly correlated amongst themselves.

Keywords: Quality of curriculum delivery, observation, positive youth development program.

[*] Correspondence: Professor Daniel TL Shek, PhD, FHKPS, BBS, JP, Chair Professor of Applied Social Sciences, Department of Applied Social Sciences, The Hong Kong Polytechnic University, Hunghom, Hong Kong. E-mail: danielshek@inet.polyu.edu.hk

Introduction

To promote holistic development among adolescents in Hong Kong, a two-tier positive youth development program entitled Project P.A.T.H.S. (**P**ositive **A**dolescent **T**raining through **H**olistic **S**ocial Programmes) was initiated and financially supported by The Hong Kong Jockey Club Charities Trust in 2005. The overall objective of the Project P.A.T.H.S. is to develop a quality curriculum promoting positive youth development in students in the junior secondary years. Based on systematic literature review and researchers' experiences in program construction, the Tier 1 Program is developed for all Secondary 1 to Secondary 3 students, with 20 hours of training at each grade. With the essential features of strong theoretical underpinnings, professional training for teachers and social workers, flexible teaching schedule and combination of units as well as a rigorous quality assurance process, healthy development and effective developmental outcomes of the participating students are expected.

Based on the principle of triangulation, there are several lines of evidence supporting the effectiveness of the Tier 1 Program of Project P.A.T.H.S. both in the Experimental Implementation Phase (EIP) and Full Implementation Phase (FIP). Objective outcome evaluation using both experimental and quasi-experimental designs (1,2) as well as subjective outcome evaluation collected from the program participants and implementers (3-9) showed that the program was beneficial to the participants. Apart from quantitative evaluation, qualitative findings including focus group interviews (10,11), analyses of the students' weekly diaries (12) and case studies (13,14) also showed that both program participants and implementers had positive perceptions of the program and regarded it as helpful to the students' overall development. While the outcomes of a program are important to consider, it is equally important to appreciate the fact that the outcomes of an intervention program are contingent on the quality of the process of program implementation. As such, it is crucial to conduct process evaluation which can provide answers to the questions of "what happened during the implementation and why did it happen that affected the program's ability to achieve its outcomes?"

According to Summerfelt (15), well-implemented process evaluation can lead to a more generalizable "understanding of the links between theory and practice, practice and outcome, and ultimately, theory and outcome" (p.56). Nearly every school-based program provides a set of guidelines for proper implementation, yet everyday practicalities (e.g., limited time and/or resources) and school politics may interfere with ideal program delivery in schools. Western findings like the studies of Dusenbury et al (16) and Lillehoj, Kenneth and Richard (17) consistently showed that school-based prevention or intervention programs fail to provide services in a manner consistent with the program expectations, thus resulting in reduced program effect. In addition, contextual factors such as inefficiency, low administrative support and low staff morale would also create program failure. Hence, guaranteeing its implementation as designed and delivery in its entirety at the classroom level is an essential factor for the effective school-based programs.

One of the most commonly used methods to evaluate implementation is an assessment of delivery quality and adherence to an intervention protocol through classroom observation. In Project P.A.T.H.S., findings of the systematic classroom observation conducted in both the Experimental Implementation Phase (18,19) and Full Implementation Phase (20) indicated that the quality of implementation and program adherence were high. Such findings were consistent with the data collected from other strategies such as the workers' perceptions of program implementation under interim evaluations (21,22,23). Generally speaking, the existing evaluation findings are very positive showing that different stakeholders have favorable perceptions of the program and its effectiveness.

Instead of simply understanding the actual delivery of an existing program (i.e., outcome evaluation), process evaluation can be used to serve as guidance for refinement of a developing program as well as response to the needs of practitioners. The latter functions of process evaluation were particularly important for Project P.A.T.H.S. in the Experimental Implementation Phase (January 2006 to August 2008), a phase with the objectives of accumulating experience in program implementation, and familiarizing front-line workers with the program design and philosophy. With the aim of providing ongoing support and guidance to the participating schools, the Research Team has launched a "Co-Walker Scheme" since December 2006. In this scheme, colleagues of the project served as co-walkers to take care of the participating schools in the format of providing consultation and support, school visits, and observations. All these efforts were made with the purpose to enhance the quality of program implementation, to examine the feasibility of implementing the program in schools, and to promote the morale of the front-line workers.

It is argued that classroom observation conducted by co-walkers is highly informative because it adopts an empathetic stance with respect to the views and needs of the implementers. Meeting or discussion over school's and implementers' concerns would usually be held before and/or after the classroom observation. Therefore, while the previous systematic classroom observation aims to examine the implementation quality and effectiveness of Tier 1 Program, the co-walkers' observation targets at providing guidance and feedback for implementation. Furthermore, data collected from the co-walkers' observation rating forms can provide an additional perspective to examine the implementation quality of the Tier 1 Program.

Against this background, the present study intends to examine the implementation quality of the Secondary 2 Curriculum in the Experimental Implementation Phase. With respect to the developmental characteristics of Secondary 2 students, such as adjustment to puberty, cognitive maturation, rapid expansion of social circle, increased stress, encountering higher levels of social expectations, and gradual detachment from the family, the Secondary 2 Curriculum was designed to focus more on cultivating the students' development in the individual and society domains, such as encouraging students to live a meaningful life and to participate in healthy community activities. As such, it is necessary to utilize the data of co-walkers' observation to act as another mirror to reflect on how the Secondary 2 Curriculum was delivered in classrooms in the Experimental Implementation Phase.

Methods

Participants

There were 49 schools joining the Secondary 2 Curriculum of the Project P.A.T.H.S. in the EIP in the 2006/07 academic year. Among these schools, 21 adopted the 20-hour full program that involves 40 teaching units and 28 adopted the 10-hour core program that involves 20 teaching units. Due to school rejection and time constraint, only 10 schools joined the observation study conducted by the co-walkers. Among the 10 observed schools, four schools adopted the 20-hour full program and 6 schools adopted the 10-hour core program. The average number of students per class was 35.53 and the average number of instructors per class was 2.07. The average duration of observation was 32 minutes.

Procedures

For each school joining the co-walker observation study, systematic observations of one or two teaching units were conducted. The 15 units under observation covered 6 positive youth development constructs, including cognitive competence, behavioral competence, moral competence, prosocial norms, spirituality, clear and positive identity, and one conclusion session. The observer for each school was the designated co-walker who was a registered social worker. During observation, the observer observed how the units were implemented and was required to complete an observation form covering four major areas, including basic information, implementation mode of units, program fidelity and adherence, and quality of program delivery in an independent manner. For program fidelity and adherence, the observer rated the degree of adherence in percentages and recorded the time used to implement the unit. For the quality of program delivery, student interest, student participation and involvement, classroom control, use of interactive delivery method, use of strategies to enhance student motivation, use of positive and supportive feedbacks, instructors' familiarity with the students, opportunity for reflection, degree of achievement of the objectives, time management, quality of preparation, overall implementation quality, and success of implementation were rated on a 7-point scale.

As shown in Table 1, seven out of the 15 observed units were implemented by the schools adopting the 20-hour full program and the remaining eight units were implemented by the schools adopting the 10-hour core program. Considering the implementation mode, among the seven units implemented by the schools adopting the full program, five of them were incorporated into the formal curriculum and only two were implemented outside formal curriculum. In view of all the observed units, 60% (i.e. 9 units) were incorporated into the formal curriculum and 40% (i.e. 6 units) were implemented outside formal curriculum.

Table 1. The percentage of observed Tier 1 Program units implemented in different modes for schools adopting 10 hours and 20 hours of implementation

Different Mode	Hours of Implementation		
	10-hour	20-hour	Total
Incorporated into the formal curriculum	4 (50%)	5 (71.4%)	9 (60%)
Outside formal curriculum*	4 (50%)	2 (28.6%)	6 (40%)
Total	8 (100%)	7 (100%)	15 (100%)

Note. *Outside formal curriculum refers to the implementation after school, during holidays, teachers' periods, post-exam days, assembly or camps.

Results

The average overall adherence to the curriculum manuals was 81.9% (range=50%-100%), which was generally high (see Table 2). Results in Table 2 also revealed that the overall quality of implementation as assessed by the co-walkers was very high (5.60 on a 7-point rating scale). An examination of the different areas showed that the mean ratings were generally

high, except that the opportunity for reflection was relatively lower, which was only 4.80, as compared to other dimensions of the program implementation quality. In particular, the observers rated highly positive in the quality of lesson preparation by the instructors with an average score of 5.93.

Table 2. Average rates of overall adherence and observed units of curriculum delivered

Quality of Curriculum Delivery	Mean	Standard Deviation
1. Student interest	5.33	1.35
2. Student participation and involvement	5.40	1.35
3. Classroom control	5.47	1.13
4. Interactive delivery method	5.40	1.06
5. Strategies to enhance student motivation	5.33	0.82
6. Use of positive and supportive feedback	5.33	1.18
7. Instructors' familiarity with the students	5.07	1.39
8. Opportunity for reflection	4.80	1.08
9. Degree of achievement of the objectives	5.53	1.13
10. Time management	5.20	1.37
11. Lesson preparation	5.93	0.96
12. Overall implementation quality	5.60	1.06
13. Success of implementation	5.40	0.99
Overall Adherence = 81.87% (range=50%-100%)		

Internal consistency of the curriculum delivery scale was tested by calculating Cronbach's alpha, inter-item and corrected item-total correlations. The alpha coefficient for the total rating scale was very high (0.95) and would be further increased by omitting the items "strategies to enhance student motivation" and "lesson preparation" (see Table 3). Almost all items had high corrected item-total correlation, except the strategies to enhance student motivation ($r = 0.29$) and lesson preparation ($r = 0.28$) which had weak correlations. The mean inter-item correlation of the scale was 0.57.

Pearson inter-item correlation coefficients among the items of curriculum delivery are shown in Table 4. Most of the items were positively inter-correlated, ranging from 0.54 to 0.94, except "strategies to enhance student motivation" and "lesson preparation" which showed insignificant correlations to most of the items. It is noteworthy that the significant correlation coefficients can be regarded impressive in view of the small sample size involved.

Table 3. Reliability test of the Qualities of Curriculum Delivery Scale

Quality of Curriculum Delivery	Corrected item-total correlation	Total alpha if item is deleted
1. Student interest	0.917	0.940
2. Student participation and involvement	0.862	0.942
3. Classroom control	0.789	0.944
4. Interactive delivery method	0.780	0.944
5. Strategies to enhance student motivation	0.293	0.955
6. Use of positive and supportive feedbacks	0.780	0.944
7. Instructors' familiarity with the students	0.849	0.942
8. Opportunity for reflection	0.828	0.943
9. Degree of achievement of the objectives	0.715	0.946
10. Time management	0.868	0.941
11. Lesson preparation	0.276	0.956
12. Overall implementation quality	0.764	0.945
13. Success of implementation	0.920	0.941
Cronbach's alpha = 0.95.		

Discussion

This paper attempts to examine the adherence and overall implementation quality of the Tier 1 Program (Secondary 2 Curriculum) of the Project P.A.T.H.S. in the second year of the EIP based on co-walkers' observation. The present study showed that the overall degree of adherence to the teaching units assessed by the co-walkers was on the high side, with the mean program adherence of 81.9%. This finding was generally consistent with the process evaluation findings on the Tier 1 Program (Secondary 2 Curriculum) in the EIP (2006/07 school year) (19). These findings are very encouraging as studies showed that program adherence in related intervention programs was not high in the West.

Practically speaking, the findings suggested that the need for modifying the units in the implementation process was not high. These findings challenge the common belief that manual-based positive youth development programs cannot be easily used and significant modifications must be made for different adolescent populations. Such a myth is not uncommon among in program implementers of positive youth development programs. In fact, Mowbray, Holter, Teague and Bybee (24) stressed that high quality treatment effectiveness research should utilize a program manual for training and supervising intervention staff and for monitoring program quality and performance, helping to ensure fidelity to the model being researched.

The second major conclusion of the study is that different aspects of the program delivery were perceived to be very positive. These aspects include (a) student interest and involvement (item 1 and 2), (b) management and teaching strategies used by the instructors (items 3, 4, 5, 6, and 10), (c) instructors' relationship with the students (item 7). Moreover, the co-walkers perceived that the objectives of the units implemented could be achieved (item 9) and the overall quality of implementation was high (item 12).In particular, the co-walkers had very high appreciation on instructors' effort in preparing the lesson (item 11). This finding was consistent with the subjective outcome evaluation on the Tier 1 Program (Secondary 2 Curriculum) in the EIP (2006/07 school year) (8,9), which revealed the opinions of both participants and program implementers that the instructors were well prepared for the lessons. Most important of all, the implementation was regarded as successful by the observers (item 13). Of course, one should be cautious when attempting to generalize the present findings to other school contexts.

Nevertheless, the degree of reflection (item 8) was the lowest among the items. There are four possible explanations. First, the time allocated to implement the units was generally tight in most participating schools and thus little opportunities were provided for students' reflection. As reflected in the interim evaluation findings on the Tier 1 Program (Secondary 2 Curriculum) in the EIP (2006/07 school year) (23), 11.8% of the worker respondents commented that the implementation time was pressing and insufficient for running all activities. Second, reflection is not extensively introduced in Hong Kong school context. In the Hong Kong culture, teaching is still primarily didactic rather than interactive in nature. Third, since the study was conducted in the EIP, the instructors might be less familiar with the use of reflection when implementing the program during this adapting period. In fact, reflective learning is not the mainstream learning method adopted by teachers in Hong Kong. Fourth, some instructors who took part in implementing the program were social workers of the school (13 units out of 15 units). As the social workers were less acquainted with the students, this might make the running of reflection session less smooth. In general, the pretest finding based on co-walkers' observation provided an additional information in revealing the program delivery phenomena in schools.

In relation to the reliability of the thirteen items assessing the program implementation quality, the Cronbach's alpha was 0.95 (see Table 3). This revealed that the thirteen aspects of the program implementation quality had a very high internal consistency and they altogether formed a highly reliable instrument in evaluating and measuring the implementation qualities. Regarding the corrected item-total correlations, almost all of the correlation coefficients were high ($r > 0.72$), except the "strategies to enhance student motivation" ($r = 0.29$) and "lesson preparation" ($r = 0.28$) which showed low correlation coefficients. This could be explained by the small sample size of the study since only 10 schools joined this study (about one-fifth of all participating schools) and totally only 15 units were observed under this study. In the public health context, assessment of the process of implementing health education programs is important. Obviously, the instrument developed in this study is helpful to researchers implementing similar programs on positive youth development.

With reference to the inter-item correlations of the thirteen dimensions of the program implementation quality (see Table 4), most of the qualities were positively inter-correlated, except "strategies to enhance student motivation" and "lesson preparation". Although lesson preparation had the highest rating among the thirteen dimensions of the program implementation, it did not correlate with success of implementation and most of the other qualities. One possible explanation is that well-preparation does not guarantee good program implementation. Actually, high input of curricula preparation might not mean that the program implementers had equipped themselves with professional and adequate skills in implementing the program. This assumption was consistent with and supported by the interim evaluation findings on the Tier 1 Program (Secondary 2 Curriculum) in the EIP (2006/07 school year) (23), 9.1% of the worker respondents reported that the content was too much and some topics were difficult to handle. Moreover, 6.8% of them revealed that instructors did not acquire adequate skills to run the activities. Furthermore, as the range of scores was small in the high scores in preparation, this would result in lower correlation coefficients with other variables.

Besides, "strategies to enhance student motivation" was not correlated with other program implementation qualities. This might be due to the similarity of the activity formats and the complexity of the curricula content which could not arouse students' motivation to learn. In fact, the workers' opinions on the Secondary 2 Curriculum requiring improvement in the interim evaluation findings on the Tier 1 Program (Secondary 2 Curriculum) in the EIP (2006/07 school year) (23) had supported this argument - 13.7% of the worker respondents reflected that the activities were too many or too complex or too shallow or could not arouse students' interests. In addition, 11.8% of the worker respondents indicated that some activity formats were similar. Another possibility is that the program implementers might lack skills in motivating the students.

There are several limitations of the study. First, due to school rejection and time constraint, only 10 schools participated in this study. It would be desirable to include more schools with different characteristics to participate in the study. Second, the cooperation of the students and the strong motivation of the instructors might be due to the observation of visitors or outsiders. They might be an exception, not the norm for implementation of the P.A.T.H.S. program curriculum. Third, the characteristics of Secondary 2 students might also affect the results. For Secondary Two students, they probably had got used to the secondary school life after a year of adaptation. That would make a difference in the implementation of the program. Fourth, of the 15 units being observed, most of them (13 units) involved the participation of school social workers in the implementation of the program. Some students might not participate actively in the P.A.T.H.S. program because they did not get acquainted with the school social workers. In this case, it might be difficult to carry out the interactive mode of curriculum delivery. Actually, this fact was reflected in the interim evaluation findings on the Tier 1 Program (Secondary 2 Curriculum) in the EIP (2006/07 school year) (23). 2.3% of the worker respondents expressed that the social workers did not get acquainted with the students.

Fifth, this study only based on adherence and the quality of implementation in understanding the quality of the program implementation process. Sixth, as there was only one co-walker observed each lesson, the subjectivity of the co-walker should be taken into account. Finally, the findings only described the implementation situation in Hong Kong school culture. It might not be applicable to other cultures' school contexts. Despite these limitations, the existing research findings suggested that the quality of implementation of the Tier 1 Program was high and they constituted some insights into effective implementation of the P.A.T.H.S. program curriculum.

Table 4. Inter-correlations among items of the Curriculum Delivery Assessment

Item	1	2	3	4	5	6	7	8	9	10	11	12	13
1. Student interest	1.00												
2. Student participation and involvement	0.94^{**}	1.00											
3. Classroom control	0.69^{**}	0.62^{*}	1.00										
4. Interactive delivery method	0.86^{**}	0.93^{**}	0.43	1.00									
5. Strategies to enhance student motivation	0.35	0.45	-0.03	0.50	1.00								
6. Use of positive and supportive feedbacks	0.87^{**}	0.94^{**}	0.58^{*}	0.81^{**}	0.47	1.00							
7. Instructors' familiarity with the students	0.87^{**}	0.86^{**}	0.67^{**}	0.81^{**}	0.23	0.86^{**}	1.00						
8. Opportunity for reflection	0.79^{**}	0.64^{**}	0.79^{**}	0.51	0.32	0.62^{*}	0.68^{**}	1.00					
9. Degree of achievement of the objectives	0.58^{*}	0.46	0.81^{**}	0.41	-0.13	0.34	0.57^{*}	0.62^{*}	1.00				
10. Time management	0.85^{**}	0.72^{**}	0.81^{**}	0.58^{*}	0.19	0.66^{**}	0.71^{**}	0.89^{**}	0.76^{**}	1.00			
11. Lesson preparation	0.07	-0.09	0.49	-0.04	-0.06	-0.17	0.16	0.54^{*}	0.63^{*}	0.39	1.00		
12. Overall implementation quality	0.65^{**}	0.62^{*}	0.65^{**}	0.67^{**}	0.17	0.46	0.65^{**}	0.55^{*}	0.85^{**}	0.60^{*}	0.47	1.00	
13. Success of implementation	0.81^{**}	0.78^{**}	0.79^{**}	0.73^{**}	0.36	0.68^{**}	0.71^{**}	0.75^{**}	0.82^{**}	0.83^{**}	0.41	0.85^{**}	1.00

$^{**}p < 0.05$, $^{*}p < 0.01$

The present findings also throw lights on future research and practices. To better understand the quality of the program implementation process, it is suggested that using ethnographic strategies with prolonged engagement and observations would be helpful in ensuring the reliability of the study findings. Moreover, process evaluation with reference to other dimensions, such as context of the implementation and the involvement of other stakeholders (25), would help the program developers to further understand the quality of the program implementation process. With reference to the comment of Linnan and Steckler (26), that "a number of gaps in current knowledge about process evaluation must be addressed if the field is to move forward" (p. 8), it is suggested that future studies should refine the concept of process, and the related assessment and interpretation methods.

Some recommendations could be made to improve the success of the program implementation. First, the participating schools should be encouraged to increase their level of adherence to the planned curriculum. Researchers (27-30) increasingly recognize the importance of ensuring that prevention programs are implemented as designed and delivered in their entirety, both in research and in non-research contexts, in order to ensure intervention effectiveness. Second, strengthening the opportunity for reflection and interactive delivery of curriculum could help increasing the implementation efficacy. For example, according to Wilson et al (31), each of the planned activities and group processes such as team building, social skill development, Photovoice, critical dialogue, democratic decision making, and participating in social action, reflection, and self-evaluation contributed to individual and group efficacy in Nance's YES! intervention model.

Third, based on the experiences in the EIP, it is advised that the co-walkers could provide more relevant skills and support to the instructors to increase the implementation effectiveness, especially on how to provide opportunities for students' reflection, in the Full Implementation Phase. Shek et al (19) stressed that reflection is an invaluable part in the learning process that encourages students to evaluate one self and one's values, which in turn enables their growth and development, and therefore it should be further emphasized in subsequent instructors' training. Finally, the program implementers could consider prolonging the activity time from half an hour to one hour so as to improve the quality of implementation of reflection. In addition, in order to strengthen the qualities of reflection and interactive delivery of program curriculum, it is suggested that the program implementers could consider using some material reward and most importantly, arousing students' intrinsic motivation, to encourage students to actively participate in class activities.

Acknowledgments

The preparation for this paper and the Project P.A.T.H.S. were financially supported by The Hong Kong Jockey Club Charities Trust.

References

[1] Shek DTL. Effectiveness of the Tier 1 Program of the Project P.A.T.H.S.: preliminary objective and subjective outcome evaluation findings. ScientificWorldJournal 2006;6:1466-74.

[2] Shek DTL, Siu AMH, Lee TY, Cheung CK, Chung R. Effectiveness of the Tier 1 Program of Project P.A.T.H.S.: objective outcome evaluation based on a randomized group trial. ScientificWorldJournal 2008;8:4-12.

[3] Shek DTL, Ma HK. Subjective outcome evaluation of the Project P.A.T.H.S.: findings based on the program participants. ScientificWorldJournal 2007;7: 47-55.

[4] Shek DTL, Siu AMH, Lee TY. Subjective outcome evaluation of the Project P.A.T.H.S.: findings based on the perspective of the program implementers. ScientificWorldJournal 2007;7:195-203.

[5] Shek DTL, Sun RCF. Subjective outcome evaluation of the Project P.A.T.H.S.: qualitative findings based on the experiences of program implementers. ScientificWorldJournal 2007;7:1024-35.

[6] Shek DTL, Sun RCF. Subjective outcome evaluation of the Project P.A.T.H.S.: qualitative findings based on the experiences of program participants. ScientificWorldJournal 2007;7:686–97.

[7] Shek DTL. Evaluation of the Tier 1 Program of Project P.A.T.H.S.: secondary data analyses of conclusions drawn by the program implementers. ScientificWorldJournal 2008;8:22-34.

[8] Shek DTL, Sun RCF, Chan CWY. Evaluation of Project P.A.T.H.S. (Secondary 2 Program) by the program participants: findings based on the Experimental Implementation Phase. ScientificWorldJournal 2008;8:526-35.

[9] Shek DTL, Sun RCF, Lung DWM. Evaluation of Project P.A.T.H.S. (Secondary 2 Program) by the program implementers: findings based on the Experimental Implementation Phase. ScientificWorldJournal 2008;8:536-46.

[10] Shek DTL, Lee TY, Siu A, Lam CM. Qualitative evaluation of the Project P.A.T.H.S. based on the perceptions of the program participants. ScientificWorldJournal 2006;6:2254-63.

[11] Shek DTL, Lee TY. Qualitative evaluation of the Project P.A.T.H.S.: findings based on focus groups with student participants. Int J Adolesc Med Health 2008;20(4):449-62.

[12] Shek DTL, Sun RCF, Lam CM, Lung DWM, Lo SC. Evaluation of Project P.A.T.H.S. in Hong Kong: utilization of student weekly dairy. ScientificWorldJournal 2008;8:13-21.

[13] Shek DTL, Sun RCF. Implementation of a positive youth development program in a Chinese context: the role of policy, program, people, process, and place. ScientificWorldJournal 2008;8:960-96.

[14] Shek DTL, Chak YLY, Chan CWY. School-related factors in the implementation of a positive youth development project in Hong Kong. ScientificWorldJournal 2008;8:997-1009.

[15] Summerfelt WT. Program strength and fidelity in evaluation. Appl Dev Sci 2003;7(2):55-61.

[16] Dusenbury L, Rosalind B, Mathea F, William BH. A review of research on fidelity of implementation: implications for drug abuse prevention in school settings. Health Educ Res 2003;18(2):237-56.

[17] Lillehoj CJ, Kenneth WG, Richard S. Program provider and observer ratings of school-based preventive intervention implementation: agreement and relation to youth outcomes. Health Educ Behav 2004;31(2):242-57.

[18] Shek DTL, Ma HK, Lui JHY, Lung DWM. Process evaluation of the Tier 1 Program of the Project P.A.T.H.S. ScientificWorldJournal 2006;1:300-9.

[19] Shek DTL, Lee TY, Sun RCF. Process evaluation of the Implementation of the Secondary 2 Program of Project P.A.T.H.S. in the Experimental Implementation Phase. ScientificWorldJournal 2008;8:83-94.

[20] Shek DTL, Ma HK, Sun RCF, Lung DWM. Process evaluation of the Tier 1 Program (Secondary 1 Curriculum) of the Project P.A.T.H.S.: findings based on the Full Implementation Phase. ScientificWorldJournal 2008;8:35-46.

[21] Shek DTL, Sun RCF. Implementation of the Tier 1 Program of the Project P.A.T.H.S.: interim evaluation findings. ScientificWorldJournal 2006;6: 2274–84.

[22] Shek DTL, Ma HK, Sun RCF. Interim evaluation of the Tier 1 Program (Secondary 1 Curriculum) of the Project P.A.T.H.S.: first year of the Full Implementation Phase. ScientificWorldJournal 2008;8:47-60.

[23] Shek DTL, Sun RCF, Siu AMH. Interim evaluation of the Secondary 2 Program of Project P.A.T.H.S.: insights based on the Experimental Implementation Phase. ScientificWorldJournal 2008;8:61-72.
[24] Mowbray CT, Holter MC, Teague GB, Bybee D. Fidelity criteria: development, measurement, and validation. Am J Eval 2003;24:315-40.
[25] Saunders RP, Evans MH, Joshi P. Developing a process-evaluation plan for assessing health promotion program implementation: a how-to guide. Health Promot Pract 2005;6:134-47.
[26] Linnan L, Steckler A. Process evaluation for public health interventions and research: an overview. In: Steckler A, Linnan L, editors. Process evaluation for public health interventions and research. San Francisco: Jossey-Bass, 2002:1-23.
[27] Domitrovich CE, Greenberg MT. The study of implementation: current findings from effective programs that prevent mental disorders in school-aged children. J Educ Psychol Cons 2000;11:193-221.
[28] Spoth R. Challenges in defining and developing the field of rural mental disorder preventive intervention research. Am J Community Psychol 1997;25:425-48.
[29] Durlak J. Why program implementation is important. J Prev Interv Community 1998;17:5-18.
[30] Greenberg M, Domitrovich C, Graczyk P, Zins J. The study of implementation in school-based prevention interventions: theory, research, and practice. In Report to Center for Mental Health Services (CMHS). Substance Abuse Mental Health Services Adminstration, U.S. Department of Health and Human Services, 2005:13.
[31] Wilson N, Minkler M, Dasho S, Wallerstein N, Martin AC. Getting to social action: the youth empowerment strategies (YES!) Project. Health Promot Pract 2006;1:1-9.

Submitted: January 02, 2009.
Revised: January 30, 2009.
Accepted: February 15, 2009.

In: Public Health Yearbook 2009
Editor: Joav Merrick
ISBN: 978-1-61668-911-7

Chapter 32

Evaluation of Positive Youth Development Programs That Help Secondary 2 Students with Greater Psychosocial Needs

Daniel TL Shek, PhD, FHKPS, BBS, JP*[*1,2,3] and Rachel CF Sun, BSocSc, PhD[4]

[1]Department of Applied Social Sciences, The Hong Kong Polytechnic University, Hong Kong, PRC, [2]Department of Sociology, East China Normal University, Shanghai, PRC, [3]Kiang Wu Nursing College of Macau, Macau, PRC and [4]Department of Social Work, The Chinese University of Hong Kong, Hong Kong, PRC

Abstract

The Tier 2 Program of the Project P.A.T.H.S. is designed and implemented primarily by school social workers which attempts to help adolescents with greater psychosocial needs. After completion of the Tier 2 Program in the Experimental Implementation Phase (Secondary 2 level), 1,898 Secondary 2 students in 49 schools responded to the Subjective Outcome Evaluation Form (Form C) to assess their views on the program, instructors and perceived effectiveness of the program. Results showed that a large proportion of the respondents had positive perceptions of the program and the instructors and roughly four-fifths of the respondents regarded the program as helpful to them. Pearson correlation analyses showed that perceptions of the program and instructors were significantly correlated with perceived effectiveness of the program. Participants joining programs that adopted both adventure-based counseling approach and volunteer training activities generally perceived higher levels of program effectiveness and had better global

* Correspondence: Professor Daniel TL Shek, PhD, FHKPS, BBS, JP, Chair Professor of Applied Social Sciences, Department of Applied Social Sciences, The Hong Kong Polytechnic University, Hunghom, Hong Kong. E-mail: danielshek@inet.polyu.edu.hk

views on the program than did participants attending programs adopted either approach only.

Keywords: Secondary prevention, subjective outcome evaluation, volunteer training and services, adventure-based counseling.

INTRODUCTION

Positive Adolescent Training through Holistic Social Programmes (Project P.A.T.H.S.) is a two-tier program that aims to promote positive youth development in junior secondary school students in Hong Kong (1, 2). The Tier 1 Program is a manual-based curriculum designed by the Research Team to provide 20-hour training for Secondary 1 to 3 students of the participating schools on a universal basis, whereas the Tier 2 Program is a selective prevention program designed by social services agencies to address the unique needs of students who display greater psychosocial needs in each participating school. Although evaluation studies based on different evaluation strategies and data sources have shown the effectiveness of the Tier 1 Program in both Experimental Implementation Phase (3-11) and Full Implementation Phase (12-19), evaluation findings supporting the effectiveness of the Tier 2 Program are sparse (20, 21). In addition, although the existing studies have shown that a large proportion of the respondents had positive perceptions of the programs, instructors and program benefits (20, 21), they are limited to the Tier 2 Program at the Secondary 1 level. As the Tier 2 Program is also provided to Secondary 2 students of the Experimental Implementation Phase, there is a need to examine the participants' perceptions of the Tier 2 Program at the Secondary 2 level.

Because the Tier 2 Program is tailor-made to suit the specific needs of students in the unique school context, the program contents varies among schools. Nonetheless, some similarities of the program modes can be delineated as the social services agencies are requested to design the programs with reference to the 15 positive youth development constructs covered in the project as well as goals and objectives covered in this project (22). With reference to the positive youth development constructs of "resilience" and "prosocial involvement", adventure-based counseling approach and volunteer training and services were found to be the two commonly adopted approaches in the Tier 2 Program (20, 21).

Adventure-based counseling (ABC) is a kind of counseling intervention, which engages participants in challenging and adventure activities and aims to enhance adolescents' cohesiveness, communication, problem-solving and decision-making skills in the process, and to foster their growth needs, such as courage, resilience, responsibility, belonging, mastery, autonomy and altruism (23, 24). Apart from incorporating therapeutic or developmental elements, the ABC activities also serve as metaphors for real-life issues with reference to the experiential learning theory (25). Carlson and Cook (26) noted that adolescents who could successfully overcome the challenges in the program and transfer the experiences to other life challenges in the present or future may result in new behavioral and cognitive patterns. Although there is a paucity of literature documenting the effectiveness of the adventure-based counseling programs, some existing studies showed that such programs had created positive changes in different target groups, such as seriously ill adolescents (26) and delinquent youth (27). Nevertheless, there are arguments pointing out that the positive effects of ABC may not be sustainable over time.

On the other hand, volunteer training and services are means to engage students in community services that aim to contribute to their learning and growth. There are different types of volunteer training and services requiring different levels of student involvement. For example, some programs require students being volunteers and offering help to the needy within their capabilities, and these volunteers were found to have higher levels of empathy and altruism after participating in the programs (28). Some programs require the "helpers" to be trained in advance and offer volunteer services to the helpers under supervision, such as "Teen Outreach" (29) and Teen Hot Line programs (30, 31), which were found to benefit not only the needy in the community, but also the youth volunteers themselves in terms of a higher level of acceptance and fewer problem behaviors. In addition, some programs allow youths to participate in voluntary associations and provide opportunities to them to practice interpersonal skills or organizing skills, and these programs were found to facilitate youth's bonding with healthy people (32) and citizenship in adulthood (33). In general, programs related to volunteer training and community services were found to produce positive changes in adolescents.

A survey of the literature shows that there are many factors influencing the implementation and effectiveness of a program. One of them is program characteristics, such as comprehensiveness, relevance to the needs of students and diversity of training modes (34, 35). Research studies showed that programs were rated as effective in fostering students' positive outcomes if the programs were characterized by high peer interaction (36) and high peer involvement (37). Another critical determinant influencing teaching effectiveness is professional teaching skills, such as the amount of information transmitted, presentation style, arousal of student interest, and rapport with students (38). Thus, it is believed that program implementers having such teaching skills, together with caring and responsible characteristics could greatly facilitate program success (34, 35). Moreover, as positive relationships among program characteristics, program implementers' characteristics and perceived program effectiveness were found in Secondary 1 Program of the Project P.A.T.H.S. (21), it was hypothesized that there would be positive relationships among these three domains in the Secondary 2 Program.

The findings of a subjective outcome evaluation study based on the perspective of the participants of the Tier 2 Program (Secondary 2 level) implemented in the Experimental Implementation Phase are presented in this paper. Besides describing the profile of responses based on subjective outcome evaluation, the relationships among program characteristics, program implementers' characteristics and perceived program effectiveness were examined. Furthermore, whether participants joining different programs differed in their evaluation of the program were examined. As documentation on practice research was rare in the local social work literature (3), the purpose of this paper is to systematically document the effectiveness of youth programs designed by the social services agencies in the Tier 2 Program of the Project P.A.T.H.S..

Methods

Participants and procedures

A total of 49 schools joined the Secondary 2 Program of the Project P.A.T.H.S. in the Experimental Implementation Phase (2006-07 school year). In these schools, there were 2,542 participants joining the Tier 2 Program. Among these participants, 2,439 were students identified by teachers, parents and/or via self-administered questionnaires as having greater psychosocial needs and they were invited to join the Tier 2 Program. The other participants were 103 parents and teachers of those identified students. The mean number of participants joining the Tier 2 Program per school was 51.88 (ranged from 17 to 240 participants). The average number of sessions provided per school (normally one and a half hours to three hours per session) was 22.63 (ranged from 1 to 62 sessions).

A total of 1,898 participants (mean=38.73 participants per school, ranged from 8 to 199) responded to the Subjective Outcome Evaluation Form (Form C) developed by the Research Team (40), usually immediately after completion of the Tier 2 Program. The overall response rate was 74.67%. There are three plausible reasons for this response rate: 1) some participants withdrew from the Tier 2 Program before completion; 2) some participants were absent in the last session and did not complete the evaluation form; 3) some schools did not invite the adult participants to respond to the evaluation form as Form C was primarily designed for students.

On the day of data collection, the purpose of the evaluation and the principle of confidentiality were explained to the participants, and their "passive" informed consent was obtained. Adequate time was provided for the participants to complete the questionnaire in a self-administration format and in anonymous manner. To facilitate program evaluation, the Research Team developed an evaluation manual with standardized instructions for collecting the subjective outcome evaluation data (40). In addition, adequate training was provided to the social workers during the 20-hour training workshops on how to collect and analyze the data collected using the Form C.

Instruments

The Subjective Outcome Evaluation Form (Form C) was designed by Shek and Siu (39) which aims to measure the perceptions of the Tier 2 Program. There are seven parts in this evaluation form:

- Participants' perceptions of the program, such as program design, quality of service, appropriateness of the program, and interaction among the participants (8 items).
- Participants' perceptions of the workers, such as the preparation of the workers, professional attitude and knowledge, and interaction with the participants (8 items).
- Participants' perception of the effectiveness of the program, such as resilience and overall personal development (8 items).
- Things that the participants appreciated most (open-ended question).
- Opinions about the workers (open-ended question).
- Things that the participants learnt from the program (open-ended question).
- Areas that require improvement (open-ended question).

After collecting the data, social work service providers were requested to input the data in an EXCEL file developed by the Research Team which would automatically compute the frequencies and percentages associated with the different ratings for an item. When the providers submitted the reports, they were also requested to submit the soft copy of the consolidated data sheets. The data from all service providers were then aggregated to "re-construct" the overall profile by the Research Team. Because the Tier 2 Program was designed according to the various needs and the contextual situations of different schools, two trained research assistants (one with a Bachelor Degree in Social Work and has front-line social work experiences for adolescents and one with a Bachelor Degree in Social Sciences) categorized the program contents strictly according to the program proposal together with the actual activities indicated in the program reports.

RESULTS

Reliability analysis with the schools as the unit of analyses showed that the Form C was internally consistent: 8 items related to the program (alpha=.99, mean inter-item correlation=.92), 8 items related to the worker (alpha=.99, mean inter-item correlation =.90), 8 items related to the effectiveness (alpha=.99, mean inter-item correlation =.94), and 24 items based on whole Form C (alpha=.99, mean inter-item correlation =.88).

Table 1. Summary of the program characteristics and effectiveness

Main Program Approach	Clientele	Average No. of Participants	Average Program Attendance (%)	Average No. of Program Aims Indicated in the Reports	Average No. of Constructs Indicated in the Reports	Mean of Overall Effectiveness
Adventure Based Counseling Approach and Volunteer Training and Services (Type A) (N=20)	a(N=17)	39.76	84.49	2.35	6.06	4.87
	b(N=2)	28.50	84.50	3.50	6.00	4.58
	d(N=1)	168.00	78.80	2.00	5.00	4.45
Adventure Based Counseling Approach Only (Type B) (N=11)	a(N=11)	46.64	73.97	1.91	5.00	4.54
Volunteer Training and Services Only (Type C) (N=12)	a(N=8)	69.13	85.26	2.00	6.50	4.41
	c(N=1)	63.00	90.00	2.00	2.00	4.82
	d(N=3)	67.33	90.00	3.33	7.00	4.30
Other Approaches (Type D) (N=6)	a(N=5)	48.00	84.82	1.40	4.80	4.59
	d(N=1)	70.00	91.67	2.00	10.00	4.32

Note:
a=Only students involved
b=Students and parents involved
c=Students and teachers involved
d=Students, parents and teachers involved

Results of the content analyses showed that three major types of program elements were identified, namely, element based on adventure-based counseling approach, element based on volunteer training and services, and element based on other program types. A program would be classified as containing the adventure-based activities and counseling (ABC) elements if activities matched with theory of adventure-based counseling identified. Similarly, a program would be classified as containing volunteer training and services elements if it is related to program-planning skills and organizing volunteer services. The most popular volunteer services found in the Tier 2 Program were visiting elderly and providing services for mentally handicapped people. Finally, programs without elements of ABC or volunteer training and services were classified as "others", and this category included groups promoting personal growth and/or emotion management, programs related to adolescents' love affairs and communication with opposite sex, and workshops related to installation art and broadcasting.

Table 2. Comparison of the positive views towards Tier 2 Program among different program approaches

	Participants with positive responses in different program approach									
	ABC Approach and Volunteer Training and Services[1]		ABC Approach[2]		Volunteer Training and Services[3]		Others[4]		Overall	
	N (total response)	%	N (total response)	%	N (total response)	%	N (total response)	%	N (total response)	%
1. The activities were carefully planned.	608 (669)	90.88	331 (391)	84.65	509 (670)	75.97	145 (160)	90.63	1593 (1890)	84.29
2. The quality of the service was high.	622 (670)	92.84	345 (391)	88.24	495 (669)	73.99	142 (160)	88.75	1604 (1890)	84.87
3. The service provided could meet the participants' needs.	617 (668)	92.37	343 (388)	88.40	517 (666)	77.63	142 (160)	88.75	1619 (1882)	86.03
4. The service delivered could achieve the planned objectives.	628 (668)	94.01	339 (389)	87.15	522 (669)	78.03	150 (160)	93.75	1639 (1886)	86.90
5. Participants could get the service they wanted.	611 (670)	91.19	334 (390)	85.64	494 (667)	74.06	138 (159)	86.79	1577 (1886)	83.62
6. Participants had much interaction with other participants.	623 (670)	92.99	345 (387)	89.15	537 (668)	80.39	145 (160)	90.63	1650 (1885)	87.53

	Participants with positive responses in different program approach									
	ABC Approach and Volunteer Training and Services[1]		ABC Approach[2]		Volunteer Training and Services[3]		Others[4]		Overall	
7. Participants would recommend others who have similar needs to participate in the program.	610 (668)	91.32	330 (387)	85.27	485 (667)	72.71	141 (158)	89.24	1566 (1880)	83.30
8. On the whole, participants were satisfied with the service.	637 (670)	95.07	346 (391)	88.49	524 (666)	78.68	147 (160)	91.88	1654 (1887)	87.65

Note:

[1]The program contents related to both adventure-based counseling approach and volunteer training and services were indicated in the Tier 2 Program reports.

[2]The program contents related to adventure-based counseling approach were indicated in the Tier 2 Program reports.

[3]The program contents related to volunteer training and services were indicated in the Tier 2 Program reports.

[4]Except adventure-based counseling approach and volunteer training and services, other program contents were indicated in the Tier 2 Program reports.

Table 3. Comparison of the positive views towards Tier 2 Program workers among different program approaches

	Participants with positive responses in different program approach									
	ABC Approach and Volunteer Training and Services[1]		ABC Approach[2]		Volunteer Training and Services[3]		Others[4]		Overall	
	N (total response)	%	N (total response)	%	N (total response)	%	N (total response)	%	N (total response)	%
1. The worker(s) had professional knowledge.	635 (670)	94.78	351 (388)	90.46	560 (669)	83.71	148 (160)	92.50	1694 (1887)	89.77
2. The worker(s) demonstrated good working skills.	638 (670)	95.22	352 (385)	91.43	549 (670)	81.94	147 (159)	92.45	1686 (1884)	89.49
3. The worker(s) were well prepared for the program.	639 (668)	95.66	354 (385)	91.95	551 (666)	82.73	153 (160)	95.63	1697 (1879)	90.31

Table 3. (Continued)

	Participants with positive responses in different program approach									
	ABC Approach and Volunteer Training and Services[1]		ABC Approach[2]		Volunteer Training and Services[3]		Others[4]		Overall	
4. The worker(s) understood the needs of the participants.	627 (667)	94.00	341 (388)	87.89	540 (667)	80.96	147 (160)	91.88	1655 (1882)	87.94
5. The worker(s) cared about the participants.	642 (669)	95.96	352 (386)	91.19	549 (670)	81.94	145 (159)	91.19	1688 (1884)	89.60
6. The worker(s)' attitudes were very good.	639 (669)	95.52	346 (386)	89.64	559 (666)	83.93	151 (160)	94.38	1695 (1881)	90.11
7. The worker(s) had much interaction with participants.	624 (668)	93.41	338 (386)	87.56	524 (665)	78.80	147 (160)	91.88	1633 (1879)	86.91
8. On the whole, participants were satisfied with the worker(s).	642 (667)	96.25	343 (385)	89.09	564 (669)	84.30	151 (160)	94.38	1700 (1881)	90.38

Note:
[1]The program contents related to both adventure-based counseling approach and volunteer training and services were indicated in the Tier 2 Program reports.
[2]The program contents related to adventure-based counseling approach were indicated in the Tier 2 Program reports.
[3]The program contents related to volunteer training and services were indicated in the Tier 2 Program reports.
[4]Except adventure-based counseling approach and volunteer training and services, other program contents were indicated in the Tier 2 Program reports.

As shown in Table 1, the Tier 2 Programs were further categorized into four types in terms of the main types of program elements used or program approaches adopted. They are: 1) adventure-based counseling (ABC) approach together with volunteer training and services (Type A, 40.82%); 2) ABC only (Type B, 22.45%); 3) volunteer training and services only (Type C, 24.49%); and 4) other approaches (Type D, 12.24%). An analysis of the programs delivered showed that ABC approach and volunteer training and services were the two major program elements adopted for the Tier 2 Program, and about 88% of all programs delivered by 49 secondary schools contained at least one of these two elements.

Table 4. Comparison of the positive views towards Tier 2 Program effectiveness among different program approaches

	Participants with positive responses in different program approach									
	ABC Approach and Volunteer Training and Services[1]		ABC Approach[2]		Volunteer Training and Services[3]		Others[4]		Overall	
	N (total response)	%	N (total response)	%	N (total response)	%	N (total response)	%	N (total response)	%
1. The service has helped participants a lot.	604 (654)	92.35	318 (383)	83.03	498 (656)	75.91	141 (158)	89.24	1561 (1851)	84.33
2. The service has enhanced participants' growth.	614 (654)	93.88	326 (381)	85.56	514 (656)	78.35	139 (158)	87.97	1593 (1849)	86.15
3. In the future, participants would receive similar service(s) if needed.	606 (654)	92.66	326 (383)	85.12	474 (655)	72.37	136 (158)	86.08	1542 (1850)	83.35
4. Participants have learnt how to help themselves through participating in the program.	626 (655)	95.57	330 (380)	86.84	526 (654)	80.43	146 (158)	92.41	1628 (1847)	88.14
5. Participants have had positive change(s) after joining the program.	603 (654)	92.20	330 (382)	86.39	510 (656)	77.74	140 (157)	89.17	1583 (1849)	85.61
6. Participants have learnt how to solve their problems through participating in the program.	614 (651)	94.32	327 (382)	85.60	521 (650)	80.15	146 (158)	92.41	1608 (1841)	87.34

Table 4. (Continued)

	Participants with positive responses in different program approach									
	ABC Approach and Volunteer Training and Services[1]		ABC Approach[2]		Volunteer Training and Services[3]		Others[4]		Overall	
7. Participants' behavior has become better after joining this program.	592 (654)	90.52	317 (380)	83.42	485 (653)	74.27	137 (158)	86.71	1531 (1845)	82.98
8. Those who knew the participants agree that this program has induced positive changes in them.	589 (653)	90.20	309 (380)	81.32	475 (653)	72.74	136 (156)	87.18	1509 (1842)	81.92

Note:
[1]The program contents related to both adventure-based counseling approach and volunteer training and services were indicated in the Tier 2 Program reports.
[2]The program contents related to adventure-based counseling approach were indicated in the Tier 2 Program reports.
[3]The program contents related to volunteer training and services were indicated in the Tier 2 Program reports.
[4]Except adventure-based counseling approach and volunteer training and services, other program contents were indicated in the Tier 2 Program reports.

Table 5. Inter-correlations among different domains in subjective outcome evaluation

Variables / Items	Views about program	Views about instructors
Views about program	1	0.94**
Views about instructors	0.94**	1
Perceived effectiveness of the program:		
1. The service has helped participants a lot.	0.94**	0.87**
2. The service has enhanced participants' growth.	0.96**	0.89**
3. In the future, participants would receive similar service(s) if needed.	0.93**	0.87**
4. Participants have learnt how to help themselves through participating in the program.	0.96**	0.89**
5. Participants have had positive change(s) after joining the program.	0.93**	0.89**
6. Participants have learnt how to solve their problems through participating in the program.	0.91**	0.87**
7. Participants' behavior has become better after joining this program.	0.91**	0.87**
8. Those who knew the participants agree that this program has induced positive changes in them.	0.87**	0.80**

Note: A Bonferroni adjustment to the alpha level (17 pairs of correlations) was used. $^{**}p < 0.003$.

Table 6. Comparison of the views about Tier 2 program among different program approaches

Variable	Program Approach	Mean (Standard Deviation)	F-value
Comparison between Adventure-Based Counseling Approach-related Programs and Others			
Views about program	1	4.74 (0.33)	2.76 n.s.
	2	4.55 (0.47)	
Views about instructors	1	4.91 (0.30)	1.73 n.s.
	2	4.78 (0.43)	
Perceived effectiveness of the program	1	4.72 (0.39)	2.75 n.s.
	2	4.51 (0.47)	
Global views	1	4.79 (0.33)	2.54 n.s.
	2	4.61 (0.45)	
Comparison between Volunteer Training and Services-related Programs and Others			
Views about program	3	4.69 (0.42)	0.22 n.s.
	4	4.63 (0.36)	
Views about instructors	3	4.89 (0.38)	0.67 n.s.
	4	4.81 (0.29)	
Perceived effectiveness of the program	3	4.70 (0.44)	1.47 n.s.
	4	4.54 (0.40)	
Global views	3	4.76 (0.41)	0.74 n.s.
	4	4.66 (0.34)	

Table 6. (Continued)

Comparison between Programs Adopting Two Program Approaches and Others			
Views about program	5	4.79 (0.28)	3.64 n.s.
	6	4.58 (0.44)	
Views about instructors	5	4.97 (0.27)	2.86 n.s.
	6	4.79 (0.39)	
Perceived effectiveness of the program	5	4.82 (0.32)	6.08*
	6	4.53 (0.46)	
Global views	5	4.86 (0.28)	4.38*
	6	4.63 (0.42)	

Note: * $p < 0.05$; n.s. = non-significant; 1=Adventure-Based Counseling Approach-related Programs (Group A and Group B); 2=Others (Group C and Group D); 3=Volunteer Training and Services-related Programs (Group A and Group C); 4=Others (Group B and Group D); 5=Programs adopting 2 program approaches (Group A); 6=Programs adopting 1 program approach or other approaches (Group B and Group C and Group D).

The mean overall effectiveness of all Tier 2 Programs ranged from 4.30 to 4.87 on a six-point scale towards the positive side. The average number of positive youth development constructs indicated in the reports for each type of programs ranged from 2 to 10 and the mode was 3.

Based on the quantitative data derived from the closed-ended questions, several observations can be highlighted from the findings. First, over 80% of the respondents perceived that they participated in a positive manner in the Tier 2 Program (see Table 2). For example, 87.65% of the participants indicated that they were satisfied with the service; 87.53% indicated that they had much interaction with other participants.

Second, a very large proportion of the participants had positive evaluation of the social workers implementing the program (see Table 3). For example, 90.38% of the respondents were satisfied with the worker(s); 90.31% indicated that the worker(s) were well-prepared for the program; 90.11% indicated that the attitudes of worker(s) were very good; 89.77% indicated that the worker(s) had professional knowledge. Third, as shown in Table 4, about four-fifths of the respondents perceived that the program had induced positive changes in them. For example, the participants had learnt how to help themselves (88.14%) and how to solve their problems (87.34%) through participating in the program, and perceived that the services had promoted their growth (86.15%).

Furthermore, Table 5 shows that various domains of the subjective outcome evaluation were inter-related - the overall views about the program and the overall views about the instructors were significantly correlated with each other, and both of them were positively correlated with all eight aspects of the perceived effectiveness of the program. Hence, the hypotheses outlined in the earlier part of the paper were supported.

Comparisons between different program approaches were carried out. Two sets of analyses were carried out to address the questions of whether there were differences in the subjective outcome evaluation ratings between (i) programs with and without adventure-based counseling elements and (ii) programs with and without volunteer training and services.

As shown in Table 6, analyses showed that the two types of programs did not differ in each category. A third set of analyses was carried out to examine whether there were differences in the subjective outcome evaluation ratings between programs adopting two approaches and programs adopting one approach or others. The results showed that participants attending programs that adopted both ABC approach and volunteer training and services had significantly better views about the program effectiveness and global views of the program than those attending programs adopting either one approach only or other approaches (Table 6).

DISCUSSION

The present study was conducted to systematically evaluate the Tier 2 Program of the Project P.A.T.H.S. designed by social services agencies. Several points could be highlighted from the present findings. First, results showed that the various measures derived from Form C were internally consistent in the present study and across studies (21). As it is important to use standardized assessment tools for conducting client satisfaction survey, the present findings form the basis of providing reliable information for further analyses.

Second, the present study showed that adventure-based counseling and volunteer training and services were two dominant program approaches used by social workers working with adolescents and young people in Hong Kong, as they covered 87.8% of all delivered Tier 2 Programs. About 22-25% of the delivered programs adopted either Type B program (adventure-based counseling approach only) or Type C program (volunteer training and services only), and about 41% adopted Type A program (a mixture of Types B and C). Although different programs had unique aims to cater the students' needs of different schools, they all shared common ultimate goals of creating positive changes in students and enhancing their positive development.

Third, a large proportion of the participants perceived the program in a positive light, as nearly 90% of the respondents had favorable perceptions of the program and workers implementing the program and roughly four-fifths of the respondents perceived the program to be beneficial to their own development. These findings were consistent with those gathered from the Secondary 1 level (20, 21), and suggested that the Tier 2 Program of the Secondary 2 level was also helpful to the program participants. Nonetheless, these positive findings should be viewed together with the limitations of subjective outcome evaluation, such as demand characteristics, halo effect and positive bias.

Fourth, consistent with hypotheses, there were positive relationships among program characteristics, program implementers' characteristics and perceived program effectiveness. The present findings further support the thesis that quality of the program and program implementers are intimately related to perceived benefits of the program. As there are very few studies in this area, the present findings can be regarded as pioneering additions to the literature.

Finally, the present findings give some insights on the differences in subjective outcome evaluation findings across different programs. There are two interesting observations deserving our attention. First, there were no differences between programs utilizing and not utilizing adventure-based counseling approach, as well as between programs with and without voluntary training and services. Second, participants joining programs that adopted both approaches perceived higher levels of program effectiveness than did participants joining programs adopted one approach only. These findings suggest that programs combining multi-components would be perceived as more helpful and beneficial by Secondary 2 students and their parent or teacher participants. In the domain of adolescent prevention and positive development programs, there are increasing research findings suggesting that multi-level intervention or interventions involving multiple intervention elements are more powerful in changing adolescent behavior than do programs utilizing a single approach or element. The present findings basically concur with such views.

It is noteworthy that there are several limitations in the present study.

First, only 74.67% of the program participants responded to Form C and some adult participants might not complete the evaluation form. Although this is not a low response rate, effort should be made to maintain higher response rates in future studies. Second, as the present findings were "re-constructed" from the evaluation reports submitted by the social work agencies, the units of analyses were schools instead of individuals. Hence, the power of the statistical analyses would become low and individual variations were lost in the process. This may explain why there were few significant differences among the different modes of Tier 2 Programs. Finally, the limitations of subjective outcome evaluation utilizing quantitative findings should be realized and triangulation with qualitative findings would be helpful.

Despite these limitations, the present study showed that the Tier 2 Program designed by the social services agencies were perceived positively and were regarded as helpful by Secondary 2 students participating in the Tier 2 Program.

Acknowledgments

The preparation for this paper and the Project P.A.T.H.S. were financially supported by The Hong Kong Jockey Club Charities Trust.

References

[1] Shek DTL. Adolescent developmental issues in Hong Kong: relevance to positive youth development programs in Hong Kong. Int J Adolesc Med Health 2006;18:341-54.

[2] Shek DTL. Construction of a positive youth development program in Hong Kong. Int J Adolesc Med Health 2006;18(3):299-302.

[3] Shek DTL. Effectiveness of the Tier 1 Program of the Project P.A.T.H.S.: preliminary objective and subjective outcome evaluation findings. ScientificWorldJournal 2006; 6:1466-74.

[4] Shek DTL, Ma HK. Subjective outcome evaluation of the Project P.A.T.H.S.: findings based on the perspective of the program participants. ScientificWorldJournal 2007;7:47-55.

[5] Shek DTL, Siu AMH, Lee TY. Subjective outcome evaluation of the Project P.A.T.H.S.: findings based on the perspective of the program implementers. ScientificWorldJournal. 2007;7:195-203.

[6] Shek DTL, Sun RCF. Subjective outcome evaluation of the Project P.A.T.H.S.: qualitative findings based on the experiences of program implementers. ScientificWorldJournal 2007;7:1024-35.

[7] Shek DTL, Sun RCF. Subjective outcome evaluation of the Project P.A.T.H.S.: qualitative findings based on the experiences of the program participants. ScientificWorldJournal 2007;7:686-97.

[8] Shek DTL, Ma HK, Lui JHY, Lung DWM. Process evaluation of the Tier 1 Program of the Project P.A.T.H.S. ScientificWorldJournal 2006;6:2264-73.

[9] Shek DTL, Sun RCF. Implementation of the Tier 1 Program of the Project P.A.T.H.S.: interim evaluation findings. ScientificWorldJournal. 2006;6:2274-84.

[10] Shek DTL, Lee TY, Siu A, Lam CM. Qualitative evaluation of the Project P.A.T.H.S. based on the perceptions of the program participants. ScientificWorldJournal 2006;6:2254-63.

[11] Shek DTL, Sun RCF, Lam CM, Lung DWM, Lo SC. Evaluation of Project P.A.T.H.S. in Hong Kong: utilization of student weekly dairy. ScientificWorldJournal 2008;8:13-21.

[12] Shek DTL, Siu AMH, Lee TY, Cheung CK, Chung R. Effectiveness of the Tier 1 Program of Project P.A.T.H.S.: objective outcome evaluation based on a randomized group trial. ScientificWorldJournal 2008;8:4-12.

[13] Shek DTL, Sun RCF. Evaluation of Project P.A.T.H.S. (Secondary 1 Program) by the program participants: findings based on the Full Implementation Phase. Adolesc 2008;43(172):807-22.

[14] Shek DTL, Ma HK. Evaluation of Project P.A.T.H.S. (Secondary 1 Program) by the program implementers: findings based on the Full Implementation Phase. ScientificWorldJournal 2008;8:492-501.

[15] Shek DTL, Ma HK, Sun RCF, Lung DWM. Process evaluation of the Tier 1 Program (Secondary 1 Curriculum) of the Project P.A.T.H.S.: findings based on the Full Implementation Phase. ScientificWorldJournal 2008;8:35-46.

[16] Shek DTL, Ma HK, Sun RCF. Interim evaluation of the Tier 1 Program (Secondary 1 Curriculum) of the Project P.A.T.H.S.: first year of the Full Implementation Phase. ScientificWorldJournal 2008;8:47-60.

[17] Shek DTL, Lee TY. Qualitative evaluation of the Project P.A.T.H.S.: findings based on focus groups with student participants. Int J Adolesc Med Health 2008; 20(4):449-62.

[18] Shek DTL, Sun RCF. Implementation of a positive youth development program in a Chinese context: the role of policy, program, people, process, and place. ScientificWorldJournal 2008;8:960-96.

[19] Shek DTL, Chak YLY, Chan CWY. School-related factors in the implementation of a positive youth development project in Hong Kong. ScientificWorldJournal 2008;8:997-1009.

[20] Shek DTL, Lee TY, Sun RCF, Lung DWM. Positive youth development programs targeting students with greater psychosocial needs: subjective outcome evaluation. ScientificWorldJournal 2008;8:73-82.

[21] Shek DTL, Sun RCF. Helping students with greater psychosocial needs: evaluation of a positive youth development program. ScientificWorldJournal 2008;8:515-85.

[22] Catalano RF, Berglund ML, Ryan JAM, Lonczak HS, Hawkins JD. Positive youth development in the United States: research findings on evaluations of positive youth development programs. Prev Treatment 2002. Accessed 2008 Aug 1. URL: http://aspe.hhs.gov/hsp/PositiveYouthDev99/

[23] Brendtro LK, Strother MA. Back to basics through challenge and adventure. Reclaim Children Youth 2007;16(1):2-6.

[24] Carns AW, Carns MR, Holland J. Learning the ropes: challenges for change. TCA J 2001;29(1):66-71.

[25] Fletcher TB, Hinkle JS. Adventure based counseling: an innovation in counseling. J Couns Dev 2002;80(3):277-85.

[26] Carlson KP, Cook M. Challenge by choice: adventure-based counseling for seriously ill adolescents. Child Adolesc Psychiatr Clin North Am 2007;16:909-19.

[27] Glass JS, Myers JE. Combining the old and the new to help adolescents: individual psychology and adventure-based counseling. J Mental Health Couns 2001;23(2):104-14.

[28] Ornum WV, Foley JM, Burns PR, DeWolfe AS, Kennedy EC. Empathy, altruism, and self-interest in college students. Adolescence 1981;16(64):799-808.

[29] Allen JP, Philliber S, Herrling S, Kuperminc GP. Preventing teen pregnancy and academic failure: experimental evaluation of a developmentally based approach. Child Dev 1997;64(4):729-42.

[30] Dolan B. A teen hot line. Adolesc 1995;30(117):195-200.

[31] Schondel C, Boehm K, Rose J, Marlowe A. Adolescent volunteers: an untapped resource in the delivery of adolescent preventive health care. Youth Soc 1995;27(2):123-35.

[32] O'Donnell J, Michalak EA, Ames EB. Inner-city youths helping children after-school programs to promote bonding and reduce risk. Soc Work Educ 1997;19:231-42.

[33] McFarland DA, Thomas RJ. Bowling young: how youth voluntary associations influence adult political participation. Am Sociol Rev 2006;71:401-25.
[34] Nation M, Crusto C, Wandersman A, Kumpfer KL, Seybolt D, Morrissey-Kane E, Davino K. What works in prevention: principles of effective prevention programs. Am Psychol 2003;58:449-56.
[35] Weissberg RP. Improving the lives of millions of school children. Am Psychol 2000;55:1360-73.
[36] Harachi TW, Abbott RD, Catalano RF, Haggerty KP, Fleming CB. Opening the black box: using process evaluation measures to assess implementation and theory building. Am J Community Psychol 1999;27:711-31.
[37] Peterson L, Rigby K. Countering bullying at an Australian secondary school with students as helpers. J Adolesc 1999;22:481-92.
[38] Marques TE, Lane DM, Dorfman PW. Towards the development of a system for instructional evaluation: is there consensus regarding what constitutes effective teaching? J Educ Psychol 1979;71(6):840-9.
[39] Shek DTL, Siu AMH, Lui JHY, Lung DWM. P.A.T.H.S. to Adulthood: A Jockey Club Youth Enhancement Scheme (Evaluation Manual). Hong Kong: Soc Welfare Pract Res Centre, Chinese Univ Hong Kong, 2006.

Submitted: January 10, 2009.
Revised: February 25, 2009.
Accepted: March 8, 2009.

Section four
Sport and adolescence

In: Public Health Yearbook 2009
Editor: Joav Merrick
ISBN: 978-1-61668-911-7

Chapter 33

Psychosocial Considerations in Youth Sports: An American Perspective

Donald E Greydanus**, MD and Helen D Pratt, Ph D
Department of Pediatrics and Human Development, Michigan State University College of Human Medicine, East Lansing, Michigan, United States of America

Abstract

This article identifies various psychosocial factors influencing children and adolescents who are involved in sports. The emphasis is on lessons learned from being part of highly organized sports programs in the United States which have a primary emphasis on winning. We start with developmental issues and then proceed to the effects of (over) training, chronic illness or disability and intrinsic or extrinsic influences on sport participation experience by youth. This review also considers such concepts as psychological reactions to injury, stress and anxiety, depression and suicidal ideation, substance use and aggression. We conclude that sports participation by children and adolescents can have beneficial effects. However, these effects can be lifelong and potential adverse results of a highly competitive system must also be understood. This article reviews some of the psychosocial issues observed in American youth participation in highly organized sports programs. It is hoped that the lessons learned may be of help to others who develop and expand these programs for their children and adolescents.

Keywords: Adolescence, sport, psychosocial.

---

* Correspondence: Professor Donald E Greydanus, MD, Pediatrics and Human Development, Michigan State University College of Human Medicine, Pediatrics Program Director, Michigan State University/Kalamazoo Center for Medical Studies, 1000 Oakland Drive, Kalamazoo, MI 49008-1284 United States. E-mail: Greydanus@kcms.msu.edu

Introduction

Physicians, parents, educators, coaches, and adolescents acknowledge and promote the health benefits of regular physical activity in shaping the lives of young people (1). In the United States, the increased focus on involving youth in sport activities through their schools and communities has shifted from being spontaneous and fun to being highly organized and competitive. Proponents having youth adopt a competitive attitude towards their sport participation justify their actions by saying that competition is a helpful tool for teaching these youth how to make physical activity part of a lifelong strategy to stay physically fit and also, to teach them many important things about participation in life -- how to win and even more important, how to lose but maintain a winning attitude.

Additional cited benefits include the development of the following skills: a) frustration tolerance, b) strategic planning skills that will be useful in later life, c) pro-social skills, d) friendship making and maintaining, e) emotional coping, f) good work and academic habits, g) good self-esteem, h) ability to work as part of a team, and i) the ability to integrate these skills into the school and community (2-7). Some parents state they experience personal benefits from having their children participate in sport activities by using practice sessions and events as a means of personal socialization and status.

However, experience from many decades of highly organized sports programs for children and adolescents in the United States show these competitive sports programs may also create emotional stress, and poor self-esteem for youth who can not meet performance expectations of themselves or the significant adults in their lives (4,6-10). Also, considerable stress can be noted in athletes "successfully" involved in competitive sports (11).

As the adolescent is experiencing physical, cognitive, social, and emotional changes due to the normal process of adolescence, it is imperative that parents, coaches, physicians, and others remember that they may be placing increased pressures on the adolescent to perform and practice; this is noted even though the efforts of engaging them in sport activities may be well intentioned. Problems can arise when adults place expectations that exceed the adolescent's capabilities, leading him or her to experience self-doubt, internal conflict, and stress; in addition, this can result in responses by the adolescent athlete that are frequently difficult for adults to understand - arguments, refusal to participate in sports, and angry outbursts (2,4,5).

Adolescent development

Early adolescence

At this stage of development (10-14 years of age) adolescents are preoccupied with rapidly changing events of puberty, beginning of symbolic movement away from the home environment, comparison with peers, worry over perceived physical abnormalities, establishment and maintenance of same-sex friendships, and the development of initial abstract thought (1,12,13). Their thinking is concrete; they understand what is and is not expected of them (basic rules of behavior, techniques and social rules of sports) but usually cannot generalize these rules from one situation to another. They may not connect consistent daily practice with performance on game day, since behavior and consequences are processed based on the here and now. They tend to attribute success or failure to their uniqueness rather than to the team effort (12). Peer acceptance is important but the approval and support from family are guiding forces. These adolescents are also able to enjoy and take pride in increasingly complex accomplishments and begin to improve their self-image. Those adolescents who experience consistent successes often develop a positive self-image, while those who experience repeated failures may develop a poor self-image (2,3,5).

Growth, physical skill and development vary widely among youth and may result in awkwardness and increase concerns about body image (4,14). Mismatches in team sports often occur when participation is based on age or grade level alone, without concern for pubertal development (4). Normal comparisons between self and peers may cause the adolescent to be either distressed or feel superior (2,4).

Middle adolescence

During middle adolescence (14-18 years) adolescents demand increased levels of independence from their parents and authority; they begin to rely on peers for their frames of reference versus parents and family members (1,12). They use peer feedback to set personal goals and rules of conduct (4). They are developing increasing levels of inductive and deductive reasoning ability, even reflecting on the thought process itself (11,12). They use their enhanced cognitive abilities to fantasize in developing theories about life and who they will grow up to be.

Adolescents at this stage of development will increasingly become altruistic and the coach becomes a very important role model at this stage. The adolescent by now has determined his or her sexual identity and will need support if that choice does not fit the expectations of family, peers or community (12). During middle adolescence feelings are very intense and risk taking behavior can cause conflict with parents and authority figures. Factors, such as chronic illness, physical or psychological trauma, that impair normal development may retard self acceptance (4).

Late adolescence

During late adolescence (19 to 21 + years) most issues of emancipation should be essentially resolved, and final pubertal changes have occurred. Abstract thinking and empathy skills are well developed and personal values clearer and well defined. The older adolescent athlete at this stage is better able to deal with pressures from parents, coaches, and society, as well as personal failures (4). The well adjusted, mentally and physically healthy adolescent has developed a secure, acceptable body image and gender role; he or she is able to maintain mutually giving and caring adult relationships, including sexual relationships (1,12,13). He or she has a more realistic view of the role of sports in the overall scheme of his or her life (12)

Puberty

Precocious puberty

Adolescents who are early developers may be stronger, faster and have developed better motor coordination compared to their peers, resulting in superior athletic performance; such youth are often called “superstars." These adolescents may become accustomed to considerable attention and praise from others, especially their coaches. However, we must prepare them for the inevitable time when their peers catch up with them developmentally and they may be no longer out performing others; then, inevitable frustration and disappointment might be experienced by these youth, their families and their coaches. We must remember that only one-fourth of these "superstars" will remain in this category through middle as well as late adolescence and beyond. Be prepared to recognize and treat youth who experience depression, anxiety, or even act out during this transition period. Provide encouragement for the development of the teen's other abilities (music, art, scholarship, others) in preparation of loss of “superstar” status and as an important aspect of all human development.

Delayed puberty

Adolescents who are smaller, weaker and less coordinated may experience the frustration, anxiety, and disappointment of not being able to meet performance expectations when playing sports (14). They may even be ignored by peers as well as coaching staffs. Provide these adolescents with encouragement to continue to engage in activities that will help them build strength, endurance and skills as they continue to mature physically and mentally. Point out that they will eventually grow and be more competitive with their peers. Encourage the development of other skills as well.

Overtraining

Over training can also result in overall negative mood disturbances in youth. Some youth may train harder and become more stressed because the training does not produce the desired outcomes encouraged by competitive sports; these youth may develop more negative attitudes about participation and then, performance deteriorates. Adolescents who are allowed appropriate rest may develop more positive attitudes towards participation (15). Over training can also result in more injuries to the athlete.

Chronic illness and disability

Adolescents with physical disabilities or chronic illness may be denied participation in sports or may perceive themselves as being incapable of participation. However, they should be provided developmentally, physically, and age appropriate outlets for engaging in physical activities (4). Physically challenged adolescents especially should be able to participate in sport activities and allowed to be a contributing part of modified or special groups. By participation in sports the physically challenged youth can derive all the same physical and psychosocial benefits as for other adolescents (16).

Intrinsic factors that influence sport participation experience

Whether or not an adolescent participates in sport activities is influenced by many factors, including gender, class, race, and age relations as well as political, economic, social and cultural factors (5). Historically, American females have participated at a lower rate than their male peers. The influence of coaches, parents, teachers, academic grades, access to activities, and transportation may be additional factors. The adolescent is not in total control of whether or not he or she plays. Adults, especially coaches, define who has the skills and capabilities that are noteworthy and valuable, selecting those who are then allowed to participate.

In general as children move through adolescence, they become less physically active. If the adolescent sees him or herself physically competent or skilled in a particular sport, he or she will have a more positive attitude toward participation and will enjoy such activities (16). Adolescents are increasingly likely to develop lifelong habits of physical activity if they perceive sport participation as beneficial to their physical fitness, as a way to maintain or improve skills, and as a means to improve appearance, muscular strength, endurance and flexibility. Those adolescents who see participation as a barrier, or perceive other factors as barriers to engaging in sport activities (such as peer rejection, time, level of fitness, weight, poor health, or access) will tend not to participate nor remain committed to engaging in sport activities. Other factors that affect participation include whether or not the parents are physically active and supportive of participation, and whether or not the adolescent has access to activities (transportation, money for equipment, convenient play spaces, and sport equipment) (16).

The adolescent's beliefs about the purpose and causes of success in sport are also important. Those who believe the purpose of sport participation is for personal development, status, and lifetime health, are better at coping with psychological issues associated with sport participation. Athletes who are focused on pro-social and adaptive achievement beliefs about sport participation are more likely to facilitate adaptive cognitive and affective patterns in competitive sports during adolescence (17,18).

Youth learn about competitive behavior as children; those who develop a "win at all costs" attitude may find it difficult to deal with failure. They learn to place value on a particular accomplishment and learn a means of achieving that goal. When they discover that someone else also values the same accomplishment or object and is willing to work equally as hard (or harder) to attain it, they learn about competition.

The idea of being a "former winner" (i.e., a "current loser") may affect how they approach similar situations in the future. The manner in which they cognitively process the inability to accomplish that task or obtain that object, may determine how he or she will function in the future in similar situations (12,19).

Adolescents who perform poorly in sport activities may experience negative consequences of the socialization process (embarrassment, rejection, criticism, ridicule, and punitive intervention) (2). Those who engage in sports beyond his or her physical capabilities (due to late physical maturation, cognitive deficits or chronic illness) may experience physical and psychological trauma. Adolescents who are inexperienced, lack innate abilities, or have a poorly developed body sense (i.e., eye-hand coordination, gross motor skills, attention skills, socialization skills) are also vulnerable to suffering physical and psychological trauma from sport participation (2-5,12).

Additional social deficits (such as excessive restlessness, talkativeness, bossiness, and attention-getting behaviors) may also be a risk. Adolescents who perceive that they are not meeting the expectations of coaches, parents, or peers (because of their repeated failures in competition) can suffer as well (2-4,12).

Extrinsic factors that influence sport participation experience

Sport participation may be viewed as a social process that many see as a way to link themselves and their children to the larger social world in which it occurs (2). Socialization is tied to selection, and ignoring this fact makes it difficult to understand sport participation.

In the best case scenario, sport participation enhances the socialization process by bringing the adolescent prestige that leads peers and significant others to treat him or her more seriously as a worthy human being, and wanting to establish personal peer relationships (2,20). When participation causes young people to be noticed by those who can positively influence their academic lives, positive changes are then more likely. Sport participation may not always lead to creating attributes, connections or reputations which facilitate achievement in non-sport activities (2-5).

Parents

Parents have a greater influence with children less than 10-12 years than in the older teens. By this later age the child's values about winning have been developed and fixed. At each stage of development, all adolescents are better able to develop a positive self-esteem if they are nurtured by a stable home life with caring parents, stable peer groups and academic success, along with some proficiency in their chosen sport (2,4). Parents who are involved, encouraging, and making suggestions may have a more positive effect on their child's character development. However, if parents are too enthusiastic or overbearing they can have a detrimental effect on the athlete's values about winning (14). Most parents expect their adolescent to excel and be recognized by his or her peers and the parent's peers. If parents invest time, money, and friendships in their child's sport participation, they may experience (and exert) more pressure for their child to perform and play well (2-5,12).

Coaches

The roles of coaches and other adults and sports heroes can become very important to help set personal limits and develop a stable life image (4,5,14). As athletes mature, the coach becomes the most significant source of influence. The coach's techniques are crucial factors in the way an individual player views himself or herself in the sport and ultimately in society. An adept coach will use positive techniques while carefully and rarely using punitive measures to motivate and teach athletes. He or she will help shape competence and increased performance though feedback and training, and also help what is ultimately of great importance---the athlete's self-concept and self-esteem (5).

Parents and coaches have a significant influence on the means and responses selected by the adolescent, depending on the stage of development the adolescent has attained. Coaches are involved in the development of winning or losing attitudes; as the level of competition increases, the significance of winning also increases (5). Development of character and morals are most strongly influenced by parents and family. However, the influence coaches do have is more related to the coach's and individual adolescent's interactions than as an inherent value of sports (2).

Peers

Peer acceptance may wax and wane with the performance of an athlete. Some athletes may experience rejection and criticism from peers for lack of skill, competence or performance during a specific time; however winning and elite athletes may also experience rejection, jealously and criticism from peers (2,21). Teammates tend to be more accepting and complimentary to each other when they win and more rejecting and critical when they lose. The athlete must decide what level of personal recognition and social acceptance are necessary to his or her survival. It is important that the individual athlete understand this dynamic (5).

Media

The American media has much to do with the positive image given to sports heroes in the United States. Professional sports heroes earn tremendous salaries, and command enormous respect from all levels of our society (22). Many youth dream of becoming superstars in their favorite sport and this dream is common in American youth. If a youth is considered a good athlete by peers, parents and others, much goodwill is automatically afforded to this fortunate individual. It is normal for youth to seek to excel and for parents to expect this performance. All forms of the media regularly participate in considerable coverage of sports events and can transform a player of any age into a superstar. The media coverage of winners may reinforce the message that winning at all costs is success while losing is always a failure (2,3). The media projects the idea that success in sports means success in life, and that not being number one means limited achievements or overt failure in life. Adolescents can develop an unhealthy attitude that winning is more important than fairness and fun (1).

Psychological effects of injury

The risk of injury increases with longer practice time and the degree of difficulty of routines. Repetitive stress on the developing musculoskeletal system can result in injuries. The pressure to practice and compete while injured compounds the risk of further musculoskeletal injuries. Athletes who have low coping skills and poor social support are more likely to be vulnerable to poor outcomes when dealing with the stresses of sports injury (23-26). Although the adolescent may initially minimize or deny the extent of his or her injury, the realization that they can not play or perform at previous levels may result in feelings of anger, isolation, and loneliness. The periods of absence from practice and competition may be overwhelming to athletes who are accustomed to the intensity and demands of their normal routine (though a few athletes may even welcome this post-injury phase).

The challenges faced during recovery may often combine pain with failure to perform to certain personal expectations. The athlete may find that he or she cannot complete exercises to stay fit. Following recovery, the athlete may not being able to perform to a level achieved prior to the injury. Some may find a new emotion, that of fear of re-injury. As the adolescent recovers from the injury and regains strength and stamina, the depression should lift and acceptance and hope follow. The physician can be a key "player" in motivating the adolescent to work toward recovery by explaining that depression and anger are normal outcomes of injury, the healing process, and the therapeutic process. Cognitive-behavioral techniques combined with appropriate physical therapy and medical interventions can help the athlete move toward recovery (6,10,24-27).

Competitive stress and anxiety

Stress and anxiety can have both a positive or negative impact on children and adolescents (4,6,7,10,28-30). Sports activity can teach the athlete that, stress is a natural part of sports participation. Sports participation may teach the athlete how to handle competition, performance anxiety and even defeat. It may also teach the youth about physical fitness, how to develop social skills and friendships, and the importance of team play in sports and in life. Anxiety appears to act differently than other emotions on sport performance. Higher levels of anxiety are associated with an individual's best performance and interventions to reduce pre-competition anxiety may actually worsen the performance (29). Although a certain amount of arousal or stress is necessary to performing, stress can also impede performance and cause health problems in children (3,28). Events such as pre-game situations, losing games, and fear of failure have been identified as increasing the emotional stress levels of young athletes (3,6,7).

Stress can be a hazard on the playing field, having an adverse affect on performance and increasing injury (7,10). Cognitive-behavioral techniques (relaxation response, stress inoculation training, biofeedback, mediation, counseling by psychologists, yoga, deep muscle relaxation, self- hypnosis, visualization, breath control, time management and multi-dimensional relaxation training) have been shown to be effective in enhancing sport performance, improving recovery from injury, and preventing sport injury (26-33).

The stress of trying for a team and not making it can be a positive experience (if handled well) or a very negative one. Negative consequences to overwhelming stress are many, including chronic fatigue ("athletic burnout syndrome")--with rapid loss of previous skills. Such "burnout" can also result from over training by over-zealous teens (as well as their parents or coaches). Children and teens should enjoy their sports participation and not be forced into specializing in one sport or another too soon --- in the hopes of producing another famous, wealthy superstar. Teens who do excel at one sport may feel sad or anxious when "off-season." Encouraging other (perhaps non-competitive) sports, interests (i.e., music or art) and social activities may help such youth.

Parents can be counseled to avoid joining the current milieu of victory at any cost, which is characteristic of highly organized sports programs in the United States. School personnel and parents can seek to have sports participation by children and adolescents which develop positive goals. These goals can include learning the joy of physical activity and a sense of competence. Our teens should not be placed under overwhelming pressure to win, despite the "price of victory." Parents should not push their children beyond abilities or teach their children that self-esteem comes only from winning. Some youth feel that they are loved and valued only if they do well in sports. Counseling against such attitudes should start early by the trusted clinician. It is educational for clinicians to go to a sports event at an elementary or junior/ high school event in the United States and observe the yelling parents who are rude to their children, coaches, umpires and fellow parents-in a vain attempt to teach love only through victory and victory at any cost.

Depression and suicidal ideation

Athletes who limit their socialization to social groups who are only related to a particular sport may experience periods of depression, sadness, anxiety, restlessness, and irritability when they are off season; therefore it is important for coaches, parents, teachers and physicians to encourage adolescents to develop social and athletic activities during these off seasons." These athletes should engage in additional sport activities simply for fun and exercise and be encouraged to develop friendships and relationships with individuals and groups that are involved in other physical and social activities (34).

Substance abuse

There are increasing reports of recreational and performance enhancing drug and alcohol use by many American athletes (35-38). There is a negative relationship between sport participation and smoking in adolescents (35). Decreased substance use is associated with adolescents who increased their aerobic fitness following an aerobic training program. A study of former college athletes revealed they are more likely to use tobacco and alcohol than non-athletes in later life; runners were least likely to smoke; although female runners consumed alcohol at the same rates as male runners and non-runners, they were more likely to have chronic alcohol use than non-runners (35).

A three year prospective study of 1,245 American adolescents aged 12-16 years found that 33% of these athletes had never smoked cigarettes, consumed alcohol nor used marijuana; 25% of students reported smoking in the past 30 days, 52% reported alcohol use in the past year and 13% reported marijuana use in the past year (35). White students reported more cigarette smoking and alcohol consumption compared to non-whites (35). Increasing age is associated with increases in the prevalence of all reported substance use (36). Lower socioeconomic status was associated with higher reported use of marijuana while higher socioeconomic status was associated with lower reported use of cigarettes. Males who participated in competitive athletics were significantly more likely than non-athletes to initiate alcohol use while the most active or most fit females were likely to initiate cigarette smoking (35). In contrast the most active males (those who participated in competitive athletics) appeared more at-risk for initiating alcohol consumption than their less active counterparts.

Aggression and violence

Current research has not empirically established a relationship between media coverage of sports and violent behavior and little is known about how people integrate their exposure to media coverage of sports into the rest of their lives (2,22). A survey of 2,436 high school students found no significant differences for violent or delinquent behavior between athletes and non-athletes (45). However it did show that non-contact sport athletes (male and female) were less likely to engage in various violent and delinquent behaviors than were contact sport athletes and non athletes (45).

Rates of deviant behavior among male/female athletes are similar or lower than rates among non-athletes. No differences in violence between racial groups and social class backgrounds across sports have been observed. Short-term differences in delinquency rates for all athletes and non athletes were proven non-significant over time. A three year follow-up showed that racial, social, and athlete versus non athlete differences in deviant behavior were not present (22). Sports related violence has become a critical social problem in many countries. Documented events of violent disturbances have occurred in European countries, Australia, Central and South America, Asia, and North America (22). Media coverage may exploit participant violence in sport by promoting a view that this is a natural and unchangeable ordering of a world in which men compete violently together. Media shows may contribute to a social climate that is conducive to violent behavior. Sport is a cultural practice that embodies a climate of toughness, aggression, and physical dominance especially in angry males. (22)

Conclusion

Adolescents' unique experiences in sports and physical fitness require special approaches (5). Participation in normal spontaneous sports activity can facilitate growth in a variety of ways for athletes: character development, social adjustment, positive personality traits and attitudes, emotional control, sports-man like behavior, leadership skills, empathy, cooperation, a more outgoing and socially well adjusted personality, self-discipline, self-confidence, initiative, courage, loyalty, and self expression (19,34,46). Youth who (including those with physical disabilities and those who have a chronic illness) participate in spontaneous sports activities display both physiologic and psychological benefits. Most experts believe that teaching a healthy life style has its greatest chance of being adopted if the skills are learned and practiced in childhood and through adolescence. However, the increased pressure to engage youth in competitive sport activities increases the likelihood that adolescents will experience psychosocial stressors related to sports participation. (47-50) Lessons learned about psychosocial issues related to the highly organized American sports programs with a relentless drive for victory at all costs is reviewed.

References

[1] Greydanus DE, ed. Caring for your adolescent: ages 12 -21. New York: Bantam, 1991:251-66.

[2] Coakley J. Sport and Socialization. Exerc Sport Sci Rev 1993;21:169.

[3] Patel DR, Greydanus DE, Pratt HD. Psychosocial aspects of youth sports. In: Patel DR, Greydanus DE, Baker RJ, eds. Pediatric practice: Sports medicine. New York: McGraw-Hill, 2009:26-37.

[4] Farrell E. Sports medicine: psychological aspects. In: Greydanus DE, Wolraich, ML, eds. Behavioral pediatrics. New York: Springer, 1992:425-34.

[5] Gegler-Bentz, B. Psychological aspects. In: Stanitski CL, ed. Pediatric and adolescent sports medicine. Philadelphia: WB Saunders, 1994:77-93.

[6] Smoll FL, Smith RE. Stress and the adolescent athlete. Adolesc Med 1991;2 (1):47-64.

[7] Smoll FL, Smith RE. Psychology of the young athlete: stress-related maladies and remedial approaches. Pediatr Clin North Am 1990;37(5):1021.

[8] American College of Sports Medicine. ACSM guidelines for exercise testing and prescription, 8th ed. Philadelphia: Lippincott Williams Wilkins, 2010.

[9] Patel DR, Pratt HD, Greydanus DE. Adolescent growth, development and psychosocial aspects of sports participation: an overview. Adolesc Med 1998;9(3):425-40.

[10] Smith RE, Smoll FL. Behavioral research and intervention in youth sports. Behav Ther 1991;22(3):329.

[11] Luckstead EF, Greydanus DE. Medical care of the adolescent athlete, Los Angeles, CA: Pract Manage Inf Corp, 1993.

[12] Greydanus DE, Pratt HD. Adolescence: A continuum from childhood to adulthood, 3rd ed. Des Moines, IA: Iowa Dept Public Health, 1995.

[13] Greydanus DE. Adolescence: a perspective. In: Ziai M, ed. Pediatrics, 4th Ed. Boston, MA: Little Brown, 1990:68-478.

[14] Patel DR, Greydanus DE. The adolescent athlete. In: Hofmann AD, Greydanus DE, eds. Adolescent medicine. Stamford: Appleteon-Lange, 1997:607-38.

[15] McCann S. Overtraining and burnout. In: Murphy SM, ed. Sport psychology interventions. Champaign, IL: Human Kinetics, 1995:347-68.

[16] Brenner JS. Overuse injuries, overtraining, and burnout in child and adolescent athletes. Pediatrics 2007;119(6):1242-5.

[17] Treasure DC, Roberts GC. Cognitive and affective concomitants of task and ego goal orientations during the middle school years. J Sport Exerc Psychol 1994;16:15.

[18] Weinberg RS. Goal setting and performance in sport and exercise settings: a synthesis and critique. Med Sci Sports Exerc 1993;469: 1993.

[19] United States Public Health Service. Healthy People 2000. Washington, DC: US Gov Printing Office, DHHS Publication 91:50212, 1991.

[20] Dyment PG. The adolescent athlete. In: Hofmann AD, Greydanus DE, eds. Adolescent medicine, 2nd ed. Norwalk, CT: Appleton Lange, 1989:417-30.

[21] Butt DS. Psychological motivation and sports performance in world class women field hockey players. Int J Women Studies 1985; 8(4):328.
[22] Young K. Sport and collective violence. Exerc Sport Sci Rev 1991;19:539.
[23] Smith R E, Smoll FL, Ptacek JT. Conjunctive moderator variables in vulnerability and resiliency research life stress, social support and coping skills, and adolescent sport injuries. J Pers Soc Psychol 1990;58(2):360-70.
[24] Rostella RJ. Psychological care of the injured athlete. In: Kulund DN, ed. The injured athlete. Philadelphia, PA: Lippincott-Raven, 1988:151-62.
[25] Duffy FM. Psychological characteristics of the chronically injured athlete. In: Hoerner EF, ed. Head and neck injuries in sports. Philadelphia, PA: Am Soc Test Materials,1994.
[26] Weinberg RS, Comar W. The effectiveness of psychological interventions in competitive sport. Sports Med 1994;18(6):406.
[27] Petruzzello SJ, Landers DM, SalazarW. Biofeedback and sport/exercise performance: applications and limitations. Behav Ther 1991;22(3):371.
[28] Strasburger VC, Reeve A. The adolescent with chronic pain: basic principles of psychosomatic medicine. Adolesc Med 1991;23:677.
[29] Raglin JS. Anxiety sport performance. Exerc Sport Sci Rev 1992;20:243.
[30] Wilks B. Stress management for athletes. Sports Med 1991;11(5):289.
[31] Begel D. The psychotherapist and the adolescent athlete. Sports Psychiatr 1998;7(4):867-77.
[32] Hardy L, Jones G. Sport psychology. In: Harries M, Williams C, Stanish WD, Micheli LJ, eds Oxford textbook of sports medicine. New York: Oxford Univ Press, 1994:118-36.
[33] Hellstedt JC. Invisible players: a family systems model. In: Murphy SM, ed. Sport psychology interventions. Champaign, IL: Human Kinetics, 1995:117-46.
[34] Baum AL. Suicide in athletes: A review and commentary. Clin Sports Med 2005;24(4):853-9.
[35] Bovard RS. Risk behaviors in high school and college sports. Curr Sports Med Rep 2008;7(6):359-66.
[36] Heischober BS, Hofmann AD. Substance abuse. In: Hofmann AD, Greydanus DE, eds. Adolescent medicine, 3rd ed. Stamford, CT: Appleton Lange, 1997:703-39.
[37] Lescohier I, Gallagher SS. Unintentional injury. In: DiClemente RJ, Hansen WB, Ponton LE, eds. Handbook of adolescent health risk behavior. New York: Plenum, 1991:224.
[38] Johnson WA, Landry GL. Nutritional supplements: Fact vs fiction. Adolesc Med 1998;9(3):501-13.
[39] Greydanus DE, Patel DR. Doing in the adolescent athlete: the hope, hype, and hyperbole. Pediatr Clin North Am 2002;59.
[40] Golden NH. Eating disorders: Anorexia nervosa and bulimia nervosa in the adolescent. In: Greydanus DE, Patel DR, Pratt HD, eds. Essential adolescent medicine. New York: McGraw-Hill, 2006:635-50.
[41] Comerci GD, Greydanus DE. Eating disorders: anorexia nervosa and bulimia. In: Hofmann AD, Greydanus DE, eds. Adolescent medicine 3rd ed. Stamford, CT: Appleton Lange, 1997:683-702.
[42] Davis C, Kennedy SH, Ravelski E, Dionne M. The role of physical activity in the development and maintenance of eating disorders. Psychol Med 1994;24:957.
[43] Reddy V, Reid L. Anorexia nervosa and bulimia nervosa. In: Greydanus DE, Patel DR, Pratt HD, Calles JL Jr, eds. Behavorial pediatrics, 3rd ed. New York: Nova Science, 2009.
[44] Tofler IR, Stryer BK, Micheli LJ, Herman LR. Physical and emotional problems of elite female gymnasts. N Engl J Med 1996;335(4):381.
[45] Levin DS, Smith EA, Caldwell LL, Kimbrough J. Violence and high school sports participation. Pediatric Exercise Science 1995;7:379.
[46] Pratt HD, Patel DR, Greydanus DE. Sports and the development of the child and adolescent. In: DeLee JC, Drez D, Miller MD, eds. Orthopaedic sports medicine. Philadelphia, PA: Saunders Elsevier, 2003:624-62.
[47] Stryer BK, Tofler IR, Lapchick R. A developmental overview of child and youth sports. Soc Sport Psychiatr 1998;7(4).
[48] Tofler IR, Knapp PK, Drell MJ. The achievement by proxy spectrum in youth sports: historical perspective and clinical approach to pressured and high-achieving children and adolescents. Sport Psychiatr 1998;7(4),809-20.

[49] Weiss MR, Chaumeton N. Motivational orientations in sport. In: TS Horn, ed. Advances in sport psychology. Champaign, IL: Human Kinetics, 1992:61-100.

[50] Greydanus DE, Patel DR, Luckstead EF, eds. Office orthopedics and sports medicine. Adolesc Med 1998:9(3):425-63.

Submitted: May 01, 2009.
Revised: June 15, 2009.
Accepted: June 21, 2009.

In: Public Health Yearbook 2009
Editor: Joav Merrick

ISBN: 978-1-61668-911-7

Chapter 34

SPORTS DOPING: USE OF DRUGS AND SUPPLEMENTS TO ENHANCE PERFORMANCE

Donald E Greydanus**, MD
and Dilip R Patel, MD, FAAP, FACSM, FAACPDM, FSAM

Department of Pediatrics and Human Development, Michigan State University College of Human Medicine, East Lansing, Michigan, United States of America

ABSTRACT

Use of different drugs and supplements is a world-wide phenomenon in athletics. Drugs and nutritional supplements are used for many reasons, in hopes of feeling good, promoting good health, preventing illness, improving overt illness, reducing fatigue or enhancing muscle development, strength and appearance. Though unproven to be effective, various substances are popular with adolescent athletes of all types--cyclists, distance runners, soccer players, weight lifters, figure skaters, judo athletes, tennis players, football players and many others. A society which emphasizes winning over positive benefits of sports activity sets up its youth to try various chemicals to enhance sports performance as well as to relieve the stress that such pressure for winning inevitably brings. Much is not really known about how these substances affect the health of our youth, since research is often limited and typically only adult males in competitive sports are studied. Relating a known effect of drugs can also be difficult because there are multiple confounding variables found in the research studies and minimal information is available regarding long term effects of these drugs, especially in adolescents. This article reviews selected drugs and supplements used for doping by young athletes. It is important

* Correspondence: Professor Donald E Greydanus, MD, Pediatrics and Human Development, Michigan State University College of Human Medicine, Pediatrics Program Director, Michigan State University/Kalamazoo Center for Medical Studies, 1000 Oakland Drive, Kalamazoo, MI 49008-1284 United States. E-mail: Greydanus@kcms.msu.edu

to note that the popularity and use of different substances change over time, sometimes rapidly, as new ones come to the market and old ones fade out of fashion. Also popular agents may vary in different countries and sports setting in which the athlete participates.

Keywords: Doping, anabolic steroids, creatine, protein, amino acids.

INTRODUCTION

The use of various substances to improve sports performance has been attempted for thousands of years--at least since the Greek and Roman Olympics, when athletes tried mushrooms and opioids. The availability of numerous nutritional chemicals has complicated this phenomenon to a considerable extent in current times. Manufacturers often provide attractive claims about their products, emphasizing that their chemicals improve lean body mass and strength while reducing fat, increase energy, improve aerobic capacity, enhance motor skills, provide antioxidant effects and other impressive results; use of performance enhancing agents by athletes raises complex medical and ethical questions (1-7).

Doping in sports is defined "as the use by an athlete of a substance or method banned by the International Olympic Committee (IOC) or prohibited by an International Sports governing body" (8). According to the World Anti-Doping Agency (WADA), doping is defined as "the occurrence of one or more of the anti-doping rule violations" as set forth in its code (9). The aims of prohibiting doping are to protect an athlete's rights to compete on a level playing field without the use of performance enhancing drugs, prevent harmful side effects, and to ensure the safety of the athletes (8). Doping is also believed to "undermine the fundamental spirit and the collective pursuit of human and sporting excellence" (8).

The first cohesive step in this direction was with the creation of a medical commission by the IOC in 1967, which introduced a list of prohibited substances and anti-doping regulations (10). Screening for prohibited agents was implemented in the 1972 Munich Olympic Games. WADA was created in 1999 and since then is the main agency, which establishes the Anti-doping code to facilitate worldwide harmonization of implementation of anti-doping regulations (10). The World Anti-Doping Code has published The 2009 Prohibited List that lists the different categories of prohibited substances or methods used for doping (11) (see table 1). There is a separate list of substances prohibited in competition and also in specific sports.

ANABOLIC ANDROGENIC STEROIDS (AAS)

In 1935 testosterone was isolated and developed as a chemical to improve metabolism. Since then, a variety of synthetic testosterone derivatives or anabolic steroids have been developed, that include oxymetholone, stanozolol, and nandrolone decanoate, and others.

The belief that AAS will improve muscle development, strength and personal appearance has resulted in a high level of use by adolescent and adult athletes around the world. In the United States, 5-11% of high school males and up to 2.5% of high school females uses these drugs; 50% start under age 16 years and about 33% of teens who use AAS are not athletes (12,13-16). These drugs are often used with various other chemicals as well.

Athletes who consume AAS in high amounts may develop a gain in lean muscle mass, strength, and body weight (with some water retention), if they also engage in marked resistance exercise-training at the same time (3,4,6). Anabolic steroid use without appropriate training and adequate protein intake may not result in such changes. Sports with athletes at high risk for using these chemicals include body building, wrestling, football, sprinting, discus throwing, shot putting and others. High doses are used and vary with the specific drug used and some athletes are involved with steroid stacking, using many drugs simultaneously. The female athlete seeks a dose which allows increase in muscle mass and strength, but below masculinization effects, which are however difficult to avoid. Side effects of anabolic steroids are many, as listed in table 2 (3,17,18).

Table 1. Prohibited substances and methods

Main categories of prohibited substances	Anabolic agents Hormones and related substances (growth hormone, IGF1, insulin, erythropoietin) Beta-2-agonists Hormone agonists and modulators Diuretics and other masking agents
Main categories of prohibited methods	Enhancement of oxygen transfer Chemical and physical manipulation Gene doping

Table 2. Side effects of anabolic steroids

Masculinization of females • Hirsutism • Clitoromegaly Alopecia (males also) Fluid retention Growing athletes • Acceleration of maturation • Early epiphyseal closure • Shortened ultimate adult height Psychologic changes with rise in: • Aggressiveness • Irritability • Depression Gastric ulcers	Hyperglycemia Acne vulgaris (can be severe) Decrease in glycoproteins (FSH and LH) with: • Decreased sperm • Decreased testosterone levels • Reduction in testicular size Increase in tendon injuries Increase in liver function tests Hepatic neoplasms (including a hepatocellular carcinoma) • Peliosis hepatitis Prostatic enlargement Reduction in high density lipoprotein (HDL) • Potential rise in cardiovascular disorders Wilms tumor (at least one case reported)

Human Chorionic Gonadotropin (HCG) hormone may be taken intramuscularly, in attempts to counteract the steroid-induced effect of testicular size reduction; though this reduction is reversible, germinal element defects may persist for many weeks (19). HCG or

Human Growth Hormone (hGH) may also be used to increase the effect of steroids on muscle tissue, and are especially abused by power and speed athletes (20).

The source of these substances may not be the best, and impurities can cause unknown and unexpected adverse effects, for example Creutzfeld-Jacobs disease with hGH (21). Other peptide hormones (HCG, ACTH, EPO [erythropoietin]) may be used as anabolic agents with or without anabolic steroids (19,20,22). ACTH (corticotrophin) increases blood levels of endogenous corticosteroids and has a euphoric effect.

Dehydroepiandrosterone (DHEA)

DHEA is a precursor to testosterone and estrogen used by athletes. It is marketed in nutrition stores as a natural androgenic hormone which is derived in the adrenal glands and also found in wild yams. Many unsubstantiated claims are provided by the manufacturers of this chemical, including increased longevity, prevention of heart disease and cancer, improvement of immunity, reduction in depression, increased libido and many more (3,19). Some athletes use DHEA as a safe substitute for anabolic steroids, either as a pill or intramuscular agent at a dose of 50-100 mg per day over 6 to 12 months. The urine will test positive for testosterone and side effects similar to anabolic steroids are noted. Hirsutism in females and irreversible gynecomastia in males are reported in doses which exceed 100 mg per day. A potential link between development of prostatic and endometrial cancer has been postulated in adults who take DHEA in hopes it is a fountain of youth.

Androstenedione

Androstenedione is a tesosterone precursor found in Scotch pine tree pollen (3). It is taken at a dose of 100 to 200 mg per day, one hour before the sports activity. It may increase testosterone in short episodes, though the testosterone-estrogen ratios are normal within one day (3,19). The popularity of this chemical increased after reports of various superstar athletes using it. Since then reports of its less then stellar effects for athletes and its many side effects have contributed to its declining popularity.

Creatine

Creatine is an essential amino acid synthesized from arginine and glycine in the liver, pancreas and especially, the kidneys; it is found in muscle tissue (3,23,24). Claims from magazine advertisements and from sellers of creatine is that it is a natural product (readily available in milk, meat, fish and other foods) which can increase power for short-term activities and augment muscle mass. Studies do suggest there may be a 5-15% improvement in short-term, repetitive, intermittent, high intensity exercise, including in power-related sports (as sprinting or American football) (23,24). Increased weight may result, due to fluid retention versus increased protein synthesis and increased muscle mass. There is no improvement seen in long-term endurance activities. Supplementation can increase the total creatine by 10-25%; the greatest amount of uptake is during the first 4 days of creatine loading, followed by a plateau of creatine levels (3). Glucose can increase the uptake of creatine, while caffeine antagonizes the effect of creatine.

A loading dose of 20 gm per day for one week is often used, followed by 10-15 gm per day. An increase of 0.7 to 3 kg in body weight in one month has been reported. Weight gain can be maintained on 5 grams per day of creatine during a 10 week period of detraining and continued four weeks after the creatine is stopped (3,23,24). Though creatine is considered safe, there are side-effects and risks: weight gain (due to water retention), nausea, abdominal pain, diarrhea, muscle cramps, muscle strains, dehydration in hot and humid weather, potential renal function deterioration, suppression of endogenous synthesis, and cardiac muscle hypertrophy (25-28). Long term (i.e., over 1 year) effects are unknown and no controlled studies are done in adolescents.

PROTEIN AND AMINO ACIDS

The use of protein and amino acid supplements have sparked a long-lasting debate regarding their efficacy in sports performance (25-29). The recommended daily dietary intake for most individuals for protein is 0.8 g/kg/day. Though athletes do need more protein than their non-exercising peers, most athletes take enough protein from their diets and probably do not benefit from extra protein. If the teen has a deficient diet, supplements may help. Wrestlers, gymnasts, dancers and others may have poorly balanced diets and seek to lower their weights. Evaporated milk and protein powder (egg or soy) are low cost supplements that can be recommended. The use of branched-chain amino acids and others which may increase the production of growth hormone has not been proven to be of benefit to adolescent athletes. High doses of protein or amino acid supplements can lead to gastrointestinal symptoms.

HMB (beta-hydroxy beta-methylbutyrate) is a metabolite of leucine and is not an essential nutrient (27). It is present in breast milk, citrus fruits and cat fish. Its role in humans is unclear, including its claimed role as a sports performance enhancing agent. Increased muscle mass may result along with decreased protein breakdown and enhanced muscle repair processes (32). It is used as an anabolic supplement during strength training and given at a dose of 3 grams per day. As noted with the other substances and nutrients, more study is necessary to identify any ergogenic potential as well as short-term and long-term side-effects.

L-Carnitine is an essential amino acid which is synthesized from lysine and methionine in the liver and kidneys; it is found in meat and dairy products (28). L-carnitine is the physiologically-active form. Most of the carnitine in the body is in the muscle tissue. It is used by athletes in an attempt to improve endurance activities at a dose of 2 grams per day (1). Its effectiveness is unproven and it may induce diarrhea in some; it is usually taken in an impure state (mixed with d-carnitine).

L-tryptophan is an essential amino acid which, in the 1980s, was linked to the eosinophilia myalgia syndrome and deaths (due to impurities found in the product) (3,25,26). Tryptophan undergoes enzymatic change to become 5-hydroxytryptophan and then serotonin. An increase in serotonin may lead to some analgesia, a sense of less pain and delayed fatigue with muscle activity and thus prolonged exercise tolerance. However, it may cause drowsiness and studies confirming its sports performance enhancing potential remain inconclusive.

Arginine is an essential amino acid which stimulates Human Growth Hormone and insulin secretion while increasing creatine stores (29). Amounts such as 2-10 grams per day are linked with increased muscle mass and strength when combined with resistance training. Glutamine is a non-essential amino acid and is the most abundant amino acid in human muscle and plasma. It is found in peanuts, soybeans and almonds. It induces release of hGH and ACTH. It is claimed to increase high intensity resistance training effects. Conjugated linoleic acid (CLA) is found in treated cheese, milk, yogurt, beef and venison. Linoleic acid is a non-essential amino acid, has been claimed to increase in lean body mass and serve as an antioxidant agent (3,25,26). It is also claimed to enhance immune status and bone mineral status.

Antioxidants

Antioxidants are marketed to reduce damage from exercise-induced free radicals. The major readily available and widely marketed antioxidants include alpha tocopherol (vitamin E), beta carotene (precursor of vitamin A),and ascorbic acid (vitamin C) (3,30). Their role in enhancing sports performance is unproven (30-31). They may have a role in smokers, mountain climbers, and athletes with diets poor in antioxidants, individuals with diabetes mellitus and those exposed to polluted air. However, very large doses of vitamin C and beta carotene may cause adverse side effects.

The United States Olympic Committee guideline suggests the following daily intake: Beta-carotene: 3-20 mg (5000-33,340 IU); Vitamin C: 250-1000 mg; and Vitamin E: 100-400 IU.

Some of the other substances with antioxidant properties include linoleic acid, copper, zinc, manganese, selenium and iron. Athletes in endurance sports (as running) may have increased dietary iron requirements over the non-athlete, partially due to an increased loss of iron in the gastrointestinal tract (less in the sweat and urine).

Minerals

Several trace elements and mineral have been used by athletes to enhance performance (31,32). Iron has not been shown to have ergogenic properties and there is no clear evidence to provide routine iron supplementation to athletes. A multivitamin with iron is suggested for vegetarian athletes as well as female adolescents with increased menstrual blood loss and low consumption of red meat. Overall, iron deficiency anemia is the most common form of anemia in the world, and anemia can adversely affect sports performance, especially endurance sports. However excess iron may lead to various side effects and toxicity.

Chromium is an essential trace element which is a cofactor for insulin and is found in mushrooms, nuts, whole grain breads, cereals, brewer's yeast, asparagus, wine, beer, prunes and others (32). The intake of chromium is poor in the general population and it is lost in urine during exercise. It does increase protein synthesis and thus may lead to a gain in muscle mass. Evans has noted an increase in lean body weight with decreased body fat in individuals on chromium (32). Other studies have not confirmed this finding and the overall usefulness of this trace element as a sports performance enhancing agent remains unsubstantiated (3,31,32). There is no established daily dietary requirement for chromium, and a daily intake in the range of 50 to 200 mcg/day is suggested. Side effects of excess chromium supplements include gastrointestinal intolerance, anemia, cognitive impairment, chromosomal damage, interstitial nephritis and others. Chromium picolinate can be taken as part of a multi-vitamin tablet--daily amounts of chromium should not exceed 200 mcg/day.

Vanadium is a non-essential trace mineral found in shellfish, parsley, mushrooms and other foods. There is no known deficiency state in humans. Vanadium has an insulin-like action and can increase muscle mass. Vanadyl sulfate is marketed as a muscle builder and athletes use up to 60 mg per day orally for 3 months. However, there are no studies to support actual anabolic effects. Side effects include diarrhea, gastrointestinal cramps, green tongue and others.

Boron is a substance essential for plants, but not humans. It is present in foods of plant origin, non-citrus fruits, leafy vegetables, nuts and legumes. Though sold to increase muscle mass, there are no studies to support increased lean body mass, total testosterone or strength.

MISCELLANEOUS SUBSTANCES

Blood doping ("blood packing" or "bloodboosting") uses the athlete's own blood to augment aerobic performance (22). Currently used laboratory tests do not identify the athlete who uses blood doping and thus its exact prevalence is not known. The oxygen carrying capacity of the athlete is increased and the hemoglobin may rise to 19 to 20 g/100 ml. However, the increased blood viscosity also increases the risk for cerebrovascular accidents, myocardial infarctions, seizures, and sudden death. EPO (erythropoietin), also used by endurance athletes, stimulates red blood cell production and can lead to these side effects as well.

Various stimulants (as amphetamine, ephedrine or caffeine) have been used to mask pain and allow continued participation (33). Stimulants can lead to increased aggressiveness along with anxiety, tremor, hypertension, tachycardia, dehydration, cerebrovascular accidents and other side effects. They are also banned in the Olympics, since they may give the athlete an unfair advantage. If the athlete has medically-documented asthma, some medications are acceptable to the Olympic medical committee, such as terbutaline or salbuterol (versus ephedrine).

Caffeine has been used to increase athletic performance by decreasing the perception that the athlete is becoming tired. Some studies have observed that 2 to 3 cups of coffee may allow cyclists to continue on bicycle ergometers beyond what they could without the added caffeine (3,33). This xanthine derivative increases lipid metabolism, enhances free fatty acid release from adipocytes and also increases catecholamine stimulation. If too much caffeine is taken, the athlete's performance may be reduced by the resultant increased diuresis and sympathomimetic stimulation. An Olympic athlete is banned if found with a urine caffeine level over 15 mcg/ml.

Sodium bicarbonate has also been used to prolong exercise by reducing acidosis-induced fatigue during bouts of exercise. Non-steroidal anti-inflammatory drugs (NSAIDs) have been used as pain relievers to encourage athletes to augment their sports activity in the face of painful injuries (35). Unfortunately, more severe, even permanent injuries may result. Side effects of NSAIDs include loss of blood in the gastrointestinal tract, reduction of renal perfusion, salt and water retention, reduction of platelet aggregation, and/or heat illness from defects of thermal regulation. Beta-blockers (as propranolol) have been used to reduce performance anxiety by controlling hand tremor, tachycardia and hypertension. They are banned in some Olympic sports.

Diuretics are often used by athletes to cause weight loss and also dilute urine to mask doping with various substances. Side effects of diuretics include weight loss, weakness, dehydration, electrolyte imbalance and cardiac arrhythmias. The weakened athlete may be at risk for injury, as observed in wrestling, for example. There is a report of pulmonary embolism in a high school wrestler using diuretics (4).

Conclusion

Athletic youth and adults are enticed to take a wide variety of drugs, chemicals and nutrients in a never-ending battle to seek the best possible sports performance. Anabolic steroids and creatine are currently widely popular doping agents used by these youth and elite athletes. The drive to victory at any cost has contributed to this sports doping phenomenon in many teenage and adult athletes in this milieu. Unfortunately, many compound this issue by abusing various illicit drugs as well. The pediatric consultant as well as the general medial practitioner providing medical care to adolescents should be vigilant with regards to the use of drugs and supplements in the context of sports or otherwise. It should be routine practice during office visits to inquire about such use of drugs and nutritional supplements and to provide correct information and guidance regarding their risks and purported benefits.

Acknowledgments

Thanks to Kim Douglas for help with the preparation of this manuscript.

References

[1] Jenkinson DM, Harbert AJ. Supplements and sports. Am Fam Physician 2008;78(9):1039-46.

[2] Catlin DH, Fitch KD, Ljungqvist A. Medicine and science in the fight against doping in sport. J Intern Med 2008;264(2):99-114.

[3] Smith DV, McCambridge TM. Performance-enahancing substances in teens. Contemp Pedaitr 2009;26(20):36-45.

[4] Greydanus DE, Patel DR. Sports doping in the adolescent athlete: the hope, hype, and hyperbole. Pediatr Clin North Am 2002;49:829-55.

[5] Catlin DH, Murrya TH. Performance enhancing drugs, fair competition, and Olympic sport. JAMA 1996;276(3):231.

[6] Clarkson PM, Thompson HS. Drugs and sport: research findings and limitations. Sports Med 1997;24(4):366.

[7] Johnson WA, Landry GL. Nutritional supplements: facts vs. fiction. Adolesc Med 1998;9(3):501-14.
[8] http://www.cces.ca/pdfs/CCES-PUB-Substance Classification-E.pdf. Accessed on March 8, 2009.
[9] http://www.wada-ama.org/rtecontent/document/code _V2009_En.pdf. Accessed on March 8, 2009.
[10] Barroso O, Mazzoni I, Rabin O. Hormone abuse in sports: The antidoping perspective. Asian J Androl 2008;10(3):391-402.
[11] http://www.wada-ama.org/rtecontent/document/ 2009_Prohibited_List_Eng_Final_20_Sept_08.pdf. Accessed March 8, 2009.
[12] Faigenbaum AD, Zaichkowsky LD, Gardne DE, et al. Anabolic steroid use by male and female middle school students. Pediatrics 1998;101(5):E6.
[13] Tanner SM, Miller DW, Alongi C. Anabolic steroid use by adolescents: Prevalence, motives and knowledge of risks. Clin J Sports Med 1995;5108.
[14] Graham MR, Davies B, Grace FM, Kicman A, Baker JS. Anabolic steroid use: patterns of use and detection of doping. Sports Med 2008;38(6):505-25.
[15] Sjöqvist F, Garle M, Rane A. Use of doping agents, particularly anabolic steroids, in sports and society. Lancet 2008;371(9627):1872-82.
[16] Castillo EM, Comstock RD. Prevalence of use of performance-enhancing substances among United States adolescents. Pediatr Clin North Am 2007;54(4):663-75.
[17] Casavant MJ, Blake K, Griffith J, Yates A, Copley LM. Consequences of use of anabolic androgenic steroids. Pediatr Clin North Am 2007;54(4):677-90.
[18] Kanayama G, Hudson JI, Poipe HG Jr. Long-term psychiatric and medical consequences of anabolic-androgenic steroid abuse: A looming public health concern? Drug Alcohol Depend 2008;98(1-2):1-12.
[19] Smurawa TM, Congeni JA. Testosterone precursors: Use and abuse in pediatric athletes. Pediatr Clin North Am 2007;54(4):787-96.
[20] Rickert VI, Pawklak-Morello C, Sheppard V, et al. Human growth hormone: a new substance of abuse among adolescents? Clin Pediatrics 1992;31(12):723.
[21] Geyer H, Parr MK, Koehler K, Mareck U, Schänzer W, Thevis M. Nutritional supplements cross-contaminated and faked with doping substances. J Mass Spectrom 2008:43(7):892-902.
[22] Pommering TL. Erythropoietin and other blood-boosting methods. Pediatr Clin North Am 2007;54(4):691-9.
[23] Juhn MS, Tarnopolsky M. Oral creatine supplementation and athletic performance: A critical review. Clin J Sport Med 1998;8:286-97.
[24] Lattavo A, Koperud A, Rogers PD. Creatine and other supplements. Pediatr Clin North Am 2007;54(4):735-60.
[25] Nemet D, Walach B, Eliakim A. Protein and aminoacid supplements in sports: Are they really necessary? Isr Med Assoc J 2005;7(5):328-32.
[26] Krieder RB, Miriel V, Bertun E. Amino acid supplements and exercise performance: analysis of the proposed ergogenic value. Sport Med 1993;16(3):190-223.
[27] Palisini D, Stachy JJ. Beta-hydroxy-beta-methylbutyrate and its use in athletics. Curr Sports Med Rep 2005;4(4):220-3.
[28] Brass EP. Carnitine and sports medicine: use or abuse? Ann NY Acad Sci 2004;1033:67-78.
[29] Campbell BI, LaBounty PM, Roberts E. The ergogenic potential of arginine. J Int Soc Sports Nutr 2004;1(2):35-8.
[30] Armstrong LE, Maresch CM. Vitamin and mineral supplements as nutritional aids to exercise performance and health. Nutri Rev 1996;53:S149- 58.
[31] Volpe SL. Minerals as ergogenic aids. Curr Sports Med Rep 2008;794):224-9.
[32] Evans GW. The effect of chromium picolinate on insulin controlled parameters in humans. Int J Biosocial Med Res 1989;11163-90.
[33] Burke LM. Caffeine and sports performance. Appl Physiol Nutr Metab 2008;33(6):1319-34.
[34] Bohn AM, Khodaee M, Schwenk TL. Ephedrine and other stimulants as ergogenic aids. Curr Sport Med Rev 2003;2(4):220-5.

[35] Alaranta A, Alaranta H, Helenius I. Use of prescription drugs in athletes. Sports Med 2008;38(6):449-63.

Submitted: May 05, 2009.
Revised: June 16, 2009.
Accepted: June 21, 2009.

In: Public Health Yearbook 2009
Editor: Joav Merrick

ISBN: 978-1-61668-911-7

Chapter 35

ABUSE OF GROWTH HORMONE BY ATHLETES

Manmohan Kamboj**, MD
and Dilip R. Patel, MD, FACSM, FAAP, FAACPDM, FSAM
Division of Pediatric Endocrinology and Department of Pediatrics and Human Development, Michigan State University College of Human Medicine, East Lansing, Michigan, Michigan State University Kalamazoo Center for Medical Studies, Kalamazoo, Michigan, United States of America

ABSTRACT

Doping in sports brings up not only ethical issues of fairness in competition, but also highlight the health hazards that the athletes may be at risk for. Many substances have been used for doping in sporting competitions since the ancient times. Growth hormone has been in use by elite athletes for the last several decades. Easy accessibility coupled with inadequate methods of detection available has made human growth hormone a logical option for doping in sports. Recent research work has established methodologies for detection of doping with growth hormone possible and ongoing work continues to refine these procedures.

Keywords: Doping, Recombinant Human Growth Hormone (rhGH), athletes, Human Growth Hormone (hGH).

* Correspondence: Associate professor Manmohan Kamboj, MD, Division of Pediatric Endocrinology, 1000 Oakland Drive, Kalamazoo, Michigan 49008, United States. E-mail: kamboj@kcms.msu.edu

Introduction

About 5% of high school students in the United States revealed in a survey to having used growth hormone (GH) (1). Human growth hormone (hGH) has been used by elite athletes for doping in sports for several decades. Potential benefits that may be expected from use of GH are based on the normal physiologic effects of GH. These include augmentation of height, changes in body composition, increased muscle mass, and decreased fat mass (2-5). Although lipolytic effects are documented in growth hormone deficient patients who are treated with hGH, no studies to date have clearly shown the lipolytic effects of the hGH in healthy, trained athletes (5-8).

Tall stature may offer an advantage in some sports. The limitation here is understandably absence of this benefit in older adolescents once their growing epiphyses are fused. The most useful benefit of hGH is probably that of protein anabolism and increased muscle mass. Multiple studies demonstrate the usefulness of hGH in children and adolescents who have growth hormone deficiency in improving muscle mass, muscle strength, exercise capacity, pulmonary ventilation, oxygen uptake, cardiac muscle mass, and cardiac output (2-5,9-11). GH also increases the blood volume and improves erythropoesis in individuals with growth hormone deficiency (12). However, no studies thus far have demonstrated these effects of recombinant hGH (rhGH) in healthy individuals or athletes who have no growth hormone deficiency.

hGH abuse includes GH derived both from natural as well as recombinant sources. Insulin like growth factor1 (IGF1) is responsible for many of the physiological actions of hGH and has also been used to achieve the effects of GH for doping. IGF1 has been available commercially for the last several years as well. Newer pharmacologic options that are theoretically possible for abuse in the future include the use of growth hormone secretogogues (GHS). GHS are GH releasing peptides that stimulate endogenous GH release. These are still not available commercially but have the potential of being abused in sports once approved for use in different GH deficiency states (13).

Physiology

The Hypothalamo-Pituitary-Growth Hormone–IGF-1 Axis (HPG-IGF-1 Axis)

Growth hormone or somatotropin is secreted by the somatrophs in the anterior pituitary gland. The secretion of GH is regulated by two hypothalamic hormones, which act in opposite ways. The growth hormone releasing hormone (GHRH) stimulates the secretion of GH by increasing transcription of GH-mRNA. Somatropin release inhibiting hormone (SRIH or somatostatin) lowers the frequency and amplitude of GH pulses without directly interfering with its synthesis. hGH secreted by the pituitary somatotrophs stimulates the liver to produce IGF1. Seventy to 80% of IGF1 in circulation is bound to IGF binding protein 3 (IGFBP-3) and acid labile subunit (ALS) in a ternary 150-kDA protein complex with a long half life, and therefore does not show wide fluctuations in blood levels (14,15). The growth and metabolic effects of GH are predominately carried out via IGF-1, although GH also has direct effects as well.

Human Growth Hormone (hGH)

hGH is a single chain polypeptide which has multiple isoforms including the 22-kDA form (comprising 65% to 80% of total GH), 20-kDA form (5 to 10%), and other inactivated forms (16-18). The spontaneous GH secretion is pulsatile with diurnal variation, with most secretion occurring at night. GH and IGF-1 exert a negative feedback at the level of the hypothalamus and pituitary somatotrophs and decrease GH secretion. GH secretion may be stimulated either by increasing GHRH or by lowering SRIH. Some of the common factors, which stimulate GH secretion are summarized in table 1, and its metabolic effects are listed in table 2 (19).

Table 1. Factors causing stimulation of growth hormone

Increase Growth Hormone Releasing Hormone	Decrease Somatostatin (GH) Release Inhibiting Hormone
Sleep	Fasting
Fasting	Cysteamine
Exercise	Pyridostigmine
L-dopa/dopamine agonists	Arginine
Adrenergic agents	Clonidine
Serotonergic agents	Insulin - hypoglycemia
Hyperthyroidism	Glucagon
Gamma-Aminobutyric Acid	Propranolol
Opioids	Growth Hormone Related Peptide
Corticotropin Releasing Hormone	Gamma-Aminobutyric Acid
GH secretagogues	
Vasopressin	
Neuropeptide Y	
Prostaglandins E_1, E_2	
Prostacyclin PGI_2	

ADVERSE EFFECTS OF GH USE AND ABUSE

The experience with physiologic replacement doses of rhGH in children and adolescents is fairly extensive since 1985. The availability of longitudinal data in the GH registries, have facilitated long term follow-up for adverse effects. The use of rhGH in children to treat growth hormone deficiency or for other therapeutic indications within recommended guidelines has been found to be relatively safe. Adverse effects of GH treatment with recommended therapeutic doses are well-documented (see table 3) (19).

Table 2. Metabolic effects of growth hormone

Growth	Increases growth by stimulation of cartilage growth at the epiphysis

Effect on protein synthesis	• Positive nitrogen balance
	• Increase amino acid transport into cells
	• Increase mRNA
	• Decrease urea production and blood urea nitrogen (BUN)
	• Laboratory findings in hGH deficiency:
	  • High/normal BUN
	  • Low serum phosphorus
	  • Low alkaline phosphatase

Effect on Bone/Mineral Metabolism (12, 13)	• Increase calcium absorption • Increase urinary calcium excretion • Decrease urinary phosphorus excretion • Increase vitamin D (1,25 dihydroxy) • Increase osteocalcin • Increase bone density by increasing bone mass by increasing both osteoclastic and osteoblastic function
Effect on Fat Metabolism	• Inhibit maturation of adipocytes • Increase lipolysis
Effect on Carbohydrate Metabolism (11)	• In infants – maintains normal glucose homeostasis • In older children/adults – prevents hypoglycemia by reducing insulin sensitivity • During long term GH treatment – GH causes hyperinsulinemia and insulin resistance

Table 3. Adverse effects of growth hormone with therapeutic use

Creutzfeld-Jacob Disease (CJD)	Reported in patients who received human pituitary derived GH. Not seen with the recombinant, biosynthetic GH used today.
Tumor formation	Since GH is mitogenic, there exists a theoretical risk of tumor formation. Multiple studies have thus far allayed this fear (14). The increased risk of tumor formation with GH treatment seems to be only in patients at high risk for malignancy prior to treatment (15). However, ongoing surveillance is very important to screen for this important theoretical risk factor.
Pseudotumor cerebri (benign intracranial tension)	Usually due to fluid shifts in the central nervous system (CNS). The condition usually resolves after stopping GH temporarily for a few days and then resuming it at a lower dose.
Slipped capital femoral epiphysis	The exact cause of slipped capital femoral epiphysis (SCFE) in patients receiving growth hormone is not clear. May be related to either rapid growth or changes in bone structure with GH. Patients should be followed for pain in the knee or hip and monitored for any painful walking or limping.
Hyperinsulinemia and insulin resistance	The data is still not clear regarding the incidence of insulin resistance, its relationship with the GH dose, and its reversibility with discontinuation of GH therapy.

The benefits that may be perceived in athletes doping GH versus those effects seen in individuals treated with rhGH for growth hormone deficiency or other medical indications may be due to the difference in the doses used. For doping, doses as high as 10 to 20 times the normal physiologic doses may be used by athletes (5). Acute and long-term effects from use of growth hormone and related substances at much higher doses by athletes are difficult to ascertain because of insufficient data.

Large doses of hGH as used in doping may cause some of the complications as have been well demonstrated in patients with acromegaly including hypertropic cardiomyopathy, systemic hypertension, diabetes mellitus, and increased risk of breast and colon cancer (20-23). The post-treatment GH level is the main determinant of the risk of morbidity and mortality in acromegaly (22). With the advent of rhGH, the risk of Creutzfeld Jacob Disease (CJD) has been virtually eliminated, but the cadaveric GH still remains available and being cheaper may be a more practical option, thus predisposing some athletes to the risk of CJD. The ongoing risk of diseases such as hepatitis and human immunodeficiency virus infection remains possible with needle sharing for the subcutaneous administration of GH. One study demonstrated cardiovascular effects including left ventricular hypertrophy and increased cardiac output within four weeks of supraphysiologic doses of GH (20,23).

DETECTION OF HGH DOPING

The detection of hGH doping has been challenging for several reasons. hGH secretion is pulsatile with diurnal variation; therefore, random blood or urine levels of hGH are not reliable tests for doping. Stress and exercise are stimulants of hGH secretion. Athletes are subjected to both these stimuli especially around the time of competition, and thus the GH levels measured following exercise are not reliable. The endogenous hGH secreted by the pituitary is predominantly the 22-kDA molecule, which is structurally similar to the rhGH and the cadaveric GH used for GH treatment. Therefore, GH levels in blood will not be able to differentiate the source of GH. Urine testing for GH is also not reliable because only small amount of hGH is secreted in the urine.

Large scale screening for doping of any substance in athletes preferably needs to be an easy, reliable, fairly rapid with high specificity and sensitivity. In general, urine testing is a preferred method of screening. The ideal test for detection should preferably cover a fairly wide window of opportunity for detection of the drug after having been administered. It has been very challenging to develop an adequate test for detection of hGH doping. Two main groups of researchers have been instrumental in devising two different approaches to the testing. The first approach is based on the ability to differentiate between different isoforms of hGH and was pioneered by Strasburger and Bedlingmaier (24). The second approach was developed later by the GH-2000 team lead by Sonksen (25,26). This method is based on the effect of hGH on hGH-dependent markers, and the ability to measure these markers reliably.

The isoform method (The differential immunoassay method)

The hGH secreted by pituitary exists in different isoforms, namely, the 22-kDA form (about 70%), 20- kDA form (about 5 to 15%), and other forms (such as dimers, oligomers, fragmented, acylated, acidic and desaminated isoforms) making up the rest. Recombinant GH is however only 22-kDA. When hGH is administered in large quantities, the endogenous GH secretion by the pituitary gland is suppressed. Therefore, these individuals will have a higher proportion of the 22-kDA hGH form versus the proportion seen normally. However, administration of cadaveric GH will not exhibit this difference in the isoforms of GH. It is also important to remember that if there is abuse with a GH secretagogue (GHS), which will stimulate and increase the endogenous pituitary hGH secretion, the composition of hGH will also be like normal as well.

The German method uses one assay to measure 22-kDA isoform and a second assay to measure all other hGH isoforms (i.e., the permissive assay). Normally the ratio of 22-kDA hGH to total GH is less than 1. In GH abuse the ratio is greater than 1 (27,28). The Australian-Japanese consortium utilizes separate assays to measure 22-kDA and 20-kDA isoforms (29).

Subcutaneously administered rhGH has a short half life and is cleared from circulation rapidly. This limits the window of opportunity for reliable testing to about 36 hours with spontaneous hGH secretion returning to normal in about 48 hours. Therefore, an individual who may be abusing hGH for a prolonged period of time and who then discontinues it several days before the event will not be detected (30,31). The second category for caution includes athletes using cadaveric GH/or GH secretagogues who will go undetected as their hGH secretion pattern and hGH isoforms proportions will be normal (32).

The levels and proportion of isoforms are not affected by age, sex, ethnicity or other factors (32,33). Exercise causes a transient increase in the 22-kDA fraction and therefore there may be a compromised sensitivity if the test were done soon after the sporting event (33). This method is a good test for random testing to detect hGH abuse. It has lower sensitivity when used after the sporting event. It will also not be useful if cadaveric GH or GHS are abused (34,35).

The growth hormone dependent marker measurement method

This method is based on the work of GH-2000 and GH-2004 projects and multiple studies have been done to delineate reference ranges of the markers measured, with acceptable sensitivity and specificity (39). This method involves the measurement of GH dependent markers namely IGF-1 and pro-collagen type 3 (P-III-P). These markers are chosen as their levels remain fairly constant with very little diurnal or day to day variability (36). Following exercise level of IGF-1 may increase by 20% and P-III-P by 10.2%, compared with a 300% elevation after GH administration. Therefore, sporting events would not interfere significantly with measurements following the event (37,38).

The administration of hGH leads to changes in multiple growth factors and serum proteins called GH dependent markers. Therefore, measurement of these markers and comparison with expected reference ranges would be able to detect GH administration especially in supraphysiologic doses as in doping. Many such markers have been investigated and narrowed down to the selection of IGF-1 and P-III-P for the purposes of testing for GH doping (32,33).

IGF-1 and P-III-P levels have a long half life and more stability of levels, and therefore offer a wider window of opportunity for testing to be done. Detailed studies have established consistent worldwide reference ranges (32). Using more than one marker such as IGF-1 and P-III-P offers improved sensitivity and specificity. The significantly marked increase observed in IGF-1 and P-III-P following the administration of hGH offers clear differentiation between individuals receiving hGH and those who are not (32,33,39).

Sporting injuries may cause P-III-P levels to increase by about 20% (2 to 3 weeks) after an injury while IGF-1 levels remain unchanged (32). However, no false positives have been reported because of injury (32).

Conclusion

Doping with hGH continues to be a challenge in the sporting world. The extent of abuse of growth hormone and related agents by young athletes is difficult to ascertain. However, significant risks associated with growth hormone doping have been recognized based on reports from athletes who have used growth hormone in the past. What is known thus far may be the tip of the iceberg. There are no long term trials of use of supraphysiologic GH doses to be able to accurately gauge the adverse effects for obvious reasons. It is unlikely that safety data for use of supraphysiological, doping doses of GH on long term basis will ever be obtained because of the ethical issues involved in conduction of such scientific trials. Any significant adverse effects may only be noted retrospectively on random reporting by individuals with history of GH doping in the past.

Two main procedures have been defined and clearly delineated for detection of GH, namely, the isoform method, and the GH dependent marker method. Work is ongoing to try to further refine the methodologies, and reference ranges so that these testing measures may be used successfully at a commercial level for detection of GH hormone doping. Newer investigative procedures are being looked into to refine these procedures further as well as using other technologies such as surface Blasmon resonance and mass spectrometry (33,40, 41). Well defined reference ranges, and cut off levels to clearly delineate between positive and negative for GH doping are needed before routine use in sporting events can be implemented (5).

References

[1] Rickert VI, Pawlak-Morello C, Sheppard V, Jay MS. Human growth hormone: A new substance of abuse among adolescents? Clin Pediatr (Phila) 1992;31(12):723-6.

[2] Jørgensen JO, Vahl N, Hansen TB, Thuesen L, Hagen C, Christiansen JS. Growth hormone versus placebo treatment for one year in growth hormone deficient adults: Increase in exercise capacity and normalization of body composition. Clin Endocrinol (Oxf) 1996;45(6):681-8.

[3] Gibney J, Wallace JD, Spinks T, Schnorr L, Ranicar A, Cueno RC, Lockhart S, Burnand KG, Salomon F, Sonksen PH, Russell-Jones D. The effects of 10 years of recombinant human growth hormone (GH) in adult GH-deficient patients. J Clin Endocrinol Metab 1999;84(8):2596-602.

[4] Jørgensen JO, Thuesen L, Müller J, Ovesen P, Skakkebaek NE, Christiansen JS. Three years of growth hormone treatment in growth hormone-deficient adults: Near normalization of body composition and physical performance. Eur J Endocrinol 1994;130(3):224-8.

[5] Bidlingmaier M, Wu Z, Strasburger CJ. Problems with GH doping in sports. J Endocrinol Invest 2003;26(9):924-31.

[6] Crist DM, Peake GT. Loftfield RB, Kraner JC, Egan PA. Supplemental growth hormone alters body composition, muscle protein metabolism and serum lipids in fit adults: Characterization of dose-dependent and response-recovery effects. Mech Ageing Dev 1991;58(2-3):191-205.

[7] Yarasheski KE, Zachweija JJ, Angelopoulos TJ, Bier DM. Short-term growth hormone treatment does not increase muscle protein synthesis in experienced weight lifters. J Appl Physiol 1993;74(6):3073-6.

[8] Dean H. Does exogenous growth hormone improve athletic performance? Clin J Sport Med 2002;12(4):250-3.

[9] Janssen YJ, Doornbos J, Roelfsema F. Changes in muscle volume, strength, and bioenergetics during recombinant human growth hormone (GH) therapy in adults with GH deficiency. J Clin Endocrinol Metab 1999;84(1):279-84.

[10] Nass R, Huber RM, Klauss V, Müller OA, Schopohl J, Strasburger CJ. Effect of growth hormone (hGH) replacement therapy on physical work capacity and cardiac and pulmonary function in patients with hGH deficiency acquired in adulthood. J Clin Endocrinol Metab 1995;80(2):552-7.

[11] Cittadini A, Cuocolo A, Merola B, Fazio S, Sabatini D, Nicolai E, et al. Impaired cardiac performance in GH-deficient adults and its improvement after GH replacement. Am J Physiol 1994;267(2 Pt 1):E219-25.

[12] Christ ER, Cummings MH, Westwood NB, Sawyer BM, Pearson TC, Sönksen PH, Russell-Jones DL. The importance of growth hormone in the regulation of erythropoiesis, red cell mass, and plasma volume in adults with growth hormone deficiency. J Clin Endocrinol Metab 1997;82(9):2985-90.

[13] Thevis M, Schänzer W. Emerging drugs: Potential for misuse in sport and doping control detection strategies. Mini Rev Med Chem 2007;7(5):531-7.

[14] Jones JI, Clemmons DR. Insulin-like growth factors and their binding proteins: Biological actions. Endocr Rev 1995; 6(1):3-34.

[15] Ranke MB, Elmlinger M. Functional role of insulin-like growth factor binding proteins. Horm Res;48 Suppl 4:9-15.

[16] Leung KC, Howe C, Gui LY, Trout G, Veldhuis JD, Ho KK . Physiological and pharmacological regulation of 20-kDA growth hormone. Am J Physiol Endocrinol Metab 2002;283(4):E836-43.

[17] Cooke NE, Ray J, Watson MA, Estes PA, Kuo BA, Liebhaber SA. Human growth hormone gene and the highly homologous growth hormone variant gene display different splicing patterns. J Clin Invest 1988;82(1):270-5.

[18] DeNoto FM, Moore DD, Goodman HM. Human growth hormone DNA sequence and mRNA structure: Possible alternative splicing. Nucleic Acids Res 1981;11,9(15):3719-30.

[19] Allen DB, Rose SR, Reiter EO. Normal growth and growth disorders. In: Kappy MS, Allen DB, Geffener ME, eds. Principles and practice of pediatric endocrinology. Springfield, IL: Charles C Thomas, 2005.

[20] Diamanti-Kandarakis E, Tsilakis D, Lazarides S, Kandarakis H, Bergele A. Hormones in sports: Growth hormone abuse. Hormones (Athens) 2004;3(1):37-45.

[21] Bengtsson BA, Edén S, Ernest I, Odén A, Sjögren B. Epidemiology and long-term survival in acromegaly. A study of 166 cases diagnosed between 1955 and 1984. Acta Med Scand 1988;223(4):327-35.

[22] Orme SM, Mcnally RJ, Cartwright RA, Belchetz PE. Mortality and cancer incidence in acromegaly: A retrospective cohort study. United Kingdom Acromegaly Study Group. J Clin Endocrinol Metab 1998;83(8):2730-4.

[23] Cittadini A, Berggren A, Longobardi S, Ehrnborg C, Napoli R, Rosén T, et al. Supraphysiological doses of GH induce rapid changes in cardiac morphology and function. J Clin Endocrinol Metab 2002;87(4):1654-9.

[24] Bidlingmaier M, Wu Z, Strasburger CJ. Doping with growth hormone. J Pediatr Endocrinol Metab 2001;14(8):1077-83.

[25] Healy ML, Dall R, Gibney J, Bassett E, Ehrnborg C, Pentecost C, et al. Toward the development of a test for growth hormone (GH) abuse: A study of extreme physiological ranges of GH-dependent markers in 813 elite athletes in the post-competition setting. J Clin Endocrinol Metab 2005;90(2):641-9.

[26] Erotokritou-Mulligan I, Bassett EE, Kniess A, Sönksen PH, Holt RI. Validation of the growth hormone (GH)-dependent marker method of detecting GH abuse in sport through the use of indpendent data sets. Growth Horm IGF Res 2007;17(5):416-23.

[27] Bidlingmaier M, Wu Z, Strasburger CJ. Problems with GH doping in sports. J Endocrinol Invest 2003;26(9):924-31.

[28] Wu Z, Bidlingmaier M, Dall R, Strasburger CJ. Detection of doping with human growth hormone. Lancet 1999;13 353(9156):895.

[29] Momomura S, Hashimoto Y, Shimazaki Y, Irie M. Detection of exogenous growth hormone (GH) administration by monitoring ratio of 20kDa- and 22kDA-GH in serum and urine. Endocr J 2000;47(1):97-101.

[30] Wu RH, St Louis Y, DiMartino-Nardi J, Wesoly S, Sobel EH, Sherman B, Saenger P. Preservation of physiological growth hormone (GH) secretion in idiopathic short stature after recombinant GH therapy. J Clin Endocrinol Metab 1990;70(6):1612-5.

[31] Keller A, Wu Z, Kratzsch J, Keller E, Blum WF, Kniess A, et al. Pharmacokinetics and pharmacodynamics of GH: Dependence on route and dosage of administration. Eur J Endocrinol 2007;156(6):647-53.

[32] Holt RI. Beyond reasonable doubt: Catching the growth hormone cheats. Pediatr Endocrinol Rev 2007;4(3): 228-32.

[33] Holt RI, Sönksen PH. Growth hormone, IGF-I and insulin and their abuse in sport. Br J Pharmacol 2008;154(3):542-56.

[34] Wallace JD, Cuneo RC, Bidlingmaier M, Lundberg PA, Carlsson L, Boguszewski CL, et al. Changes in non-22-kilodalton (kDa) isoforms of growth hormone (GH) after administration of 22-kDa recombinant human GH in trained adult males. J Clin Endocrinol Metab 2001;86(4):1731-7.

[35] Wallace JD, Cuneo RC, Bidlingmaier M, Lundberg PA, Carlsson L, Boguszewski CL, et al. The response of molecular isoforms of growth hormone to acute exercse in trained adult males. J Clin Endocrinol Metab 2001;86(1):200-6.

[36] McHugh CM, Park RT, Sönksen PH, Holt RI. Challenges in detecting the abuse of growth hormone in sport. Clin Chem 2005;51(9):1587-93..

[37] Wallace JD, Cuneo RC, Lundberg PA, Rosén T, Jørgensen JO, Longobardi S, et al. Responses of markers of bone and collagen turnover to exercise, growth hormone (GH) administration, and GH withdrawal in trained adult males. J Clin Endocrinol Metab 2000;85(1):124-33.

[38] Wallace JD, Cuneo RC, Baxter R, Orskov H, Keay N, Pentecost C, et al. Responses of the growth hormone (GH) and insulin-like growth factor axis to exercise, GH administration, and GH withdrawal in trained adult males: A potential test for GH abuse in sport. J Clin Endocrinol Metab 1999; 84(10):3591-601.

[39] Nelson AE, Ho KK. A robust test for growth hormone doping – present status and future prospects. Asian J Androl 2008;10(3):416-25.

[40] Chung L, Clifford D, Buckley M, Baxter RC. Novel biomarkers of human growth hormone action from serum proteomic profiling using protein chip mass spectrometry. J Clin Endocrinol Metab 2006;91(2):671-7..

[41] Barroso O, Mazzoni I, Rabin O. Hormone abuse in sports: The antidoping perspective. Asian J Androl 2008; 10(3):391-402.

Submitted: April 28, 2009.
Revised: June 10, 2008.
Accepted: June 22, 2008.

In: Public Health Yearbook 2009
Editor: Joav Merrick

ISBN: 978-1-61668-911-7

Chapter 36

PREVENTION OF SUDDEN CARDIAC DEATH IN YOUNG ATHLETES: IMPACT AND LIMITATIONS OF PREPARTICIPATION SCREENING

Saad A. Siddiqui, MD
and Dilip R.Patel, MD, FAAP, FACSM, FSAM, FAACPDM*
Department of Pediatrics and Human Development, Michigan State University College of Human Medicine, East Lansing, Michigan, United States of America

ABSTRACT

Sudden death of a young athlete ($\leq$ 35 y of age) is always disconcerting. In the United States, the incidence of sudden cardiac death (SCD) is 2 in 100 000 among high school athletes and 1 in 65000 amongst collegiate athletes. The most common cause of SCD in a young athlete in the United States is hypertrophic cardiomyopathy (26%). Other main causes include commotio cordis (20%), anomalous origin of the coronary artery (14%), myocarditis, valvular heart disease, premature atherosclerotic heart disease, arrythmogenic right ventricular dysplasia, and aortic dilatation and rupture (5%-8% combined incidence). In athletes $\geq$ 35 years of age, coronary artery disease is the most common cause of sudden cardiac death. The pathophysiology of SCD is explained by and is a direct extension of the physiologic remodeling of the heart. Remodeling is characterized by chamber dilation and hypertrophy and precipitates fatal ventricular fibrillation. The main aim of pre-participation screening is to identify athletes at risk for

* Correspondence: Professor Dilip R Patel, MD, MD, FAAP, FACSM, FSAM, FAACPDM, Department of Pediatrics and Human Development, Michigan State University College of Human Medicine, Kalamazoo Center for Medical Studies, Kalamazoo, Michigan, MSU/ KCMS/ Pediatrics, 1000, Oakland Drive, Kalamazoo, MI 49008-1284 United States. Tel: 269-337-6450; Fax: 269-337-6474; E-mail: patel@kcms.msu.edu

SCD. In the United States, the screening is based on personal and family history and focused cardiovascular examination. In the United States, an electrocardiogram (ECG) is not recommended for mass screening of asymptomatic young athletes. Management of SCD includes prompt recognition and initiation of cardiopulmonary resuscitation (CPR), defibrillation, and early mobilization of emergency medical services (EMS). This article reviews screening and prevention of SCD in young athletes.

Keywords: Sudden cardiac death, cardiac modeling, hypertrophic cardiomyopathy, automated external defibrillator, electrocardiogram.

INTRODUCTION

The first instance of sudden death in an athlete dates back to the 490 BC, when a Greek runner died after having run from Marathon to Athens to deliver news of the victory over the Persians (1). In more recent times however there have been many reports of elite athletes in various sports having succumbed to this intriguing phenomenon. These include basketball players, figure skaters, football players, and hockey players (2). Sudden death in a previously healthy athlete is counterintuitive and especially disconcerting as this group of people is considered to be the healthiest amongst the general population and exercise has been proven to decrease the risk of life threatening cardiovascular disease (2).

Sudden cardiac death generally refers to "nontraumatic and unexpected sudden death that may occur from a cardiac arrest, within 6 hours of a previously normal state of health" (3). Based on the American Heart Association (AHA) guidelines, in the discussion that follows, an athlete refers to one who has a natural aptitude for, or is reasonably skilled in physical exercises, sports, or games; a young athlete is generally younger than 35 years of age. The term competitive athlete refers to an athlete who participates in a sport requiring systematic training and regular competition (4).

EPIDEMIOLOGY

The exact incidence and prevalence rates for SCD in young athletes are not known because of a lack of mandatory reporting and absence of a national database (2). One large study has estimated the incidence to be 1 in 200,000 among high school athletes in the United States (5). Another study suggests the incidence in collegiate athletes to be about 1 in 65,000 (6). The annual incidence of SCD in the US is between 50 and 100 (2). The incidence of cardiovascular collapse as the cause of athletic fatalities is twice that of death caused by trauma (7,8). SCD is more common in men than in women, at a ratio ranging from 5:1 to 9:1; this may be from the higher sport participation rate in men in competitive sports (9). The incidence is higher in African American athletes (10). This disparity could be from a higher number of competitive athletes (almost 40%) who are African American (2). In previous studies from Italy, the incidence of SCD in athletes was reported at 3/100 000 (32). This difference between the US and Italy, is thought to be due to the relatively younger age of the American athletes and the inclusion of a larger number of females (33). In more recent studies, the incidence of SCD in Italian athletes has been shown to be decreasing partly attributed to effective pre-participation screening that includes an electrocardiogram. In the United States the most common sports associated with SCA are football, basketball, and ice hockey, whereas it is soccer in Europe (10-12).

CAUSES OF SUDDEN CARDIAC DEATH

Physical exertion acts as a trigger for precipitation of sometimes lethal arrhythmias in the presence of underlying structural heart diseases or other susceptibilities (8). In the US the most common cause of sudden cardiac death in young athletes is hypertrophic cardiomyopathy (26%) (9-11). The second most frequent cause of sudden cardiac death in athletes is anomalous origin of the coronary artery (14%), most commonly the left coronary artery arising from the right sinus of Valsalva (9,12). This group of patients may have a completely normal ECG and exercise stress test and will first manifest symptoms with exertion while playing sport (13). Other heart related conditions that can cause sudden cardiac arrest (SCA) include myocarditis, valvular heart disease such as aortic stenosis and myxomatous mitral valve disease, premature atherosclerotic heart disease, arrythmogenic right ventricular dysplasia, and aortic dilatation and rupture (5%-8% combined incidence) (11-13). No structural abnormality of the heart is found in 2% of young athletes who suffer SCD. These athletes may have long QT syndrome, Brugada syndrome, polymorphic catecholaminergic tachycardia, Wolf-Parkinson-White (WPW) syndrome, or abnormalities of the conducting system (9,12). In athletes older than 35 years, coronary artery disease is the most common cause of sudden cardiac death (12).

In young children commotio cordis is an important cause of sudden death. Commotios cordis results from a blunt trauma to the chest by a fast moving projectile, such as a baseball or ice hockey puck (2,5). The mechanism of cardiac arrest is ventricular fibrillation. The blow should be inflicted within a very narrow window of time (within 30-40 msec, just before repolarization) at the peak of the T wave (14,25). The exact ion channel mechanism is not unknown. Commotio cordis accounts for 20% of sudden cardiac death in children on the field (14).

PHYSIOLOGY AND REMODELING

The knowledge of cardiovascular changes that result from regular exercise dates back a 100 years (16). The term athlete's heart refers to the benign increase in cardiac mass and specific circulatory and cardiac morphological alterations that result from regular exercise, and represents a physiologic adaptation to systemic training (12,15). Endurance training (dynamic, isotonic or aerobic) such as in running or swimming, and resistance training (static, isometric or anaerobic), such as in weight training induce different training effects on the cardiovascular system (see table 1) (17). In most sports, however, there is some overlap of endurance and resistance training. This is exemplified in sports such as skiing, rowing, cycling, and triathlon. It is, therefore, expected that with regular exercise training there would be some combination of chamber dilation and wall thickness increase (15).

Table 1. Effect of different types of exercise on cardiac function

Endurance training	Increased oxygen utilization Decreased peripheral vascular resistance Increased stroke volume Increased cardiac output Volume overload: ventricular dilatation
Resistance training	No change in oxygen utilization No change in cardiac output Increased peripheral vascular resistance Increased heart rate Pressure overload: ventricular hypertrophy

The cardiac remodeling associated with regular exercise training in athletes is not a uniform phenomenon. Fifty percent of athletes may show some cardiac remodeling that will include one or all of the following: increase left ventricle (LV), right ventricle (RV) or left atrium (LA) chamber size. Ventricular wall thickness may or may not be increased. These changes are usually associated with normal systolic and diastolic function. Remodeling may occur rapidly or more gradually. Most of these changes are still within normal limits when compared to an age and sex matched sedentary individual (15).

The degree of structural change in the heart may correlate with the type of sport that the athlete is involved in, but this has not been proven conclusively (18-20). The clinical variables that may play a role in influencing the degree of structural change in the heart include body size (50%), type of sport (14%), gender (7%), age (4%) and unknown factors (25%) (21). Genetics also plays a role and may be responsible for some of the unknown variables (21).

Several changes on the ECG are noted due to cardiac remodeling with regular exercise training. About 60% of athletes have a normal ECG, whereas 15% may have an ECG changes suggestive of an underlying heart disease (22). The most commonly observed ECG changes include early repolarization, increased QRS voltages, diffuse T wave inversion, and deep Q waves (22-24). The most common rhythm abnormalities in the athlete include bradycardia, 1st degree heart block, and Wenkebach phenomenon (12,24, 25). Recent studies with Holter monitor have identified more complex ventricular arrhythmias, which are usually abolished on discontinuing training and may be of no clinical significance. These may be considered part of the spectrum that constitutes the athletes heart (26,27).

Often the changes in ventricular chamber size and wall thickness seen in competitive athletes may mimic structural heart disease. A ventricular wall thickness between 13 mm and 15 mm and left ventricular end diastolic size greater ≥ 55mm but ≤ 60mm), constitute the "gray zone" of overlap between physiologic change and structural heart disease (28,29). In these cases it is often difficult to make a decision, whether to allow or not to allow continued competitive sport participation. One option is to discontinue training and serially measure these variables (30). Normalization would suggest physiological change and the athlete may be allowed to resume competitive sport participation (15).

In most athletes the changes in heart that occur with regular training and conditioning regress with deconditioning; however, in 20% of these athletes the changes may be permanent (15). There is no evidence to show that athlete's cardiac remodeling has a disabling, permanent or detrimental course (15,31).

PRE-PARTICIPATION CARDIOVASCULAR SCREENING

Pre-participation screening of competitive athletes refers to the "systematic practice of medically screening large populations of athletes before participation in sports for the purpose of identifying abnormalities that could provoke disease progression or sudden death" (40,41). The main objective of such screening is to identify athletes who have cardiovascular risk factors and selectively restrict their participation in competitive sport (or treat them) to avoid SCD on the field (34). This is especially important, as some recent studies of automated external defibrillator (AED) use on the athletic field have indicated that outcomes have generally been poor and that prevention is the best strategy (42). Early recognition of risk is important for all age ranges of the population. Thirty to 50% of all SCDs are first clinical events and up to 67% occur either as first events or among those with identified disease considered to be at low risk for SCD (53).

History and physical examination (H&P)

The current American Heart Association (AHA) recommendations for cardiovascular screening of competitive young athletes consist of a review of 12 items (8 for personal and family history and 4 for physical examination) (see table 2) (15,34,45). A positive response to one or more of these items is considered an indication for referral to a specialist for cardiovascular evaluation (34). For athletes older than 35 years a personal and family history of coronary artery disease should be obtained (34).

Unlike in some other countries, such as in Italy, in the US there is no mandate or law regarding preparticipation screening (15,34). The venues and institutions conducting and organizing the sports events have a responsibility to provide for such screening services (15,34). In case of a high school athlete the personal physician is expected to conduct the 12-point screening evaluation (34). At higher level of athletic participation, it is the team physician who decides appropriate medical screening procedures (34).

H&P as recommended by the AHA guidelines has long been the standard of cardiovascular screening for competitive athletes in the United States. More recently there have been several studies published that question the efficacy of the screening H&P alone. Glover et al reported a study of 134 cases of SCD who had undergone a screening H&P (39). Based on H&P, only 3 % of cases were suspected of having cardiac disease and eventually only <1% received an accurate diagnosis (39). This conferred a low sensitivity to H&P as a screening tool. Glover et al also showed that for most high school athletes, the H&P was not being administered in accordance with AHA recommendations (39).

Forty percent of states had H&P forms for high school athletes, which were judged incomplete and inadequate. A recent revaluation of the H&P forms has been more encouraging with 81% having H&P forms that are at least adequate (≥9 of 12 AHA recommended H&P points) (46). In 64% of states non-physicians could administer the H&P and 35% states allowed chiropractors to perform the H&P (34).

In case of college athletics, 25% of colleges were judged to have inadequate forms (47). The National Collegiate Athletic Association (NCAA) has a similar H&P recommendation and includes 10 out of 12 H&P points from the AHA recommendations (48).

The H&P has come under scrutiny for having low sensitive for identifying athletes with cardiovascular risk factors (34). It has also been argued that hypertrophic cardiomyopathy (HCM) is usually asymptomatic with normal findings on examination (49). Corrado et al have published data substantiating the higher efficacy of ECG in diagnosing athletes with HCM and channelopathies (35). The advantages of H&P include cost effectiveness, need for minimal resources, and efficiency in administration with reasonable sensitivity (34).

Table 2. The 12 element American Heart Association recommendations for preparticipation cardiovascular screening of competitive athletes

Medical history Parental verification is recommended for high school and middle school athletes	
Personal history	1. Exertional chest pain/discomfort. 2. Unexplained syncope/near syncope (judged not to be neurocardiogenic or vasovagal; of particular concern when related to exertion) 3. Excessive exertional and unexplained dyspnea/fatigue associated with exercise 4. Prior recognition of a heart murmur 5. Elevated systemic blood pressure
Family history	6. Premature death (sudden and unexplained, or otherwise before age 50 because of heart disease in one or more relative 7. Disability from heart disease in a close relative younger than 50 8. Specific knowledge of certain cardiac conditions in family members: hypertrophic or dilated cardiomyopathy, long-QT syndrome, or other ion channelopathies, Marfan syndrome, or clinically important arrhythmias
Physical examination	9. Heart murmur (auscultation should be performed in both supine and standing positions [or with Valsalva maneuver], specifically to identify murmurs of dynamic left ventricular outflow tract obstruction) 10. Femoral pulses to exclude aortic coarctation 11. Physical stigmata of Marfan syndrome 12. Brachial artery blood pressure (sitting position) preferably taken both arms

Electrocardiogram

The electrocardiogram (ECG) has received a lot of attention recently consequent to the Italian studies showing marked decrease in SCD rates after making ECG part of standard screening (37). The International Olympic committee and the European Sports Council require an ECG before sports participation (43,44). Japan has been subjecting all first, seventh, and tenth graders to an ECG since 1973 (52). The interest in ECG stems from the fact that 90% of patients with HCM have an abnormal ECG (51). Other ECG detectable diseases also causing SCD include arrythmogenic right ventricular dysplasia (ARVD), ion channelopathies, dilated cardiomyopathy, and Wolf-Parkinson-White syndrome (WPW) (33).

Corrado et al (35) showed that they were able to identify 22 athletes with HCM based on screening ECG, later confirmed with an echocardiogram (ECHO). Eighty two percent of the patients had abnormal ECG, while 23% had some suggestions of underlying disease based on family history (35). In an extension of the above study, Corrado et al (36,37) showed an 89% decrease in the incidence of SCD in screened athletes in Italy. A study conducted in Nevada, of more than 5,000 high school athletes, showed the sensitivity of the ECG at 78% in detecting athletes at risk; this compares to 3% sensitivity for the history and physical examination alone (54). The specificity seems to increase when ECG changes considered grossly abnormal are pursued with further studies.

In United States, routine ECG is not recommended at present as part of cardiovascular screening of young asymptomatic athletes. Reasons cited for not including ECG include cost, need for trained personnel, need for appropriate infrastructure, false positive findings warranting further unnecessary testing, and potential to cause anxiety in otherwise healthy athletes and their families (34). Current recommendations include improving the existing H&P forms improve their yield, and creating a national data registry for incidence of SCD to better assess the incidence of SCD in the US athletic population. Because SCD is a rare event in young athletes, with a large number of athletes, it is estimated that it will cost $3.4 million to save one athlete's life from SCD, and $330,000 to identify one athlete at risk for SCD (34). The sensitivity of the screening ECG depends greatly on the person reading it. The knowledge of specific ECG presentation in healthy adolescents and the knowledge of ECG changes in athletes are imperative to determine what a grossly abnormal change is (36).

There have been several questions raised regarding the Italian study that has become the basis to include ECG as a screening tool (36). One argument against that study includes that it is an observational study and not a prospective study with a control population (34). Also the incidence rates that the Italians have managed to achieve after almost 25 years of ECG screening are not significantly different from the existing SCD rates in the United States.

Myerburg et al (55) make several points in favor of including ECG for cardiovascular screening of competitive athletes. They contend that the false positive rate of 10%-25% cited in the AHA recommendations for abnormal findings on ECG is too high and according to their estimate it is about 4.8% (34,56). Myerburg et al (55) have suggested that all school athletes receive ECGs only twice during their school athletic career. This will mitigate the need for annual ECG for each athlete and will significantly bring down the cost of such a program (55). With regards to personnel, the argument is that ancillary health staff with an interest in sudden cardiac arrest (SCA) should be recruited and trained to provide for the numbers required for a functional screening strategy that includes ECG (55). Fuller et al based on their study of 5000+ high school athletes estimated including ECG in the screening protocol will cost $44000 for each life saved (54). Fuller et al report that screening 700 000 high school athletes annually results in 1080 years of life gained when an ECG is used, compared with 92 years of life gained when the AHA recommended history and physical examination alone is used (54). The average cost of screening in Japan is $8800/life saved and in Italy a similar type of program cost $15926/life saved, both include ECG (57,58).

These figures are well below the $3.4 million/life saved data presented in the AHA report. With government subsidy and with more realistic cost assessment it has been surmised that a screening program with ECG can be put in place at 20%-25% of the cost presented in the AHA update (34,55).

As is evident from the discussion above there is still no real consensus among all experts regarding whether routine ECG screening would be prudent to apply to the US athlete population. As of now the AHA report is considered the standard of care. This dilemma calls for the need of prospective studies among local communities to validate the use of the ECG with more data that may change the current policy of screening athletes.

2-Echocardiogram (ECHO)

Echocardiogram is the standard for the diagnosis of structural heart disease. Diastolic and systolic function, wall motion abnormalities, wall thickness, valve morphology, and internal chamber size can be assessed with confidence with echocardiogram. Recent studies have also validated the imaging technique for visualizing the origin of the coronary arteries (59). Including contrast and tissue Doppler greatly increases the likelihood of diagnosing ARVD while using the 2D-ECHO (60). Adding an echocardiogram to a cardiovascular screening program will confer a high likelihood of identifying structural abnormalities of the heart raising both the sensitivity and specificity of such a program. There are inherent problems with such a recommendation. These mostly include the scarcity of resources both equipment and personnel. Moreover, it will almost quadruple the cost of such a program. As it stands today an echocardiogram can be considered a good confirmatory test following the initial screening. This is unlikely to change in the near future unless the portable and cost effective devices become available and more experts capable of reading the images are readily available.

Genetics

There have been significant advances in the identification of genetic causes for cardiovascular diseases (61,62). This leads to the question of present or future methods involving identification of genetic risk factors for cardiovascular disease using genetic testing as a screening tool. Even though great progress has been made in the identification of these genetic mutations, the genotype-phenotype correlation is still poor. It cannot be reliably predicted if an identified mutation will eventually lead to an expression of disease. This may lead to a high false positive rate. With more mutations identified, the battery of tests is ever increasing and to apply the entire set to an athlete is not prudent. This brings us back to the need for a good H&P as an initial screening tool with great emphasis on family history to identify individuals at risk. Once the proband is identified the entire family can be screened for that specific mutation that has been identified (59).

Exercise stress testing

Exercise testing has been recommended in athletes older than 35 years of age. This is also part of the extended Italian recommendation for athletes >35 years old. Maximal exercise testing is an integral component to unmask arrhythmia in ARVC, familial catecholaminergic polymorphic ventricular tachycardia, and long QT syndrome. Frequent ventricular extrasystoles during exercise indicate underlying cardiac disease (59). Exercise testing is of limited value in the diagnosis of HCM, but has an important role in risk stratification. Failure of the systolic blood pressure to rise by = 20 mm Hg is one of the risk factors for SCD in HCM. Marked ST segment depression during exercise is suggestive of ischemia.

Other tests

Several other tests are available for identification of certain specific conditions (Table 3). These tests cannot be used for mass screening due to the low yield and also due to the need for expertise to successfully obtain and interpret the results. They become important after screening has raised concerns for specific problems (59).

Table 3. Additional testing available to the athlete for specific concerns

Testing available to screen athletes	Indications	Comments
Holter monitoring	Quantification of extra systoles, identification of tachy- and brady-arrhythmias.	Cost involved, need for expert interpretation.
Cardiac MRI	Arrythmogenic right ventricular dysplasia (ARVD) and anomalous origin of the coronary arteries.	Cost and need for expert image acquisition and reading.
Tissue Doppler	ARVD	Inherent proarrythmogenic risk of the medication, need for monitoring, limited application.
Sodium channel blocker challenge	Brugada syndrome	Limited application. Need for monitoring.
Adenosine challenge for pre-excitation	Familial risk of Wolf-Parkinson-White syndrome and supraventricular tachycardia but with baseline normal ECG.	

On site use of automated external defibrillators (AEDs)

AED placement at schools, NCAA venues and other sport venues is on the rise. The current perception is that the AED placed at strategic locations at public places will help in improving survival after an SCA (64). Several studies done to evaluate survival after a SCA on the athletic field with timely use of an AED device by reasonably trained personnel fail to show improved survival (42,65,66). Further studies on a larger scale need to be done to evaluate the efficacy of the AED and the EAP with regards to SCD in athletes.

CONCLUSION

SCD seems to be an issue with significant medical, public health, ethical, social, and financial ramifications. Though the etiology and pathophysiology of SCD are well researched, better studies need to be done to assess the true incidence of SCD in athletes in US. The need for a national database cannot be overemphasized. With discrepancies in the recommendations regarding screening, a new approach needs to be explored. The current screening recommendations regarding the inclusion or exclusion of the ECG in the screening protocol should be carefully debated and reconsidered. Ideally the preparticipation screening should identify all athletes at risk of SCA. But this is not the case and a certain percentage of asymptomatic athletes with no risk factors do end up having SCA on the field. It is therefore important to plan ahead for such an event (64).

REFERENCES

[1] Van Camp SP. Sudden death. Clin Sports Med 1992;11:273-89.
[2] Germann CA. Sudden cardiac death in athletes: a guide for emergency physicians. Am J Emerg Med 2005;23,504-9.
[3] Maron BJ. Triggers for sudden cardiac death in athlete. Cardiol Clin 1996; 14:195-210.
[4] Natarajan B, Kinore V. Syncope and near syncope in competitive athletes. Curr Sports Med Reports 2006;5:300-6.
[5] Maron BJ, Gohman TC. Aeppli D. Prevalence of sudden cardiac death during competitive sports activities in Minnesota high school athletes. J Am Coll Card 1998;32:1881-4.
[6] Harmon KG, Drezner JA. Management of sudden cardiac arrest in Athletes. Curr Sports Med Rep 2007;6(3):170-6.
[7] Basilico FC. Cardiovascular disease in athletes. Am J Sports Med 1999;27:108- 21.
[8] Cantu RC. Congenital cardiovascular disease: the major cause of athletic death in high school and college. Med Sci Sports Exerc 1992;24:279-80.
[9] Maron BJ, Shirani J, Poliac LC, et al. Sudden death in young competitive athletes. Clinical, demographic, and pathological profiles. JAMA 1996;276:199-204.
[10] Maron BJ, Carney KP, Lever HM. Relationship of race to sudden cardiac death in competitive athletes with hypertrophic cardiomyopathy. J Am Coll Cardiol 2003;41:974- 80.
[11] Van camp SP, Bloor CM, Mueller FO, Cantu RC, Olson HG. Non-traumatic sports. death in high schools and college athletes. Med Sci Sports Exerc 1995;27:641-7.
[12] Maron BJ. Sudden death in young athletes.N Eng J Med 2003;349:1064-75.

[13] Basso C, Maron BJ, Corrado D, Thiene G. Clinical profile of congenital coronary artery anomalies with origin from the wrong aortic sinus leading to sudden death in young competitive athletes. J Am Coll Card 2000;35:1493-1501.
[14] Link MS, Wang P, Pandian NG, Bharati S, Udelson JE, Lee MY, Vecchiotti MA, VanderBrink BA, Mirra G, Maron BJ, Estes NA 3rd. An experimental model of sudden death due to low-energy chest-wall impact (commotio cordis). N Engl J Med 1998;338:1805-11.
[15] Maron BJ, Pelliccia A. The heart of trained athletes: Cardiac remodeling and the risk of sports, including sudden death. Circulation 2006;114;1633-44.
[16] Rost R. The athlete's heart: historical perspective. Cardiol Clin 1992:197-207.
[17] Mitchell JH, Haskell W, Snell P, Van Camp SP. Task Force 8: classification of sports. J Am Coll Cardiol. 2005;45(8):1364-7.
[18] Abernethy WB, Choo JK, Hutter AM Jr. Echocardiographic characteristics of professional football players. J Am Coll Cardiol. 2003;41(2):280-4.
[19] Fagard R. Athlete's heart. Heart 2003;89(12):1455-61.
[20] Spirito P, Pelliccia A, Proschan MA, Granata M, Spataro A, Bellone P, Caselli G, Biffi A, Vecchio C, Maron BJ. Morphology of the "athlete's heart" assessed by echocardiography in 947 elite athletes representing 27 sports. Am J Cardiol 1994; 74(8):802-6.
[21] Pelliccia A, Culasso F, Di Paolo FM, Maron BJ. Physiologic left ventricular cavity dilatation in elite athletes. Ann Intern Med 1999; 130(1):23-31.
[22] Pelliccia A, Maron BJ, Culasso F, Di Paolo FM, Spataro A, Biffi A, Caselli G, Piovano P. Clinical significance of abnormal electrocardiographic patterns in trained athletes. Circulation 2000;102(3):278-84.
[23] Huston TP, Puffer JC, Rodney WM. The athletic heart syndrome. N Engl J Med 1985;313(1):24-32.
[24] Choo JK, Abernethy WB 3rd, Hutter AM Jr. Electrocardiographic observations in professional football players. Am J Cardiol 2002; 90(2):198-200.
[25] Balady GJ, Cadigan JB, Ryan TJ. Electrocardiogram of the athlete: an analysis of 289 professional football players. Am J Cardiol 1984;53(9):1339-43.
[26] Biffi A, Pelliccia A, Verdile L, Fernando F, Spataro A, Caselli S, Santini M, Maron BJ. Long-term clinical significance of frequent and complex ventricular tachyarrhythmias in trained athletes. J Am Coll Cardiol 2002;40(3):446-52.
[27] Biffi A, Maron BJ, Verdile L, Fernando F, Spataro A, Marcello G, Ciardo R, Ammirati F, Colivicchi F, Pelliccia A. Impact of physical deconditioning on ventricular tachyarrhythmias in trained athletes. J Am Coll Cardiol 2004;44(5):1053-8.
[28] Pelliccia A, Maron BJ, Culasso F, Spataro A, Caselli G. Athlete's heart in women. Echocardiographic characterization of highly trained elite female athletes. JAMA1996;276(3):211-5.
[29] Sharma S, Maron BJ, Whyte G, Firoozi S, Elliott PM, McKenna WJ. Physiologic limits of left ventricular hypertrophy in elite junior athletes: relevance to differential diagnosis of athlete's heart and hypertrophic cardiomyopathy. J Am Coll Cardiol 2002;40(8):1431-6.
[30] Maron BJ, Pelliccia A, Spirito P. Cardiac disease in young trained athletes. Insights into methods for distinguishing athlete's heart from structural heart disease, with particular emphasis on hypertrophic cardiomyopathy. Circulation 1995;91(5):1596-601.
[31] Pelliccia A, Maron BJ, De Luca R, Di Paolo FM, Spataro A, Culasso F. Remodeling of left ventricular hypertrophy in elite athletes after long-term deconditioning. Circulation 2002;105(8):944-9.
[32] Corrado D, Basso C, Rizzoli G, Schiavon M, Thiene G. Does sports activity enhance the risk of sudden death in adolescents and young adults? J Am Coll Cardiol 2003;42(11):1959-63.
[33] Corrado D, Basso C, Schiavon M, Pelliccia A, Thiene G. Pre-participation screening of young competitive athletes for prevention of sudden cardiac death. J Am Coll Cardiol 2008;52(24):1981-9.
[34] Maron BJ, et al. Recommendations and considerations related to preparticipation screening for cardiovascular abnormalities in competitive athletes: 2007 Update: A scientific statement from the American Heart Association Council on Nutrition. Physical Activity, and Metabolism: Endorsed by the American College of Cardiology Foundation. Circulation 2007;115:1643-55.
[35] Corrado D, Basso C, Schiavon M, Thiene G. Screening for hypertrophic cardiomyopathy in young athletes. N Engl J Med 1998;339(6):364-9.

[36] Corrado D, McKenna WJ. Appropriate interpretation of the athlete's electrocardiogram saves lives as well as money. Eur Heart J 2007;28(16):1920-2.

[37] Corrado D, Basso C, Pavei A, Michieli P, Schiavon M, Thiene G. Trends in sudden cardiovascular death in young competitive athletes after implementation of a preparticipation screening program. JAMA 2006;296(13):1593-601.

[38] Thompson PD, Levine BD. Protecting athletes from sudden cardiac death. JAMA 2006;296(13):1648-50.

[39] Glover DW Maron BJ. Profile of preparticipation cardiovascular screening for high school athletes. JAMA 1998;279(22):1817-9.

[40] Maron BJ, Thompson PD, Puffer JC, McGrew CA, Strong WB, Douglas PS, et al. Cardiovascular preparticipation screening of competitive athletes: A statement for health professionals from the Sudden Death Committee (clinical cardiology) and Congenital Cardiac Defects Committee (cardiovascular disease in the young), American Heart Association. Circulation 1996;94(4):850-6.

[41] Corrado D, Pelliccia A, Bjørnstad HH, Vanhees L, Biffi A, Borjesson M, et al. Study Group of Sport Cardiology of the Working Group of Cardiac Rehabilitation and Exercise Physiology and the Working Group of Myocardial and Pericardial Diseases of the European Society of Cardiology. Cardiovascular pre-participation screening of young competitive athletes for prevention of sudden death: proposal for a common European protocol. Consensus Statement of the Study Group of Sport Cardiology of the Working Group of Cardiac Rehabilitation and Exercise Physiology and the Working Group of Myocardial and Pericardial Diseases of the European Society of Cardiology. Eur Heart J 2005;26(5):516-24.

[42] Drezner JA, Rogers KJ. Sudden cardiac arrest in intercollegiate athletes: detailed analysis and outcomes of resuscitation in nine cases. Heart Rhythm 2006;3(7):755-9.

[43] IOC Medical Commission, International Olympic committee (IOC). Sudden cardiovascular death in sports: Lausanne recommendations: Preparticipation cardiovascular screening. December 10th 2004. http://multimedia.olympic.org/pdf/en_report_886.pdf

[44] Bille K, Schamasch P, Brenner JI, Kappenberger L, Meijboom FJ, Meijboom EJ. Sudden death in athletes: the basics of the "Lausanne recommendations" of the International Olympic Committee. Circulation. 2005; 112(supplement II):II-830.

[45] Glover DW, Maron BJ. Evolution over 8 years of the US preparticpitaion screening process for undetected cardiovascular disease in US high school athletes. Circulation 2006;114(suppl II):II-502.

[46] Pfister GC, Puffer JC, Maron BJ. Preparticipation cardiovascular screening for US collegiate student-athletes. JAMA 2000;283(12):1597-9.

[47] Matheson GO, Boyanian-O'Neill LA, Cardone D, Dexter W, DiFiori J, Fields KB, et al. Preparticipation physical evaluation. 3rd ed. Minneapolis: Mcgraw-Hill Med, 2005.

[48] Maron MS, Olivotto I, Zenovich AG, Link MS, Pandian NG, Kuvin JT, et al. Hypertrophic cardiomyopathy is predominantly a disease of left ventricular outflow tract obstruction. Circulation 2006;114(21):2232-9.

[49] Maron BJ. Hypertrophic cardiomyopathy: a systematic review. JAMA 2002;287(10):1308-20.

[50] Maron BJ, McKenna WJ, Danielson GK, Kappenberger LJ, Kuhn HJ, Seidman CE, et al. Task Force on Clinical Expert Consensus Documents. American College of Cardiology Committee for Practice Guidelines. European Society of Cardiology. American College of Cardiology/European Society of Cardiology clinical expert consensus document on hypertrophic cardiomyopathy. A report of the American College of Cardiology Foundation Task Force on Clinical Expert Consensus Documents and the European Society of Cardiology Committee for Practice Guidelines. J Am Coll Cardiol 2003;42(9):1687-713.

[51] deGregario C, Magliarditi A, Maguadda L. Dramatic electcrocardiographic changes in a junior athlete with unpredictable hypertrophic cardiomyopathy. Int J Cardiol 2009; Epub, May 1.

[52] Tasaki H, Hamasaki Y, Ichimaru T. Mass screening for heart disease of school children in Saga city: 7-year follow up study. Jpn Circ J 1987;51:1415-20.

[53] Myerburg RJ. Sudden cardiac death: exploring the limits of our knowledge. J Cardiovasc Electrophysiol 2001;12:369-81.

[54] Fuller CM, McNulty CM, Spring DA, Arger KM, Bruce SS, Chryssos BE, et al. Prospective screening of 5,615 high school athletes for risk of sudden cardiac death. Med Sci Sports Exerc 1997;29:1131-8.

[55] Myerburg RJ, Vetter VL. Electrocardiograms should be included in preparticipation screening of athletes. Circulation 2007;116(22): 2616-26.

[56] Pelliccia A, Culasso F, Di Paolo FM, Accettura D, Cantore R, Castagna W, et al. Prevalence of abnormal electrocardiograms in a large, unselected populationundergoing pre-participation cardiovascular screening. Eur Heart J 2007;28:2006-10.

[57] Tanaka Y, Yoshinaga M, Anan R, Tanaka Y, Nomura Y, Oku S, et al. Usefulness and cost effectiveness of cardiovascular screening of young adolescents. Med Sci Sports Exerc 2006;38:2-6.

[58] Quaglini S, Rognoni C, Spazzolini C, Priori SG, Mannarino S, Schwartz PJ. Cost-effectiveness of neonatal ECG screening for the long QT syndrome. Eur Heart J 2006;27:1824-32.

[59] Zeppilli P, dello Russo A, Santini C, Palmieri V, Natale L, Giordano A, Frustaci A. In vivo detection of coronary artery anomalies in asymptomatic athletes by echocardiographic screening. Chest 1998;114:89–93.

[60] Sen-choudary S, McKenna WJ. Sudden cardiac death in the young: a strategy for prevention by targeted evaluation. Cardiology 2006;105(4):196-206.

[61] Crispell KA, Hanson EL, Coates K, Toy W, Hershberger RE: Periodic rescreening is indicated for family members at risk of developing familial dilated cardiomyopathy. J Am Coll Cardiol 2002; 39:1503-7.

[62] Brugada R, Hong K, Dumaine R, Cordeiro J,Gaita F, Borggrefe M, et al. Sudden death associated with short-QTsyndrome linked to mutations in HERG. Circulation 2004;109:30-5.

[63] Schimpf R, Wolpert C, Gaita F, Giustetto C, Borggrefe M: Short QT syndrome. Cardiovasc Res 2005;67:357-66.

[64] Drezner JA, Courson RW, et al. Inter-Association Task Force Recommendations on Emergency Preparedness and Management of Sudden Cardiac arrest in High School and College Athletic Programs: A consensus Statement. J Athletic Training 2007; 42(1):143-58.

[65] Maron BJ, Gohman TF,Kyle SB,Estes NA 3rd, Link MS. Clinical profile and spectrum of commtio cordis. JAMA 2002; 287:1142-6.

[66] Maron Bj, Wentzel DC, Zenovich AG, Estes NA 3rd, Link MS. Death in a young athlete due to commotio cordis despite prompt external defibrillation. Heart Rhythm 2005;2:991-3.

Submitted: May 01, 2009.
Revised: June 15, 2009.
Accepted: June 21, 2009.

In: Public Health Yearbook 2009
Editor: Joav Merrick
ISBN: 978-1-61668-911-7

Chapter 37

SPORT PARTICIPATION BY ADOLESCENTS WHO HAVE HYPERTENSION

Vimal Master Sankar Raj, MD, Venu Parachuri, MD, Dilip R Patel*, MD, FACSM, FAAP, FAACPDM, FSAM and Alfonso Torres, MD

Department of Pediatrics and Human Development, Michigan State University College of Human Medicine, East Lansing, Michigan, USA, and Pediatric Residency Training Program, Michigan State University Kalamazoo Center for Medical Studies, Kalamazoo, Michigan, United States of America

ABSTRACT

The incidence of systemic hypertension among adolescents and young adults has been on the rise. Several factors have contributed to this including, obesity, physical inactivity, unhealthy food habits, drug abuse, and familial tendencies. Early onset hypertension in children and adolescents has been associated with premature atherosclerosis and subsequent cardiovascular mortality and morbidity thus placing a huge economic burden on the individual family as well as the society in general. This article reviews the beneficial effects of exercise both aerobic and resistance training on blood pressure and the current recommendations for sports participation by adolescents who have hypertension.

Keywords: Hypertension, pre-hypertension, post-exercise hypotension, state 2 hypertension.

* Correspondence: Professor Dilip R Patel, MD, MD, FAAP, FACSM, FSAM, FAACPDM, Department of Pediatrics and Human Development, Michigan State University College of Human Medicine, Kalamazoo Center for Medical Studies, Kalamazoo, Michigan, MSU/ KCMS/ Pediatrics, 1000, Oakland Drive, Kalamazoo, MI 49008-1284 United States. Tel: 269-337-6450; Fax: 269-337-6474; E-mail: patel@kcms.msu.edu

INTRODUCTION

Definitions of normal blood pressure and hypertension are summarized in table 1 (1). Blood pressure standards for children and adolescents between the ages 1 year and 17 year are based on sex, age, and height. Determination of normal or abnormal blood pressure value is based on published blood pressure standards based on normative data (1).

The prevalence of essential hypertension increases with age. The prevalence of hypertension increases from 15% among 18 to 39 years to almost 55% in men older than 55 years (2,3). It is also more prevalent in men when compared to woman. Hypertension can be classified based on etiology as primary when essentially no cause could be attributed for its occurrence and secondary when a specific cause for hypertension such as renal, cardiovascular or endocrine could be identified.

Many factors including genetic, diet, body habitus and stress plays a role in the development of essential hypertension. With increasing incidence of obesity there has been increasing occurrence of essential hypertension in adolescents. Some of the specific physical examination findings that could help identify the secondary causes for hypertension are noted in table 2.

Table 1. Definitions and classification of hypertension in children and adolescents

Category	Criteria: Systolic or diastolic blood pressure percentile for sex, age, and height measured on at least 3 separate occasions
Normal	$< 90^{th}$
Prehypertension	90th to $< 95^{th}$ or if blood pressure exceeds 120/80 mm Hg even if below 90th percentile up to $< 95^{th}$ percentile. This occurs typically at 12 years old for systolic blood pressure and 16 years old for diastolic blood pressure
Stage 1 hypertension	95th percentile to 99th percentile plus 5 mm Hg
Stage 2 hypertension	$< 99^{th}$ percentile plus 5 mm Hg

From: The fourth report on the diagnosis, evaluation, and treatment of high blood pressure in children and adolescents. U.S. Department of Health and Human Services, National Institutes of Health, National Heart, Lung, and Blood Pressure Institute. NIH Publication No 05-5267, Revised May 2005.

EXERCISE AND BLOOD PRESSURE

Beneficial effects of exercise on blood pressure reduction, both systolic and diastolic have been described in many studies. Both aerobic and resistance training have been shown to reduce blood pressures in acute phase (post-exercise hypotension) as well as over long-term. Though there are many controlled trials on the effect of aerobic exercise on blood pressure reduction, similar research on resistance training is limited. Most exercise programs generally combine both aerobic and resistance exercises.

Table 2. Examples of physical examination findings suggestive of definable hypertension*

	Finding†	Possible Etiology
Vital signs	Tachycardia	Hyperthyoidism, pheochromocytoma, neuroblastoma, primary hypertension
	Decreased lower extremity pulses; drop in BP from upper to lower extremities	Coarctation of aorta
Eyes	Retinal changes	Severe hypertension, more likely to be associated with secondary hypertension
Ears, nose, and throat (ENT)	Adenotonsillar hypertrophy	Suggests association with sleep-disordered breathing (sleep apnea), snoring
Height/weight	Growth retardation	Chronic renal failure
	Obesity(high BMI)	Primary hypertension
	Truncal obesity	Cushing syndrome, insulin resistance syndrome
Head and neck	Moon facies	Cushing syndrome
	Elfin facies	Williams syndrome
	Webbed neck	Turner syndrome
	Thyromegaly	Hyperthyroidism
Skin	Pallor, flushing, diaphoresis	Pheochromocytoma
	Acne, hirsuitism, striae	Cushing syndrome, anabolic steroid abuse
	Café-au-lait spots	Neurofibromatosis
	Adenoma sebaceum	Tuberous sclerosis
	Malar rash	Systemic lupus erythematosus
	Acanthrosis nigricans	Type 2 diabetes
Chest	Widely spaced nipples	Turner syndrome
	Heart murmur	Coarctation of the aorta
	Friction rub	Systemic lupus erythematosus (pericarditis), collagen-vascular disease, and end stage renal disease with uremia
	Finding†	Possible Etiology
	Apical heave	Left ventricular hypertrophy/chronic hypertension
Abdomen	Mass	Wilms tumor, neuroblastoma, pheochromocytoma
	Epigastric/flank bruit	Renal artery stenosis
	Palpable kidneys	Polycystic kidney disease, hydronephrosis, multicystic-dysplastic kidney, mass (see above)
Genitalia	Ambiguous/virilization	Adrenal hyperplasia
Extremities	Joint swelling	Systemic lupus erythematosus, collagen vascular disease
	Muscle weakness	Hyperaldosteronism, Liddle syndrome

BMI, body mass index; BP, blood pressure.

*Adapted from Flynn, JT. Evaluation and management of hypertension in childhood. *Prog Pediatr Cardiol* 2001;12:177-88.

† Findings listed are examples of physical findings and do not represent all possible physical findings.

From: The fourth report on the diagnosis, evaluation, and treatment of high blood pressure in children and adolescents. U.S. Department of Health and Human Services, National Institutes of Health, National Heart, Lung, and Blood Pressure Institute. NIH Publication No 05-5267, Revised May 2005.

The phenomenon of the acute reduction of blood pressure after exercise is called post-exercise hypotension, which occurs in both individuals with normal blood pressure as well as those with elevated blood pressure, with higher reduction in hypertensive individuals (4-11).

Average blood pressure reduction in hypertensive individuals is around 8 to 10 mm Hg when compared to 6 to 7 mm Hg in pre-hypertensive individuals and 3 mm Hg in individuals with normal blood pressure (12). Seventy five percent of individuals with elevated blood pressure show the post exercise hypotension effect with the rest showing no change, which is roughly the same kind of response with any pharmacological therapy (13).

A 20-minute bout of acute exercise at 40% intensity has been shown to elicit post exercise hypotension effect with much higher drop in blood pressure with increasing intensity of exercise (14-17). The post exercise hypotension effect after a single bout of acute aerobic exercise can last up to 24 hours with the maximal reduction in the first five hours (14,15,18). Intermittent shorter duration exercise sessions at different times during the day show a more sustained effect on reducing blood pressure when compared to one continuous session (19). Some studies suggest that the chronic effects on blood pressure reduction with regular exercise may be the result of accumulation of the acute effects over a long period of time. Blood pressure generally returns back to its pre-exercise level within 2-4 weeks of cessation of regular exercise (20,21).

There are few controlled trials on the acute effect of resistance training on blood pressure. There are few observational studies with varying results. One study showed a reduction in diastolic blood pressure an hour after 11 to 18 minutes of static exercise without much change in systolic blood pressure, and another study showed an acute elevation of systolic blood pressure for up to 15 minutes after acute resistance exercise with no significant change in diastolic blood pressure (22,23). There is no real consensus on the acute effect of resistance training on blood pressure. Regular resistance exercise over a period of 5 to 8 weeks has been shown to reduce both the systolic and diastolic blood pressure with greater reduction in individuals who have hypertension. In one trial on hypertensive individuals, reductions ranging from 16 to 43 mm Hg for systolic and 2 to 24 mm Hg for diastolic blood pressure has been reported (24). In normotensive individuals the magnitude of such an effect is much less, with a 5 mm Hg reduction in diastolic blood pressure without significant change in systolic blood pressure (25).

Mechanism of reduction of blood pressure with exercise

Most of the proposed mechanisms for the beneficial effect of exercise on reducing blood pressure involve regulation of sympathetic nervous activity which in turn affects vascular resistance and subsequent reduction in blood pressure. Also cardiopulmonary baroreceptors have a greater inhibitory effect after exercise. Effects of regular exercise on vasoactive substances including a reduction in vasoconstrictive endothelin 1, and an increase in vasodilators like nitric oxide also play a major role in exercise-related reduction in systemic blood pressure (26-28). Regular endurance training has been shown to increase arterial compliance and lumen diameter, both likely contributing to the long-term reduction in systemic blood pressure associated with regular exercise (29,30).

Blood pressure reduction in exercise can also be secondary to the fact that exercise affects a number of other risk factors that contribute to hypertension including abdominal adiposity and insulin resistance, which are independent risk factors for hypertension. Exercise also lowers the level of inflammatory cytokines which by means of endothelial dysfunction can be a risk factor for hypertension (31).

Even though beneficial effects of exercise on blood pressure both acutely and in long term have been documented by various studies, individuals who exhibit an abnormal or exaggerated hypertensive response to exercise with systolic blood pressure > 200 mm Hg may be at an increased risk for left ventricular systolic dysfunction (32). Strenuous weight training in unconditioned individuals can cause sudden reduction in central arterial compliance; therefore exercise intensity should be increased gradually (33). Exercise programs of moderate intensity, which incorporate both aerobic and resistance training of at least 20 to 30 minutes duration for most days in a week tend to have the most favorable effect on blood pressure.

RECOMMENDATIONS FOR SPORTS PARTICIPATION AND EXERCISE

The 36th Bethesda Conference task force on systemic hypertension recommendations for exercise and sport participation by individuals who have hypertension are summarized in table 3 (34).

Table 3. 36th Bethesda conference recommendations for exercise by athletes who have hypertension

Stage of hypertension	Recommendation
Pre-hypertension	Modify lifestyle No restriction from physical activity
Sustained hypertension	Echocardiography Those with true left ventricular hypertrophy (LVH) should limit participation until blood pressure is controlled with appropriate drug therapy
Stage 1-hypertension in the absence of target organ damage including LVH or concomitant heart disease	Allow full sport and exercise participation Monitor blood pressure frequently once exercise program is begun
Stage 2-hypertension even without target organ damage	Restricted exercise and sport participation, especially from high static sports, until hypertension is well-controlled
Hypertension and concomitant another cardiovascular disease	Sport and exercise participation based on type and severity of the associated condition

Based on Kaplan NM, Gidding SS, Pickering TG, Wright JT. Task force 5: Systemic hypertension. JACC 2005;45(8):1346-8.

Individuals who would like to take part in competitive sports should have a thorough pre-participation evaluation done. If the initial blood pressure ranges between high normal to pre-hypertensive range, repeat measurements in the office at different times over a period of 3 to 4 weeks or recording blood pressure outside office settings like ambulatory blood pressure monitoring will help in ruling out white coat hypertension (34). With persistently elevated blood pressure, a complete evaluation to ascertain the etiology, risk factors, and any target organ damage must be done (1,35,36). A study on hypertensive men in the presence of risk factors showed an increase in cardiovascular morbidity with vigorous training programs that involved intensity levels > 60% (37).

Prevention and Public Health Perspective

With the increasing prevalence of obesity and its association with hypertension, weight loss could be a very effective method in controlling and preventing hypertension (38). Regular physical activity of moderate intensity for at least 30 to 60 minutes a day in addition to restricting sedentary activity to < 2 hours is generally recommended (1,39). Dietary changes including reduction of total caloric and fat intake and increasing fiber, fresh fruit and vegetable intake should be adopted by the whole family and involving a nutritionist if necessary will help in weight loss and preventing future hypertension (1).

In adolescents the ill effects of smoking, alcohol and drugs should be discussed by the parents, teachers, and physicians on a regular basis. Smoking cessation has a major role in preventing cardiovascular morbidity. Regular screening for hypertension should be done by checking blood pressure in the office when adolescents come for their examination. Proper techniques for measuring blood pressure including using appropriate cuff size are important to avoid spuriously high or low blood pressure measurements. Use of ambulatory blood pressure monitoring may be indicated in some settings such as white coat hypertension and sometimes might unmask hypertension in certain individuals whose blood pressure is normal in clinical settings but might be elevated otherwise (40).

Early detection and treatment of hypertension by instituting life style modification and drug therapy can prevent target organ damage. With most deaths in the United States being secondary to cardiovascular diseases and with hypertension being one of the main risk factors, prevention can have a huge impact on public.

Conclusion

Prevalence of obesity and hypertension in adolescents is increasing. It is important to identify those who are at risk and intervene early in order to prevent long term morbidity and mortality. The beneficial effects of exercise in reducing blood pressure both acutely as well as in long term has been documented in various studies thus making it one of the most effective yet underutilized therapeutic option. Screening for high blood pressure should be a part of annual adolescent health maintenance visits and the task of the physician in addressing the need for weight loss and regular exercise during each visit cannot be oversemphasized. Hypertensive athletes who wish to participate in competitive sports should be monitored closely and advised to follow the recommendations for sports participation depending on their stage of hypertension and their overall health.

ACKNOWLEDGMENTS

Thanks to Kim Douglas for assistance in preparation of this manuscript.

REFERENCES

[1] The fourth report on the diagnosis, evaluation, and treatment of high blood pressure in children and adolescents. Bethesda, MD: US Dept Health Hum Serv, Natl Inst Health, Natl Heart Lung Blood Pressure Inst, NIH Publication No 05-5267, Revised May 2005.
[2] Watkins D, McCarron P, Murray L, Cran G, Boreham C, Robson P, McGartland C, Davey Smith G, Savage M. Trends in blood pressure over 10 years in adolescents: analyses of cross sectional surveys in the Northern Ireland Young Hearts project. BMJ 2004;329(7458):139.
[3] Fagard RH. Athletes with systemic hypertension. Cardiol Clin 2007;925:441-8.
[4] Pescatello LS, Franklin BA, Fagard R, Farquhar WB, Kelley GA, Ray CA. Exercise and hypertension. American College of Sports Medicine Position Stand. Med Sci Sports Exer 2004;36(3):533-53.
[5] Coats, AJS. Systemic and forearm vascular resistance changes after upright bicycle exercise in man. J Physiol 1989;413:289-98.
[6] Fleg JL, Lakatta EG. Prevalence and significance of postexercise hypotension in apparently healthy subjects. Am J Cardiol 1986;57:1380-4.
[7] Bennett T, Wilcox RG, MacDonald IA. Post exercise reduction of blood pressure in hypertensive men is not due to acute impairment of baroreflex function. Clin Sci 1984;67:97-103.
[8] Brownley KA. Acute aerobic exercise reduces ambulatory blood pressure in borderline hypertensive men and women. Am J Hypertens 1996;9:200-6.
[9] Kenney MJ, Seals DR. Post exercise hypotension: key features, mechanisms and clinical significance. Hypertension 1993;22:653-4.
[10] Pescatello LS, Qulikowich JM. After effects of dynamic exercise on ambulatory blood pressure. Med Sci Sports Exerc 2001;33:1855-61.
[11] Thompson PD, Crouse SF. The acute versus the chronic response to exercise. Med Sci Sports Exerc 2001;33:S438-45,S452-3.
[12] Fagard RH. Prescription and results of physical activity. J CardioVasc Pharmacol 1995;25(suppl 1):20-7.
[13] Volker K. Physical activity, hypertension and cardiac and circulatory system. Med Clin (Munich) 2006;101(suppl 1):61-5.
[14] Brownley KA, West SG. Acute aerobic exercise reduces ambulatory blood pressure in borderline hypertensive men and women. Am J Hypertens 1996;9:200-6.
[15] Thompson PD, Crouse SF. The acute versus the chronic response to exercise. Medsci Sport Exerc 2001;33(suppl 6):438-45.
[16] Wallace JP, Bogle PG. The magnitude and duration of ambulatory blood pressure reduction following acute exercise. J Hum Hypertens 1999;13:361-66.
[17] Quinn TJ. 24 hour, ambulatory blood pressure responses following acute exercise: impact of exercise intensity. J Hum Hypertens 2000;14:547-53.
[18] Hagberg JM, Park JJ. The role of exercise training in the treatment of hypertension: an update. Sports Med 2000;30:193-206.
[19] Park S, Rimk LD. Accumulation of physical activity leads to greater blood pressure reduction than a single continuous session in prehypertension. J Hypertens 2006;24:1761-70.
[20] Meredith IT, Jennings GL, Esler MD, Dewar EM, Bruce AM, Fazio VA, Korner PI. Time course antihypertensive and autonomic effects of regular endurance exercise in human subjects. J Hypertens 1990;8(9):859-66.

[21] Motoyama M, Sunami Y, Kinoshita F, Kiyonaga A, Tanaka H, Shindo M, et al. Blood pressure lowering effect of low intensity aerobic training in elderly hypertensive patients. Med Sci Sports Exerc 1998;30:818-23.
[22] Hill DW, Collins MA. Blood pressure response after weight training exercise. J Appl Sports Sci Res 1989;3:44-47.
[23] O'Connor PJ, Bryant CX. State anxiety and ambulatory blood pressure following resistance exercise in females. Med Sci Sports Exerc 1993;25:516-21.
[24] Kiveloff B, Huber O. Brief maximal isometric exercise in hypertension. J Am Geriatr Soc 1971;19:1006-12.
[25] Ray CA, Carrasco DI. Isometric handgrip training reduces arterial pressure at rest without changes in sympathetic nerve activity. Am J Physiol Heart Circ Physiol 2000;279:H245-9.
[26] Maeda S, Miyauchi T, Kakiyama T, Sugawara J, Iemitsu M, Irukayama-Tomobe Y, et al. Effects of exercise training of 8 weeks and detraining on plasma levels of endothelium derived factors, endothelin-1 and nitric oxide, in healthy young humans. Life Sci 2001;69(9):1005-16.
[27] Jungersten L, Ambring A, Wall B, Wennmalm A. Both physical fitness and acute exercise regulate nitric oxide formation in healthy humans. J Appl Physiol 1997;82(3):760-4.
[28] Kingwell BA, Sherrard B, Jennings GL, Dart AM. Four weeks of cycle training increases basal production of nitric oxide from the forearm. Am J Physiol 1997;272(3 pt 2):H1070-7.
[29] Cameron JD, Dart AM. Exercise training increases total systemic arterial compliance in humans. Am J Physiol 1994;266(2 pt 2):H693-701.
[30] Huonker M, Halle M, Keul J. Structural and functional adaptations of the cardiovascular system by training. Int J Sports Med 1996;Suppl.3:S164-72.
[31] Abramson JL, Vaccarino V. Relationship between physical activity and inflammation among apparently healthy middle aged and older US adults. Arch Intern Med 2002;162(11):126-92.
[32] Mottram PM, Haluska B. Patients with hypertensive response to exercise have impaired systolic function without diastolic dysfunction or left ventricular hypertrophy. J Am Col Cardiol 2004;43:848-53.
[33] Miyachi M, Kawano H. Unfavorable effects of resistance training on central arterial compliance: a randomized intervention study. Circulation 2004;110:2858-63.
[34] Kaplan NM, Gidding SS, Pickering TJ, Wright JT. Task force 5: systemic hypertension. JACC 2005;(45):1346-8.
[35] Joint national committee on detection, evaluation and treatment of high blood pressure. The 6th report of the JNC on detection, evaluation and treatment of high BP (JNC VI) Arch Intern Med 1997;157:2413-46.
[36] Vanhees L, Defoor JG, Schepers D, Lijnen P, Peeters BY, Lacante PH, Fagard RH. Effects of bisoprolol and atenolol on endurance, exercise capacity in healthy men. J Hypertens 2000;18:35-43.
[37] Shaper AG, Wannamethee G, Walker M. Physical activity, hypertension and risk of heart attack in men without evidence of ischemic heart disease. J Hum Hypertens 1994;8:3-10.
[38] Sinaiko AR, Steinberger J. Relation of insulin resistance to blood pressure in childhood. J Hypertens 2002;20:509-17.
[39] Krebs NF, Jacobson MS. Prevention of pediatric overweight and obesity. Pediatrics 2003;112:424-30.
[40] Stabouli S, Kotsis V. White coat and masked hypertension in children associated with target organ damage. Ped Nephrol 2005;20:1151-55.

Submitted: May 02, 2009.
Revised: June 27, 2009.
Accepted: July 04, 2009.

In: Public Health Yearbook 2009
Editor: Joav Merrick
ISBN: 978-1-61668-911-7

Chapter 38

BACK PAIN IN ADOLESCENT ATHLETES

Donald E Greydanus*, MD
and Dilip R Patel, MD, FAAP, FACSM, FAACPDM, FSAM
Department of Pediatrics and Human Development, Michigan State University College of Human Medicine, East Lansing, Michigan, United States of America

ABSTRACT

Back pain in adolescent athletes is common. The most common cause of acute low back pain in adolescent athletes is musculotendinous injury. It is also the most common cause of back pain overall. The most common identified structural anomaly is in adolescents who present with chronic or recurrent activity related low back pain is spondylolysis. In all adolescents with back pain psychosomatic disorder must be considered in the differential diagnosis. Other significant causes of low back pain in adolescent athletes include scoliosis, kyphosis, diskitis, slipped disk, and inflammatory spondyloarthropathies. Evaluation is mostly based on history and physical examination. Imaging studies are indicated in some cases based on findings on history and examination. Management is non-operative in most cases and includes a short period of rest from sports, followed by physical therapy and conditioning. This articles reviews common causes of low back pain in adolescent athletes such as musculotendionus injuries, psychosomatic pain, spondylolysis, diskitis, scoliosis, kyphosis, and ankylosing spondylitis.

Keywords: Low back pain, musculotendinous strain, psychosomatic pain, spondylolysis.

* Correspondence: Professor Donald E Greydanus, MD, Pediatrics and Human Development, Michigan State University College of Human Medicine, Pediatrics Program Director, Michigan State University/Kalamazoo Center for Medical Studies, 1000 Oakland Drive, Kalamazoo, MI 49008-1284 United States. E-mail: Greydanus@kcms.msu.edu

Introduction

Back pain is a common manifestation of spinal disorders, including sport-related injuries. Spinal injuries may occur at an incidence of 10-15% in athletes and spinal injuries associated with neurologic complications at 0.6% to 1% (1). This article reviews a number of these disorders, including muscular back strain, psychosomatic back pain, a variety of structural spinal disorders (spondylolysis, spondylolisthesis, scoliosis, kyphosis), slipped spinal disc, discitis, osteomyelitis, spinal tumors and ankylosing spondylitis (2-10).

Musculotendinous and Ligamentous Injury

The incidence of low back pain in youth is approximately 30%, in contrast to 60-80% often reported in adults; its incidence approximates that of adults by 16 years of age (11-16). Low back pain in the adolescent is usually due to paravertebral muscle spasm, often of a traumatic origin (3). There may be a history of an acute stress (falling, hit during sports, improper lifting technique, others) with or without such additional factors as obesity, soft bed, poor general posture, heavy back packs, use of shoes which do not fit well, change in height of the shoe heels, or failure to properly warm-up before athletic activities. Low back pain has been linked to the adolescent growth spurt and asynchronous growth; muscular and ligamentous growth may lag behind bone growth, contributing to low back pain (10). Some activities can lead to muscular strain, as noted in musicians. For example, bass players are prone to back pain due to their position while playing, whereas harpists may develop back pain while moving their heavy instrument (16-18).

Prevention of muscular back pain should be part of anticipatory guidance, especially after any pain episodes. Youth should be instructed in proper posture and lifting techniques. Teens should know they must lift objects while bending both knees and not to use back packs which are over 20% of their weight. School packs should have wide straps which are padded and have a hip strap for heavy weights.

Since there are a number of conditions which can cause low back pain (see table 1), a thorough history with examination of the entire spine and associated nerve roots is important to determine what studies are necessary to pinpoint the correct underlying disorder (1-15). Back pain, which radiates down the hips and into the lower extremities, may suggest a ruptured disk. Roentogenographic studies may include back x-rays, computed tomography scan, and magnetic resonance imaging (MRI). A bone scan and electromyogram (EMG) may be helpful. Seronegative spondyloarthropathy must be considered in patients with an elevated erythrocyte sedimentation rate (ESR), positive rheumatoid factor, positive HLA-B27, and characteristic x-rays.

Relative rest and use of medications (analgesics and muscle relaxers) are initially recommended for acute back pain due to muscle strain (2,8,19). Several days of bed rest have not been shown to be superior to a few days (19). Antiinflammatory medications are often used, such as ibuprofen, ketoprofen, naproxen sodium, naproxen, mefenamic acid and others. Muscle relaxants, sometimes used, include baclofen, carisoprodol, cyclobenzaprine, dantrolene, methocarbamol, orphenadrine and others. The use of narcotic analgesics is discouraged, except for severe pain and only for a limited time. Physical therapy is often helpful after the acute pain episode to restore low back muscle strength and conditioning. Hyperextension exercises may improve the strength of paravertebral muscles while isometric flexion exercises may strengthen lumbar and abdominal muscles (2,19,21). A supportive (hard) mattress is recommended for all these patients, while weight reduction is recommended for the obese patient.

Table 1. Common causes of back pain in adolescents

– Psychosomatic back pain
– Postural back pain
– Acute and chronic muscle, tendon and ligament injuries
– Injuries of the spine
– Painful scoliosis and kyphosis
– Inflammatory spondyloarthropathies
– Diskitis and osteomyelitis
– Hypermobility syndrome
– Slipped or ruptured disk
– Benign and metastatic tumors
– Referred pain from abdominal, pelvic and genitourinary conditions

Psychosomatic back pain

In a study of 167 children between 2 and 20 years of age (with an average age of 13.7 years) who had back pain, psychosomatic disorder was the most common diagnosis in 57% who did not have an organic disorder (4). Indeed, behavioral or psychological underpinnings to chronic pain syndromes (including chronic back pain) in adolescents are well-know to clinicians and researchers (8,22,23). Humans are susceptible to the pressures of stress and emotional factors, and pain in various body parts can result, whether in the head, abdomen, chest, extremities or back. The impact of divorce, incest, rape, family dysfunction, societal chaos, litigation, depression, anxiety, death of family members or friends, war and others can result in a variety of psychosomatic disorders, including chronic pain syndrome.

A careful medical and psychological evaluation may reveal evidence of physiologic or behavioral pathology in the youth who presents with chronic back pain. Clues may be found in the evaluation, including a positive family or patient history for somatic complaints, evidence of family dysfunction, history of multiple visits to different clinicians, presence of la belle indifference, and other features (23). A number of findings are suggestive of an organic etiology for the back pain, such as pain which awakens the patient from sleep, weight loss, fever, chills, worsening pain, nausea, emesis and pain associated with menstruation or urination (2,3,5,7).

Management of chronic back pain syndrome starts with early recognition by the clinician of the possibility of a psychosomatic disorder. An evaluation which looks at both physiologic and behavioral factors from the beginning can be very helpful to the patient and family that such a possibility exists, and indeed, is quite common. Thus, a thorough psychological assessment should be part of the evaluation process. A variety of treatments are available for the adolescent with a psychosomatic back pain disorder, once the correct diagnosis is considered and confirmed. These plans include individual therapy, family therapy, relaxation training, and biofeedback.

Obtaining important information from the adolescent often depends on establishing adequate rapport with the patient (see table 2) (24). The clinician's attitude toward the adolescent and parents is critical; a genuine attitude of concern is important to convey. It is vital that the all relevant information about the pain syndrome be obtained in order to make the correct diagnosis and to develop a beneficial management plan. The historian must be an active listener as he or she seeks to identify what factors have contributed to the youth's pain syndrome. The active listener observes the patient's body language, voice characteristics (as tone, inflection and volume), facial features, rate of speech, and body position. Allow the teen to speak uninterrupted, while the historian maintains eye contact and sits with arms at the side as well as with open hands.

Table 2. Establishing rapport

- Introduce yourself. Shake hands. Make eye contact. Smile. Use a firm but gentle hand shake. Greet each person in the room individually.
- Explain the sequence of events for your interaction. Tell the adolescent what's going to happen.
- Present a pleasant and accepting demeanor.
- Monitor your body language. A stern, "parental" look on the face, crossed arms, or very close physical proximity may communicate negative non-verbal messages.
- Use active listening and ask open-ended questions.
- Remain non-judgmental

From: Greydanus DE, Pratt HD: Manual on adolescent health care. Adolescence: A continuum from childhood to adulthood. 3rd ed. Des Moines, Iowa: Iowa Health Dept Publ, 1996.

Structural defects of the spine

Spondylolysis and spondylolisthesis

Spondylolysis and spondylolisthesis are the most common structural abnormalities which lead to low back pain in adolescents, including athletes (25-27). Spondylolysis refers to a defect of the pars interarticularis (degenerative or deficient, congenital or acquired) (25). Spondylolysis in adolescent athletes generally represents a stress fracture of the pars interarticularis due to repetitive stress. Risk factors for spondylolisthesis and spondylolysis include the growth spurt, positive family history, (excessive) sports activity and repetitive use of back muscles (involving flexion, extension and rotation motions) (25,26). Spondylolysis causes up to 50% of significant low back pain in teens, especially gymnasts (9). Spondylolysis with back pain is increased in teens involved in over 15 hours of competitive sports activity: weightlifting (highest rates), baseball, golf, gymnastics, racketball, volleyball, rowing and others (25-27).

Spondylolisthesis is noted in 5% to 6% of humans and refers to subluxation (forward slippage) of a vertebra, most commonly in the lumbar spine. Usually there is anterior displacement of the L5 (fifth lumbar vetebra) on S1 (25). The next most common one is L4 on L3, followed in sequence by L3 on L2 and L2 on L1. The types of spondylolisthesis are listed in table 3. A positive family history may be noted, especially for dysplastic spondylolisthesis. This latter type has an elongation of the pars interarticularis, while the isthmic type results from a fatigue (stress) fracture of the pars interarticularis. Isthmic spondylolisthesis is usually noted in adolescent athletes whose sport involves forced rotation and extension of the lumbar spine; thus rowers, football players, cyclists, dancers and gymnasts are at risk for this disorder (27).

These teens usually present with back pain that often improves with forward bending. In some cases, sciatica may develop with the back pain moving to lateral aspects of one or both thighs (due to lumbosacral nerve root pressure). There is worsening lordosis of the lumbar spine ("step-off" deformity of the spine), and tight hamstring muscles (25). In severe cases there may be reduced strength and sensation in the lower limbs. An oblique x-ray of the lumbosacral spine is most useful to identify spondylolysis; whereas, a lateral x-ray reveals the spondylolisthesis, and in 40%, scoliosis. Radionuclide scanning, especially a single photon emission CT bone scan, can allow an early diagnosis of spondylolysis (7,27). Further evaluation may be necessary, such as a MRI or electromyogram for neurologic dysfunction.

Table 3. Sub-types of spondylolisthesis

- Isthemic
- Dysplastic
- Traumatic
- Degenerative
- Pathologic

Fortunately, most of these youth have mild pain and respond well to a plan which strengthens the back muscles and allows optimal low back posture (25). These athletes may continue with their sports if the symptoms are not aggravated. Analgesics and appropriate physical therapy are often beneficial. Some protocols use back brace to provide sufficient immobilization until the defect is healed. Uncommonly, spinal fusion is needed for progressive spondylolisthesis, intolerable back pain, significant gait disturbance and other compromising complications (26).

Scoliosis

Ramirez noted that 23% of teens with idiopathic scolioisis presented with back pain and 9% continued with back pain at follow-up (28). Though back pain may be present with idiopathic scoliosis, other types of scoliosis should be considered when back pain develops in adolescents who have scoliosis (see table 4) (28-31). Painful spinal curvature in the adolescent may be due to congenital abnormalities (usually detected at birth or during childhood) as well as various muscle and nerve disorders (3-9). Untreated, progressive scoliosis from any cause may lead to degenerative arthritis, chronic back pain, severe cardiopulmonary compromise (with pulmonary hypertension and cor pulmonale) and other sequelae.

Adolescents should be screened for scoliosis during their growth phases, especially during rapid growth changes. The patient is inspected from the side (checking for kyphosis) and from the back while standing (with both feet placed together); he or she then bends to at least 90 degrees (Adams forward-bending test). The forward bending test assesses spinal flexibility as well as possible asymmetry of the thoracic and lumbar vertebrae (7). A non-idiopathic type of scoliosis is suggested by observing changes in the thoracic spine with a left convexity (versus the right convexity of idiopathic scoliosis), angular defects (usually sharp and short), spasm of the paravertebral muscles, any painful curvatures, hemangiomas, spinal dermal sinus, nerve root irritation, legs of unequal lengths, nevi, café au lait spots, and others.

Imaging studies may be indicated to measure the degree of the scoliosis and when pathologic cause for scoliosis is suspected.

Table 4. Types of scoliosis

Infantile idiopathic scoliosis	Ages 0-3; left thoracic curve; mostly males; 20% are progressive
Juvenile idiopathic scoliosis	Ages 3-10; equal male-female ratio
Adolescent idiopathic scoliosis	Most common type seen in adolescents
Functional scoliosis	Compensatory spinal curve due to structural defect other than in the spine; e.g., a shortened leg
Congenital scoliosis	Congenital vertebral anomalies-hemivertebrae, failure of segmentation; 25%-50% also have renal anomalies; cardiac anomalies also noted
Neuromuscular scoliosis	Cerebral palsy, poliomyelitis, spinal muscle atrophy, muscular dystrophy, childhood paraplegia, arthrogryposis, amyotonia congenita, diastematomyelia, others
Neurofibromatosis	Short, angular thoracic scoliosis that may produce paraplegia
Miscellaneous	Spinal cord tumors (osteoid osteoma, lipoma, others) Marfan's syndrome Morquio's disease Ehlers-Danlos syndrome Juvenile rheumatoid arthritis Fractured vertebra Post-irradiation Postburn Prader-Willi syndrome Riley-Day syndrome Syrinx Tethered cord

Reprinted with permission from: Greydanus DE. The musculoskeletal system. In: Hofmann AD, Greydanus DE, eds. Adolescent medicine, 3rd ed. Stamford, CT: Appleton Lange, 1997:291.

Depending on the indication any of the various radiographic techniques can be obtained that include anteroposterior, lateral, and oblique films of the spine, magnetic resonance imaging, computerized tomography scan, and bone scan. Treatment is dependent on the exact findings, but can involve observation, bracing, and a variety of surgical procedures (28-31).

There is no evidence that electrospinal orthosis (nocturnal electrical stimulation of back muscles), megavitamins, or dietary management are beneficial. Exercises neither prevent nor correct scoliosis.

Kyphosis

Kyphosis (sagittal plane malalignment) is considered normal if mild in the cervical, thoracic or lumbar regions of the spine. Overt kyphosis in adolescents can represent either postual kyphosis (95% of kyphosis in teens) or Scheuermann disease (dorsum rotundum; adolescent round back) (9). Chronic slouching may lead to the postual form, whether due to habit, embarrassment over breast development or conscious effort to control one's posture. Back pain can be develop in both of these conditions. Rigidity of the kyphosis and back pain with forward flexion suggests Scheuermann disease. Diagnosis and identification of underlying spinal structural deformities is aided by a roentgenographic evaluation of the spine. Management of postural kyphosis involves exercise and physical therapy to improve abdominal and back muscle strength. Good posture is important and may be encouraged with such activities as dance exercises (i.e., ballet or various modern dance styles) and with such sports as tract and weightlifting. Attention to any associated behavioral issues is also beneficial. Treatment of Scheuermann disease depends on its severity and may involve observation, upper back exercising (hyperextension), bracing (early in the disease course), and, for severe disease, surgery (7).

OTHER CAUSES OF BACK PAIN

Slipped spinal disc

A slipped intervertebral disc may present with vague back pain symptoms, possibly including transient sciatic discomfort (7). A straight leg raise (SLR) test may induce pain due to stretching of a nerve root (suggesting the possibility of a herniated disc); however, teens with a excessive flexibility (as ballet dancers and other athletes) may not always demonstrate a positive SLR test in this situation (7). When herniation develops, there is often more constant low back pain, spasm of paravertebral muscles with reduced range of motion with or without radiculopathy. Movement of the disc into the spinal canal can lead to compression of nerve roots with reflexes, sensation and muscle strength all reduced; atrophy of involved muscles may be seen. Confirmation of this uncommon diagnosis in adolescence is with magnetic resonance imaging (MRI) or computerized tomography (CT) scan (7). Modification of activities, relative rest, and physical therapy are initially recommended. If this fails, in a small percentage of cases surgery may be necessary.

Discitis and osteomyelitis

Septicemia may lead to an infection of the intervertebral disc space (discitis) or vertebral bacterial infection (osteomyelitis) (7,15). A urinary tract or respiratory tract infection may be the precipitating factor, allowing bacterial sepsis (often due to Staphylococcus aureus). Vertebral osteomyelitis is found in intravenous drug users and patients with sickle cell disease. Patients develop fever with back pain which may extend to the hip or leg, bony tenderness, involuntary muscle contractures, abdominal pain or gait disturbances. An increased white blood count and erythrocyte sedimentation rate, suggest a bacterial infection. Plain x-rays often eventually reveal disc space narrowing; while radionuclear bone scan is positive, and magnetic resonance imaging is diagnostic (7). Blood cultures are positive in half or less of the cases, while a needle biopsy (with culture and sensitivities) can be diagnostic and helpful regarding the correct antibiotics to use. After 10 to 14 days, x-rays may show a narrowed disc space and end plate changes (irregularities, erosions); there may or may not be non-specific soft tissue abnormalities. Eventually, spinal roentgenograms demonstrate fraying and then collapse of the involved vertebral body. Management includes bed rest, spine immobilization, antibiotics (oral and intravenous), and sometimes surgery (as open biopsy and anterior spinal fusion).

Spinal tumors

A number of different tumors, though rare, may be found in the spine that will cause back pain, including osteoid osteoma, osteoblastoma, aneurysmal bone cyst, Ewing tumor, leukemia, lymphoma and metastatic lesions (3,5,7). A variety of symptoms can be observed, including constant back pain, spinal tenderness and rigidity, and involuntary muscle contractions; scoliosis may be also noted. Abnormalities of the neurological system may occur, including reduced lower limb sensation, reduced muscle strength, and even foot deformity. Loss of bladder and bowel function may also develop. Management of benign tumors involves excision and bone grafting while treatment of malignant tumors is dependent on the type and extent of spread (2,5,7).

Ankylosing spondylitis (Marie Strümpell spondylitis)

Rheumatic diseases should be considered in the evaluation of adolescent athletes who present with chronic or recurrent back pain (32,33). Ankylosing spondylitis is a chronic inflammatory disorder involving sacroiliitis and a variety of features, as outlined in table 5 (32,33). The spine is involved, usually in an ascending fashion, as well as other joints (knee, hip, shoulder). The etiology is not known and it is classified with other seronegative spondyloarthropathies (Reiter's syndrome, post bacterial dysentery arthritis, arthritis with inflammatory bowel disease and psoriatic arthritis). Ankylosing spondylitis is usually diagnosed in males between 15 and 30 years.

Table 5. Features of ankylosing spondylitis

- Bony ankylosis of the posterior intervertebral, costovertebral, and sacroiliac joints
- Ossification of the spinal ligaments and intervertebral disk margins
- Rigid, immobile bony thoracic cage (chest pain develops due to involvement of the manubrosternal joint)
- Peripheral joint swelling, tenderness, and motion restriction of various joints, including hip, shoulder, knee, wrists, metacarpophalangeal joints, and metatarsophalangeal joints. Joint damage is especially noted in the hips and shoulders
- Achilles tendonitis
- Nongranulomatous anterior uveitis (25%)
- Cardiac defects
  - Aortic insufficiency (root of aorta and aortic valve affected)
  - Conduction defects noted on ECG: increased PR interval, bundle branch block, and complete AV dissociation
  - Mitral insufficiency
  - Myopericarditis
- Apical pulmonary fibrosis (a late complication characterized by bronchiectasis, cavity formation, fibrosis, and aspergilloma)
- Cauda equina syndrome (urinary incontinence, muscle wasting, pain, and sensory loss due to involvement of the cauda equina)
- Secondary renal amyloidosis

Reprinted with permission from: Greydanus DE. The musculoskeletal system. In: Hofmann AD, Greydanus DE, eds: Adolescent medicine, 3rd ed. Stamford, CT: Appleton Lange, 1997:295.

A careful history often reveals family members with psoriasis, reactive arthritis or inflammatory bowel disease.

The patient usually presents with chronic low back pain (or ache) with morning stiffness which may improve after arising from sleep and moving about. Other symptoms can include pain and stiffness in the thoracic area, fatigue, anorexia (with weight loss), and fever. Examination demonstrates reduced low back flexion and restricted lumbar spine movement. Laboratory evaluation may reveal anemia (hypochromic), negative rheumatoid factor, positive anti-nuclear antibody (ANA), and increased erythrocyte sedimentation rate; the histocompatibility antigen HLA B27 is present. Roentgenographic studies show the classic bilateral, symmetric sacroiliitis, unless the patient has an immature spine. A diagnosis of ankylosing spondylitis is made with x-ray evidence of bilateral sacroiliitis along with 2 of these 3 findings: history of pain at the lumbar spine or dorsolumbar junction, reduced movement of the lumbar spine in all three planes and limitation of chest expansion of one inch or less (at fourth intercostal space).

Management centers around physical therapy, exercising (especially swimming), medication and sleeping on a firm mattress. Physical therapy is used to prevent joint contractures, reduce muscle weakness and improve back movement. Medications used include aspirin and nonsteroidal anti-inflammatory drugs. Other treatment modalities include steroid injection into inflammed joints and as a last resort, spinal radiotherapy.

Conclusion

Back pain is a common complaint among teenagers, including athletes. Though trauma is a major etiologic factor, a careful search is recommended to look for a wide variety of causes. Though sports activity may lead to very severe complications, early diagnosis and active treatment will benefit most teens who present with back pain (2,3,33). More research is recommended to identify risk factors behind back pain in our children and youth (34).

References

[1] Patel DR, Rowe D. Thoracolumar spine injuries, In: Patel DR, Greydanus DE, Baker RJ, eds. Pediatric practice: Sports medicine. New York: McGraw Hill Med, 2009:377-95.
[2] Curtis C, d'Hemecourt P. Diagnosis and management of back pain in adolescents. Adolesc Med 2007;18(1):140-64.
[3] Standaert CJ. Low back pain in the adolescent athlete. Phys Med Rehabil Clin N Am 2008;19(2):287-304.
[4] Combs JA, Caskey PM. Back pain in children and adolescents: A retrospective review of 648 patients. South Med J 1997; 90(8):789-92.
[5] Kim HJ, Green DW. Adolescent back pain. Curr Opin Pediatr 2008;20(1):37-45.
[6] Payne WK III, Ogilvie JW. Back pain in children and adolescents. Pediatr Clin North Amer 1996;43(4): 899-917.
[7] Richards BS, McCarthy RE, Akbarnia BA. Back pain in childhood and adolescence. AAOS Instructional Course Lectures 1999;48:525-541.
[8] Glancy FL. The diagnosis and treatment of back pain in children and adolescents: an update. Adv Pediatr 2006;53:227-40.
[9] Stanitski CL. Conditions of the spine. Adolesc Med 1998;9(3):515-32.
[10] Jeffries LJ, Milanese SF, Grimmer-Somers KA. Epidemiology of adolescent spinal pain: a systematic review of the research literature. Spine 2007;32(23):2630-7.
[11] Olsen TL, Anderson RL, Deanwater SR, Kriksa AM, Cauley JA, Aaron DJ, et al. The epidemiology of low back pain in an adolescent population. Am J Publ Health 1992;82:606-8.
[12] Jones GT, Macfarlane GJ. Epidemiology of low back pain in children and adolescents. Arch Dis Chil 2005;90(3):312-6.
[13] McCleary MD, Congeni JA. Current concepts in the diagnosis and treatment of spondylolysis in young athletes. Curr Sports Med Rep 2007;6(1):62-6.
[14] DePalma MJ, Bhargava A. Nonspondylolytic etiologies of lumbar pain in the young athlete. Curr Sports Med Rep 2006;5(1):44-9.
[15] King HA. Back pain in children. Orthoped Clin North Amer 1999; 30:467-74.
[16] Fishbein M. Medical problems among ICSOM musicians. Med Probl Perform Art 1988; 3(1):1-14.
[17] Brandfonbrener AG. Epidemiology of the medical problems of performing artists. In: Sataloff RT, Alice G Brandfonbrener AG, Lederman RJ, eds: Textbook of performing arts medicine. New York: Raven, 1991: 25-69.
[18] Bejjani FJ, Kaye GM, Benham M. Musculoskeletal and neuromuscular conditions of instrumental musicians. Arch Phys Med Rehabil 1996;77:406-13.
[19] Chilton MD, Nisenfeld FG. Nonoperative treatment of low back injury in athletes. Clin Sport Med 1993;12 (3):547-56.
[20] Atlas SJ, Volinn E. Classics from the spine literature revisited: A randomized trial of 2 days versus 7 days of recommended bed rest for acute low back pain. Spine 1997; 22:2331-7.
[21] Ippolito E, Versari P, Lezzerini S. The role of rehabilitation in juvenile back disorders. Pediatr Rehabil 2006;9(3):174-84.

[22] Prins Y, Crous L, Louw QA. A systematic review of posture and psychosocial factors as contributors to upper quadrant musculoskeletal pain in children and adolescents. Physiother Theory Pract 2008;24(4):221-42.
[23] Sherry DD, McGuire T, Mellins E, et al. Psychosomatic musculoskeletal pain in childhood: Clinical and psychological analysis of 100 children. Pediatrics 1991;88(6):1093-9.
[24] Greydanus DE, Pratt HD. Manual on adolescent health care. Adolescence: A continuum from childhood to adulthood, 3rd ed. Des Moines, Iowa: Iowa Health Dept Publ, 1996.
[25] Cavalier R, Herman MJ, Cheung EV, Pizzutillo PD. Spondylolysis and spondylolisthesis in children and adolescents: I Diagnosis, natural history, and nonsurgical management. J Am Acad Orthop Surg 2006;14(7):417-24.
[26] Cheung EV, Herman MJ, Cavalier R, Pizzutillo PD. Spondylolysis and spondylolisthesis in children and adolescents: II Surgical management. J Am Acad Orthop Surg 2006;14(8):488-98.
[27] Stinson JT. Spondylolysis and spondylolisthesis in the athlete. Clin Sport Med 1993;2(3):517-28.
[28] Ramirez N, Johnston LE, Browne RH. The prevalence of back pain in children who have idiopathic scoliosis. J Bone Joint Surg 1997;79A:364-8.
[29] Bleck EE. Adolescent idiopathic scoliosis. Dev Med Child Neurol 1991;33(2):167-73.
[30] McLain RF, Karol L. Conservative treatment of the scoliotic and kyphotic patient. Brace treatment and other modalities. Arch Pediatr Adolesc Med 1994;48(6):646-51.
[31] Maruyama T. Bracing adolescent idiopathic scoliosis: a systematic review of the literature of effective conservative treatment looking for end results 5 years after weaning. Disabil Rehabil 2008;30(10):786-91.
[32] Jennings F, Lambert E, Fredericson M. Rheumatic diseases presenting as sport-related injuries. Sports Med 2008;38(11):917-30.
[33] Brent LH. Inflammatory arthritis: an overview for primary care physicians. Postgrad Med 2009;121(1):148-62.

Submitted: May 06, 2009.
Revised: June 17, 2009.
Accepted: June 22, 2009.

In: Public Health Yearbook 2009
Editor: Joav Merrick

ISBN: 978-1-61668-911-7

Chapter 39

EVALUATION AND TREATMENT OF ANKLE SPRAINS

Donald E Greydanus**, MD
and Dilip R Patel, MD, FAAP, FACSM, FAACPDM, FSAM
Department of Pediatrics and Human Development, Michigan State University College of Human Medicine, East Lansing, Michigan, United States of America

ABSTRACT

Ankle is a complex joint with many ligaments stabilizing the joint. Ankle sprains are commonly seen in sports in which jumping and landing, and sudden cutting are involved, as exemplified by American football, soccer, volleyball and gymnastics. The majority of ankle sprains are to the lateral ligaments resulting from an inversion type injury. Clinical assessment mainly depends up on history of the mechanism of injury and initial symptoms, and a careful physical exam of the ankle as well as for any associated injuries. Routine use of X-rays is not always useful. Treatment is generally conservative with early ice, rest, elevation, and protective weight bearing, followed by complete rehabilitation with physiotherapy. Delayed recovery and chronic pain should prompt further investigation and orthopedic consultation.

Keywords: Ankle sprain, inversion sprain, syndesmosis sprain.

* Correspondence: Professor Donald E Greydanus, MD, Pediatrics and Human Development, Michigan State University College of Human Medicine, Pediatrics Program Director, Michigan State University/Kalamazoo Center for Medical Studies, 1000 Oakland Drive, Kalamazoo, MI 49008-1284 United States. E-mail: Greydanus@kcms.msu.edu

Introduction

A sprain is an injury to a ligament while a strain represents an injury to any part of the musculotendinous unit. Ankle sprains are the most common ankle injury, representing 15% of all athletic injuries (1-5). Main risk factors for ankle sprains in young athletes include previous ankle injuries (especially with limited recovery), limited flexibility of the Achilles tendon, increased ligament laxity in general, and increased weight (2,3).

In the ankle joint, the tibia and fibula are connected to the talus and calcaneus. The ankle is stabilized by three ligament groups, the medial, lateral and interosseous ligaments (1,3). The lateral group consists of 3 separate ligaments: anterior talofibular, calcaneofibular, and posterior talofibular. The lateral ligaments are involved in over 85% of ankle sprains (1). The medial (deltoid) ligament is a large, thick and strong structure which is involved in 5% of ankle sprains (1). There is also a ligamentous connection between the tibia and fibula over the entire length, the tibiofibular syndesmosis, which is involved in approximately 10% of ankle sprains (6).

Mechanisms of Ankle Sprain

Most ankle sprains are caused by inversion (turning the joint in or under) with plantar flexion (downward motion) of the foot which leads to the sprain of the lateral ankle ligaments (1,3). The anterior talofibular ligament is the first one to be disrupted. With continued progression of inversion and plantar flexion with more force, the calcaneofibular ligament and then the posterior talofibular are injured (1-5). Eversion (turning the joint out) and dorsiflexion (upward motion) of the foot can disrupt the deltoid ligament and also the syndesmotic ligament (6). This can be caused by sudden deceleration, landing from a jump or suddenly changing direction. External rotation can lead to a "high" ankle strain or disruption of the syndesmotic ligament (6-9). There is a greater incidence of bone injury with disruption of the deltoid and the tibiofibular ligaments. Sports in which ankle sprains are more commonly seen are listed in table 1.

Table 1. Sports with an increased risk for ankle sprains

American football
Basketball
Baseball
Dancing
Gymnastics
Hockey
Martial arts
Rugby
Running
Soccer
Volleyball
Wrestling

EVALUATION

History

The history includes questions about the mechanism of injury, history of previous ankle injury and the degree of pain and swelling which has developed (3). It is helpful to ask about the foot position at the time of injury and whether the athlete can now bear weight. The athlete may have rolled or fell on a stretched ankle – often noted with soccer injuries. Others state that it feels as though they stepped off a curb or stepped into a hole. The history of ankle locking is a worrisome feature, as is a "popping" or "snapping" sensation with rapid or severe ankle swelling. An Achilles tendon rupture leads to a sensation of being kicked in the heel. History of previous ankle injury is a significant risk factor for recurrence of sprain.

Examination

The athlete with an ankle sprain should be evaluated for the pain, swelling, and ecchymosis (3). The vascular integrity of the injured ankle should be assessed as well. There can be minimal swelling if ice was immediately applied. Ecchymosis is a common yet non-specific and often delayed finding. It is helpful to localize the area of tenderness and which ligaments are involved. The anterior talofibular ligament is palpated 2 to 3 fingerbreadths in front of and below the lateral malleolus. The calcaneofibular ligament is palpated 1 to 2 fingerbreadths below and downward to the lateral malleolus. However, significant ankle swelling often makes localization of tenderness difficult. The range of motion at the ankle joint (with and without resistance) should be assessed.

A number of specific tests have been used to assess the ligamentous integrity, such as anterior drawer test, inversion (stress) test, and the squeeze test (1-9). The anterior drawer test is used to evaluate the integrity of the anterior talofibular ligament. With the foot in the neutral position, one hand is placed above the ankle (holding the leg steady), while the examiner's other hand is around the heel, move the heel forward. Slight movement represents a +1, moderate movement +2 and marked movement is a +3. Increased forward motion compared to uninjured ankle and soft end point to the movement indicates a positive sign.

Inversion stress test is useful to assess sprain of the calcaneofibular ligament, with or without associated injury to the anterior talofibular ligament. With one hand over the lower leg just above the ankle, the examiner steadies the leg. With the other hand the examiner turns the foot inwards (inversion). This is compared to the uninjured ankle. With sprain of the calcaneofibular ligament there is increased pain or laxity depending up on the degree of tear.

The squeeze test is used to assess for syndesmotic injury. The examiner places the hand about 6 inches below the knee with thumbs on the fibula and fingers on the medial aspect of the tibia. Then the examiner squeezes the leg. If pain is elicited in the diatal leg or ankle, it suggests syndesmotic injury.

Imaging studies

Roentgenographic evaluation is often indicated in growing athletes to rule out growth plate injuries (1,2). Their use in the skeletally mature athletes is much more limited. When ordered, they include anteroposterior, lateral and mortise views.

The Ottawa rules recommendations include pain in the area of the malleoli, inability to bear weight right after the injury and unable to take four steps while being examined; or other localized bony tenderness as indications for X-rays (10). These criteria may be applicable in older adolescents; children and younger adolescents with ankle injuries need individual clinical judgement. Other possible indications for x-rays are listed in table 2.

Table 2. Indications for X-rays in ankle sprains

Ottawa ankle rules criteria met
Rapid onset of swelling
Joint instability
Localized bone tenderness
Eversion sprains
Syndesmotic sprains
Severe pain
Deformity

Stress films are not recommended by most experts when dealing with acute ankle injuries in teenagers. Some experts suggest stress films are helpful for chronic ankle instability and before surgical repair of ligaments. Tomograms or MRI can be used to detect occult fractures (11). A foot series is recommended for an inability to bear weight and or pain over the mid-foot (anterior process of the calcaneous, base of the fifth metatarsal, navicular, cuboid, cuneiforms). In chronic pain and instability further evaluation with computed tomography scan or magnetic resonance imaging may be indicated.

Associated injuries

A number of conditions can be associated with ankle sprains that can cause chronic or recurrent ankle pain (see table 3) (1,4,12-15). Fractures can occur, especially over the distal fibula and proximal fifth metatarsal (12). A Jones fracture is especially difficult to heal. Increased side to side movements of the foot with anterior tenderness suggests syndesmotic injury, especially with eversion sprains (7). Fifteen percent of complete ligament tears have an associated fracture, mostly involving the talus fifth metatarrsal fibula or tibia. Bony tenderness in teenagers with open epiphysis suggests a fracture, even with negative x-rays; it is classified as a non-displaced physeal fracture or Salter-Harris Type I fracture. Eversion sprains may also be associated with bimalleolar and proximal fibular fractures.

Table 3. Conditions associated with ankle sprains

Distal fibular physis fracture
Talar dome fracture
Avulsion fracture at base of the 5th metatarsal
Jones Fracture
Fibula fracture (proximal or shaft)
Syndesmotic injuries
Disruptions of peroneal or Achilles tendons
Malleolar fractures

MANAGEMENT

Most ankle sprains are not characterized by ankle instability or other injuries and respond rapidly to the PRICE method of management: Protection, rest, ice, compression, elevation (4,16-19). Ice should be applied immediately with a compression dressing (see table 4). Crushed ice in a plastic bag or other container is applied in a cycle of 15 to 20 minute intervals, separated by 20-45 minutes for at least four times a day.

Table 4. Phases of cryotherapy

Cold sensation: 1-3 minutes
Painful stage (burning, aching): 2-7 minutes
Anesthesia stage: numbness which decreases pain
Deep tissue reflex vasodilation phase:
12-15 minutes into the cryotherapy

A towel over the skin (along with appropriate compression coverage) will prevent frostbite. This can be applied as long as there is swelling. An ice-water whirlpool can also be used. Application of heat is not effective in the recovery process especially during the first 72 hours. Non-steriodal anti-inflammatory drugs can also be used in the recovery period for the management of pain and possibly decrease inflammation. These medications do not affect the recovery.

Elevation of the injured leg is useful in the early phase of recovery, especially during the first 2 to 3 days and as long as there is swelling. Prolonged rest is not recommended since it will hinder a rapid recovery. Early, protected weight bearing (depending on the pain tolerance of the athlete and the severity of the injury) facilitates recovery. Crutches may be used for as short a time as needed. Different types of compression methods are available, such as Ace wraps or ankle braces. Air Stirrups orthosis prevent inversion and eversion and are used for a lateral sprain injury without medial or syndesmotic ligament injury.

Athletes with medial ligament or syndesmotic injuries, and associated injuries, especially when a fracture is suspected, suggest need for an orthopedic consultation (6,8). Also if the athlete with an uncomplicated lateral ankle sprain is not improved within two weeks of the PRICE treatment, further evaluation and orthopedic consultation are indicated.

Recovery of an uncomplicated ankle sprain typically takes 2 to 6 weeks. The goal of management is full recovery of the ankle joint and not just pain relief. Cryotherapy should always be applied after exercising. Range of motion exercises are begun as tolerated. If the adolescent with an uncomplicated ankle sprain is improved after two weeks (sooner if an athlete) resistance training exercises can begin. When developing an injury rehabilitation program, treatment adherence by the adolescent athlete is crucial to maximize recovery. The teen should understand the nature of his or her injury and the specific steps of the rehabilitation program and why the steps are necessary. The clinician or trainer can write down each step of the program and have the adolescent check off each part as recovery occurs.

Range of motion exercises includes activities such as foot circles (tracing small circles in the air), using the large toe to trace letters of the alphabet or picking up marbles with the toes (2,4,17). Achilles tendon (heel cord) stretching exercises are very useful. General ankle stretching exercises can be done in the sitting position with knees flexed. The athlete can grab his or her foot and move the ankle in various motions.

Swimming and biking (as tolerated) can be an important part of the rehabilitation process to preserve cardiovascular conditioning and prevent muscle disuse atrophy. Progressive strength training exercises can be recommended under the direction of a sports trainer or physical therapist, if available. Proprioception training is then added to the rehabilitaion program using a balanced board or beam exercises.

The final stages of rehabilitation are aimed toward helping the athlete regain coordination and agility skills. Alternate jogging and running, as well as running figures of "8" or zig-zag cutting can be recommended. Ankle taping may help with needed support in the late recovery phase. Careful evaluation by the clinician and trainer is important to detect additional complications of ankle sprain, such as chronic ankle instability. In general, athletes are not allowed back into competitive activity until at least 90% of functional recovery has occurred. Causes of delayed recovery and chronic ankle pain are listed in table 5 (4,5,12-17).

CONCLUSION

Ankle injuries are common in youth sports. The most common injury is a sprained ankle. Most ankle sprains are inversion sprains affecting the lateral ligaments of the ankle.

Table 5. Common causes of delayed recovery or chronic pain

Incomplete rehabilitation program
Significant scaring
Occult fracture
Tibiofibular diastasis
Chronic synovitis
Soft tissue impingement
Inadequate training and conditioning
Mechanical or functional instability

Although most sprains are not associated with other injuries, significant neurovascular or bony injuries should be ruled out at the initial evaluation. Radiographic evaluation is often indicated in acute sprains, especially to rule out growth plate injuries. Initial treatment is based on the PRICE principle. Early mobilization is strongly encouraged and it has been shown to shorten the recovery time. For competitive adolescent athletes management of ankle sprains should include a complete rehabilitation program, because inadequate rehabilitation is the most common cause of recurrent sprains. Most athletes will recover in 2-6 weeks and will be able to return to sports.

REFERENCES

[1] Safran MR, Benedetti RS, Bartolozzi, et al. Lateral ankle sprains: a comprehensive review: Part I Etiology, pathoanatomy, histopathogenesis, and diagnosis. Med Sci Sports Exer 1999;31:S429-37.

[2] Safran MR, Zachazewski JE, Benedetti RS, et al. Lateral ankle sprains: A comprehensive review: Part II Treatment and rehabilitation with emphasis on the athlete. Med Sci Sports Exer 1999:S438-47.

[3] Patel DR, Janiski C. Ankle sprains in young athletes Part I How to evaluate, manage, and prevent. Contemp Pediatr 2005;22(12):65:75.

[4] Patel DR. Ankle sprains in young athletes Part II How to evauate, manage, and prevent: Contemp Pediatr 2005;22(12):76-82.

[5] Fong DT, Hong Y, Chan LK, Yung PS, Chan KM. A systematic review on ankle injury and ankle sprain in sports. Sports Med 2007;37(1):73-94.

[6] Rammelt S, Zwipp H, Grass R. Injuries to the distal tibiofibular syndesmosis: an evidence-based approach to acute and chronic lesion. Foot Ankle Clin 2008;13(4):611-33.

[7] Williams GN, Jones MH, Amendola A. Syndesmotic ankle sprains in athletes. Am J Sports Med 2007;35(7):1197-207.

[8] Jones MH, Amendola AS. Acute treatment of inversion ankle sprains: immobilization versus functional treatment. Clin Orthop Relat Res 2007;455:169-72.

[9] Lin CF, Gross ML, Weinhold P. Ankle syndesmosis injuries: anatomy, biomechanics, mechanism of injury, and clinical guidelines for diagnosis and intervention. J Orthop Sports Phys Ther 2006;36(6):372-84.

[10] Stiell IG, Greenberg GH, McKnight D, Nair RC, McDowell I, Reardon H, et al. Decision rules for the use of radiography in acute ankle injuries: refinement and prospective validation. JAMA 19913;269:1127-32.

[11] Bencardino J, Rosenberg ZS, Delfault E. MR imaging in sports injuries of the foot and ankle. MRI Clin N Am 1999;7(1):131-49.

[12] Lee JC, Calder JD, Healy JC. Posterior impingement syndromes of the ankle. Semin Musculoskelet Radiol 2008;12(2):154-59.

[13] Umans HR, Cerezal L. Anterior ankle impingement syndromes. Semin Musculoskelet Radio 2008;12(2):146-53.

[14] Sanders TG, Rathur SK. Impingement syndromes of the ankle. Magn Reson Imaging Clin North Am 2008;16(1):29-38.

[15] van Rijn RM, van Os AG, Bernsen RM, Luijsterburg PA, Koes BW, Bierma-Zeinstra SM. What is the clinical course of acute ankle sprains? A systematic review of literature Am J Med 2008;121(4):324-31.

[16] Holmes A, Delahunt E. Treatment of common deficits associated with chronic ankle instability. Sports Med 2009;39(3):207-24.

[17] Hubbard TJ, Hicks-Little CA. Ankle ligament healing after an acute ankle sprain: an evidence-based approach. J Athl Train 2008;43(5):523-9.

[18] Kerkhoffs GM, Handoll HH, de Bie R, Rowe BH, Struijs PA. Surgical versus conservative treatment for acute injures of the lateral ligament complex of the ankle in adults. Cochrane Database Syst Rev 2007;18(2):CD000380.
[19] Jones MH, Amendola A. Syndesmosis sprains of the ankle: a systematic review. Clin Orthop Relat Res 2007;455:173-5.

Submitted: May 03, 2009.
Revised: June 17, 2009.
Accepted: June 21, 2009.

In: Public Health Yearbook 2009
Editor: Joav Merrick
ISBN: 978-1-61668-911-7

Chapter 40

KNEE INJURIES IN ADOLESCENT ATHLETES

Dilip R Patel*, MD, FAAP, FACSM, FAACPDM, FSAM
Department of Pediatrics and Human Development, Michigan State University College of Human Medicine, East Lansing, Michigan, United States of America

Abstract

The knee is the most commonly injured joint from sport participation. Estimates of knee injuries range from 10-60% in various sports, and 50% of adolescent athletes present with sport-related knee pain. Most injuries in the adolescent athlete are due to overuse. Idiopathic anterior knee pain, Osgood-Schlatter disease, patellar tendinitis, osteochodritis dissecans, pathologic plicae, and bursitis are some of the many causes of chronic or recurrent symptoms. Referred pain from the hip, spine, abdomen, or pelvic pathology should always be considered in any athlete presenting with knee pain. Acute trauma is less common and can result in ligament injuries, meniscal tears, and fractures. In the adolescent athlete with acute trauma, injuries of the distal femoral and proximal tibial physes should also be considered in the differential diagnosis. This article reviews common overuse and acute injuries in young athletes.

Keywords: Overuse injuries, osteochondritis dissecans, idiopathic anterior knee pain, anterior cruciate ligament tear, Osgood-Schlatter disease

* Correspondence: Professor Dilip R Patel, MD, MD, FAAP, FACSM, FSAM, FAACPDM, Department of Pediatrics and Human Development, Michigan State University College of Human Medicine, Kalamazoo Center for Medical Studies, Kalamazoo, Michigan, MSU/ KCMS/ Pediatrics, 1000, Oakland Drive, Kalamazoo, MI 49008-1284 United States. Tel: 269-337-6450; Fax: 269-337-6474; E-mail: patel@kcms.msu.edu

Introduction

In adolescent athletes, knee is the most commonly involved joint in sports injuries. Estimates of acute and overuse knee injuries range from 10 % in ballet, to as high as 60% in American football. Acute and overuse injuries of the knee together constitute about 15% of all sports related injuries, and in practice knee problems resulting from sports participation may account for half of all patient visits (1-4).

In most cases the primary care physician is the first contact for the athlete who typically presents following an acute injury, pain due to overuse, acute or chronic swelling, locking sensation, or giving away sensation. In the setting of an acute trauma, a history of significant direct impact to the knee, difficulty to bear weight, rapid onset of swelling, instability, and localized bony tenderness should prompt consideration of acute fracture or dislocation and neurovascular injury must be ruled out (2,3). In the adolescent athlete presenting with an acute trauma, neurovascular symptoms or signs distal to knee, inability to fully extend the knee, gross instability, deformity, and tense hemarthrosis need orthopedic consultation (see table 1).

Table 1. Indications for orthopedic surgical consultation

Main conditions

- Complete tear of anterior or posterior cruciate ligaments
- Complete tear of medial or lateral collateral ligaments
- Torn meniscus
- Patellar dislocation
- Fracture in and around knee
- Ruptured or avulsed quadriceps or patellar tendon
- Intra-articular loose body
- Osteochondritis dessicans
- Osteomyelitis
- Pyogenic arthritis

Main clinical features

- Chronic or recurrent pain with swelling
- Loose body sensation
- Locking
- Sense of knee or leg giving away
- Neurovascular signs
- Acute hemarthrosis
- Gross intability
- Deformity

Gradual onset of pain that is recurrent or chronic, a history of loose body sensation, recurrent locking, and deformity suggest overuse injuries (1,2). The differential diagnosis of acute knee injuries is listed in table 2, and chronic or recurrent pain and injuries is listed in table 3 (1-6).

Table 2. Acute injuries of the knee

Anterior cruciate ligament injuries
Medial collateral ligament injuries
Lateral collateral ligament injuries
Patellar dislocation and subluxation
Medial meniscal tears
Lateral meniscal tears
Dislocation of the knee
Tears of quadriceps tendon
Tears of the patellar tendon
Injuries of the distal femoral or proximal tibial physes
Patellar fractures
Femoral and tibial fractures

Table 3. Intrinsic causes of chronic or recurrent pain in knee

Anterior

Idiopathic anterior knee pain
Quadriceps tendinitis
Patellar stress fracture
Patellofemoral osteochondrits dissecans
Sindig-Larsen-Johanssen syndrome
Patellar tendinitis
Patellar subluxation
Chondromalacia patella
Hoffa syndrome

Posterior
Hamstring strains and tendinitis
Poterolateral corner injuries
Symptomatic Baker or popliteal cyst

Medial
Pes anserine bursitis and tendinitis
Medial collateral ligament sprain
Medial meniscus injury
Pathologic medial plica
Osteochondritis dissecans

Lateral
Popliteus tendinitis
Iliotibial band friction syndrome
Lateral meniscus injury
Lateral collateral ligament sprain

Main indications for x-ray are listed in table 4. In addition to antero-posterior and lateral views, a tangential view (sunrise view or Merchant's view) is recommended for evaluation of the patella (7).

Table 4. Indications for x-rays

A history of significant direct impact to the knee
Difficulty to bear weight
Rapid onset of swelling
Instability on examination
Localized bony tenderness
Apparent deformity
A history of loose body sensation
Recurrent locking
Chronic or recurrent effusion
Chronic or recurrent pain

Overuse injuries

Overuse injuries of the knee are far more common then the acute injuries of the knee, and their diagnosis and management fall well within the purview of the primary care physician. Chronic or recurrent activity related knee pain is the most common presenting symptom of overuse injuries and causes of which are listed in table 3. High intensity and high volume activities consistently contribute to this type of injuries. By definition an overuse injury implies response of the normal tissue to excessive stress. Overuse injuries in the adolescent can affect tendons, epiphysis, apophysis, bones, joint, and articular cartilage. Idiopathic anterior knee pain is the most common overuse injury of the knee.

Idiopathic anterior knee pain

A number of specific injuries can cause anterior knee pain in a young athlete. However in many athletes the exact etiology of the pain cannot be conclusively established. Although patellofemoral syndrome is a most common cause of anterior knee pain in adolescents, the terms are not synonymous (7).

Mechanism

The most consistent factor leading to the anterior knee pain is intense physical activity overloading the patellofemoral mechanism (7-12). The patellofemoral unit provides the mechanism for knee extension and deceleration. Soft tissue attachments and the bony supporting structures provide the static stability for the patella in the femoral groove. Some authors consider malalignment and abnormal tracking of patella to be a major factor contributing to the development of patellofemoral pain (7,9). Vastus medialis obliquus plays an important role in providing dynamic stability to the patella and its proper tracking in the femoral groove. Dysfunction and weakness of vastus medialis is noted in some athletes with patellofemoral syndrome. Many anatomical factors have been postulated to explain the syndrome of patellofemoral pain. These include abnormal position of the patella, abnormal quadriceps angle, muscle imbalance, hyperpronated feet, ligamentous laxity, genu varum or valgus, and chondromalacia (1,7-12). Chondromalacia patellae is a pathologic diagnosis indicating softening and erosion of the cartilage of the patellofemoral joint, and in some athletes is a cause of severe anterior knee pain (7).

Diagnosis

Anterior knee pan is typically seen in a young active athlete who presents with activity related knee pain. Pain is typically gradual in onset, unilateral or bilateral, and exacerbated by a recent increase in physical activity (1,7). The pain is aggravated after prolonged sitting (theater sign), going up and coming downstairs, and prolonged squatting. Usually the athlete presents following several weeks of pain. The athlete might have tried pain medications intermittently. When the severity of pain adversely affects the performance, the athlete seeks medical attention. Some athletes may give a history of the knee catching, locking or giving away. Swelling is uncommon.

Examine the athlete for the presence of gait abnormality, increased lumbar lordosis, asymmetry of hips or lower extremities, hyperpronated feet, and atrophy and weakness of the quadriceps muscles by comparing to the normal side. Decreased flexibility of the hamstrings and quadriceps is a common finding in many athletes with anterior knee pain. Lateral patellar deviation can be detected by placing a row of three dots in a straight line while the knee is relaxed (one several inches above the knee in the midline, one several inches below and one at mid patellar point) and determining for lateral displacement of the patellar dot on isometric quadriceps contraction. In some athletes tenderness may be elicited by exerting pressure on the articular margins of the patella while displacing it medially or laterally (Perkin sign) (1,7). A crepitus may be felt in some athletes. In some patients pain is elicited when the quadriceps is contracted and the examiner holds the patella down preventing its upward movement (Clarke sign) (1).

Radiographs are not indicated routinely. Abnormal tilt of the patella may be associated with maltracking. This is seen best with a tangential view at 45 degree of flexion of the knee. In many cases the examination and X-rays are normal and the diagnosis is based solely on symptoms.

Treatment

Conservative treatment consists of relative rest, local ice, and judicious use of medications to help control the pain (7). Extended periods of sitting, squatting, and climbing up or going down stairs and full arc knee extension exercises should be avoided (1,7). Non-impact activities such as cycling with a proper fit, swimming, and walking are strongly recommended. Idiopathic anterior knee pain is a benign condition, and resolves in most cases over a period of few months to up to 2 years (1,7,10,12). The majority of athletes can continue sports participation. Complete rest and immobilization are not recommended. The most effective treatment involves closed kinetic chain exercise regimen (where the foot is in contact with the ground, e.g. step downs, lunges, partial squats, leg presses) for the quadriceps, hamstrings, gastrocnemius, and soleus muscles. Focus should be on strengthening, flexibility, endurance and neuromuscular retraining of these muscles (1,4,7-9). The effectiveness of different kinds of taping techniques and knee braces varies considerably and their use should be individualized (13). Surgical intervention is rarely necessary. This may be indicated in athletes with chronic, recurrent pain of severe nature, to possibly correct anatomical abnormalities contributing to the pain.

Osgood-Schlatter disease

Osgood-Schlatter disease is an overuse injury affecting the tibial tubercle apophysis (1,3,14). Osgood-Schlatter disease is commonly seen during Tanner stage 2 or 3. It is more common in adolescent boys (1,14). The incidence is higher in athletes compared to non-athletes, 21 % in athletes compared to 4.5 % in non-athletes in one study (9,14).

Mechanism

Rapid growth and increased physical activity predisposes to the development of this condition during early adolescence. The immature patellar tendon-tibial tubercle junction is highly susceptible to submaximal, repetitive tensile stress resulting from high intensity sport activity (4,14). The underlying pathology is suggestive of minor avulsions at the site and subsequent inflammatory reaction.

Diagnosis

Symptoms are bilateral in 20 to 30 % of patients (4). Anterior knee pain is the most common presentation. The pain is aggravated by sports involving jumping, squatting, and kneeling, and is relieved by a period of rest. Localized tenderness and sometimes swelling over the tibial tubercle are noted on examination. X-ray may show fragmentation of tibial tubercle and sometimes an ossicle in the patellar tendon.

Treatment

Treatment is conservative. Decreased activity and rest will result in significant improvement in pain. In some athletes it is not uncommon for recurrent pain to last up to two years before complete resolution (1,4,14). Osgood-Schlatter disease is a benign, self-limited condition and over treatment should be avoided. The adolescent should be allowed to participate in all sports as tolerated. Hamstrings and quadriceps stretches should be done on a regular basis to improve and maintain flexibility.

The most common complication is a persistent localized swelling, which may only be of cosmetic concern. Ossicle formation in the patellar tendon may be source of chronic pain in some athletes and removal of such an ossicle may be indicated. Presence of Osgood-Schlatter disease does not necessarily predispose the athlete for complete avulsion of the patellar tendon from the tibial tuberosity. This is only a potential concern during rapid growth phase just prior to fusion of the tublercle to tibia (4).

Sinding-Larsen-Johansson syndrome

This overuse injury affects the junction of the inferior pole of the patella and the insertion of the patellar tendon (4,8).

Mechanism

Repetitive traction at the inferior pole of the patella is believed to be the main mechanism that leads to Sinding-Larsen-Johansson syndrome (1,4). The immature inferior pole of the patella is especially vulnerable to repetitive traction injury. Chronic excessive traction leads to calcification and ossification at the junction of the inferior pole and patellar tendon.

Diagnosis

Anterior knee pain of gradual onset is the most common presentation. Pain is aggravated by jumping and running activities. It is localized over the inferior pole of the patella and proximal insertion of the patellar tendon.

Usually there is no history of direct trauma to the area. On palpation, point tenderness is elicited at the patella-patellar tendon junction. Calcification and ossification at the patella-patellar tendon junction is seen on plain films. This should be differentiated from a bipartite patella or a patellar sleeve fracture.

Treatment

Overtreatment should be avoided. No long term complications have been reported form Sinding-Larsen Johanssen syndrome. Sport participation is allowed as tolerated, with some modification in activity intensity and volume.

In some athletes, the recurrent pain may persist for 12 to 18 months before spontaneous resolution occurs (1,4). Local ice massage is recommended. Because decreased flexibility of hamstrings is a common finding in many athletes, regular hamstrings stretches should be done. Local injection of corticosteroid into and around the patellar tendon is contraindicated, and may predispose to tendon weakness and rupture.

Osteochondritis dissecans (OCD) of knee

OCD is an important cause of knee pain in the adolescent, both in the athlete and the non-athlete (1,4,6). OCD is characterized by delamination of the subchondral bone, with or without the involvement of the articular cartilage. In the knee, it most commonly affects the medial condyle, and this accounts for 75% of all OCD cases (4). OCD is four times more common in males than in females and the lesion is bilateral in 10%-20% of the cases (4).

Mechanism

The exact etiology or mechanism leading to the OCD lesion has not been elucidated; however, intense activity and repetitive trauma are considered to be significant factors.

Diagnosis

The athlete presents with a history of gradual onset of knee pain. These athletes are usually very active in sports. The pain is typically located over anterior knee, and is characterized as aching sensation, worse during activity. There may be a history of intermittent knee swelling following practice or game participation.

On examination mild effusion may be noted. Range of motion may or may not be affected. In early stages of the lesion the articular cartilage over the femoral condyle is intact and findings on examination are non-specific. In late stages, the articular cartilage is eroded; the fragment may separate and become an intra-articular loose body. Findings on examination at this stage may include effusion, locking, and loss of motion. In lesions of medial femoral condyle, pain is elicited, when the athlete flexes the internally rotated leg, from full extension to about 30 degrees. On x-rays of the knee the lesion appears as a well demarcated radiolucent area.

Treatment

In most cases, early recognition and a period of 8-12 weeks of rest from sports typically allows for the OCD lesion to heal, when the lesion is still in early stages (4). Later in the course when the lesion is more advance with disruption of the cartilage with or without separation of the subchondral fragment, immobilization and orthopedic evaluation are indicated.

Acute knee injuries

Acute knee injuries are seen both in contact sports such as soccer, rugby, hockey, kabaddi and American football, as well as non-contact sports such as basketball and volleyball (2,3). Mechanism of injury is most useful in suspecting the injured structure. Sudden change in direction, especially with foot planted can result in injury of the anterior cruciate ligament (ACL) and the meniscus (2). Landing off balance may also result in anterior cruciate ligament injury. Collateral ligaments are typically injured as a result of a direct impact to the medial or lateral aspect of the knee. A direct impact against tibia when the knee is flexed is associated with isolated sprain of the posterior cruciate ligament.

A pop or a snap felt at the time of injury is usually associated with an anterior cruciate tear. Rapid onset of swelling following trauma indicates an acute hemarthrosis, which is generally associated ACL tear, patellar dislocation, or a fracture. With meniscal injury the swelling is minimal and gradual, although a peripheral meniscal tear can cause significant hemarthrosis. A meniscal injury or an intra-articular loose body can cause locking of the knee. History of knee or leg giving away indicates joint instability typically associated with a complete tear of the anterior cruciate ligament. The athlete feels immediate pain at the time of a ligamentous injury, dislocation or a fracture.

The first task in an acutely injured knee is to assess for neurovascular injury. Radiation of pain, numbness, paresthesias, and sensation of cold, distal to knee may suggest neurovascular involvement and need for emergent consultation. Similarly on examination, any gross deformity, pallor, poor arterial pulse, decreased sensation or paralysis distal to the knee need further assessment and emergent treatment. Once a neurovascular injury is ruled out further assessment is directed to diagnose specific injuries to other structures.

On examination assess the extent of intra-articular effusion, look for deformity, and assess active and passive range of motion at knee. The examiner should attempt to accurately localize tenderness over bony or soft tissue structures. This will greatly help narrow down the anatomic diagnosis. Always compare findings to the uninjured knee.

Medial collateral ligament injuries

Medial collateral ligament sprains result from a valgus or external rotation stress to the knee with foot planted. Athlete has medial knee pain and is able to walk with some discomfort. There is usually no effusion and the flexion and extension motions are normal. A valgus stress at 30 degrees knee flexion increases the medial knee pain. In complete tear, increased laxity may be noted. There is localized tenderness over the ligament on the medial aspect of the knee. Uncomplicated sprains of the medial collateral ligament resolve with a period of relative rest of few days to weeks. A hinged brace allows early range of motion, strengthening, and endurance exercises to continue during healing phase. The athlete may return to full sports participation when asymptomatic and has a normal examination.

Anterior cruciate ligament injuries

Anterior cruciate ligament sprain commonly results from a twisting or hyperextension force to the knee. Athlete feels immediate pain and sometimes a sensation of popping at the time of the tear. There is a rapid onset of hemarthrosis. The Lachman test is positive. Perform Lachman test with athlete supine, knee flexed at 15 degree; stabilize the femur with one hand and move the tibia forward. Feel for increased forward motion of tibia over femur and for the end-point of the movement. In anterior cruciate ligament sprain there is a soft end point and increased forward motion of tibia over femur. These injuries should be should be referred to an orthopedic surgeon. In an active young athlete treatment is usually surgical reconstruction of the ligament followed by aggressive post-operative rehabilitation.

Medial meniscus tear

A medial meniscus tear may either be an isolated injury or may be associated with other ligamentous injuries (2,3). A deceleration force with twisting motion leading to compression is the usual mechanism causing tearing of the meniscus. The athlete may present with knee pain, minimal swelling, and locking. There is medial joint line tenderness. The athlete may have a positive McMurray test. In this test the patient is supine with hip and knee flexed. The examiner holds the knee with one hand and the foot with the other. Then the examiner extends the knee simultaneously externally rotating the leg. The athlete may feel pain or the examiner may feel the torn posterior horn of the medial meniscus. Meniscal tears have poor potential for healing and most young athletes may need arthroscopy and repair.

Patellar dislocation

A direct impact to the patella or a forceful quadriceps contraction during a cutting motion can result in acute patellar dislocation (2,3). In most cases the patella is dislocated laterally. The athletes presents with acute onset severe pain, rapid onset of swelling, obvious deformity, restriction of motion and significant tenderness. Athlete resists attempts to push patella laterally (Apprehension test). Initial treatment consists of closed reduction and immobilization of the knee in extension. This is followed by a rehabilitation program that includes strengthening exercises. Closed reduction is achieved with quadriceps and hamstrings relaxed athlete supine with leg flexed at the hip and knee, followed by gentle extension of the knee while maintaining pressure over patella directed from lateral to medial direction. One should carefully rule out associated fracture or rupture of the quadriceps (2).

Conclusion

Acute and chronic knee injuries are common in sports. The primary care physician being the first contact person bears the burden of appropriate diagnosis, triage, and further consultation as needed for these athletes. Some specific conditions need referral, however many problems can be managed by the primary physician.

References

[1] Patel DR, Lyne DE. Overuse injuries of knee. In: Patel DR, Greydanus DE, Baker RJ, eds. Pediatric practice: Sports medicine. New York: McGraw Hill Med, 2009:330-41.

[2] Cline S. Acute knee injuries. In: Patel DR, Greydanus DE, Baker RJ, eds. Pediatric practice: Sports medicine. New York: McGraw Hill Med, 2009:342-360.
[3] Siow HM, Cameron DB, Ganley TJ. Acute knee injuries in skeletally immature athletes. Phys Med Rehabil Clin North Am 2008;19(2):319-45.
[4] Stanitski CL, DeLee JC, Drez D. Pediatric and Adolescent Sports Medicine. Philadelphia, PA: WB Saunders, 1994.
[5] McGuine T. Sports injuries in high school athletes: A review of injury-risk and injury-prevention research. Clin J Sport Med 2006;16(6):488-99.
[6] Roach JW. Knee disorders and injuries in adolescents. Adolesc Med 1998;9(3):589.
[7] Mann G, Constantini N, Hetsroni I, Meiden O, Dolev E, Morgenstern D, et al. Anterior knee-pain syndrome. Adolesc Med 2007;18(1):192-220.
[8] Galanty HL, et al. Anterior knee pain in adolescents. Clin J Sports Med 1994;4(3):176.
[9] Fulkerson JP. Dignosis and treatment of patients with patellofemoral pain. Am J Sports Med 2002;30:447-56.
[10] Sandow MJ, Goodfellow JW. The natural history of anterior knee pain in adolescents. J Bone Joint Sur 1985;67-B(1):36.
[11] Milgrom C, Finestone A, Shlamkivitch N, Giladi M, Radin E. Anterior knee pain cause by overactivity: a long-term perspective. Clin Orthop Relat Res 1996;331:256-60
[12] Blond L, Hansen L. Patellofemoral pain syndrome in athletes: A 5.7 year retrospective follow-up study of 250 athletes. Acta Orthopaedica Belgica 1998;64:393.
[13] Paluska SA, McKeag DB. Using patellofemoral braces for anterior knee pain. Phys Sportsmed 1999;27(8):81.
[14] Gholve PA, Scher DM, Khakharia S, Widmann RF, Green DW. Osgood-Schlatter syndrome. Curr Opin Pediatr 2007;19(1):44-50.

Submitted: May 01, 2009.
Revised: June 15, 2009.
Accepted: June 21, 2009.

In: Public Health Yearbook 2009
Editor: Joav Merrick
ISBN: 978-1-61668-911-7

Chapter 41

CRICKET INJURIES

Dilip R Patel*, MD, FAAP, FACSM, FAACPDM, FSAM
Department of Pediatrics and Human Development, Michigan State University College of Human Medicine, East Lansing, Michigan, United States of America

Abstract

Cricket is a popular sport worldwide. It is a non-contact sport, with moderate dynamic and low static demands on the energy systems. Many children and adolescents begin playing cricket at an early age and continue to participate for a number of years with increasing level of intensity. The incidence of injuries varies depending upon the age of the player and level of competition. Between 30% and 50% of the players report some injury during peak season. The most common significant injury in cricket is to the thoraco-lumbar spine in fast bowlers, because of repetitive, rotation, extension, and lateral flexion movements. Other acute injuries include soft tissue contusions, abrasions, and eye injuries from impact with the ball. Overuse injuries include shoulder impingement, elbow overuse injuries, patellar tendinitis, and stress fractures. This article reviews the epidemiology, mechanisms and prevention of cricket injuries in youth.

Keywords: Cricket, fast bowling, lumbar spondylolysis, thrower's shoulder.

Introduction

Cricket is one of the most popular sports in the world and its origin dates back to 1150 in England (1). Marylebone Cricket Club in England is the official governing body for cricket. Cricket is a ball and bat field sport played by two opposing teams with 11 players each. The bat is made of wood, the length not exceeding 38 inches, and the ball is hard, has a cork

* Correspondence: Professor Dilip R Patel, MD, MD, FAAP, FACSM, FSAM, FAACPDM, Department of Pediatrics and Human Development, Michigan State University College of Human Medicine, Kalamazoo Center for Medical Studies, Kalamazoo, Michigan, MSU/ KCMS/ Pediatrics, 1000, Oakland Drive, Kalamazoo, MI 49008-1284 United States. Tel: 269-337-6450; Fax: 269-337-6474; E-mail: patel@kcms.msu.edu

foundation covered with leather. There are two wickets, one each at either end of the pitch, consisting of three stumps, each 28 inches high placed side by side. Each team can play two innings, and tournament matches last for three days or five days. One day matches with limited overs are also popular. In many countries it is a national pastime, and is played in organized tournaments, as well as recreationally by children and adults alike in streets and parks. In spite of such popularity of the sport, especially among children and adolescents, only limited data have been published regarding injuries in cricket in general, and in youth in particular.

Demands of the sport

Cricket is a non-contact sport, with moderate dynamic and low static demands on the energy systems. Depending up on the level of competition, many cricketers sustain high level of stress, especially during season, accounting for an increased incidence of overuse injuries (2). It is mostly outdoor sport, however indoor cricket is especially popular in New Zealand and Australia. Energy expenditure in college players has been estimated to range from 700-1,000 kJ/m2/hour (3). During the play of the game there are repeated periods of short (lasting less than 20 seconds) high intensity activity utilizing anaerobic energy pathways (3).

Many children and adolescents begin playing cricket at an early age, and continue to participate for a number of years, with increasing level of intensity. The most common and significant overuse injury is to the thoraco-lumbar spine in fast bowlers, due to repetitive, rotation, extension, and lateral flexion movements during bowling (1,4-9). The peak ground reaction forces (when the foot hits the ground during running) can be as high as four to nine times the body weight of the bowler, and this load is transmitted to the spine (10). Fast bowlers are particularly prone to developing back pain and lumbar stress injury leading to spondylolysis and other spine abnormalities (4,5,7,8,10-12). Bartlett et al in their review of the biomechanics of fast bowling presented a detailed analysis of the three types of fast bowling techniques namely, side-on, front-on, and mixed types (10). This and other studies suggest that the mixed type technique used by many fast bowlers is the most stressful to the spine, leading to back pain and thoracolumbar abnormalities. Other factors contributing to back and spine overuse injuries in bowlers include bowling too many overs, poor lumbar and hamstring flexibility, poor lower body strength, poor bowling technique, greater release height, obesity, and poor pre-season conditioning (13).

Stretch has reviewed the biomechanics, kinematics, and kinetics of batting in cricket (3). Batting requires highly developed neuromotor skills, dynamic interceptive abilities, and visual-spatial processes.

Epidemiology

Perhaps the first documented injury resulting in death in cricket was that of Frederick, Prince of Wales, who died of complications from a ball hitting his head, in 1751 (13-15). Fatalities are fortunately very rare in cricket. Stretch reported on the seasonal incidence and nature of musculoskeletal injuries in schoolboy cricketers in South Africa (16). The author noted seasonal incidence of injuries in all players to be 49%. In this study the most common injuries were to the back and trunk (33.3%); followed by upper extremities (24.6%), and lower extremities (22.8%). Bowlers were the most likely to be injured (47.6%), compared to the batsmen (29.8%), and fielders (22.8%). There was no difference in the number of injuries sustained during practice or match. A significant number of injuries were recurrent injuries (36.8%). Back injuries were most common in bowlers, while those to upper extremities in fielders, and to head and face in batsmen. The incidence of injuries in schoolboy cricketers was similar to that for club and provincial cricketers (16, 17).

Finch reported that cricket injuries accounted for 4% of all sports-related injuries seen in the hospital emergency departments in Australia; making it the eighth commonest cause of sports-related injuries seen in emergency departments (13). These were acute musculoskeletal injuries requiring emergency visit, and thus do not account for many injuries not seen as emergencies, and the vast majority of cricket injuries are not severe.

Acute injuries can result from direct impact from a ball or bat, collision with another player, or a fall and hitting the ground (13,16,17). Some of the risk factors that contribute to increased likelihood of acute direct impact trauma include young age, low level of skill, novice player with little experience, and failure to use appropriate protective equipment (13). The incidence of recurrent injuries range from 20% to 30 % in some studies, suggesting a need for proper rehabilitation of initial injuries (16,18). The recovery time for the majority of typical musculoskeletal injuries range from 1 to 7 days (16). During a given season relatively more injuries tend to occur during early part when players are not best conditioned, as well as toward the end of the season when there are too many matches scheduled over a short period of time (16).

Injuries

A wide range of injuries, from acute to overuse, and mild to severe, has been recognized in cricket; overuse injuries, especially in fast bowlers have been studied most extensively, while most other injuries have been described largely as case reports (see table 1). Lumbar spondylolysis, seen commonly in fast bowlers, can be career limiting or career ending for the fast bowler. It is even more significant in the adolescent players during their growth period. Many authors have reported on this and other spinal abnormalities in fast bowlers (1,4,6-9,19). Hardcastle studied a group of 16 to 18 year old fast bowlers, and found a high incidence of back pain associated with radiological abnormality; pars interarticularis defect in 54%, and disc degeneration in 63% (19). Annear examined former fast bowlers and found a significantly higher incidence of spondylolysis and disc degeneration detected on radiological imaging (4). Bowling also stresses the shoulder and many players develop overuse injury of shoulder, often referred to as the “thrower’s shoulder” (11). The underlying pathophysiology involves rotator cuff inflammation, edema, and impingement, often associated with glenohumeral instability. The bowler complaints of activity related shoulder pain, particularly throwing or other overhead activity. There is a loss of throwing length, and overarm throwing may be too painful to continue (11).

Other overuse injuries are less common. Overuse injuries of the lower extremities, such as, shin splints, anterior knee pain, patellar tendinitis, and stress fractures of tibia, fibula or metatarsals, may result from considerable amount of running involved (13,20). The wicketkeeper may develop knee pain, tendinitis, and patellofemoral syndrome from standing for long hours in squatting position; and chronic injury to hands from catching the balls (20). Splitting or chronic abrasive injury of the skin over the fingers has been described in bowlers, resulting from repeated friction and pressure from the seam of the ball in spin bowlers (13,21).

Table 1. Cricket injuries

Acute	Overuse	Other
Rotator cuff tear Finger and hand injuries (contusions, lacerations, finger fractures and dislocations) Fracture of forearm (radius or ulna) Shoulder dislocation Acute musculotendionus tears (quadriceps, hamstrings, supraspinatus, gastrocnemius) Eye injuries (detached retina, orbital fracture, ruptured globe, traumatic iritis, hyphaema, corneal abrasion, laceration, eyeball contusion, chronic glaucoma)	Lumbar spondylolysis and spondylolisthesis Disc degeneration Nonspecific anterior knee pain Patellar tendinitis Tibial stress syndrome (shin splints) Stress factures (tibia, fibula, metatarsals) Talotibial exostoses Heel contusions Shoulder impingement Glenohumeral instability Rotator cuff tendinitis Biceps tendinitis Elbow overuse injuries	Blunt chest trauma Head trauma Facial fractures Temperomandibular dislocation Splenic rupture Pneumomediatinum Splitting or wearing of the finger skin Osteoarthritis of finger joints and knee

Data from Refs. [1, 4-9,13,16-30,33,34].

Acute injuries can occur from impact with another player, ground, ball or bat. Head injury, eye injury, facial fractures, and dental injuries can result from direct impact from the ball (22-25). The batsman is especially vulnerable to these types of injuries. Eye injuries, though not common, are some of the most serious injuries in cricket, particularly in indoor cricket (5,22,24,26). Blunt impact to the chest causing death from cardiac arrhythmias and myocardial infarction have been reported (27). Ball impact to abdomen resulting in intra-abdominal injuries, and traumatic splenic rupture from impact to the ground or from ball can occur (28). Injuries to testis can occur from ball impact. Finger injuries including contusions, abrasions, lacerations, fractures, and dislocations have been reported, more commonly in indoor cricket (29). Acute musculotendionus strains (such as hamstring, quadriceps, gastrocnemius) can occur while running between wickets, and suddenly stopping (13). Acute sprains of ligaments of ankle and knee are seen associated with running. Such injuries are more common in indoor cricket. Rare case reports of pneumothorax and pneumomediastinum have been found in literature (30).

Prevention

General, non-specific preventive measures, applicable to many sports and exercise activities, should also be followed by cricketers. These include maintaining overall conditioning; including cardiovascular, as well as muscular strength, flexibility, and endurance (13,31). Proper warm-up, and stretching should be routinely done. Appropriate development of skills is especially important for the young cricketers. Robertson has described a special program for children; developed in Australia, called Kanga cricket (32). This type of cricket is modified to suit the needs of beginner children. The ball is softer and smaller, and the bat and stumps are also modified to be lightweight. Rules have also been modified. Preventive measures specifically for the fast bowlers should include correct bowling technique, limitation of number of overs during a specified time, avoiding mixed style of bowling, and early and prompt recognition and treatment of back pain or underlying spinal problem. Appropriate use of mouth-guards, visors, boxes, gloves, helmets, padding, and testicular cups is recommended to prevent injuries, however, children and adolescents playing cricket in an informal setting are less likely to use protective equipment and thus may be more vulnerable to preventable injuries. Thus proper awareness and education in this area will be useful.

Conclusion

Cricket is a widely popular sport played by youth in many countries at various levels of tournaments. It is generally a safe sport and many players begin at an early age. Fortunately severe injuries are rare. However a number of overuse and acute injuries have been reported in cricket. Back pain and spinal problems are common and significant injuries in fast bowlers. Many general and specific measures can be taken to prevent cricket injuries.

Acknowledgments

This article is adapted from author's previous works: Patel DR, Stier B, Luckstead EF. Major international sport profile. Pediatr Clin N Am 2002;49:769-792. Used with permission.

References

[1] Hardcastle P. Lumbar pain in fast bowlers. Aust Fam Physician 1991;20:943.

[2] Bartlett RM. The science and medicine of cricket: an overview and update. J Sports Sci 2003;21(9):733-52.

[3] Stretch RA, Bartlett R, Davids K. A review of batting in men's cricket. J Sport Sci 2000;28:931.

[4] Annear PT, Chareka TMH, Foster DH, Hardcastle PH. Pars interarticularis stress and disc degeneration in cricket's potent strike force: the fast bowler. Aust NZ J Surg 1992;62:768.

[5] Engstrom CM, Walker DG. Pars interarticularis stress lesions in the lumbar spine of cricket fast bowlers. Med Sci Sports Exerc 2007;39(1):28-33.

[6] Elliott B, Khangure M. Disk degeneration and fast bowling in cricket: an intervention study. Med Sci Sports Exerc 2002;34(11):1714-8.

[7] Orchard JW, James T, Portus M, Kountouris A, Dennis R. Fast bowlers in cricket demonstrate up to 3- to 4-week delay between high workloads and increased risk of injury. Am J Sports Med 2009;37:6.
[8] Burnett AF, Khangure MS, Elliott BC, Foster DH, Marshall RN, Hardcastle PH. Thoracolumbar disc degeneration in young fast bowlers in cricket: a follow-up study. Clin Biomech 1996;11(6):305-10.
[9] Foster D, John D, Elliott B, Akland T, Finch K.Back injuries in fast bowlers in cricket: a prospective study. Br J Sports Med 1989;23:150.
[10] Bartlett RM, Stockill NP, Elliot BC, Burnett AI. The biomechanics of fasting bowling in men's cricket: a review. J Sport Sci 1996;14:403.
[11] Drescher WR, Falliner A, Zantop T, Oehlert K, Petersen W, Hassenpflug J. Br J Sports Med 2004;38(4):E14.
[12] Elliott BC. Back injuries and the fast bowler in cricket. J Sports Sci 2000;18:983.
[13] Finch CF, Elliott BC, McGrath AC. Measures to prevent cricket injuries. Sports Med 1999;28:263.
[14] Stretch RA. Cricket injuries: A longitudinal study of the nature of injuries to South African cricketers. Br J Sports Med 2003;37(3):250-3.
[15] Brasch R. How sports begin. Longman, UK: Camberwell, 1971.
[16] Stretch RA. Seasonal incidence and nature of injuries in schoolboy cricket. S Afr Med J 1995;85:1182.
[17] Stretch RA. The incidence and nature of injuries in first-league and provincial cricketers. S Afr Med J 1993;83:339.
[18] Smith C. Sports injuries encountered on a first class international cricket tour. Sports Med 1991;6:10.
[19] Hardcastle P, Annear P, Foster DH, Chakera TM, McCormick C, Khangure M, Burnett A. Spinal abnormalities in young fast bowlers. J Bone Joint Surg 1992;74B:421.
[20] Corrigan AB. Cricket injuries. Aust Fam Physician 1984;13:558.
[21] Agosta J. Epidemiology of podiatric sports medicine clinic. Austr Podiatrist 1994;28:93.
[22] Aburn N. Eye injuries in indoor cricket at Wellington Hospital: A survey from January 1987 to June 1989. NZ Med J 1990;103:454.
[23] Fong LP. Sports-related eye injuries. Med J Aust 1994;160:743.
[24] Forward GR. Indoor cricket injuries. Med J Aust 1998;148:560.
[25] Lim LH, Moore MH, Trott JA, David DJ. Sports-related facial fractures: A review of 37 patients. Aust N Z J Sug 1993;63:784.
[26] Jones NP, Tullo AB. Severe eye injuries in cricket. Br J Sports Med 1986;20:178.
[27] Heymann TD. It's not cricket! Myocardial infarction following non-penetrating blunt chest trauma. Br J Clin Pract 1994;48:338.
[28] Du Toit DF, Rademan F. Splenic rupture caused by a cricket ball: A case report. S Afr Med J 1987;71:796.
[29] Sadleir LG, Horne G. Indoor cricket finger injuries. NZ Med J 1990;103:3.
[30] Clements MR, Hamilton DV. Pneumomediastinum as a complication of fast bowling in cricket. Postgrad Med J 1982;58:435.
[31] Antoun JS, Lee KH. Sports-related maxillofacial fractures over an 11-year period. J Oral Maxillofac Surg 2008;66(3):504-8.
[32] Robertson I. Aussie sports and organized sport. Canberra, Aust: Aust Sports Commission, 1982.
[33] Bell P. Cricket: Injury in long trousers. Br J Sports Med 1999;33:151.
[34] Wani AA, Ramzan AU, Tariq R, Kirmani AR, Bhat AR. Head injury in children due to cricket ball scenario in developing countries. Pediatr Neurosurg 2008;44(3):204-7.
[35] Orchard JW. Newman D, Stretch R, Frost W, Mansingh A, Leipus A. Method for injury surveillance in international cricket. Br J Sports Med 2005;39(4):E22.

Submitted: May 02, 2009.
Revised: June 17, 2009.
Accepted: June 21, 2009.

In: Public Health Yearbook 2009
Editor: Joav Merrick

ISBN: 978-1-61668-911-7

Chapter 42

MARTIAL ARTS INJURIES IN YOUTH

Dilip R Patel*[*], MD, FAAP, FACSM, FAACPDM, FSAM
Department of Pediatrics and Human Development, Michigan State University College of Human Medicine, East Lansing, Michigan, United States of America

ABSTRACT

Martial arts are becoming increasingly popular among children and adolescents in many countries. Thousands of young children and adolescents are involved in taekwondo, karate, mixed martial arts, and other less well-known disciplines. Increasing media coverage has drawn attention to this growing trend and its potential benefits for youth. Proponents cite many benefits from participation, including self-defense, cardiovascular fitness, flexibility, improved self-esteem, and improved concentration. Some studies have reported on the role of martial arts in treating psychological and behavioral disorders. Injury rates have decreased with increasing awareness and preventive measures, such as padded floors and mandatory equipment. This article provides an overview of medical aspects of martial arts participation, injuries, and prevention strategies.

Keywords: Alolescence, martial arts, taekwondo, concussion, karate.

---

[*] Correspondence: Professor Dilip R Patel, MD, MD, FAAP, FACSM, FSAM, FAACPDM, Department of Pediatrics and Human Development, Michigan State University College of Human Medicine, Kalamazoo Center for Medical Studies, Kalamazoo, Michigan, MSU/ KCMS/ Pediatrics, 1000, Oakland Drive, Kalamazoo, MI 49008-1284 United States. Tel: 269-337-6450; Fax: 269-337-6474; E-mail: patel@kcms.msu.edu

INTRODUCTION

Millions of children and adults participate in martial arts, and the trend is evident for increasing participation. In the United States 1.5 to 2 million Americans participate in martial arts, of whom approximately 20% are children (1,2).

There are many styles of martial arts, which have had their origins in different countries, and their popularity varies in different parts of the world, for instance, tae kwon do and hap ke do in Korea, judo in Japan, and kung fu in China (2-5). Taekwondo is popular among youth, the average age of competitors being 16-17 years (3). Reasons cited for training in the varied disciplines include self defense, cardiovascular fitness, flexibility, improved self-esteem and concentration.

DEMANDS OF THE SPORT

Most martial arts have some common physiologic, neuromuscular, and biomechanical demands. Both, aerobic and anaerobic energy pathways are important. In typical tournament settings each round can last 2 (tae kwon do) to 3 (karate) minutes with either single or double elimination fights. There may also be three consecutive rounds each lasting 2 minute or 3 minute (4,5). Martial arts is demanding in terms of constant practice and disciplined training. Concentration, speed, visual perceptual abilities, flexibility, and neuromuscular coordination are all critical attributes for martial arts participants (5).

INJURIES

Martial arts injuries have been documented in medical literature since the late sixties, when Streeton reported (6) a case of haemoglobinuria after karate exercises involving considerable trauma to the hands. Potential determinants of injuries in martial arts include: lack of appropriate supervision, inadequate and incorrect training, inappropriate aggression, male sex, younger age, inexperience, and improper use of equipment (1,3,5-13). In his study of trauma epidemiology in the martial arts, Birrer (13) made several observations: minor contusions of the upper and lower extremities, particularly of the digits, are the most common; lower belt ranks and younger ages are associated with increased risk of injury; the use of protective equipment reduces the number and severity of injuries; and men have higher injury rates and severity than women (13). His data included injuries from all types of martial arts activities, supervised and informal unsupervised sparring.

Fatal injuries, though rare in youth, have been reported in adults. The first reported deaths occurred in three trainees secondary to anterior chest wall trauma (14). Since then several fatalities have been documented (9-15). A number of life-threatening injuries have also been reported, including some associated with prolonged disability (16-18). The most common injuries are minor acute soft tissue injuries (see table 1). In addition, many unusual acute and chronic injuries have been documented as listed in table 2 (19-38).

Table 1. Most common martial arts injuries

– Concussions
– Acute soft tissue contusion of extremities
– Overuse tendinitis
– Sprains and dislocations of fingers
– Abrasions

Injuries occur more frequently and are more severe in tournaments (10,12,39-41). Injuries occur in nearly 1 of every 4 matches in the competition setting, and preventive techniques have been shown to reduce this rate (42,43). Zemper estimated that the magnitude of severity increased 3 to 20 times in tournaments (12). In tournament matches, head and neck injury rates increase dramatically equaling and often outnumbering injuries to the extremities and trunk (10,13,39,41,43-45). This injury pattern is the opposite in non-tournament settings where extremity injury (especially lower extremity) predominates (3,13,46). Some studies suggest that the risk for significant head injury in competitive situations approaches or exceeds the rate for other sports such as American football (12,42). A clear association exists between repeated concussions and a decline in the ability to process information efficiently; the full significance of these findings on the adolescent or pre-adolescent athlete have not been fully elucidated (2,5,8,48-51).

Several investigators have identified younger age and inexperience as risk factors for injury in the martial arts (9,13,15,39,41,52). Incidence and severity of injuries increase in frequency throughout the first two years of participation (13).

The incidence of injuries varies across studies, and studies are difficult to compare, mainly because of methodological differences. In 1988, Birrer reported an injury rate of 16.9 per 100,000 participants per year placing it eighth among various sports (basketball = 188, American football =16, aquatic=46, lacrosse=39.5, wrestling=26, sledding=24.6, dancing=18.8) (1). In 1996, Birrer again suggested that martial arts injuries compared favorably with other sports, with injury rates less than that for golf or common exercise (13).

The average injury rate in martial arts of 3.5 injuries per 1000 participants per year, was less than golf (5.4), general exercise (6.9), gymnastics (15.6), wrestling (22.9) and American football (74.6) (13). Zemper and Pieter found that the 'time loss' injury rates among college students placed taekwondo third for both males and females (12).

In the United States, data from the National Electronic Injury Surveillance System (NEISS) estimated the incidence of injury to be 8.2 per 100,000 population per year based on injuries presenting to emergency facilities (15). Peak injury rates occurred in post-pubertal males and females in the 5-14 (16.5 injuries/ 100,000 population/ year) and 15-24 (19.2 injuries/ 100 000 population per year) year age groups. Birrer and the NEISS collected surveillance data that included all forms of martial arts (13,15).

Table 2. Relatively less frequent martial arts injuries

Head, neck, and face	• Severe head and neck injuries (19) • Scalp lacerations, skull fractures • Epistaxis • Tooth avulsions • Corneal abrasions • Stroke from neck-holding maneuver (17) • Carotid artery occlusion following a punch (16) • Blinding choroidal rupture (20) • Orbital blowout fractures (55) • Malar fractures
Upper extremity	• Fractures of thumb and fingers (13,21,46) • Nail avulsions (9) • Displaced type I coronoid fracture of left elbow (22) • Coracoid process fracture (23) • Segmental perineural and interfascicular fibrosis of the dorsal branch of the ulnar nerve • "Karate-kid finger" (24) • Dorsal dislocation of the distal end of the ulna (25) • Long thoracic nerve and dorsal scapular nerve injuries (26) • Shoulder dislocation (26) • Multiple aneurysms of both hands (27) • Kienbock's disease (28) • Lateral epicondylitis and overuse syndromes (29)
Lower extremity	• Metatarsal fractures (10) • Growth plate injuries • Sequential stress fractures of tibia (30) • Complete avulsion of hamstring tendons (38) • Osteochondral fracture of lateral femoral condyle (31) • Pelvic fracture (32) • Calcaneal apophysitis (33) • Anterior compartment syndrome • Peroneal nerve injury
Chest, abdomen, and groin	• Anterior chest impact and death (13,14) • Abdominal contusions • Winding blow to the solar plexus (55) • Liver laceration (34) • Posttraumatic recurrent hepatic alveolar echinococcosis (35) • Spleen rupture (14) • Total transection of the pancreas • Costochondritis • Rib fractures • Pneumothorax • Mediastinal emphysema (36) • Superficial thrombophlebitis of the chest wall (37) • Testicular injury

PREVENTION OF INJURIES

Recommendations for prevention of injuries in the martial arts have focused on two areas, namely, protective equipment and improved training techniques. As early as 1977, McLatchie showed that the appropriate use of protective equipment reduced the frequency of injury from 1 in 4 to 1 in 22 (43,54) The use of extensive equipment has been considered by some to be too restrictive for the participants and less appealing to the spectators (42). Over the past two decades numerous studies of various types of protective equipment have shown them to be highly effective in reducing the number and severity of injuries to martial arts participants (13,39,42,43). In fact, most injuries occur while neither the attacker nor the defender is wearing the protective gear (13). As a result, certain types of protective equipment have become standard, while the use of others remains optional for the individual participant.

Protective equipment changes the character of injuries sustained in the martial arts, for instance, use of knuckle pads reduced finger and hand injuries, decreased the severity of head injuries, and increased the frequency of minor head injuries (42). Schwartz reported that padded extremities may promote an increased use of force by the attacker (50). Based on this finding, a number of authors have raised the concern that protective equipment such as gloves and foot pads may protect the attacker more than the defender (3,9,13).

The use of head gear seems to protect the soft tissues and bones of the face (13,39,42). One of the largest insurers of the martial arts in the United States requires the use of headgear if insurance is to be in force during free-sparing (11). Since repeated head trauma, even apparently minor, could have lasting neuropsychological consequences, head contact is not recommended in children (9,10).

Other suggested ways to make martial arts safer include padded floors and mandatory use of a mouth protector because it reduces internal mouth and tooth injuries, and also the severity of concussions from blows to the mouth and jaw (8-10,55,56).

The other area receiving interest in preventing injuries is the level and method of training. Several studies suggest that inexperience (especially less than one year) and younger age were associated with the highest rates and severity of injury (9,10,13,41,42). Inexperience is thought to increase the risk of injury for several reasons, including poor attacking and blocking techniques (10).

Other factors also influence injury rates during informal sparring and competitions. Unsupervised activity is associated with increased injuries. Improved medical care, including prefight clearance guidelines, standards for return to activity after injury, and required medical coverage for tournaments would maximize safety. Uniform standards for instructors, referees, and physicians have also been recommended (13).

CONCLUSION

The various forms of martial arts are becoming increasingly popular among children and adolescents in many countries. Despite the large number of participants, there is only limited information available on the risks and benefits for youth participants. Minor musculoskeletal injuries are common, while head injuries pose the greatest risk of permanent harm (2,4,5,56,57). Deaths from participation have been reported. There is an increasing anecdotal evidence that martial arts training improves both cardiovascular fitness and psychological well-being, but standardized, prospective trials studying its effects on common problems such as aggression and attention disorders are lacking. Appropriately supervised participation in martial arts is relatively safe, and few injuries result, most are of minor nature. Interested children and adolescents, therefore, should be supported in their participation, and will benefit from it. At the same time they should be educated about proper injury prevention strategies.

Acknowledgments

This article is adapted from author's previous works: Patel DR, Stier B, Luckstead EF. Major international sport profile. Pediatr Clin North Am 2002;49:769-92. Used with permission.

References

[1] Birrer RB, Halbrook SP. Martial arts injuries: The results of a five year national survey. Am J Sports Med 1988;16:408.
[2] Pieter W. Martial arts injuries. Med Sport Sci 2005;48:59-73.
[3] Zetaruk MD, Violan MA, Zurakowski D, Micheli LJ. Injuries in martial arts: a comparison of five styles. Br J Sports Med 2005;39:29-33.
[4] Buse GJ. No holds barred sport fighting: A 10-year review of mixed martial arts competition. Br J Sports Med 2006;40:169-72.
[5] Terry CM. The martial arts. Phys Med Rehabil Clin North Am 2006;17(3):645-76.
[6] Streeton JA, Melb MB. Traumatic hemoglobinuria caused by karate exercise. Lancet 1967;2:191.
[7] Chuang TY, Lieu DK. A parametric study of the thoracic injury potential of basic tae kwon do kicks. J Biomech Eng 1992;114:346.
[8] Barua N, Roosen A. Martial arts injuries prevention and management. Ramsbury, UK: Crosswood Press, 2005.
[9] Oler M, Tomson W, Pepe D, Yoon D, Branoff R, Branch J. Morbidity and mortality in the marital arts: A warning. J Truama 1991;31:251.
[10] Pieter W, Zemper ED. Incidence of reported cerebral concussions in adult tae kwon do athletes. J R Soc Health 1998;118:272.
[11] Yard EE, Knox CL. Pediatric martial arts injuries presenting to emergency departments. United States 1990-2003. J Sci Med Sport 2007;10(4):219-26.
[12] Zemper ED, Pieter W. Injury rates during the 1988 U.S. Olympic teams trials for tae kwon do. Br J Sports Med 1989;23:161.
[13] Birrer RB. Trauma epidemiology in the martial arts: the results of an eighteen-year international survey. Am J Sport Med 1996;24:S72.
[14] Schmidt RJ. Fatal anterior chest trauma in karate trainers. Med Sci Sport Exerc 1975;7:59.
[15] National Electronic Injury Surveillance System. Washington, DC: US Consumer Safety Commission, Volumes 2-18, 1979-1994.
[16] Blumenthal DT, Riggs JE. Carotid occlusion following a karate punch to the neck. Mil Med 1996;161:562.
[17] McCarron MO, Patterson J, Duncan R. Stroke without dissection from a neck holding maneuver in martial arts. Br J Sports Med 1997;31:346.
[18] Wos W, Puzio J, Opala G. Traumatic internal carotid artery thrombosis following karate blow. Pol Przegl Chir 1977;49:1271.
[19] Aotsuka A, Kojima S. Furamoto H, et al. Punch drunk syndrome due to repeated karate kicks and punches. Rinsho Shinkeigaku 1990;30:1243.

[20] Mars JS, Pimenides D. Blinding choroidal rupture in karate. Br J Sports Med 1995;29:273.
[21] Crosby AC. The hands of karate experts: Clinical and radiological findings. Br J Sports Med 1985;19:41.
[22] Liu SH, Henry M, Bowen R. Complications of type 1 coronoid fractures in competitive athletes: a report of two cases and review of the literature. J Shoulder Elbow Surg 1996;5:223.
[23] Cottalorda J, Allard D, Dutour N, Chavrier Y. Fracture of the coracoid process in an adolescent. Injury 1996;27:436.
[24] Chiu DTW. "Karate kid" finger. Plast Reconstr Surg 1993;91:362.
[25] Russo MT, Maffuli N. Dorsal dislocation of the distal end of the ulna in a judo player. Acta Orthop Belg 1991;57:442.
[26] Jerosch J, Castro WHM, Geske B. Damage of the long thoracic and dorsal scapular nerve after traumatic shoulder dislocation: case report and review of literature. Acta Orthop Belg 1990;56:625.
[27] Vayssairat M, Priollet P, Capron L, Hagege A, Housset E. Does karate injure blood vessels of the hand? Lancet 1984;2:529.
[28] Szabo RM, Grennspan A. Diagnosis and clinical findings of Kienbock's disease. Hand Clin 1993;9:399.
[29] Tondeur M, Haentjens M, Piepsz A, Ham HR. Muscular injury in a child diagnosed by 99mTc-MDP bone scan. Eur J Nuc Med 1989;15:328.
[30] Ariyoshi M, Nagata K, Kubo M, Sato K, Inoue A. Three stress fractures at different sites in the same tibia: a case report. Acta Orthoped Scand 1997;68:406.
[31] Mbubaegbu CE, Percy AJL. Femoral osteochondral facture: a non-contact injury in martial arts? A case report. Br J Sports Med 1994;28:203.
[32] Birrer RB, Robinson T. Pelvic fracture following karate kick. NY State J Med 1991;11:503.
[33] Wirtz PD, Vito GR, Long DH. Calcaneal apophysitis (Sever's disease) associated with tae kwon do injuries. Am J Podiatr Med Assoc 1988;78:474.
[34] Cantwell JD, King Jr. JT. Karate chops and liver lacerations. JAMA 1973;224:1424.
[35] Sato N, Namieno T, Takahashi H, Yamashita K, Matsuhisa T, Uchino J. A long surviving patient with recurrences of hepatic alveolar echinococcosis after traumatic intra-abdominal rupture. J Gastroent 1996;31:885.
[36] Matsushima T, Yoneyama H, Yano T. Spontaneous mediastinal emphysema caused by strained utterance: Is it characteristic of the Japanese? Chest 1995;108:885.
[37] Schleuter AJ, Al-Jurf AS, Lentz SR. Kung fu phlebitis: An unusual presentation of Mondor's disease. Am J Hematol 1996;52:66.
[38] Kurosawa H, Nakasita K, Nakasita H, et al. Complete avulsion of the hamstring tendons from the ischial tuberosity: a report of two cases sustained in judo. Br J Sports Med 1996;30:72.
[39] McLatchie GR. Analysis of karate injuries sustained in 295 contests. Injury 1976;8:132.
[40] Siana JE, Borum P, Kryger H. Injuries in tae kown do. Br J Sports Med 1986;20:165.
[41] Stricevic MV, Patel MR, Okazaki T, et al. Historical perspective and injuries sustained in national and international tournament competitions. Am J Sports Med 1983;11:320.
[42] Johanssen HV, Noerregaard FOH. Prevention of injury in karate. Br J Sports Med 1988;22:113.
[43] McLatchie GR, Morris EW. Prevention of karate injuries: A progress report. Br J Sports Med 1977;11:78.
[44] Tuominen R. Injuries in national karate competitions in Finland. Scan J Med Sci Sports 1995;5:44.
[45] Noerregaard FOH, Johannsen HV. Pattern of injuries in Danish karate championships. Ugeskr Laeger 1986;148:1785. [Danish]
[46] Hirata K. Injuries of karate in Japan. Jpn J Educ Med 1967;3:123.
[47] Zemper ED, Pieter W. Injury rates in junior and senior national tae kwon do competition. Proceedings of first IOC World Congress in Sports Science. Colorado Springs: USOC; 1989:219-20.
[48] Gronwall D, Wrightson P. Delayed recovery of intellectual function after minor head injury. Lancet 1974;2:605.
[49] Rimel RW, Giordani JT, Barth JT, Boll TJ, Jane JA. Disability caused by minor head injury. Neurosurg 1981;9:221.

[50] Schwartz ML, Hudson AR, Fernie GR, et al. Biomechanical study of full-contact karate contrasted with boxing. J Neurosurg 1986;64:248.
[51] Zemper ED, Pieter W. Cerebral concussions in tae kwon do athletes. In: Hoerner EF, ed. Head and neck injuries in sports. Philadelphia, PA: Am Soc Test Materials, 1994.
[52] Birrer RB, Birrer CD. Unreported injuries in martial arts. Br J Sports Med 1983;17:131.
[53] Pieter W, Zemper ED. Injury rates in children participating in tae kwon do competition. J Trauma 1997; 43:89.
[54] McLatchie GR, Davies JE, Caulley JH. Injuries in karate: A case for medical control. J Trauma 1980;20:956.
[55] McLatchie GR. Karate and karate injuries. Br J Sports Med 1981;15:84.
[56] Woodward TW. A review of the effects of martial arts practice on health. WMJ 2009;108(1):40-3.
[57] Burke DT, Al-Adawi S, Lee YT, Audette J. Martial arts as sport and therapy. J Sports Med Phys Fitness 2007;47(1);96-102.

Submitted: May 01, 2009.
Revised: June 15, 2009.
Accepted: June 21, 2009.

In: Public Health Yearbook 2009
Editor: Joav Merrick
ISBN: 978-1-61668-911-7

Chapter 43

Overuse Injuries in Adolescent Athletes

Dilip R Patel*, MD, FAAP, FACSM, FAACPDM, FSAM

Department of Pediatrics and Human Development, Michigan State University College of Human Medicine, East Lansing, Michigan, United States of America

Abstract

Musculoskeletal overuse injuries result from excessive stress to normal connective tissues and supporting structures. These injuries can affect bone, tendon, muscle, joint, bursa, and growth cartilage. Sport-related overuse injuries are the most common injuries seen in adolescents and account for half of all sport-related injuries in this age group. Rapid increase in the intensity and volume of physical activity is the most consistent risk factor for overuse injury. Data on other risk factors such as anatomical variations are equivocal. Most athletes present with pain localized to the affected area. Diagnosis is generally obvious based on clinical findings and routine laboratory or imaging studies are not indicated. Modification of the level of physical activity is the most important element of treatment. Other considerations in the treatment include use of anti-inflammatory and analgesic medications, therapeutic exercises, physical therapy modalities, and identification and modification of risk factors. This article reviews the general principles of diagnosis and management of overuse injuries in adolescents.

Keywords: Overuse injuries, physical therapy, apophysitis, phonophoresis.

* Correspondence: Professor Dilip R Patel, MD, MD, FAAP, FACSM, FSAM, FAACPDM, Department of Pediatrics and Human Development, Michigan State University College of Human Medicine, Kalamazoo Center for Medical Studies, Kalamazoo, Michigan, MSU/ KCMS/ Pediatrics, 1000, Oakland Drive, Kalamazoo, MI 49008-1284 United States. Tel: 269-337-6450; Fax: 269-337-6474; E-mail: patel@kcms.msu.edu

Introduction

Musculoskeletal overuse injuries result from excessive stress applied to normal tissue that most likely lead to local inflammation (1-3). Overuse injury can affect any connective or supporting structure of the body. Common injuries are listed in table 1 (1-12).

Musculoskeletal overuse injuries are the most common injuries accounting for half of all sport-related injuries in adolescents. Adolescent growth spurt affects body size, weight, height, muscle mass, and muscle strength, with direct implications for the biomechanics and mechanisms of injuries (1,8,13,14). Musculoskeletal flexibility also decreases during adolescence.

Table 1. Common overuse injuries

Injury	Examples
Apophysitis (sites of tendon attachment)	Osgood-Schlatter disease (tibial tubercle) Sever disease (posterior calcaneal) Iselin disease (5th metatarsal) Iliac crest apophysitis
Articular cartilage and subchondral bone	Juvenile osteochondritis dissecans (medial condyle of femur, patella, talus, capitellum)
Bone (stress fractures)	Low risk stress fractures (medial tibia, fibula, ribs, radius, 2nd and 3rd metatarsals) High risk stress fractures (femoral neck, anterior tibia, patella, medial malleolus, talus, tarsal navicular, 5th metatarsal, pars interarticularis)
Bursa	Subacromial bursitis, olecranon bursitis, pre patellar bursitis, pes anserine bursitis
Growth plate stress injury	Distal radial physis (Gymnast's wrist) Proximal humeral physis (Little Leaguer's shoulder)
Tendons	Rotator cuff tendonitis, iliotibial band friction syndrome, patellar tendonitis, Achilles tendonitis
Other	Lateral epicondylitis (tennis elbow) Scheueremann's disease (vertebral endplates) Idiopathic anterior knee pain Sinding-Larsen-Johansson syndrome (distal pole of patella) Medial tibial stress syndrome (shin splints) Chronic exertional compartment syndromes of the leg Plantar faciitis

Growth of the bone generally precedes that of connective tissue during adolescence resulting in a transient period of myo-osseous disproportion that contributes to relative decrease in flexibility (1,5). Bone is also still undergoing maturation and more vulnerable to stress. Overuse injuries are common in highly trained as well as the poorly conditioned beginner athlete. Also unique to adolescents is the presence of growth cartilage at the growth plate, articular surface, and apophysis, which are sites of overuse injuries.

Numerous factors have been implicated in the causation of overuse injuries (5,7,9,15,16). A rapid increase in the intensity and volume of the physical activity are the most consistent factors associated with the development of overuse injury. Other factors that may contribute to overuse injury include, inadequate sport specific training and conditioning, incorrect sport-specific techniques, and inappropriate equipment. Hard playing surface and anatomic variations of lower extremities are less consistently associated with development of overuse injuries.

DIAGNOSIS

Pain is the most common symptom and localized tenderness the most common sign of an overuse injury. In addition to the onset, duration, course, severity, character, localization, and modifying factors of the pain, the history should include information about limitation of activity and deterioration of sport performance. Inquire about other symptoms such as swelling, ability to continue to play, and need to take pain medication. Note any recent increase in the intensity, frequency and duration of the activity. Untreated an overuse injury is progressive with continued physical activity. Its clinical course is better understood in terms of increasing severity from grade 1 to grade 4 (see table 2) (2,3,7,9).

Laboratory or imaging studies are indicated rarely to rule out other causes of musculoskeletal symptoms (see table 3) (2-4,7-10,14).

Table 2. Clinical presentation of overuse injuries

Clinical feature	Severity			
	Grade 1	Grade 2	Grade 3	Grade 4
Pain onset	Several hours Following the Activity	Immediately Following the Activity	During the Activity	At the onset Of activity; Continuous
Pain duration	< 2 wk	2-3 wk	> 3 wk	> 4 wk
Tenderness	Diffuse soreness	Poorly localized	Localized to affected area	Localized to affected area
Resolution with rest	Rapid	Longer	Several weeks	May take ≥ 8 wk
Other	Athletes continue to play with pain	Most present at this stage	Deterioration of performance	Functional disability

Table 3. Differential diagnosis of overuse injuries

Bone neoplasms	Benign: Most detected as incidental findings on plain radiographs e.g. aneurysmal bone cysts, fibrous dysplasias, non-ossifying fibromas. Some present with localized pain, e.g. osteoid osteoma Malignant: Bone pain of gradual onset, dull aching, present at rest and during night highly suggestive in adolescents
Chronic pain	Chronic, intermittent, variable pain that affect many areas of the

syndromes	body. Most seen in older children and adolescents. Family history ofhypermobility syndrome may be present
Infections	Fever and other constitutional symptoms of acute onset may be present. Affected area show acute inflammatory signs
Metabolic bone disease	Constitutional signs such as poor growth, recurrent fractures, and progressive joint deformities; poor nutrition
Muscle disease	Insidious onset, progressive muscle weakness; deep tendon reflexes may be diminished; sensation preserved (except in sensory-motor diseases)
Orthopedic conditions	Signs and symptoms specific to the condition and affected areas, often characteristic
Peripheral neuropathy	Neuropathic pain and sensory and motor disturbances in the distribution of affected nerve
Psychosomatic	Multiple psychosomatic symptoms. Always a consideration in adolescents
Rheumatic diseases	Generally gradual onset. Inflammatory arthritis affecting one or more joints or other connective tissues; may present with systemic symptoms such as fever, fatigue, or weight loss. Family history may be positive.
Systemic disease	Many systemic diseases affect musculoskeletal system, usually associated with other signs and symptoms typical of the disease.
Vasculitis	Symptoms and signs vary depending upon the affected area and the extent of involvement and may include fever, petechiae, palpable purpura, abdominal pain.

Musculoskeletal ultrasonography is a useful and practical imaging modality in the evaluation of overuse injuries. In selected cases magnetic imaging resonance (MRI) scan, such as when a high risk stress fracture is suspected (17).

Management

A reduction or cessation of sport participation or physical activity is the essential first step in the treatment of overuse injury. Depending up on the severity of the injury a complete rest from sport participation from several days to weeks may be necessary. Some alternative activities not directly affecting the injured area may be continued.

Pain and inflammation are often best alleviated by local application of crushed ice (18). Crushed ice is usually applied for 15-20 minute at a time and repeated application at 30-45 minute intervals. Routine use of non-steroidal anti-inflammatory (NSAIDs) for extended periods of time remains debatable. Depending up on the severity of pain, short term use of NSAIDs is often useful. In addition to NSAIDs, physical therapy modalities can be used effectively to control pain and inflammation (18). An individualized rehabilitation program is developed and implemented by sports physical therapist or athletic trainer. Common physical therapy modalities are listed in table 4 (18).

Table 4. Therapeutic modalities

- Deep heat by ultrasound
- Iotophoresis
- Neuromuscular electrical stimulation
- Phonophoresis (application of ultrasound using anti-inflammatory or analgesic drug)
- Superficial cold such as application of crushed ice or immersion in cold water
- Superficial heat application such as moist pack or whirlpool
- Therapeutic exercises
- Transcutaneous electrical nerve stimulation

Failure to respond to conservative treatment should prompt careful assessment to rule out other causes of symptoms, and specialist consultation as appropriate. Main preventive measures include sport-specific training and conditioning, appropriate level and progression of physical activity, and identification and correction of contributing factors (3,5,7-9,19).

Conclusion

Overuse injuries are the most common sport-related injuries seen adolescents. Certain aspects of adolescent somatic and psychosocial growth and development have implications in the pathophysiology of overuse injuries seen in this age group. Diagnosis is mainly based on clinical findings. With early recognition and intervention most injuries resolve fully allowing the athlete to return to sports. Modification of the level of activity is the main consideration in treatment.

References

[1] Patel DR, Baker RJ. Musculoskeletal injuries in sports. Prim Care 2006;33:545-79.

[2] Cassas KJ, Cassettari-Wayhs A. Childhood and adolescent sports-related overuse injuries. Am Fam Physician 2006;73(6):1014-22.

[3] Adirim TA, Cheng, TL. Overview of injuries in the young athlete. Sports Med 2003;33:75-81.

[4] Cassas KJ, Cassettari-Wayhs A. Childhood and adolescent sports-related overuse injuries. Am Fam Physician 2006;73:1014-22.

[5] Emery CA. Risk factors for injury in child and adolescent sport: a systematic review of the literature. Clin J Sport Med 2003;13:256-68.

[6] Bijur PE, Trumble A, Harel Y, Overpeck MD, Jones D, Scheidt PC. Sports and recreational injuries in US children and adolescents. Arch Pediatr Adolesc Med 1995;149:1009-16.

[7] McKeag DB. Concept of overuse: the primary care aspects of overuse syndromes in sports. Prim Care 1984;11:43.

[8] Pommering TL, Kluchurosky L. Overuse injuries in adolescents. Adolesc Med State Art Rev 2007;18(1):95-120.

[9] DiFiori JP. Overuse injuries in children and adolescents. Phys Sportsmed 1999;27:75-89.
[10] Hogan KA, Gross RH. Overuse injuries in pediatric athletes. Orthop Clin North Am 2003;34:405-415.
[11] Taylor DC, Krasinski KL. Adolescent shoulder injuries: consensus and controversies. J Bone Joint Surg Am 2009;91(2):462-73.
[12] Jones GL. Upper extremity stress fractures. Clin Sports Med 2006;25(1):159-74, xi.
[13] Caine D, DiFiori J, Maffulli N. Physeal injuries in children's and youth sports: reasons for concern? Br J Sports Med 2006;40(9):749-60.
[14] Snyder RA, Koester MC, Dunn WR. Epidemiology of stress fractures. Clin Sorts Med 2006;25:37-52.
[15] Wilder RP, Shikha S. Overuse injuries: tendinopathies, stress fractures, compartment syndrome, and shin splints. Clin Sports Med 2004;23:55-81, vi.
[16] Verna RB, Sherman O. Athletic stress injuries: part I. History, epidemiology physiology, risk factors, radiology, diagnosis and treatment. Am J Orthop 2001;30:789-806.
[17] Koh ES, Lee JC, Healy JC. MRI of overuse injury in elite athletes. Clin Radiol 2007;62(11):1036-43.
[18] Chapman BL, Liebert RB, Lininger MR, Groth JJ. An introduction to physical therapy modalities. Adolesc Med 2007;18:11-23.
[19] Hergenroeder AC. Prevention of sports injuries. Pediatrics 1998;101:1057-63.

Submitted: May 02, 2009.
Revised: June 17, 2009.
Accepted: June 21, 2009.

In: Public Health Yearbook 2009
Editor: Joav Merrick

ISBN: 978-1-61668-911-7

Chapter 44

ANTERIOR CRUCIATE LIGAMENT INJURY AND LOWER EXTREMITY STRESS FRACTURES IN YOUNG FEMALE ATHLETES

Erin C Duchan, MD and
Dilip R Patel*, MD, FAAP, FACSM, FAACPDM, FSAM

Department of Pediatrics and Human Development, Michigan State University College of Human Medicine, East Lansing, Michigan and Pediatric Residency Training Program, Michigan State University Kalamazoo Center for Medical Studies, Kalamazoo, Michigan, United States of America

ABSTRACT

The objective was to investigate the differences between sexes in the two most common injuries in the young female athlete: anterior cruciate ligament injury and lower extremity stress fracture. Design: PubMed was searched for articles in the last fifteen years, from 1994-2009, with the terms "sport injuries in females," "anterior cruciate ligament injury in females," "lower extremity stress fracture," and "stress fracture in female athletes." Data: Young female athletes have a significantly increased risk of noncontact ACL injury and lower extremity stress fractures over male athletes. Studies over the last fifteen years have focused on identifying the differences between male and female athletes in mechanism of injury, biomechanics of injury, treatment and prevention strategies. Conclusion: As female participation in competitive sports increases, the physician needs to be aware of the underlying causes of increased ACL injury and lower extremity fractures and prevention strategies for these athletes.

* Correspondence: Professor Dilip R Patel, MD, MD, FAAP, FACSM, FSAM, FAACPDM, Department of Pediatrics and Human Development, Michigan State University College of Human Medicine, Kalamazoo Center for Medical Studies, Kalamazoo, Michigan, MSU/ KCMS/ Pediatrics, 1000, Oakland Drive, Kalamazoo, MI 49008-1284 United States. Tel: 269-337-6450; Fax: 269-337-6474; E-mail: patel@kcms.msu.edu

Keywords: Female athlete, anterior cruciate ligament, lower extremity stress fracture.

Introduction

The rise of female athletics over the last several decades and the passage of Title IX in the United States has contributed to increased participation of adolescent females in recreational sports. Female athletes face unique challenges that differ from their male counterparts and this can be compounded by a growing and developing body. This article reviews the two most common injuries of young female athletes: anterior cruciate ligament (ACL) injury, specifically non-contact injury, and lower extremity stress fractures.

Search strategy

A PubMed search was conducted using the key words: sport injuries in females, anterior cruciate ligament injury in females, lower extremity stress fracture, and stress fracture in female athletes. The articles were limited to English language published in the last fifteen years, between 1994 and 2009. Relevant articles were reviewed. Additional relevant articles found in the bibliography of the original articles were also reviewed.

Anterior cruciate ligament injury

Incidence

The ACL is an intra-articular ligament that functions to stabilize the knee joint by restricting excessive anterior displacement of the tibia relative to the femur and limiting rotation of the knee. Seventy percent of ACL tears are related to sports participation with the highest incidence of ACL injury occuring in sports that involve pivoting, such as soccer, basketball, and volleyball (1,2). Injury to the ACL occurs eight times more frequently in the adolescent female athlete than male adolescent athletes; the highest injury rates occur in young women aged fifteen to twenty-five years (1). Epidemiologic studies estimate that 1 of every 100 high school female athletes will sustain an ACL injury and, among collegiate athletes, this number rises to 1 in 10 (1).

Mechanism of injury

Understanding the mechanism of injury, which is similar in males and females, is necessary to understand the gender differences in injury rates. There is not a significant difference in the rate of contact ACL injuries between male and female basketball players, 0.05 and 0.02 respectively. However the rate of noncontact ACL injuries was 0.21 in female and 0.04 in male basketball players (3). In noncontact injuries, following a jump, the "position of no return" has been identified as a high-risk landing position. In addition to landing on one foot, the "position of no return" is characterized by adducted and internally rotated hips, a less flexed knee in valgus position, and an externally rotated tibia (3). In this position, the gluteus maximus and hamstrings are unable to protect the ACL. Noncontact ACL injury that does not involve jumping typically involves a sudden change of direction and deceleration with the knee extended and the foot fixed and flat (4).

Biomechanics of injury

There has been much research devoted to elucidating the reasons for the increased incidence of ACL injury in young female athletes; however, the most promising results seem to come from biomechanical differences between males and females. There are significant differences between male and female athletes when comparing hamstring strength relative to quadriceps strength (5,6). Additionally, among female athletes, those with a relative weakness of the hamstrings compared to the quadriceps were more likely to sustain an ACL injury than female athletes with decreased quadriceps strength but hamstring strength similar to male athletes (7). As the hamstrings serve to reduce the load on the ACL by reducing tibial movement, this relative weakness, compared to the quadriceps, may increase ACL strain. Additionally, female athletes have a greater tendency to land with greater lateral trunk motion and knee abduction than male athletes (8).

Anatomically, there is a significant difference in the Q-angle between females and males (5). Females were found to have larger Q-angles, which has been associated with increased tibial internal rotation, a motion that can lead to ACL injury. Females also tend to place increased stress on knee joints and the ACL when compared to their male counterparts by landing with straighter knees and hips and their feet in a pronated and flat-footed position (9). Despite the difference in landing position, there is no significant difference in foot structure between males and females (10).

There have been many investigations into the relationship between female ovulatory hormones and ACL injury; however, the results have been inconclusive. One study showed that female hormone levels at ovulation were related to increased knee joint laxity and decreased stiffness, however a separate study revealed no significant differences between menstrual cycle and biomechanical characteristics, including knee flexion and valgus motion (11,12). A small retrospective study demonstrated a significant increase in non-contact ACL injuries during the ovulatory phase, however a separate retrospective study demonstrated a greater number of ACL injuries on days 1 and 2 of the menstrual cycle (13). At this time the role of ovulatory hormones in ACL injury is unclear.

Diagnosis

Clinical examination is typically the first step in diagnosing ACL injury. The patient will often describe an injury setting consistent with ACL injury and often relates a "popping" on injury. There are a variety of physical exam maneuvers to determine the likelihood of ACL injury, however the usefulness of these tests in variable. The anterior drawer pull test is not useful in acute conditions; however, in chronic conditions it has good sensitivity and specificity, 92% and 91% respectively (14). The pivot shift test can also be useful in diagnosing ACL injury with a specificity of 98%, however this test has a poor sensitivity of 24%, thus when positive, it is useful to rule in ACL injury (14,15).

The Lachman test is the most valid test to diagnose an ACL tear, with a sensitivity of 85% and specificity of 94%, thus the Lachman test is best for ruling out an ACL rupture (14,15). Despite this, while physical exam is as effective as magnetic resonance imaging (MRI) in diagnosing ACL injury when performed by a skilled orthopedic surgeon, agreement between specialists and primary care physicians on physical exam findings is poor, with primary care physicians tending to underdiagnose ACL injury (16,17). Additionally, females tend to have more joint laxity than males in the Lachman test, potentially making the Lachman test less useful across the sexes (18). Thus, in absence of a physician experienced in Lachman test (e.g. orthopedic surgeon or sports medicine physician), MRI has become the study of choice in diagnosing ACL injury. The MRI is also often indicated and useful in assessing associated soft tissue, cartilaginous, and osseous injuries (19).

Treatment

Long-term complications of ACL injury include recurrent instability, meniscus tears, articular cartilage damage, and/or early degenerative joint disease (20). Treatment options include both reconstructive surgery and rehabilitation or rehabilitation alone. Multiple studies have evaluated the effects of treatment options on long-term complications, and have failed to demonstrate significant difference in functional outcome between the two treatment options (21-23). Studies show that the non-operatively treated group tends to recover more quickly while the surgically treated group experiences less knee instability over time, but higher rates of osteoarthritis (21-23). The Cochrane Database, however, has suggested that further randomized trials need to be conducted to confidently determine the outcome differences between surgery versus conservative treatment (21,24).

Prevention

ACL injury prevention programs are emerging throughout the United States. The basis of these programs is to teach proper biomechanics for sports, including jumping, squatting, and landing techniques. While a few studies confirmed that injury-reduction training programs significantly reduced ACL tear rate in soccer players, studies of basketball players failed to show a decrease in injury rate (25). Despite this, strength training with a focus on hamstrings may be a beneficial adjuvant to any training program (1).

Lower Extremity Stress Fractures

Incidence

Stress fractures are injuries that result from repeated application of stress that is less than that required to fracture the same bone in a single load but greater than the bone's ability to repair it through osteoblastic remodeling. These are most likely to occur following an increase in activity intensity or when transitioning into a different sport, however technique errors may also play a role in the development of stress fractures (26). Lower extremity stress fractures are the most common in skeletally immature competitive athletes; however, location of fracture varies by sport (27). The tibia, navicular, and fibula are the most common in track and field athletes and distance runners while metatarsal fractures are most common in dancers (28,29). Both tibial and fibular stress fractures tend to occur at the distal third of the long bone (26). In a large retrospective study of sports injuries presenting to a sports medicine clinic, the average age at time of stress fracture was 20.1 years; 42.6% of patients were 15-19 years of age and 34.7% were 20-24 years of age (30). In a study of National Collegiate Athletic Association (NCAA) Division 1 athletes, the incidence of stress fractures was nearly double in female athletes compared to male athletes and in college track and field athletes the incidence of stress fractures was more than four times greater in females (31,32).

Biomechanics

Anatomic and physiologic variations that may contribute to excessive microtrauma to the bone, such as leg length discrepancy, decreased lower limb muscle strength, and excessive forefoot varus have been shown to be associated with the development of lower extremity stress fractures (28,33).

Menstrual irregularities in female athletes have also been shown to increase the likelihood of developing stress fractures because low levels of estrogen lead to increased bone turnover. In a Finnish study, nearly half of the female patients with stress fractures experienced menstrual irregularities (33). A retrospective study of track-and-field athletes found that females with a history of oligomenorrhea were six times more likely to have sustained a stress fracture (34). In female athletes with menstrual dysfunction, even those with alleged normal eating behavior, bone mineral density has been found to be significantly lower in athletes with menstrual dysfunction when compared to healthy age-matched controls (35,36).

Often menstrual irregularities are closely linked to restrictive eating and low body-mass index (BMI), as negative energy balance leads to decreased estrogen production. In a study of amenorrheic athletes, body weight and duration of amenorrhea predicted bone mineral density at the femoral neck; weight alone predicted bone mineral density at the femoral shaft and tibia (36). Female track-and-field athletes who were careful about maintaining a low body weight were eight times more likely to have experienced a stress fracture (34). Physical weight-bearing activity does not completely compensate for the decreased bone mineral density in women who have amenorrhea or low body weight, and there is a threshold of physical activity beyond which the likelihood of developing a stress fracture increases (37,38).

Diagnosis

The female athlete presenting with a stress fracture will typically complain of leg pain that is associated with physical activity. There is generally bony tenderness localized over the site of the fracture. Radiographs are typically the first-line imaging modality to confirm suspicion of stress fracture, however plain films often do not show the characteristic periosteal elevation and thickening and/or bony callous until several weeks after initial onset of injury (26). Bone scintigraphy, computerized tomography (CT) scan and magnetic resonance imaging (MRI) have been used to detect a stress fracture more accurately than physical exam and earlier in the course of injury. Multiple studies have demonstrated that the sensitivity of MRI is superior to both bone scintigraphy and CT for detecting stress fractures, however bone scintigraphy is more sensitive than CT in the detection of stress injuries (39,40). Thus radiographs should be the initial study of choice as they are less expensive and are often useful in ruling out other caused of localize bone pain and tenderness. When radiographs are negative, the MRI is the study of choice in diagnosing suspected stress fractures (39,41).

Treatment

Treatment options for lower extremity stress fractures are determined by the relative risk of the stress fracture. High-risk stress fractures are those that occur at the superior aspect of the femoral neck, the anterior tibia, the patella, the fifth metatarsal (at the junction of proximal diaphysis and tuberosity), the medial malleolus, the sesmoids of the great toe, and a displaced or nonunion tarsal navicular fracture (26,42). These fractures must be managed in consultation with an orthopedic surgeon because of the increased risk of complications, including avascular necrosis, nonunion, and malunion and thus merit urgent referral to an orthopedic surgeon (26,42,43). Incomplete and nondisplaced tarsal navicular stress fractures have an 86% heal rate when treated with six to eight weeks of non-weight-bearing cast immobilization (43). Low-risk stress fractures, those occurring at all other locations in the lower extremities, can be treated conservatively with decreased to no weight-bearing until pain-free, for an average of six to seven weeks, with a gradual return to full athletic activity (27,42).

Prevention

Significantly more stress fractures occur in female athletes with disordered eating, thus physicians need to be attuned to the dietary practices and subtle weight changes in their patients. Important screening questions include asking about elimination of certain foods, intake of dairy products, and total caloric intake per day. Additionally, physicians should query female patients about their menses and physical activity level at each exam to identify at risk individuals.

The ultimate prevention strategy involves maximizing peak bone mass in the pediatric and young adult population prior to injury by maintaining adequate calcium and caloric intake as well as hormonal and energy balance. Additionally, adolescent and young adult females should perform weight-bearing exercise to optimize bone health and prevent fractures (44).

Conclusions

There are multiple areas of prevention that physicians can focus on to reduce the incidence of ACL injury and lower extremity stress fractures in young female athletes. As diagnostic modalities and treatment approaches continue to emerge for pediatric and adolescent injuries, new protocols regarding return to play and avoidance of complications will follow. Physicians need to remain vigilant in screening their female athletes for injuries with close attention to the lower extremities.

References

[1] Benjamin H. The female adolescent athlete: specific concerns. Pediatric Annals 2007;36(11):719-26.

[2] Giugliano DN, Solomon JL. ACL tears in female athletes. Phys Med Rehabil Clin N Am 2007;18(3):417-38.

[3] Ireland ML. Anterior cruciate ligament injury in female athletes: epidemiology. J Athl Train 1999;34(2):150-54.

[4] Shimokochi Y, Shultz SJ. Mechanisms of noncontact anterior cruciate ligament injury. J Athl Train 2008;43(4):396-408.

[5] Hewett TE, Myer GD, Zazulak BT. Hamstrings to quadriceps peak torque ratios diverge between sexes with increasing isokinetic angular velocity. J Sci Med Sport 2008;11(5):452-9.

[6] Palmieri-Smith RM, McLean SG, Wojtys EM. Association of quadriceps and hamstrings cocontraction with knee joint loading. J Athl Train 2009;44(3):256-63.

[7] Myer GD, Ford KR, Barber Foss KD, Liu C ,Nick TG, Hewett TE. The relationship of hamstrings and quadriceps strength to anterior cruciate ligament injury in female athletes. Clin J Sport Med 2009;19(1):3-8.

[8] Hewett TE, Torg JS, Boden BP. Video analysis of trunk and knee motion during non-contact anterior cruciate ligament injury in female athletes: lateral trunk and knee abduction motion are combined components of the injury mechanism. Br J Sports Med 2009;43(6):417-22.

[9] Griffin LY, Agel J, Albohm MJ, Arendt EA, Dick RW, Garrett WE, et al. Noncontact anterior cruciate ligament injuries: risk factors and prevention strategies. J Am Acad Orthop Surg 2000;8(3):141-50.

[10] Jenkins WL, Killian CB, Williams DS, Loudon J, Raedeke SG. Anterior cruciate ligament injury in female and male athletes: the relationship between foot structure and injury. J Am Podiatr Med Assoc 2007; 97(5):371-76.

[11] Park SK, Stefanyshyn DJ, Loitz-Ramage B, Hart DA, Ronsky JL. Changing hormone levels during the menstrual cycle affect knee laxity and stiffness in healthy female subjects. Am J Sports Med 2009;37(3):588-98.

[12] Abt JP, Sell TC, Laudner KG, McCrory JL, Loucks TL ,Berga SL, Lephart SM. Neuromuscular and biomechanical characteristics do not vary across the menstrual cycle. Knee Surg Sports Traumatol Arthrosc 2007;15(7):901-7.
[13] Slauterbeck JR, Fuzie SF, Smith MP, Clark RJ, Xu K, Starch DW, Hardy DM. The menstrual cycle, sex hormones, and anterior cruciate ligament injury. J Athl Train 2002;37(3):275-78.
[14] Benjaminse A, Gokeler A, van der Schans CP. Clinical diagnosis of an anterior cruciate ligament rupture: a meta-analysis. J Orthop Sports Phys Ther 2006;36(5):267-88.
[15] Ostrowski JA. Accuracy of 3 diagnostic tests for anterior cruciate ligament tears. J Athl Train 2006;41(1):120-21.
[16] Kocabey Y, Tetik O, Isbell WM, Atay OA, Johnson DL. The value of clinical examination versus magnetic resonance imaging in the diagnosis of meniscal tears and anterior cruciate ligment rupture. Arthroscopy 2004;20(7):696-700.
[17] Guillodo Y, Rannou N, Dubrana F, Lefevre C, Saraux A. Diagnosis of anterior cruciate ligament rupture in an emergency department. J Trauma 2008;65(5):1078-82.
[18] Medrano D Jr, Smith D. A comparison of knee joint laxity among male and female collegiate soccer players and non-athletes. Sports Biomech 2003;2(2):203-12.
[19] Moore SL. Imaging the anterior curciate ligament. Orthop Clin North Am 2002;33(4):663-74.
[20] Ireland ML, Ott SM. Special concerns of the female athlete. Clin Sports Med 2004;23(2):281-98.
[21] Linko E, Harilainen A, Malmivaara A, Seitsalo S. Surgical versus conservative interventions for anterior cruciate ligament ruptures in adults. Cochrane Database Syst Rev 2005;18(2):CD001356.
[22] Ageberg E, Thomee R, Neeter C, Silbernagel KG, Roos EM. Muscle strength and functional performance in patients with anterior cruciate ligament injury treated with training and surgical reconstruction or training only: a two to five-year followup. Arthritis Rheum 2008;59(12):1773-79.
[23] Kessler MA, Behrend H, Henz S, Stutz G, Rukavina A, Kuster MS. Function, osteoarthritis and activity after ACL-rupture: 11 years follow-up results of conservative versus reconstructive treatment. Knee Surg Sports Traumatol Arthrosc 2008;16(5):442-48.
[24] Trees AH, Howe TE, Grant M, Gray HG. Exercise for treating anterior cruciate ligament injuries in combination with collateral ligament and meniscal damage of the knee in adults. Cochrane Database Syst Rev 2007;18(3):CD005961.
[25] Prodromos CC, Han Y, Rogowski J, Joyce B, Shi K. A meta-analysis of the incidence of anterior cruciate ligament tears as a function of gender, sport, and a knee injury-reduction regimen. Arthroscopy 2007;23(12):1320-25.
[26] Logan K. Stress fractures in the adolescent athlete. Pediatric Annals 2007;36(11):738-45.
[27] Niemeyer P, Weinberg A, Schmitt H, Kreuz PC, Ewerbeck V, Kasten P. Stress fractures in adolescent competitive athletes with open physis. Knee Surg Sports Traumatol Arthrosc 2006;14(8):771-77.

[28] Bennell KL, Malcolm SA, Thomas SA, Wark JD, Brukner PD. The incidence and distribution of stress fractures in competitive track and field athletes. A twelve-month prospective study. Am J Sports Med 1996;24(2):211-17.

[29] Brukner P, Bradshaw C, Khan KM, White S, Crossley K. Stress fractures: a review of 180 cases. Clin J Sport Med 1996;6(2):85-89.

[30] Iwamoto J, Takeda T. Stress fractures in athletes: review of 196 cases. J Orthop Sci 2003;8(3):273-78.

[31] Hame SL, LaFemina JM, McAllister DR, Schaadt GW, Dorey FJ. Fractures in the collegiate athlete. Am J Sports Med 2004;32(2):446-51.

[32] Iwamoto J, Takeda T, Sato Y, Matsumoto H. Retrospective case evaluation of gender differences in sports injuries in Japanese sports medicine clinic. Gend Med 2008;5(4):405-14.

[33] Korpelainen R, Orava S, Karpakka J, Siira P, Hulkko A. Risk factors for recurrent stress fractures in athletes. Am J Sports Med 2001;29(3):304-10.

[34] Bennell KL, Malcolm SA,Thomas SA, Ebeling PR, McCrory PR, Wark JD, Brukner PD. Risk factors for stress fractures in female track-and-field athletes: a retrospective analysis. Clin J Sport Med 1995;5(4):229-35.

[35] Tomten SE, Falch JA, Birkeland KI, Hemmersbach P, Hostmark AT. Bone mineral density and menstrual irregularities. A comparative study on cortical and trabecular bone structures in runners with alleged normal eating behavior. Int J Sports Med 1998;19(2):92-97.

[36] Rencken ML, Chesnut CH, Drinkwater BL. Bone density at multiple skeletal sites in amenorrheic athletes. JAMA 1996;276(3):238-40.

[37] Pettersson U, Stalnacke B, Ahlenius G, Henriksson-Larsen K, Lorentzon R. Low bone mass density at multiple skeletal sites, including the appendicular skeleton in amenorrheic runners. Calcif Tissue Int 1999;54(2):117-25.

[38] Loud KG, Gordon CM, Micheli LJ, Field AE. Correlates of stress fractures among preadolescent and adolescent girls. Pediatrics 2005;115(4):e399-406.

[39] Gaeta M, Minutoli F, Scribano E, Ascenti G, Vinci S, Bruschetta D, et al. CT and MR imaging findings in athletes with early tibial stress injuries: comparison with bone scintigraphy findings and emphasis on cortical abnormalities. Radiology 2005;235(2):553-61.

[40] Kiuru MJ, Pihlajamaki HK, Hietanen HJ, Ahovuo JA. MR imaging, bone scintigraphy, and radiography in bone stress injuries of the pelvis and the lower extremity. Acta Radiol 2002;43(2):207-12.

[41] Berger FH, de Jonge MC, Maas M. Stress fractures in the lower extremity. The importance of increasing awareness amongst radiologists. Eur J Radiol 2007;62(1):16-26.

[42] Weinfeld SB, Haddad SL, Myerson MS. Metatarsal stress fractures. Clin Sports Med 1997;16(2):319-38.

[43] Ostlie DK, Simons SM. Tarsal navicular stress fracture in a young athlete: case report with clinical, radiologic and pathophysiologic correlations. J Am Board Fam Pract 2001;14(5):381-85.

[44] Nattiv A. stress fractures and bone health in track and field athletes. J Sci Med Sport 2000;3(3):268-79.

Submitted: May 02, 2009.
Revised: June 27, 2009.
Accepted: July 04, 2009.

SECTION FIVE
ACKNOWLEDGMENTS

In: Public Health Yearbook 2009
Editors: Joav Merrick
ISBN: 978-1-61668-911-7

Chapter 45

About the Editor

Joav Merrick, MD, MMedSci, DMSc, is professor of pediatrics, child health and human development affiliated with Kentucky Children's Hospital, University of Kentucky, Lexington, United States and the Zusman Child Development Center, Division of Pediatrics, Soroka University Medical Center, Ben Gurion University, Beer-Sheva, Israel, the medical director of the Division for Mental Retardation, Ministry of Social Affairs, Jerusalem, the founder and director of the National Institute of Child Health and Human Development. Numerous publications in the field of pediatrics, child health and human development, rehabilitation, intellectual disability, disability, health, welfare, abuse, advocacy, quality of life and prevention. Received the Peter Sabroe Child Award for outstanding work on behalf of Danish Children in 1985 and the International LEGO-Prize ("The Children's Nobel Prize") for an extraordinary contribution towards improvement in child welfare and well-being in 1987.

Contact:

Office of the Medical Director, Division for Mental Retardation, Ministry of Social Affairs, POBox 1260, IL-91012 Jerusalem, Israel.

E-mail: jmerrick@zahav.net.il

Website: www.nichd-israel.com

Home-page: http://jmerrick50.googlepages.com/home

In: Public Health Yearbook 2009
Editors: Joav Merrick
ISBN: 978-1-61668-911-7

Chapter 46

About the National Institute of Child Health and Human Development in Israel

The National Institute of Child Health and Human Development (NICHD) in Israel was established in 1998 as a virtual institute under the auspices of the Medical Director, Ministry of Social Affairs and Social Services in order to function as the research arm for the Office of the Medical Director. In 1998 the National Council for Child Health and Pediatrics, Ministry of Health and in 1999 the Director General and Deputy Director General of the Ministry of Health endorsed the establishment of the NICHD.

Mission

The mission of a National Institute for Child Health and Human Development in Israel is to provide an academic focal point for the scholarly interdisciplinary study of child life, health, public health, welfare, disability, rehabilitation, intellectual disability and related aspects of human development. This mission includes research, teaching, clinical work, information and public service activities in the field of child health and human development.

Service and academic activities

Over the years many activities became focused in the south of Israel due to collaboration with various professionals at the Faculty of Health Sciences (FOHS) at the Ben Gurion University of the Negev (BGU). Since 2000 an affiliation with the Zusman Child Development Center at the Pediatric Division of Soroka University Medical Center has resulted in collaboration around the establishment of the Down Syndrome Clinic at that center. In 2002 a full course on "Disability" was established at the Recanati School for Allied Professions in the Community, FOHS, BGU and twice a year seminars for specialists in family medicine. In 2005 collaboration was started with the Primary Care Unit of the faculty and disability became part of the master of public health course on "Children and society". In the academic year 2005-2006 a one semester course on "Aging with disability" was started as part of the master of science program in gerontology in our collaboration with the Center for Multidisciplinary Research in Aging.

Research activities

The affiliated staff has over the years published work from projects and research activities in this national and international collaboration. In the year 2000 the International Journal of Adolescent Medicine and Health and in 2005 the International Journal on Disability and Human development of Freund Publishing House (London and Tel Aviv), in the year 2003 the TSW-Child Health and Human Development and in 2006 the TSW-Holistic Health and Medicine of the Scientific World Journal (New York and Kirkkonummi, Finland), all peer-reviewed international journals were affiliated with the National Institute of Child Health and Human Development. From 2008 also the International Journal of Child Health and Human Development (Nova Science, New York), the International Journal of Child and Adolescent Health (Nova Science) and the Journal of Pain Management (Nova Science) affiliated.

National collaboration

Nationally the NICHD works in collaboration with the Faculty of Health Sciences, Ben Gurion University of the Negev; Department of Physical Therapy, Sackler School of Medicine, Tel Aviv University; Autism Center, Assaf HaRofeh Medical Center; National Rett and PKU Centers at Chaim Sheba Medical Center, Tel HaShomer; Department of Physiotherapy, Haifa University; Department of Education, Bar Ilan University, Ramat Gan, Faculty of Social Sciences and Health Sciences; College of Judea and Samaria in Ariel and recently also collaborations has been established with the Division of Pediatrics at Hadassah, Center for Pediatric Chronic Illness, Har HaZofim in Jerusalem.

International collaboration

Internationally with the Department of Disability and Human Development, College of Applied Health Sciences, University of Illinois at Chicago; Strong Center for Developmental Disabilities, Golisano Children's Hospital at Strong, University of Rochester School of Medicine and Dentistry, New York; Centre on Intellectual Disabilities, University of Albany, New York; Centre for Chronic Disease Prevention and Control, Health Canada, Ottawa; Chandler Medical Center and Children's Hospital, Kentucky Children's Hospital, Section of Adolescent Medicine, University of Kentucky, Lexington; Chronic Disease Prevention and Control Research Center, Baylor College of Medicine, Houston, Texas; Division of Neuroscience, Department of Psychiatry, Columbia University, New York; Institute for the Study of Disadvantage and Disability, Atlanta; Center for Autism and Related Disorders, Department Psychiatry, Children's Hospital Boston, Boston; Department of Paediatrics, Child Health and Adolescent Medicine, Children's Hospital at Westmead, Westmead,

Australia; International Centre for the Study of Occupational and Mental Health, Düsseldorf, Germany; Centre for Advanced Studies in Nursing, Department of General Practice and Primary Care, University of Aberdeen, Aberdeen, United Kingdom; Quality of Life Research Center, Copenhagen, Denmark; Nordic School of Public Health, Gottenburg, Sweden, Scandinavian Institute of Quality of Working Life, Oslo, Norway; Centre for Quality of Life of the Hong Kong Institute of Asia-Pacific Studies and School of Social Work, Chinese University, Hong Kong.

Targets

Our focus is on research, international collaborations, clinical work, teaching and policy in health, disability and human development and to establish the NICHD as a permanent institute at one of the residential care centers for persons with intellectual disability in Israel in order to conduct model research and together with the four university schools of public health/medicine in Israel establish a national master and doctoral program in disability and human development at the institute to secure the next generation of professionals working in this often non-prestigious/low-status field of work. For this project we need your support. We are looking for all kinds of support and eventually an endowment.

Contact

Professor Joav Merrick, MD, MMedSci, DMSc
Medical Director, Division for Mental Retardation
Ministry of Social Affairs, POBox 1260
IL-91012 Jerusalem, Israel
E-mail: jmerrick@internet-zahav.net
Website: www.nichd-israel.com;

SECTION SIX
INDEX

INDEX

B

C

D

F

G

H

I

J

K

L

M

O

P

Q

R

S

T

U

V

W

X

Y

Z